Global Occupational Health

GLOBAL OCCUPATIONAL HEALTH

Edited by
Tee L. Guidotti

Associate Editors:
Jorma Rantanen
Suvi Lehtinen
Ken Takahashi
David Koh
René Mendes
Fu Hua
Julietta Rodríguez Guzmán

Managing Editor:
Susan G. Rose

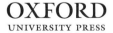

OXFORD
UNIVERSITY PRESS

Oxford University Press, Inc., publishes works that further
Oxford University's objective of excellence
in research, scholarship, and education.

Oxford New York
Auckland   Cape Town   Dar es Salaam   Hong Kong   Karachi
Kuala Lumpur   Madrid   Melbourne   Mexico City   Nairobi
New Delhi   Shanghai   Taipei   Toronto

With offices in
Argentina   Austria   Brazil   Chile   Czech Republic   France   Greece
Guatemala   Hungary   Italy   Japan   Poland   Portugal   Singapore
South Korea   Switzerland   Thailand   Turkey   Ukraine   Vietnam

Published by Oxford University Press, Inc.
198 Madison Avenue, New York, New York 10016
www.oup.com

Oxford is a registered trademark of Oxford University Press

Library of Congress Cataloging-in-Publication Data

Global occupational health / edited by Tee L. Guidotti ; associate editors,
Jorma Rantanen . . . [et al.] ; managing editor, Susan G. Rose.
      p. ; cm.
   Includes bibliographical references.
   978-0-19-538000-2 (alk. paper)
   1. Industrial hygiene. 2. World health. I. Guidotti, Tee L.
   [DNLM: 1. Occupational Health. 2. World Health. WA 400 G5625 2011]
   RC967.G654 2011
   616.9'803—dc22
                                                                2010025244

1 3 5 7 9 8 6 4 2
Printed in the United States of America
on acid-free paper

PREFACE

Global Occupational Health is a comprehensive introductory textbook designed for the preparation of professionals in occupational health. The textbook is intended for use in basic to mid-level courses, providing the reader or student with a solid foundation from which to pursue more specialized studies. The intended readership for this textbook includes technical college and university students, entry-level occupational health professionals, newly assigned government regulatory officers, and experienced health professionals and technically trained professionals who are preparing in mid-career for future work in occupational health. It is expected that this textbook will be particularly useful in "train-the-trainers" programs, providing a sound foundation for trainers who then educate others on the principles of occupational health.

The availability of this book will facilitate the preparation of occupational health professionals worldwide. It may be used as a standalone text, or it may be combined with other texts that go into greater detail on the chemistry, physics, and psychology of occupational hazards. By providing this textbook, the authors and editors also hope to create a standard for education in occupational health in the field of global health, where it is not so much neglected as completely invisible.

This textbook began as a sister work to the earlier texts *Basic Epidemiology* and *Basic Environmental Health*, all originally sponsored by the World Health Organization. Each of these textbooks has some overlapping content, in which certain fundamental topics are repeated, although from different points of view. Occupational health is discussed at length in *BEH*, and the present work, restyled *Global Occupational Health*, itself contains a lengthy discussion of epidemiology. This is necessary to make each textbook useful as a single reference and to present important principles with an emphasis on their relevance to occupational health.

The basic reference work that supports *Global Occupational Health* is the superb *ILO Encyclopaedia of Occupational Health*, which is recommended to be the standard source used for class assignments and reference. The *ILO Encyclopaedia* is currently undergoing revision for its fifth edition. Readers who wish to pursue particular topics are advised that the Internet has made reference lists, such as that provided at the end of this book, largely obsolete. In occupational health, new information becomes available every day but the basics never seem to change.

The content of this textbook is generally applicable to developing and developed economies and features a variety of case studies pertinent to different national situations. Although every effort was made to create a regional balance and diversity of authorship, some regions are represented and others are not. It is hoped that this may be remedied in future editions. The editors are aware that some readers may take exception to mention of their countries or regions in examples that suggest inadequate or unsatisfactory practices and hope that these readers will understand that it is important to provide real case studies for optimum learning but impossible to balance every bad example with a good one. Occasionally, details in the case studies have been changed for the purpose of clarifying the essential issue or making the example more useful for educational purposes. No passage in the text is intended to impugn the efforts of any government agency, country, or enterprise, and none should be considered to be an accurate record or evidence of misdeed on the part of any specific individual or enterprise. The editors also made extraordinary efforts to ensure that the problems of developing societies were addressed and given prominence throughout the text.

Global Occupational Health is divided into 31 chapters, which are organized into five basic sections. The first seven chapters deal with the basic principles of occupational health and its constituent disciplines, including epidemiology, toxicology, exposure assessment, safety, and ergonomics. The next five chapters cover different types of hazards: physical, chemical, biological, psychological, and general approaches to controlling hazards. The next six chapters deal with health-care management and health protection, beginning with four chapters on the identification and evaluation of health outcomes, with special attention to injuries, chronic musculoskeletal disorders, and occupational diseases, followed by two chapters that deal in a more general way with occupational health services in the form of fitness-to-work evaluations and prevention. Six subsequent chapters deal with various aspects of the workplace and workers, treating various industries, occupations, and types of enterprises. The final group of seven chapters deals with various aspects of occupational health services and their role in economic development and society. Almost every chapter is accompanied by boxed case studies and discussions designed for enrichment and to illustrate the points being made with concrete examples.

Each chapter in this book was originally written in draft by a lead author or authorship team. However, in the course of producing the textbook, the original drafts were greatly modified. Material has been added, deleted, and moved around between chapters. Preferred references have been substituted and definitions have been inserted. Every chapter is substantially changed from the original text as submitted by the authors. In every case, the reason for making these editorial changes was to create a more cohesive and unified book, not because the authors' submissions were deficient. Editorial problems are the responsibility of the editors.

This work was a collaborative effort over a 10-year period, from 1998 to 2008. Throughout this process, the editors have appreciated the support of the WHO staff, the International Commission on Occupational Health, the Finnish Institute of Occupational Health, Medical Advisory Services (Rockville, Maryland) and their home institutions.

ACKNOWLEDGMENTS

This text was initiated under the sponsorship of the World Health Organization. The editorial work was undertaken with the assistance of the International Commission for Occupational Health and several of its Scientific Committees. The editorial work was based at the University of Alberta in Edmonton, Alberta, Canada, until 1999 and subsequently at the George Washington University, Washington DC, United States of America, and reached its completion as an independent project in 2010. The project was initiated with a small contract from WHO, supported during its development by the Tripartite Fund for Occupational Health at the University of Alberta, supplemented by various sources including advances from the publisher, and finished with expenses support in kind by Medical Advisory Services of Rockville, Maryland (USA). Royalties from the book will go to support the Leo Noro Fund of the International Commission on Occupational Health for the benefit of members from developing countries.

The editor, Dr. Tee L. Guidotti, was responsible for commissioning chapters, editing them, and producing the completed manuscript. The associate editors contacted authors for individual chapters within their assigned area of responsibility and contributed their own. Without the dedication of Jorma Rantanen, Ken Takahashi, David Koh, Rene Mendes, Fu Hua, and Julietta Rodríguez Guzmán, this project could not have been finished.

Several experts gave valuable criticism and assisted in editing but do not appear as lead authors or editors. They include Carin Sunderström-Frisk, Peter Westerholm, Steven Markowitz, and Rene Loewenson.

The lead authors of the individual chapters produced 31 works of excellence covering almost all aspects of occupational health at a level suitable for new learners. This was a difficult assignment, and their contributions showed great thoughtfulness and care in every case.

Contributing authors assisted in various ways, providing materials for boxes, text inserted into the existing chapters, or lengthy critiques that led to revisions. Several contributing authors wrote boxed case studies to accompany the chapters. Their contribution has made the work more readable and accessible for the learner: Wai-On Phoon, Changmyung Lee, Craig Karpilow, Tsutomu Hoshuyama, and Lee Hock Siang, and the several authors who wrote boxes that accompany their own chapters. During the production of this book, Tee Guidotti changed institutions and later joined the firm of Medical Advisory Services, but maintained a continuous and active adjunct faculty position with the University of Alberta, which continues past his retirement from the George Washington University; affiliations given are those most appropriate for him at the time of the contribution.

The fine, cleanly drawn graphics in the book were drawn by Sam Motyka, of Edmonton, Alberta. Several organizations helped us to find photographs to accompany the chapters: *Saudi Aramco World* magazine (through its Saudi Aramco World Digital Image Archive, abbreviated SAWDIA in the captions), la Universidad El Bosque (Colombia), the American Industrial Hygiene Association, U.S. Prevention, the CDC Public Health Image Bank, the Finnish Institute of Occupational Health, 3M Corporation, Kemper (manufacturer of welding equipment), and sources given in individual photo credits throughout the book. Several colleagues generously provided photographs from their personal and professional collections: Earl Dotter (award-winning photographer of labor and occupational health subjects), Seifeddin Ballal (King Faisal University, Dammam, Saudi Arabia), Julietta Rodríguez Guzmán (Universidad El Bosque), Tee Guidotti (identified by affiliation at the time the photograph was taken), David Koh, and others who are identified in individual photo credits. We were assisted by many individuals in locating photographs, including Trevor Ogden (Editor of the *Annals of Occupational Hygiene*), Andrew Cutz, Katie Robert (AIHA), Donna Marie Artuso, and Suvi Lehtinen (FIOH). Sherry Selevan provided invaluable technical assistance.

A very special thanks is owed to Anthony Stones, noted British artist, for allowing us to use his superb portrait of Bernardino Ramazzini—which previously graced the printed proceedings from a regional meeting in New Zealand edited by his friend William Ivan Glass—to illustrate Box 1.1. Mr. Stones is most famous as a sculptor, with numerous works on display in public spaces, mostly in the UK. The drawing was created during a trip to Padua with Dr. Glass, who, with the enthusiastic support of Mr. Stones' wife, Lily Feng, arranged to bring Mr. Stones' artistry to a new and appreciative audience in our book.

Production staff and students at the University of Alberta and the George Washington University assisted with word processing, editing, and rewriting material for boxes: Adebola Laditan, Kathy Lassel, and Martha Embrey.

This work would not have been possible without the sustained support, interest, and occasional push provided by the staff of the World Health Organization involved in this project over its lengthy development: Carlos Corvalán, Gerry Eijkemans, Evelyn Kortum, Marilyn Fingerhut, and Ivan Ivanov, as well as Maritza Tennassee of the Pan American Health Organization. Igor Fedetov of the International Labour Organization also played an invaluable role. Medical Advisory Services, of Rockville, Maryland (USA), a consulting firm, supported Tee Guidotti during the completion of this book by allowing him to work on it as a work project, and Alan E. Burt reviewed the section on construction workers for accuracy.

Our editor at Oxford University Press, first Regan Hofmann and then Maura Roessner, showed great patience and faith in the project when we experienced unexpected delays. Finally, a special debt is owed to Susan Gail Rose, who performed a final edit and took over as managing editor for the project in the final stages of manuscript production. Sadly, Susan died in 2009, before seeing the book published. She was a fine editor, a fine lawyer, and a dedicated advocate for those injured by dangerous drugs and public health hazards.

CONTENTS

CONTRIBUTORS

Gregory Chan Chung Tsing
National University of Singapore,
 Singapore

Elizabeth Costa Dias
Federal University of Minas Gerais,
 Minas Gerais, Brazil (retired)

John Cowell
Calgary, Alberta, Canada

Igor Fedotov
International Labour Organization,
 Geneva, Switzerland

Fu Hua
School of Public Health, Fudan
 University, Shanghai, China

Tee L. Guidotti
University of Alberta, Edmonton,
 Canada
George Washington University,
 Washington DC, USA (retired)
Medical Advisory Services, Rockville
 MD, USA

Takashi Haratani
National Institute of Occupational
 Safety and Health, Japan

Harold Hoffman
Edmonton, Alberta, Canada

Tsutomu Hoshuyama
University of Occupational and
 Environmental Health, Japan

Erkki Kähkönen
Finnish Institute of Occupational
 Health, Helsinki, Finland

Pentti Kalliokoski
University of Kuopio, Kuopio, Finland

Craig Karpilow
IPA Associates, Canada

David Koh
National University of Singapore,
 Singapore

Thomas Läubli
Division of Public and Organizational
 Health
Kyoto Institute of Technology, Japan
 Leiter
University of Zurich

Changmyung Lee
Univeristy of Ulsan, Korea

Liang Youxin
School of Public Health, Fudan
 University, Shanghai, China

Jyrki Liesivuori
University of Turku, Finland

Kari Lindström
Finnish Institute of Occupational
 Health, Vantaa, Finland

Veikko Louhevaara
University of Eastern Finland
 Kuopio Campus

René Loewenson
Training and Research Support
 Centre, Harare, Zimbabwe

René Mendes
Federal University of Minas Gerais,
 Brazil (retired)

Michael Nasterlack
BASF Aktiengesellschaft,
   Ludwigshafen, Germany

Nina Nevala
Finnish Institute of Occupational
   Health
   Helsinki, Finland

Panu Oksa
Tampere Regional Institute of
   Occupational Health, Tampere,
   Finland

Rauno Pääkkönen
Tampere Regional Institute of
   Occupational Health, Tampere,
   Finland

Wai-On Phoon
Pymble Medical Consultants, Pymble,
   Australia

Jorma Rantanen
Finnish Institute of Occupational
   Health, Helsinki, Finland (retired)

Hugo Rüdiger
University of Vienna, Austria (retired)

Kai Savolainen
University of Kuopio, Finland

Lee Hock Siang
Ministry of Manpower, Singapore

Jeffrey Spickett
Curtin University, Perth, Australia

Carin Sunderström-Frisk
National Institute for Working Life,
   Solna, Sweden

Jukka Uitti
Tampere Regional Institute of
   Occupational Health, Tampere,
   Finland

E. Wallis-Long
Curtin University, Perth, Western
   Australia, Australia

Peter Westerholm
National Institute for Working Life,
   Solna, Sweden

Andreas Zober
BASF Aktiengesellschaft,
   Ludwigshafen, Germany

Global Occupational Health

1

THE PRINCIPLES OF OCCUPATIONAL HEALTH

Jorma Rantanen

Occupational health is a multi-dimensional field, encompassing science, social progress, economics, law, employment studies, and issues common to every family. The health and safety of people at work is a critical concern for all societies and all countries.

The field of occupational health touches on fundamental aspects of working life:

- making a living
- providing for a family
- staying healthy
- avoiding unnecessary risk of injury
- protecting oneself and others from harm
- creating useful products and services for societal benefit
- anticipating and preventing future problems
- sharing information
- the right to knowledge of potential health hazards
- fairness and justice in the treatment of workers
- achieving responsibility and accountability in the workplace
- minimizing the risk of necessary but hazardous work

Because occupational health issues are so fundamental to working life, they have become central social and political issues in countries with progressive policies and a tradition of social responsibility. These countries have developed systems of occupational health protection, social insurance, and medical services that reduce the burden on the worker and reduce the loss to the economy. However, these systems are not perfect, and they are often under stress. Developing countries often lack these systems or have them only in rudimentary forms. Occupational health problems are often overlooked as an obstacle to economic development when wages are low and the cost of health care is low. Occupational injuries and

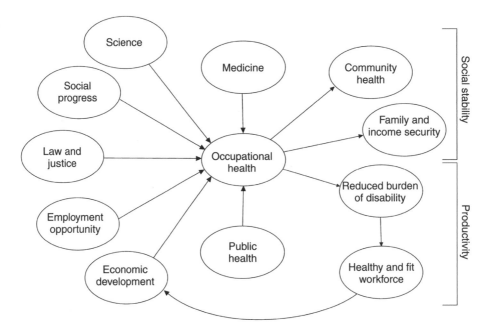

Figure 1.1 Occupational health is influenced by many factors and plays a critical role in shaping many social issues.

illness can become a significant drag on the economy, however, by reducing productivity, increasing the burden of disability and illness on people, and causing financial insecurity.

Occupational health issues are deeply embedded in society and have a profound but largely unacknowledged effect on economic development. Some of these issues include:

- the health risks that workers take to earn a living
- the consequences to their families when workers become ill or injured
- the social contract between workers and employers and the responsibility to keep the workplace safe
- the financial loss to workers and their families from a prolonged illness or disabling injury
- the cost of providing medical and rehabilitation care to injured workers
- the hidden cost to the health-care system of illnesses that are not recognized as occupational, especially those that take a long time to develop
- the cost of providing benefits and wage replacement to workers who are injured
- the loss of productivity that results from avoidable injuries and illness
- the development of new technology, the cost of production, and return on investment
- the social management of risk spreading, for example, by workers' compensation or other insurance plans
- management of and minimization of the risk of disasters

International organizations such as the World Health Organization (WHO) and the International Labour Organization (ILO) have given much attention to worker health and safety, as evidenced by the WHO Global Strategy on Occupational Health for All that was adopted by the 49th World Health Assembly in 1996 (WHO 1995) and by the ILO Convention No. 161 on Occupational Health Services (1985). The European Union includes occupational health as a part of its Employment and Social Policy Programmes. Although much effort has been made toward the worldwide implementation of those authoritative policies, much remains to be done before the WHO objective "Occupational Health for All" is achieved. In fact, out of the 3 billion workers in the world, only 10% to 15% have access to occupational health services, and these services do not necessarily correspond to the most urgent needs.

At its first session in 1950, the Joint ILO/WHO Committee on Occupational Health defined the purpose of occupational health. It revised the definition at its 12th session in 1995 to read as follows (Alli 2001):

> Occupational health should aim at the promotion and maintenance of the highest degree of physical, mental and social well-being of workers in all occupations; the prevention amongst workers of departures from health caused by their working conditions; the protection of workers in their employment from risks resulting from factors adverse to health; the placing and maintenance of the worker in an occupational environment adapted to his physiological and psychological capabilities and; to summarize: the adaptation of work to man and of each man to his job.

OCCUPATIONAL HEALTH AND DEVELOPMENT

A healthy and productive workforce is the key factor behind the social and economic development of any country. Originally, occupational health programs were designed during the advent of industrialization to prevent and treat acute and chronic illnesses and injuries among the working population. Gradually, as public health programs were developed, occupational health adopted a more specific role in the prevention and control of occupationally determined outcomes—accidents and diseases directly associated with work or working conditions. Over time, occupational health shifted its emphasis to the overall health and well-being of the working population.

Today, occupational health services in their most advanced forms are comprehensive, covering the control of hazardous factors in the work environment, promotion of work ability, and promotion of workers' general health and healthy lifestyles.

The economic costs of poor safety and health at work amount to 4% to 5% of the gross domestic product (GDP) of countries, and the bill from poor work ability is likely to be 4–5 times higher. *Work ability* is defined as the capacity to carry out one's job productively and competently so that the objectives of the work tasks are achieved without exposing the worker to physical or psychological overload. *Well-being at work* means that the criteria of work ability are met. In addition, the job generates satisfaction and the work and work community provide social support and facilitate the personal development of the worker.

Developing countries struggling to improve their standard of living should avoid the enormous loss of work ability of the workers by supporting and sustaining them and their families. Thus, supporting occupational health is an important tool for the elimination of poverty. Industrialized countries face growing problems due to the shortage of young workers and the aging of the working populations. To ensure the availability of a sufficient workforce, unnecessary losses of work ability need to be eliminated.

There are many reasons for pointing occupational health in a more comprehensive direction, due to the growing importance of work ability, work motivation, and the well-being of people in modern work life. Traditionally, occupational health was considered a service of value only to those exposed to high physical, chemical, mechanical, biological, or ergonomic exposures (i.e., the factory-level, or "blue-collar" worker). But healthy and safe working conditions now are seen to include worker well-being, good psychosocial functioning, and issues of work organization, which has expanded occupational health services to all groups of working people, starting from the factory-level blue collars up to middle and top managers (Rantanen 1999).

EQUITY AND OCCUPATIONAL HEALTH

Fairness and impartiality—under the law, in business dealings, and in the opportunity for social relationships—is the definition of the principle of *equity*. Equity in work life enables men and women of all backgrounds to obtain employment, to develop their skills at work, to fulfill multiple roles in society, and to earn the resources needed to sustain themselves and their families. It also means that no worker needs to risk health or safety while earning the necessities of life. Equitable societies value such rights as minimum basic salary, social protection, occupational health and safety, employment security, opportunity for training and education, and the right to know and right to participate.

Equity as a concept is closely related to ethics and justice. Therefore, prominent ethicists have strongly emphasized the importance of equity as both an instrument and an objective, as both a way to realize ethical principles and as an ethical goal in itself. *Distributive justice* is the principle that people should be rewarded or compensated proportionate to what they deserve, which for most practical purposes means equity. Equity in occupational health is formally considered to be an outcome of distributive justice (i.e., equal distribution of occupational health services to people without any discrimination, or compensation provided to people fairly on the basis of how badly they were injured and their living expenses).

As adverse working conditions and occupational health and safety hazards are in principle preventable, the strategies for preventing such hazards and risks, starting with high-risk occupations and the most adverse conditions, will have an equalizing impact on all occupations. Most of the differences in health outcomes are related to social and economic factors and are thus manageable with the help of social policies. This is particularly true with policies concerning occupational injuries and diseases.

Occupational health activities vary from country to country due to differences in legislation, national tradition, and medical practices. However, international organizations have identified a basic framework that is generally applicable and that works in practice.

The summary of key objectives of ILO Convention No. 161 and the related Recommendation No. 171 are collected in **Table 1.1**. The respective principles from the WHO Global Strategy on Occupational Health for All are summarized in **Table 1.2**.

TABLE 1.1

KEY OBJECTIVES OF ILO CONVENTION NO. 161 AND RECOMMENDATION NO. 171

1. Principles of national policies concerning occupational health services
2. Functions of occupational health services:
   a) Surveillance of the working environment
   b) Surveillance of workers' health
   c) Information, education, and training advice to workers and employers
   d) First aid treatment and health programs
   e) Other functions including analyzing surveillance results, reporting on occupational health service activities, and participating in research and with other services in environmental protection activities
3. Organization of occupational health services
4. Operational conditions of occupational health services including provisions for composition and competence of occupational health service teams, protection of confidential health information, and professional independence of occupational health service personnel

TABLE 1.2

THE 10 OBJECTIVES OF THE WHO GLOBAL STRATEGY ON OCCUPATIONAL HEALTH FOR ALL

1. Strengthening international and national policies for health at work and developing the necessary policy tools
2. Developing healthy work environments
3. Developing healthy work practices and promotion of health at work
4. Strengthening occupational health services
5. Establishing support services for occupational health
6. Developing occupational health standards based on scientific risk assessment
7. Developing human resources for occupational health
8. Establishing registration and data systems, developing information services for experts, effectively transmitting data, and raising public awareness through public information
9. Strengthening research
10. Developing collaborations between occupational health and other activities and services

Five basic principles have been identified as the basis for successful occupational health systems, as determined in a WHO/EURO survey of legislation in European countries concerning occupational health services (Rantanen 1990). The balance among the five principles in different economic sectors, different countries, and different enterprises may vary substantially depending on the national and local conditions, traditions, laws, and practice. The five principles are as follows.

1. *Protection and prevention.* This principle is the core of occupational health activities and includes the following:
   - identification of hazardous exposures and factors causing overload or other adverse work conditions
   - assessment of the distribution and levels of exposures, identification of exposed groups or individuals, and sources of hazards
   - assessment of risks to health and safety from exposures or adverse conditions
   - initiating, instituting, and advising on needs and means for preventive and control actions aimed at protecting workers' health and safety
2. *Adaptation.* Not all workers have equal work ability, health status, or competence. Thus, aging workers, adolescents and young workers, pregnant women, handicapped workers, migrant workers, and workers with chronic diseases may need adaptation of work, working methods, or work environment, including machinery and tools, to their special needs and abilities. Occupational health experts need to balance job demands with the special health and safety concerns of such workers, initiate and advise about work adaptations, and monitor the impact of such measures.
3. *Promotion and development.* Optimally organized work can have a positive effect on workers' health and work ability: it can develop physical, mental, and professional capacities, and it can contribute to the development of safe working practices and healthy lifestyles. This principle has become especially important for industrialized countries given their attention to maintaining work ability in aging workers, ensuring their continued participation in the workforce.
4. *Cure and rehabilitation.* In spite of efforts for prevention and protection as described in principle 1, work-related diseases, accidents, states of physical and mental overload, and acute and chronic illnesses do occur among a substantial proportion of the workforce. An aging working population suffers an increased risk of chronic disease conditions. The curative and rehabilitation principle is important to minimize the consequences of such events, to facilitate a return to original health and work ability, and, if that is not possible, to maintain the remaining work ability as much as possible.
5. *Primary health care.* Some countries and employers include a role for primary care or general practitioner-level health care as part of occupational health services. In many countries workers may not have access to anything but primary health care. In all countries, certain economic sectors, such as agriculture, small-scale enterprises, informal workers, home workers, and workers in

remote and sparsely populated areas, usually lack specialized occupational health services and depend on primary care providers. Some countries avoid overlap and have even prohibited the combination of general health services with occupational health services. They do this to emphasize a preventive approach and to keep the management of occupational injuries and illnesses without bias. However, there are many good reasons for integrating occupational health services into primary care:

- to provide primary health-care services, e.g., injury care, quickly and conveniently at the workplace or nearby
- to fill possible holes in public primary health services
- to use public services most efficiently
- to obtain a comprehensive picture of the total health of workers in the community (i.e., occupational health and general health) by capturing information at the primary care level

THE ROLE OF RESEARCH IN OCCUPATIONAL HEALTH

Occupational health practice rests on scientific knowledge, which comes largely from research. Without research, occupational health would still be backward, inefficient, inflexible, and unable to adapt to new technologies or challenges. There is a long tradition of high standards of research in the field of occupational health, oriented toward both practical problem solving and the investigation of occupational hazards to see what new knowledge can be gained for human benefit.

Occupational health practice rests on scientific knowledge, drawing from several scientific disciplines in natural sciences (physics, chemistry), biomedical sciences (biology, basic medical sciences, physiology, epidemiology), behavioral sciences (psychology, social sciences), and technology (safety technology). Applying the knowledge and methods from the basic sciences and carrying out research to produce new knowledge on the relationship between workers and the work environment are the main missions of occupational health research. Research is further divided into disciplines such as occupational/industrial hygiene, occupational medicine, occupational psychology, occupational epidemiology, safety, and ergonomics. Research may be undertaken at universities, specialized research institutes, and government agencies.

The cumulative knowledge from occupational health research is used to develop methods in occupational health practices, to train and educate occupational health experts and practitioners, and to disseminate information on work and health to numerous target groups: experts, practitioners, managers, workers and their organizations, decision and policy makers, the media, and the public at large.

THE INFRASTRUCTURE OF OCCUPATIONAL HEALTH

Occupational health is supported by a worldwide network of practitioners, public and private facilities, and institutions and organizations that are guided by laws, government agencies, and professional standards of practice. The infrastructure for occupational health protection, management of occupational injuries and illness, and compensation and public policy is called *occupational health services*.

According to international guidance, including ILO Convention 161, and national legislation, all people who take part in the workforce shall have access to occupational health services (WHO 1995). That service should be provided either at the workplace or in a nearby facility, and it should carry out a minimum set of service activities indicated in **Table 1.1**. The precise content of services may vary according to national law and practice and local conditions and needs, but a certain minimum should be found everywhere. Each worker should be provided with such services.

Occupational health services are a special, separate set of health services for workers and workplaces to prevent and control health and safety hazards at work and to promote good practice and guidance in the field of occupational health. Occupational health services should cover all workers in all workplaces, in all sectors of the economy, including industry, private and public services, agriculture, self-employment, and informal work, and cover the work done in all environments—e.g., on land, at sea, in the air (including space), underground, and even underwater. They should be available to all working people, including blue-collar workers, farmers, informal workers, middle managers, top managers, and public-sector civil servants and defense forces. In short, everyone who works should have access to an occupational health service.

Occupational health services shall be provided by competent and accredited personnel including occupational health physicians, occupational health nurses, occupational hygienists, occupational psychologists, physiotherapists, ergonomics experts, and others as defined by the national laws and regulations. Occupational health services personnel should have a certified competence in the tasks for which they are responsible.

In most countries, occupational health services apply the principle of participation—the workers and employers have a right to participate in the decisions on how the occupational health services are organized and provided. The competent authority (mostly occupational safety and health inspectors) has a right to inspect to make sure the occupational health service regulations are implemented.

According to the ILO Convention 161, the employer (where he or she exists) is responsible for financing and organizing occupational health services for his or her employees without any costs to the employee. The experts providing occupational health services are guaranteed professional independence in carrying out their activities (i.e., they make their decisions on occupational health, medical, and other services independently according to their professional competence and ethical principles).

BASICS OF A NATIONAL SYSTEM FOR OCCUPATIONAL HEALTH

The minimum structure for a national system in occupational health can be drawn from international conventions, national regulations, and international and national guidelines provided by international organizations and national legislators and authorities. Some countries have much more than this, but all should have at least this minimum structure.

The following lists the essential elements that are the minimum necessary for a national system of occupational health.

1. Legislation should set forth the basic requirements, responsibilities, and rights of authorities, employers, and workers in occupational health services.
2. Competent authorities for enforcement of legislation are often assisted and advised by a national occupational health committee appointed on a tripartite basis by the government. In most countries, the authority consists of the Ministry of Labour, Department of Occupational Health and Safety, or the Ministry of Health, Department of Occupational Health, or there may be a shared responsibility of two ministries. The enforcement functions are most often delegated to the National Board of Occupational Safety and Health, the National Board of Health, or the Occupational Safety and Health Commission with its operational units and whatever the local names for these bodies.
3. A national policy program organizes services; develops content, human resources, and conditions of operation; and plans for the development of occupational health services.
4. Infrastructures for providing services at the workplace level may utilize several options such as in-plant services, group services, private health centers, hospital-based occupational health services, or services provided by the public primary health-care units, social security institutions, etc.
5. Human resources personnel (such as personnel managers and hiring agents) should have competence, criteria, and guidelines for qualitative and quantitative aspects of the management of human resources. This includes training in how to deal with issues of compensation, insurance, accommodation, employment security, rehabilitation, and retraining.
6. Information systems should be established at several different levels:
   • normative information, laws, standards, guidelines, and instructions
   • official registries of occupational diseases and occupational accidents
   • information for experts concerning scientific and professional expert information (libraries, scientific journals, databanks, search and retrieval services, etc.)
   • practical information concerning occupational health practices, such as good practice guidelines, fact sheets, and expert journals
   • public information concerning the importance, needs, and state of occupational health
7. Support and advisory services are typically second-level services that are needed to provide specialized support to the "frontline occupational health service." Such services cover the following:
   • diagnostic services for occupational diseases (usually in polyclinics or departments of occupational medicine in hospitals)
   • analytical and measurement services for toxicology, biological monitoring, physical factors, biological agents, ergonomics, and psychology. Institutions of occupational health, university teams, or private consultancies provide such services.

- advice and consultations in work organization and workplace development
8. Occupational health is a specialized activity that requires competence in several disciplines: occupational medicine and occupational health, occupational hygiene, psychology, and others. Such competence requires special training, and many countries have set special competency-based criteria, for example, for specialists in occupational medicine. Specialist training curricula are needed at the national level to produce a sufficient number of experts needed for occupational health activities. Some international harmonization of curricula is underway at the WHO, in European Union countries, and among professional associations.
9. In addition to the contributions of experts in occupational health practices, employers, workers (treated as social partners), and their representatives need to be involved to ensure the successful implementation of occupational health at the workplace. This is carried out at the national level in the form of a tripartite (government, employers, and trade unions) national occupational health committee that is an advisory body for government policy making and implementation. Respectively, the workplace-level collaboration is organized through occupational health and safety committees, work councils, or through safety and health representatives of the enterprises.
10. The "occupational health service system" should be a part of the national general health service system infrastructure.

OCCUPATIONAL HEALTH AND ENVIRONMENTAL HEALTH

The work environment is a subset of the total environment, like the home and neighborhood. It is characterized by where people work, but workers and their families also live in the general or ambient environment, in urban, suburban, or rural settings.

Industrial, municipal, energy, agricultural, and transportation operations and facilities may have a substantial environmental impact on the health of people who live in the community. If the workers in an industry live near industrial sites (as is the case in many traditional industrial areas), they may be exposed to hazardous agents at the workplace and from the general environment, including contaminants from air, water, food, or soil.

These community exposures are almost always at lower levels than are encountered in the workplace, but they may be significant for the workers' health and are more likely to affect the health of their families and other residents. There is usually a substantial difference (often orders of magnitude) in the levels of exposure between the work environment and the general environment, due to dilution factors in the general environment.

Occupational exposures typically occur during the one-fourth to one-third of a day that is usually taken up with work. Exposures from the general environment occur over the other two-thirds of the day. Children spend 100% of their time in the home, at school, or outdoors in the general environment.

BOX 1.1

A Historical Figure in Occupational Health

The year 2000, the Millennial Year, was the third centennial of the founding of occupational medicine, the first professional specialty area to concern itself with occupational health. It began with a single book, written by an Italian physician who already had a reputation as a great teacher and scholar.

Bernardino Ramazzini's *Diseases of Workers* (*De Morbis Arteficum*) was the text that established the future medical specialty of occupational medicine and the occupational health sciences broadly. Ramazzini accumulated in one book the most relevant facts about occupational disease in his era, mostly from personal observation, and came to insights about medicine and prevention that are completely modern. His insights into the cause of occupational diseases are considered early models not only of scientific observation in occupational health but also of public health in general and pointed the way toward accurate diagnosis, compensation, and, most of all, prevention. He also came to astute conclusions about the social context of employment in his time, the nature of ethnic stereotyping, access to health care, and treatment outcomes.

Ramazzini taught at the Italian universities of Modena and Padua. He wrote fluently in Latin, in a style considered a model of elegance, and with great good humor, not hesitating to poke fun at his fellow physicians. His works are considered classics of the medical literature.

For a person of wealth and status in his society, Ramazzini was unusually understanding and dedicated toward the poor and working people of low social status. That does not mean that he was perfect: in his work one reads echoes of the prejudices of his era, but he was unusually tolerant considering his class and the times in which he lived.

It is very common to hear references to Ramazzini's early descriptions of occupational disorders expressed in terms that make it sound as if he had anticipated modern-day problems. "Ramazzini described [this or that] centuries ago and his descriptions are right on target." While Ramazzini had outstanding powers of observation and thought deeply about what he saw, he did not foretell the future.

The fact that Ramazzini's observations are relevant today is because many of the problems he described have not been solved. Many of the occupational disorders and working conditions that he described should now be eliminated, but yet they persist. The reality is that many workers still face having to choose between loss of income and safe working conditions as they did in Ramazzini's time. His work is a benchmark that tells us that we have not progressed so far as we would like to believe.

Figure 1.2 is an original drawing of Ramazzini, wearing the wig typical of his era, by Mr. Anthony Stones, who drew it as a composite sketch from portraits he found in Padua on a trip to Italy. Mr. Stones was born in New Zealand and currently divides his time between the United Kingdom and China. He is perhaps best known as a sculptor. His realistic, life-sized or greater sculptures can be seen in public collections and monuments, mostly in the UK.

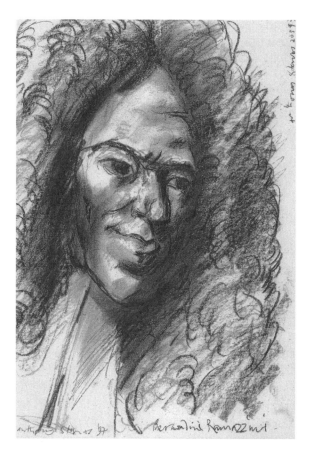

Figure 1.2 The Italian physician Bernardino Ramazzini wrote the first comprehensive treatise on occupational health in 1700. (Portrait by Anthony Stones, used with permission of the artist, supplied courtesy of William Ivan Glass, New Zealand.)

In most instances, exposures in the work environment are similar to exposures in the general environment, only more intense. For example, controlling both occupational and environmental exposures plays an important role in the prevention of chronic lung diseases such as asthma and chronic obstructive pulmonary disease. A substantial part of local environmental pollution can be controlled using the knowledge and actions of occupational health principles within the work environment. Successful examples of such approaches include, for example, successful management of lead exposure, carbon disulphide to the point where over-expsoure is now rare in developed countries, and successful control in many workplaces of solvent emissions, noise abatement, and dust controls.

For some occupations, the general environment is also a work environment and, thus, has a direct occupational health impact. Examples include agricultural work (water pollution, pesticides, and microbial agents), animal health, forestry work (environmentally active substances such as herbicides), fishery work (water pollution), and outdoor work (air pollution). In such situations, advocates of occupational and environmental health and environmental protection have good opportunities to work toward win-win solutions.

THE HISTORY OF OCCUPATIONAL HEALTH

Occupational health developed in parallel with technology and industrial activities. In the early days of industrialization, the poor social conditions of workers living in urban industrial areas were inhuman and unreasonable. The work was dangerous, full of hazardous exposures and high accident risks that often led to fatal or severe diseases and injuries. Working hours were over 12 hours a day, and child labor, without any special protections, was common. Social and housing conditions of workers were poor, communicable diseases spread epidemics, and the nutritional status of workers was poor.

By the middle of the 19th century, these conditions created concern among enlightened industrialists and physicians. Occupational health conditions were first documented in Italy by Bernardino Ramazzini (1633–1714), then in England by Percival Pott (1713–1788) and Charles Turner Thackrah (1795–1833), and spread gradually to the whole industrialized world. The main focus was in curative care and curative measures to minimize the effects of occupational hazards.

The second wave of occupational health interest started between the 19th and 20th centuries, approximately 100 years ago. In conjunction with developments in biomedicine, particularly microbiology and human cellular pathology, scientists and medical practitioners investigated singular causal factors and their relationships with single disease outcomes. Prevention and control became an important priority, particularly in the leading industrialized countries, where occupational safety and health legislation and legislation for workers' compensation for occupational injuries and diseases was passed. These activities stimulated specific prevention practices. This second wave lasted approximately 70 to 80 years. The most important focus in the work environment included machine safety, prevention of injuries from falling and slipping, prevention of explosions of pressure vessels and boilers, tool safety, and hazardous materials and explosives safety. Since World War II, occupational or industrial hygiene as a technical field has developed to measure and assess hazardous factors at work, to prioritize targets for preventive and control actions, and to design control technologies and protective equipment. Since the 1950s, occupational health services were directed toward specific preventive activities, preventive health examinations, and measurements for minimizing hazards in the work environment.

The third wave of occupational health started in the 1980s when Scandinavian scientists first considered the psychological and psychosocial aspects of work. Occupational stress, psychological hazards, workload, psychosociology at individual and group levels, and work organization became subjects of active discussion and targets for research and preventive control actions. These studies paralleled work in occupational psychology on issues of job satisfaction and work motivation. This research led to the improvement of the overall quality of work life and to health promotion, work ability, and the well-being of working people.

All three waves of occupational health history have been responses to the needs of work life in its various developmental stages. They also reflect the evolution of human work from physical, muscle-dependent manual work, through the machine power-based technology that was typical in manufacturing industries in the last century, to present-day work life, which is dominated by high information content and computer-based technology.

All three approaches are still relevant. However, the current concept of a comprehensive occupational health approach is broader than any one approach. It covers the following:

- the protection and promotion of health, work ability, and well-being of workers
- continuous improvement and development of safe and healthy work environments
- psychological, psychosocial, and organizational aspects of work, and the adoption of work and management cultures conducive to health and well-being

For occupational health services to follow such a comprehensive model requires teams with multidisciplinary expertise to address a wide range of aspects of work, including the health and work ability of workers, a healthy and safe work environment, and the organizational aspects of work. It also requires the full participation of workers and managers at the workplace to implement such practical goals in real life.

INTERNATIONAL ORGANIZATIONS

The major international occupational health organizations are part of the United Nations system or have a close working relationship to UN agencies. In addition, there are occupational health associations or societies in almost every country, usually representing certain professions and sometimes specific to certain industries.

World Health Organization (WHO)

WHO has a long tradition in occupational health dating back to the design of its constitution in 1948, which references occupational health. The famous Alma Ata Declaration (1978) called for the provision of health services in places where people work and live. The Health for All by the Year 2000 Strategy included concrete objectives for occupational health. In 1996, the 49th World Health Assembly adopted the Global Strategy on Occupational Health for All, which contains comprehensive and ambitious objectives for occupational health that are currently implemented in all WHO regions.

International Labour Organization (ILO)

ILO has worked on occupational health issues for over 80 years. One of the first health-related conventions of the ILO was Convention No. 13 in 1921 on the prohibition of white lead paint that was found to be toxic to both workers and children. In 1985, the International Labour Conference adopted Convention No. 161 and Recommendation No. 171 on occupational health services. The current Safe Work Programme consists of occupational health elements, including the Global Program for Elimination of Silicosis.

International Commission on Occupational Health (ICOH)

ICOH is a professional association of occupational health experts whose mission is to advance research, training, and information on occupational health. The ICOH has 35 scientific committees active in various fields of occupational health research. The most important ICOH document is the 1993 International Code of Ethics for Occupational Health Professionals. The Code defines the basic ethical principles for occupational health practice, obligations of health professionals, and professional independence of occupational health experts. The Code stipulates 26 different duties and obligations for occupational health professionals, guiding them in various practical activities according to ICOH's ethical principles.

These guides cover the following areas of occupational health practice:

- maintenance and upgrade of competence, including knowledge of conditions of work and scientific and technical knowledge
- advice on policies and programs for improving occupational health
- emphasis on preventive and promotion actions
- follow-up on remedial actions
- provision of information on safety and health
- protection and management of company information, healthy surveillance, workers' information on health examinations, employers' information on health examinations, and protection of confidential health data
- biological monitoring
- health promotion
- protection of community and environment
- contributions to scientific knowledge, competent scientific judgment, integrity and impartiality, professional independence, and equity
- ethics clause in employment contracts for occupational health personnel
- record keeping
- medical confidentiality
- collective health
- relationships with health professionals
- relationships with social partners
- ethics promotion
- professional audits

Other International Organizations

Other important professional organizations relate to occupational health, such as the International Occupational Hygiene Association (IOHA), the International Ergonomics Association (IEA), which produce scientific material and practical guidelines, and the International Social Security Association, in which national social insurance programs share information.

2

CHEMICAL SAFETY AND RISK ASSESSMENT

Kai M. Savolainen and Pentti Kalliokoski

Chemical safety is the general term for managing hazards associated with particular chemicals in order to prevent harm to the worker and to the community surrounding the plant or facility where the chemical is extracted, made, or used. Chemicals may cause adverse health effects and discomfort in many ways: poisoning, irritation, chemical burns, foul odor, allergies, explosions, fire and combustion products, release of heat, or induction of cold. Each type of hazard is managed differently to protect the health of the workers. (The health risks encountered by workers in the chemical industry are discussed in Chapter 23. The general field of safety is discussed in Chapter 6.)

CHEMICAL SAFETY

Residents in the vicinity of sites where chemicals are made, stored, or used or near transportation facilities may be at risk for hazardous exposure when hazardous chemicals are inadvertently released, either during normal plant operation (in which case the emissions are called *fugitive emissions*), during incidents of uncontrolled release (sometimes called industrial accidents, although the preferred term is hazardous *incident*), during transportation-related incidents, during maintenance activities (usually when the plant is started back up after extensive repairs and is not quite stable), or during incidents of abnormal operation (called *upset conditions*). A similar problem occurs when high sulfur-containing natural gas wells, compressor stations, or pipeline leaks release toxic hydrogen sulfide; in normal operation, natural gas and oil wells are not a great hazard to the community. Oil refineries can catch fire and occasionally present a hazard to the community around them, but unless upset conditions allow the release of benzene or hydrogen sulfide, their direct emissions are not highly toxic.

Concern over chemical safety has led the chemical industry in many countries to adopt policies requiring rigorous safety procedures, consultations with the community, disaster planning, and rapid communication with local residents in the

event of an incident. These programs often go by the name of Responsible Care®
(a trademark of the American Chemistry Council but used in 47 countries). Some
countries and jurisdictions have adopted "right-to-know laws" under which residents have a legal right to be told what is being stored on the sites in their
communities.

Most chemical release incidents are related to transportation incidents, often
involving derailed tanker cars on a railroad or trucking accidents. These incidents
are usually relatively minor but can be very disruptive to local communities, particularly if they block traffic or require evacuation. Major plant-related incidents
are comparatively rare but can be very serious, as for example, the 1984 incident
in Bhopal, India. A leak of methyl isocyanate gas at a pesticide manufacturing
plant killed 3,800 people and injured thousands more. By comparison, there are
hundreds of small-scale chlorine leaks every year throughout the world that
require fire department or hazardous material teams to respond in order to protect the public, creating considerable expense to the public as well as inconvenience and the risk of injury.

Multiple fatalities commonly occur in the context of a chemical release, fire, or
confined space incident. A confined space is an area that is enclosed so that air does
not circulate freely and the worker is restricted in movement, e.g., inside a tank
or down a well or in a sump (a pit or hole below ground level to collect water or
liquid runoff). Gases may collect to toxic levels in confined spaces more easily

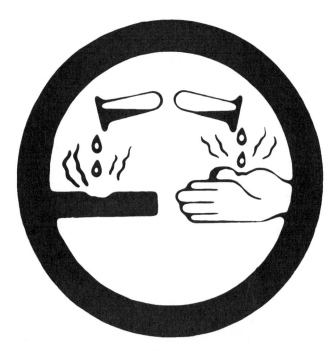

Figure 2.1 There is an international system of Chemical Safety Symbols used in most countries to identify chemical hazards; this is the symbol for a corrosive chemical that destroys
materials and damages human tissue.

than in the open atmosphere, and the restrictions of the space may make rescue difficult. If a worker (usually a male) loses consciousness, his coworkers may forget or ignore their training and attempt a rescue without using proper personal protective equipment. All too often, the result is a second (or even third) fatality and a dangerous time delay in potentially effective rescue efforts.

TOXICOLOGY

Toxicity is the preferred term to refer to the adverse effect of chemicals on the body. The word *poisoning* is usually reserved for serious systemic (total body or internal organ) toxicity and implies a potentially life-threatening or disabling level of toxicity. There are many branches of science that study the normal or desirable effects of chemicals on the body, including pharmacology (the study of medicines and the proper use of drugs) and nutrition and physiology (which use some chemicals to identify the normal functions of the body). The study of toxicity, the adverse (unwanted) effects of chemicals, and of poisonings is called *toxicology*.

The word *toxicology* originates from the Greek word *toxicon*, which means *an arrow*. In ancient times, arrows were dipped into plant poisons to increase their lethality in hunting. Today, toxicology refers to that scientific discipline that explores the deleterious effects of chemicals or of physical or biological factors on living organisms. Toxicology also explores the mechanisms whereby chemical, physical, or biological factors induce harmful effects on the organism.

There are several classifications used in toxicology. One classification is based on the target organs that are harmed by chemicals. Hence, there are terms such as neurotoxicology, lung toxicology, liver toxicology, kidney toxicology, and toxicology of the eye. Toxicology can also be divided into mechanistic toxicology, conducted mainly in university and governmental research institutions, and descriptive or regulatory toxicology that is required for classification and labeling of chemicals for registration purposes (for classifications of toxicology, see **Table 2.1**). Toxicology provides the basis for a number of regulations aimed to protect workers from potentially harmful effects. Today, toxicology has mainly a preventive function that provides information on how chemicals can be used safely.

The science of toxicology recognizes two major, and many minor, phases of a chemical's behavior in the body. The first is how the body takes in and handles the chemical: this is called *toxicokinetics*. The second, called *toxicodynamics*, addresses the effects of the chemicals on the body.

Toxicokinetics

Toxicokinetics addresses the absorption of the chemical into the body (by inhalation, ingestion, skin absorption, or an artificial route such as injection), its distribution to various organs (entrance into the bloodstream, where it goes, and where it tends to accumulate), metabolism (how the body chemically alters it), and excretion (how the body gets rid of it). The term *toxicokinetics* is also used for calculations and models that describe or predict how exposure to a chemical will result in levels in the blood and retention in various organs of the body.

TABLE 2.1

CLASSIFICATIONS OF TOXICOLOGY

Area of Toxicology	What It Covers
Mechanistic toxicology	Understanding of cellular and molecular mechanisms
Regulatory toxicology	Drafting regulations and legislation
Organ-specific toxicology	Defining organ-specific effects, defining chemically induced critical effects
Forensic toxicology	Diagnoses and fatalities
Occupational toxicology	Delineating occupational hazards and risks and prevention
Environmental toxicology	Identification of chemical hazards in the environment and their effects on humans and wildlife species
Clinical toxicology	Diagnosis and treatment of poisoning

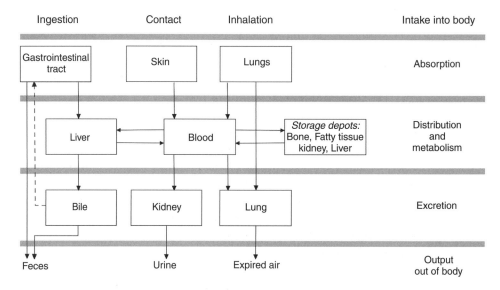

Figure 2.2 The movement of chemicals in the body can be described by the four stages of toxicokinetics: absorption, distribution, metabolism, and excretion.

Absorption is the first phase of toxicokinetics. Chemicals may enter the body through several portals, or *routes of entry*: through the lungs (inhalation), across the stomach or intestines (ingestion), across the skin (transdermal absorption), or artificially by experimental or medical routes of exposure (injection). In workplace situations, by far the most common opportunities for exposure are skin contact and inhalation of the agent. However, ingestion plays an important role in environmental exposure and in some special workplace situations, e.g., when a worker holds tools in his or her mouth or eats food in the workplace.

The route of entry is very important in determining the initial site of injury and the potential for subsequent damage. The rate at which a chemical enters the bloodstream is determined by absorption across the barrier presented by the given route of exposure, which usually reflects the degree to which the chemical is soluble in fats and oils (which make up most of cell membranes). Notably, the barrier in the lung is extremely thin, and chemicals of all kinds cross it easily, which is why inhalation usually results in much higher blood concentration than absorption by other routes.

The toxicity of the chemical may or may not involve the organ of first contact or site of entry. Many chemicals that are absorbed by ingestion damage the liver because the liver receives blood drained from the stomach and intestines. Some of these chemicals, and many others, are chemically transformed in the liver to metabolites that may be more toxic than the initial chemical. This early stage of metabolism is called *premetabolism*. Other chemicals enter the body without damage along the way but affect a distant organ. (In the case of carbon monoxide, inhalation causes no toxicity whatsoever to the lung, but the effect on the oxygen-carrying capacity of the blood may severely affect the brain.) Other chemicals may cause local toxicity without significant absorption into the body, such as strong irritants applied to the skin that cause a chemical burn. Many solvents take fat out of the skin and increase the efficiency of their own absorption across the skin and into the blood stream.

Distribution is the second phase of toxicokinetics. Once the chemical is absorbed and enters the bloodstream, it is transported in the blood to tissues throughout the body. After one pass through the circulation, the chemical is uniformly mixed in arterial blood regardless of its route of entry. The concentration in the blood peaks and then declines as the chemical is distributed to tissues throughout the body. Special barriers may act to keep the chemical from penetrating some organs, such as the *blood-brain barrier* and the placenta. Much of the chemical, however, moves into various organs; fat-soluble chemicals, in particular, move into fat-rich organs, and metals tend to locate in bone. Many chemicals, especially those that are fat-soluble, are stored in organs (storage sites are often called *depots*) and rapidly disappear from the bloodstream. Over time, some of the total amount of the chemical that is stored in organs, called the *body burden*, moves out again into the bloodstream and around the body in a process called *mobilization*.

Metabolism is the third phase of toxicokinetics. Within organs, especially the liver, many chemicals are transformed by chemical reactions into *metabolites*. These transformations may have the effect of either "detoxifying," by rendering the agent toxicologically inactive, or of "activation," by converting the native agent into a metabolite that is more active in producing the same or another toxic effect. An active chemical may be transformed into an inactive metabolite, effectively removing the agent from the body in its toxicologically active form. However, an inactive precursor may also be transformed into an active metabolite. The most complicated metabolic pathways are those for organic compounds. However, metals may also be metabolized.

Excretion is the last phase of toxicokinetics. Without excretion, the chemical or its metabolite would accumulate and remain within the body. The other components are metabolism or sequestration (storage). The kidneys are the major route of excretion for most chemicals. Chemicals that are water-soluble may be filtered or excreted unchanged. The liver, besides being an important organ for metabolism, also secretes some chemicals into bile, including heavy metals such as lead and mercury. Volatile gases are often readily excreted by the lungs because they diffuse back out from the blood, especially if they are poorly soluble.

Kinetics, often also called *toxicokinetics*, is also used to describe the elimination of chemicals from the bloodstream in mathematical terms. Metabolism and excretion define the rates of *elimination*, which is the change in the concentration of the chemical in the plasma with time. Elimination may occur because the chemical is excreted, because it is converted to something else by metabolism, or because it is stored somewhere inaccessible to the bloodstream. The description of the rates of elimination of the agent is an important tool in understanding its behavior in the body. The period required for the plasma concentration to drop by half is called the *half-life* ($t_{1/2}$), which is strictly applicable to only one type of kinetics (in which the rate of elimination is proportional to the concentration) but can also be calculated as a convenient approximation in more complicated situations. The kinetics of many chemicals in the body are very complicated and may involve many different half-lives, reflecting the different depots and rates of metabolism in different organs.

Toxicodynamics

Paracelsus (a 16th-century Swiss physician) wrote, "The dose makes the poison." He meant that everything can be toxic at a high enough exposure; it is solely the dose that matters. Chemical compounds create their toxic effects by inducing changes in cell physiology and biochemistry, thus an understanding of cellular biology is a prerequisite if one wishes to understand the nature of toxic reactions.

Toxic reactions occur by several mechanisms: activation of metabolism, production of reactive intermediates and subsequent reactions with cell macromolecules, changing receptor responses, or through abnormal defense reactions. Several compounds cause toxicity by mimicking the organism's own hormones or neurotransmitters, thereby activating the body's endogenous receptors in some non-physiological way. (See **Box 2.1** for a brief discussion of chronic lung toxicity and carcinogenicity, as they play a central role in occupational health.)

Toxicodynamics is a vast field of study that is concerned with exactly how a chemical affects the body. Chemicals may, for example, interact with molecular receptors in or on the cell to provoke reactions, they may react chemically with tissues and molecules in the body, they may change body chemistry, they may interfere with the normal action of hormones or nutrients, or they may cause irritation and inflammation in parts of the body. Toxicodynamics equally concerns itself with very specific toxic responses to chemicals (such as the responses to lead) and very general responses that are common to many chemicals, such as irritant effects. Chemicals may cause a toxic effect that gets worse with greater exposure (a *gradient* effect, such as lead poisoning), or they may cause a particular effect that does not vary but becomes more likely when exposure increases (a *stochastic* effect, such as cancer or allergies). The relationship between either the magnitude of the adverse effect or the frequency of the adverse effect and the degree of exposure to the chemical is called the *dose-response effect* (or *exposure-response effect*) and is critical to occupational health and worker protection.

A toxic reaction may take place during or soon after exposure, or it may appear only after a latency period. The longer the time interval between exposure and effect, the more difficult it is to show the relationship between them. *Acute toxicity* involves adverse effects that occur immediately or very soon after exposure. They are relatively easy to associate with the exposure, and the exposure-effect relationship can readily be demonstrated. *Chronic toxicity* usually appears after exposure of several years in humans. In chronic toxicity laboratory tests, animals are usually exposed for most or all of their lifetime.

Toxic effects often disappear after the cessation of the exposure, and if that occurs, the effects are called *reversible*. However, sometimes the damage is permanent, and these effects can be *irreversible*. Toxic chemicals that cause adverse effects in function but do not damage the structure of tissues are more likely to be reversible.

The body's ability to grow back, or *regenerate*, and replace the damaged tissue is one of the most important factors that determines reversibility of toxic effects. For example, liver tissue has a remarkable capacity to regenerate and, therefore, liver injury is often reversible. On the other hand, neuronal cells hardly regenerate at all; thus, most neuronal injury is irreversible. In particular, chronic effects tend to be irreversible.

An important mechanism of toxicity is irritation and inflammation. *Irritation* is a non-specific reaction that occurs when the physical or chemical properties (such as acidity) or chemical reactivity of the chemical causes local damage to tissue, such as on the skin or in the lung. The principal response of the body to irritation, and to many other toxic effects and immune effects (discussed below), is inflammation. *Inflammation* is a non-specific response of the body to irritation, to certain types of toxicity, to infection, to chemical signals sent by cells participating in immune responses, to foreign material in the body, and to the presence of damaged tissue. Inflammation is a complex response of the body involving specialized cells (mostly white cells from the bloodstream) that move into the local tissue to try to attack possible causes of infection and to clean up damaged tissue and debris. When visible, as on the skin, inflammation is characterized by local swelling, redness, warmth, and pain. However, inflammation can occur in any tissue and on a microscopic level. Normally, inflammation is self-limited, and its effects are reversible. Sometimes, the inflammation itself destroys normal tissue, which then must be regenerated and, to achieve a normal structure, remodeled. Other times, inflammation, particularly when severe or long lasting, results in *fibrosis*, which is the formation of scar tissue and is irreversible. Scar tissue consists of strong cords of protein that have replaced the normal structure of the tissue when the damage is too severe to be repaired by the body.

Interaction

Industrial workers are almost always exposed to several agents at the same time. The possible interactions and combined effects of these multiple exposures introduce great uncertainty into toxicology and occupational medicine. The situation is often complicated by the simultaneous presence of lifestyle factors, especially smoking and the use of alcohol and drugs, which may enhance the toxic effect of an agent.

BOX 2.1

Examples of Chronic Lung Toxicity and Carcinogenicity

Chronic damage to the lungs may be due to several subsequent exposures or due to one large dose that markedly exceeds the capacity of pulmonary defense, clearance, and repair mechanisms. Chronic pulmonary toxicity includes emphysema, chronic bronchitis, asthma, lung fibrosis, and lung cancer. The single most important cause of chronic pulmonary toxicity is tobacco smoke, which induces all types of chronic pulmonary toxicity, although not so much fibrosis.

In developed countries, where the prevalence of chronic obstructive lung diseases has increased rapidly, the finger of suspicion is often pointed at the air quality, especially that in large cities. In emphysema, the walls separating alveoli from each other disappear, which reduces the surface area for gas exchange. Chronic bronchitis is characterized by persistent cough and increased mucus secretion. In asthma, the lungs become sensitive to bronchoconstriction induced by environmental agents. In addition, asthma also involves inflammation of the airways.

Lung cancer is one of the most common cancers. In many countries, lung cancer is the most common cancer among the male population, and its incidence among females has shown a dramatic and alarming increase. The incidence of lung cancer has always carried a strong association with past smoking (i.e., the latency period of lung cancer is about 20 years after the beginning of the exposure to tobacco smoke). In addition to tobacco smoke, many chemicals can increase the risk of lung cancer. These include asbestos, radon, nickel, chromium, and beryllium. Asbestos and radon are considered to be the next most important factors causing lung cancer. Both also have a synergistic effect with smoking. The number of asbestos-related diseases has remained high (these include pleural diseases, asbestosis, and cancers), even though the use of asbestos has dramatically decreased and is now totally banned in many countries. This is due to the long latency period of asbestos-induced diseases.

At its simplest, the increased combined effect may be additive. This means that the effect of one chemical (such as a solvent) when added to that of another chemical (another solvent) produces more of the same effect (such as neurotoxicity) in proportion to the additional exposure. Because of this presumption of *additivity*, it is possible to sum up the exposure to many different solvents, taking into account their potency, and to consider the total as effectively equivalent to one exposure. This greatly simplifies regulation.

However, some combined exposures show positive interaction, also called *synergy* or *potentiation*, in which the additional effect of one chemical (e.g., the common and relatively harmless solvent MEK) is disproportionately greater in the presence of another chemical (e.g., the toxic solvent MiBK). Positive interactions may arise from the physical characteristics of the exposure: for example, exposure to dust in uranium mines greatly increases the risk of lung cancer because radionuclides in the air (radon daughters derived from the decay of uranium atoms) are adsorbed onto the surface of respirable dust particles and carried more efficiently and much more deeply into the lung than they would be otherwise. Other positive interactions occur at the cellular level. The combination of exposure to asbestos with cigarette smoking is highly synergistic in causing lung cancer.

The idea of interactions is used in occupational or industrial hygiene. The toxic effects of most organic solvents are usually considered to be additive, as noted. Industrial hygienists use the combined exposure level to assess the condition by estimating total effective exposure using a simple arithmetic calculation. It is obtained by dividing the concentration of each solvent with its occupational exposure level, or OEL, and by adding the quotients. If the sum exceeds one, the exposure is considered to be excessive. There are cases of synergism, where the toxic effects of individual exposures become greatly potentiated. In general, if the various constituents of a mixed exposure do not have known mutual interactions, the effects of different agents can be considered individually. However, few combinations of chemicals have actually been studied for synergism.

There are few examples of negative interaction, or *antagonism*, in occupational toxicology, but several examples of drugs that, if taken in combination, have less effect than the sum of the effects of either alone. The idea of antagonism has led to poorly conceived efforts to prevent exposure-related disease in the workplace by exposing workers to chemicals that reduce their risk, a strategy called *prophylaxis*. One of the few examples of antagonism in occupational toxicology was the effect of aluminum dust in reducing the effect of silica in causing the lung disease silicosis. For many years, aluminum dust was inhaled by miners in a number of countries as a preventive measure, but this was stopped when it was learned that aluminum dust causes its own health problem. Today, occupational health professionals do not consider this strategy to be ethical or effective. Modern occupational hygiene emphasizes control of exposure to the hazard itself.

Toxicity and Immunity

Toxicity is usually distinguished from immunity, including allergy, although toxicologists are sometimes interested in both. There are basic differences between toxic and immune, including allergic reactions. A toxic response disrupts the normal function or structure of the body as a consequence of a response to the chemical's own characteristics, i.e., its structure, chemical reactivity, capacity to bind with molecules in the body, etc. A toxin's effect on the body is not anticipated by the human body, nor is it remembered by the body after the exposure ceases. A toxic response will occur the first time that the body encounters the chemical, and every time the body subsequently encounters the chemical the response will develop in the same way.

An *immune reaction* is a very particular type of response in which the body's own mechanisms come into play to recognize, remember, and respond very specifically to a particular chemical. In an immune reaction, the body must first encounter a chemical and recognize it on a cellular level as foreign or distinct from itself. The chemical then becomes an *antigen*, which is simply a name for a chemical that provokes an immune response. The body keeps a memory of the chemical, or antigen, at a cellular level (specific cells in the body "remember" specific antigens) and will recognize that chemical again at the next encounter. When the body is subsequently exposed to the chemical, one of many possible immune responses may develop. These immune responses are stereotyped, meaning that they always happen in the same way and they are always triggered when the body encounters the specific chemical, even at very low levels. Immune responses are called *hypersensitivity*, and a physician will describe the condition by saying that a person has been *sensitized* or is *sensitive* to an antigen. Thus, in toxicology and medicine, the term *sensitivity* has a very specific meaning and implies an immune response, not generalized susceptibility.

Typically, cells of the immune system may produce *antibodies*, small proteins that attack and bind to the chemical antigens—vaccinations use this same response to artificially induce immunity to bacteria and viral infections. Other immune cells may directly attack the antigen, trying to destroy it as if it were a bacteria or parasite. These cells cause some damage on their own and send out chemical signals, called *cytokines*, which attract white cells from the blood and in so doing cause inflammation. Other specialized cells may react in a very specific way to antigens, triggering the release of *chemical mediators*, which in turn provoke local inflammation and reactions such as hives in the skin or asthma in the lungs. Some varieties of immune response are described in Chapter 16 on Occupational Diseases.

An allergic response is a particular type of immune reaction that is characterized by the triggering of specialized cells and the release of chemical mediators and cytokines. An allergic reaction, like other hypersensitivity responses, always requires exposure to the compound and occurs only among those individuals already sensitized after the earlier exposure. Even minute doses can elicit an allergic reaction in a sensitized individual. Common allergic responses include asthma, certain types of skin rash (eczema and urticaria, or hives), allergic rhinitis (commonly called hay fever), types of sinusitis, and food allergies (Aldridge 1996). The most serious type of allergy is called *anaphylaxis*. In this condition, exposure to the antigen may result in asthma-like wheezing, swelling that may obstruct the throat, and a drop in blood pressure. Anaphylaxis is sometimes fatal and is disproportionately triggered among people with allergies to bee stings or peanuts and among workers who handle laboratory animals.

TOXICOLOGY IN OCCUPATIONAL HEALTH

Before steps can be taken to protect the health of workers, the association between the exposure and the disease has to be established. The role of toxicology in worker protection is to identify harmful chemicals and other hazards in the first place and then to determine a safe level of exposure, if any, for their use. After toxicological research has identified exposure-effect relationships for different chemicals, limits or standards (commonly called *occupational exposure levels*, or OELs) for various industrial chemicals can be established. Workers can then be protected against excessive exposure through the measurement of exposure in the workplace, to validate the effectiveness of exposure controls and to ensure that the OELs are not violated.

Toxicology, occupational hygiene, and occupational medicine are all closely interrelated because they have a common goal—to protect workers from occupational hazards in the workplace. The role of toxicological research is to protect the worker by characterizing the biological effects of chemicals and by identifying the hazardous agents, whereas the goal of occupational hygiene is to protect workers by identifying excessive exposure levels and improving the occupational environment. Based on the insights obtained from toxicology, occupational hygienists know how to identify, evaluate, and control chemical hazards to acceptable levels. They measure levels to ensure that exposures are at a safe level and apply technology to controlling exposures if they are not. The role of occupational medicine in protecting workers from chemical toxicity is to identify early signs of adverse effects and to identify, diagnose, and treat work-related diseases.

RISK ASSESSMENT

One of the most challenging issues of toxicology has been the assessment of carcinogenic risks induced by chemicals. The concept of risk is basic to human life and is commonly applied to hazards that are encountered in such varied settings as automobile traffic, sports, health care, insurance, and financial markets. In occupational health, as with environmental health, the concept of risk has been formalized and the probabilities of risk have been quantified in a discipline called *risk assessment*. Risk assessment is a statistically based science that estimates the likelihood that a given adverse effect will occur. It is based on the principles of toxicology. While risk assessment tends to focus on single isolated risks, the management of the hazard or decision making regarding controlling the risk, a process called *risk management*, must take into account the variety of exposures humans face every day.

In risk assessment, the term *risk* implies the probability that a certain adverse health effect will take place, under defined circumstances. On the other hand, the term *security* implies the probability that no such deleterious incident will occur. First one assesses, on the basis of the weight of evidence, whether a chemical is a carcinogen or not. Secondly, one must estimate the magnitude of the risk to humans exposed to a given chemical in an occupational setting or in their general environment. The outcome of such an assessment should be an estimate of the actual number of additional cases of cancer among exposed persons. This risk assessment utilizes data from experimental animal studies, epidemiological human studies, and all available information on human exposure under different occupational and other living conditions. Risk assessment has usually been divided into four different and well-defined phases to assure that important issues will be given a fair consideration. The phases of systematic risk assessment are, in sequence:

1. hazard identification
2. hazard characterization
3. assessment of exposure
4. risk characterization

Hazard identification (step 1) concerns the identification of new chemicals or other factors that may cause harmful health effects. Previously, novel hazards were usually observed in case studies or after accidents or other excessive exposures, usually in occupational environments. Today, thorough toxicity studies are required on all pesticides, food additives, and drugs prior to human exposure. New chemicals must be studied for their potential toxic effects. In the past, hazards were mostly identified only after they had caused harmful effects in humans. Today, the vast majority of chemical products have been evaluated for their toxicity using laboratory animals. Therefore, hazard identification has evolved to a preventive procedure that is based on safety studies before a chemical compound or product reaches the market and before individuals are exposed to it.

Hazard characterization (step 2) utilizes data from toxicity studies with experimental animals. Hazard characterization includes delineating dose-effect or dose-response relationships so that the effect can be estimated for a given level of exposure. Health authorities in different countries have issued strict guidelines and regulations on the studies that must be carried out to evaluate the toxicity of pesticides, food additives, and drugs. Furthermore, the European Union, the Organisation for Economic Co-operation and Development (OECD), and the U.S. Environmental Protection Agency and Food and Drug Administration all have issued regulations to control the safety of drugs, food additives, pesticides, and other chemicals. The technical quality of the studies is governed by good laboratory practice (GLP) guidelines. **Table 2.2** lists the toxicity/safety studies required for the registration of drugs, pesticides, and food additives employing experimental animals or other test systems.

Exposure assessment (step 3) allows a risk assessor to estimate the human significance of the effects induced by high doses of a chemical in experimental animals. Exposure assessment is required for quantitative risk assessment because it allows a comparison between effects induced by high doses with those induced by low doses, and also allows one to compare how large the difference is between the dose that causes a toxic effect in an experimental animal and the human dose in an occupational setting or general environment. This is vital because, in most cases, toxicity assessment (especially for new chemicals) is based purely on experimental animal studies. Exposure assessment in the occupational environment relates the human exposure situation to the toxicity data derived from experimental animal studies. In the exposure assessment, the time-weighted average concentration of the airborne pollutants is usually determined, preferably at the breathing zone. For chemicals that may penetrate the skin, the dermal exposure should also be assessed.

The final step in risk assessment, risk characterization, aims at achieving a synthesis from the data gathered in steps 1 through 3. In risk characterization, the human exposure situation is estimated, usually from the toxicity data from animal studies. The goal of such a synthesis is quantitative risk assessment. This implies that the outcome of the process should be numerical (e.g., an estimate indicating how many extra cases of a deleterious health outcome will be produced due to exposure to a given exposure level in a given population).

When it is necessary to assess risks of compounds with carcinogenic or allergic properties, risk assessment becomes much more difficult. This applies especially to genotoxic carcinogens that have been assumed to have no safe level—thus the only safe level would be zero. In this circumstance, linear extrapolation or various mathematical models that assume the absence of a safe dose are used in human risk assessment. On these occasions, the acceptable risk level has often been set to 1/10,000,000. Linear extrapolation or mathematical models are used because the true mechanisms of chemical carcinogenesis are not known. Therefore, risk regulators, when carrying out risk assessment, are intentionally conservative in their risk assessment to guarantee the safety of exposed populations.

RISK MANAGEMENT

Risk management addresses how to manage the hazard that gives rise to the risk. The process involves a decision, often by a regulatory agency, about how to deal with the hazard. Governments have many possible alternatives for managing risks: outright bans; regulations requiring effective control technology; setting standards that limit exposure; public health advisory messages; public education; and imposing fines, taxes, or penalties for unsafe use. Industry also has many ways of dealing with hazards, including control technology, isolating or containing the hazard, substituting a less hazardous product in the production process, administrative controls to track and limit exposure of workers, educating workers, providing personal protective equipment, and good housekeeping.

TABLE 2.2

TOXICITY STUDIES FOR SAFETY/TOXICITY EVALUATION OF CHEMICALS USING EXPERIMENTAL ANIMALS AND OTHER SYSTEMS REQUIRED BY HEALTH AUTHORITIES

Name of the Study	Animal Species	Duration of Study	Reason for Study
Biotransformation	Rats/mice	1 day to weeks	Metabolism
Kinetic studies	Rats/mice	1 day to weeks	Absorption, distribution, and elimination
Acute toxicity	Rats/mice	2 weeks	Acute effects
Subacute toxicity	Rats/mice	2–3 weeks	Delayed effects, target organs
Subchronic study	Rats/mice/dogs/ rabbits	6 months	Target organs, delayed effects
Chronic studies	Rats/mice	18–24 months	Chronic effects of low exposures
Carcinogenicity	Rats/mice	18–24 months	Carcinogenic potential
Teratogenicity	Rats/rabbits	3–4 weeks	Teratogenic potential
Reproductive	Rats/mice/rabbits	Several months	Potential to affect toxicity reproduction
Irritation	Rats/rabbits	Few days	Irritation index
Sensitization	Guinea pig/rats	Few weeks	Potential to sensitize
Mutagenicity	Rats/mice/ bacterial strains/ yeasts	Few days	Potential to cause genotoxicity mutations, chromosomal damages, other genotoxic effects

Policy makers should recognize that the mere existence of a chemical hazard does not necessarily mean a risk to humans. However, risk communication is a difficult task because the concept of risk is difficult to relay and comprehend. Among lay people, especially, the familiarity of the risk (e.g., smoking vs. food additives) and the severity of the outcome of an event (e.g., airplane vs. car accident) have a major impact on the perception of risks. However, perception of risks is important because that ultimately determines how effectively the knowledge produced by toxicological research can be utilized to protect human health, both in the occupational and general environment.

If risk assessment yields reliable estimates, decision makers will be able to prioritize the health hazards and also carry out the cost/benefit analyses. Weighing health risks induced by exposure to chemical compounds against benefits or costs tends to be approached differently in different societies. The calculation is also different for occupational and environmental hazards. In the occupational environment, one deals with relatively high exposure levels compared to those normally experienced by the general public. On the other hand, the general population is much larger, and the magnitude of risk varies widely. Most workers are healthy or they would not be working, but in the general environment there are many people who are more susceptible to exposure to chemicals due to poorer health. In occupational environments, the exposure levels may be orders of magnitude higher than in the general environment, but the health effects from exposure are relatively fewer due to the lower number of exposed individuals. Also, in occupational environments, the exposed populations can be clearly defined and appropriate measures can be undertaken to prevent excessive exposure.

In addition, the present occupational exposure levels are low when compared with 20 or 30 years ago. Toxic chemicals, such as benzene and carbon disulfide, which were common causes of occupational diseases in the past, are today generally well controlled. Most of the current occupational diseases are caused by exposures that are not particularly acutely toxic but, for example, cause allergies. Even though working conditions have improved markedly during recent decades, the number of individuals suffering from occupational diseases has declined more slowly. The nature of occupational exposures and their consequences are changing; rather than causing acute poisonings, exposures are bringing about longer-term effects, such as allergies and cancers.

Solvents are an example of successful hazard control. Petroleum-based solvents were once heavily used in interior house paints and continue to be used in other industrial applications. These chemicals easily penetrate the skin. They are volatile and are therefore easily inhaled. Water-based products have increasingly replaced solvent-based paint products in many applications, such as painting, printing, and gluing. Although the water-based products may contain glycol derivatives that easily penetrate the skin, they are generally less toxic than the petroleum-based solvents they replaced.

In developing countries, exposures to chemicals like pesticides are still responsible for millions of acute poisoning cases and hundreds of thousands of fatalities every year. This is due in part to a low standard of living, poor education, failure of education to communicate the significance of preventive hygienic measures, and the hazardous effects of the compounds. Furthermore, most developing countries are situated in subtropical or tropical areas where the use of a number of chemicals, such as pesticides, is a necessity. Much more should be done to alleviate this situation, including measures to improve education and increase awareness of the toxicity of the compounds and the appropriate safety precautions.

OCCUPATIONAL EXPOSURE LIMITS

One of the most important strategies for protecting the health of workers from chemical hazards is the setting of standards, or occupational exposure limits (OEL). OELs have been set in most industrial countries to prevent excessive exposures to chemicals.

One of the most effective approaches to protecting the health of workers is to set limits on how much or what concentration of a chemical they are allowed to be in contact with and for what duration of time. Workers exposed to chemicals may experience discomfort and adverse health effects, which may develop into occupational diseases. Establishing standards of exposure limits the risk of occupational disease and limits the severity of toxic effects when they do occur.

The actual chemicals that most often cause problems include isocyanates, epoxies, and acrylic resins, which are major problems principally due to their ability to cause sensitization. Exposure to asbestos and other mineral dusts still causes numerous serious, even fatal, diseases in industrial countries. Solvents and pesticides are probably the groups of chemicals that cause the largest amount of acute poisoning-type occupational diseases.

Traditionally, the greatest occupational hazards have been considered to be inhalable chemicals. For many inhaled chemicals, the adverse effect that results over a short period of time, such as a day, is proportionate to the cumulative dose during that period. Roughly, the toxic effect is the same for any given product ($C \times t$) of concentration (C) times duration (t). A typical work shift is usually 8 hours. So, an exposure at a given level over a typical work shift is roughly equal to exposure to half that level for a double shift or twice that level for a half shift. More commonly, exposure goes up and down as the work progresses and the worker moves around. This rough relationship has given rise to the concept of a time-weighted average, in which the OEL is based on a concentration that is averaged over 8 hours. The 8-hour time-weighted average is the usual format for establishing OELs for inhaled hazards.

Time-weighted OELs are not a perfect solution, however, as there are problems with this approach. For chemicals that are rapidly metabolized or eliminated or, on the other hand, that are highly toxic (such as many toxic gases), the time-weighted average may overestimate or underestimate the true risk of toxicity. Many workers do not work regular 8-hour shifts; they may work longer shifts or overtime. Although the OEL can be recalculated for a longer work shift, the assumptions regarding concentration and duration may break down over longer periods of time. OELs do not protect all susceptible individuals and cannot protect against immune responses. Many OELs remain educated guesses, and numerous and often large changes have been made when the OEL lists have been revised.

In addition, most chemicals remain without any OEL. Only about 2,000 chemicals have an OEL, according to the International Labour Office.

For most OELs, however, the time-weighted average works acceptably well and has remained the basis for occupational exposure standards. When one compares the incidences of occupational diseases in industrialized countries with the frequency of OEL violations, a good correlation is observed. This indicates that these OELs do protect the health of workers.

OELs are ultimately based on experimental animal and epidemiological studies. Most new agents have been subjected to extensive toxicological testing. For the older chemicals, epidemiological data is often available. Key to establishing an OEL is to know, approximately, at what level toxicity begins or, for stochastic diseases such as cancer, at what level an excess risk is observed. In animal studies, one seeks to identify the highest dose that does not cause any toxicity to rodents, which is called the *no observable adverse effect level* (NOAEL). Sometimes all that is available is the lowest dose that has been observed to cause toxicity to rodents, which is called the *lowest observable adverse effect level* (LOAEL). The NOAEL or, if necessary, the LOAEL establishes a benchmark, or reference dose, around which there is great statistical uncertainty and which cannot itself be considered a safe level of exposure.

Animal studies are indispensable in evaluating chemical hazards, but the findings must be interpreted and recalculated to approximate human exposure. Human exposure is extrapolated taking into account body surface area and routes of exposure. There are differences between species to take into account, particularly with regard to metabolism. Because animal studies are conducted on relatively small numbers of animals, usually rats, there is statistical uncertainty when extrapolating to humans. Epidemiological studies have the advantage of describing the human response to chemical exposure directly. However, they may be statistically uncertain, especially if the studies are small and/or contain potential biasing factors.

Many OELs are based on sensory irritation, which has the most easily definable values. It has also been found that the OELs for sensory irritants can be experimentally evaluated with a standardized mouse test (ASTM E 981-84 bioassay) where the concentration that causes a 50% decrease in respiratory rate is determined (RD_{50}). The OELs for these chemicals are, on average, 3% of RD_{50}.

Usually, a safety margin approach is utilized by applying a safety factor to the reference dose, NOAEL, or LOAEL. This safety margin is needed to account for uncertainties and individual variation in the susceptibility of animals and humans to the effects of the exposure. Usually, the assumption is that humans are more sensitive than experimental animals. To ensure a reasonable margin of safety, the *safety factor* usually takes into consideration two aspects: first, the differences in biotransformation within a species (human), usually 10, and secondly, the differences in the sensitivity between species (e.g., rat vs. human), usually also 10. For example, if the NOAEL is 100 mg/kg, this dose is divided by the combined safety factor of 100. The safe dose level for humans would then be 1 mg/kg. This approach is used in deterministic toxicological effects, such as target organ toxicity (neurotoxicity, kidney toxicity). This approach also requires the assumption of a threshold in the effect—that there is a safe dose below which no harmful effects occur. Thus, this approach assumes that a chemical compound expresses a typical sigmoid dose-effect curve in its toxic effects.

A particularly strict exposure control policy is applied for carcinogenic chemicals. The OELs are usually lowered considerably, even when a chemical is only suspected of being a carcinogen. When the evidence becomes stronger, the OELs are usually tightened further. Vinyl chloride provides a good example; its OEL was first lowered to 20 ppm (parts per million) from 500 ppm and then further to 3 ppm in Sweden in 1974–1975, when it was discovered to cause a very rare type of cancer, angiosarcoma of the liver. The rarity of the disease made it possible to identify the association without doubt. On the other hand, the practical impact of this causal link remains rather low. It has been estimated that fewer than 400 angiosarcoma cases will appear worldwide due to vinyl chloride exposure (in comparison to the number of occupational cancers caused by asbestos, which is about 1,000-fold higher).

After the use of a chemical becomes widespread, new deleterious effects on human health may be observed. Usually, this new information is gained concerning the long-term effects. In such situations, the occupational limit values may need to be modified. Thus, the OELs tend to decrease over time as information accumulates on the toxicity of a chemical.

3

OCCUPATIONAL EPIDEMIOLOGY

Panu Oksa and Jukka Uitti

Epidemiology is the science that studies the distribution and determinants of health-related states and events in populations and how this knowledge can be applied to controlling health problems. From a practical point of view, epidemiology is the branch of public health that attempts to discover causes for diseases in order to enable disease prevention. Epidemiologists study the factors or determinants that influence health on the level of populations and communities, rather than individuals. It is a discipline that studies the occurrence of human illness.

During the 20th century, the scope of epidemiology broadened from an early emphasis on the study of infectious disease epidemics to include all phenomena related to health in populations. The range of topics may include acute and chronic diseases, mental health problems, states of health or well-being, the quality of health care, etc. As the focus of epidemiological studies has broadened, so has the methodology. It can be used in clinical, experimental, or prognostic studies; in the evaluation of preventive methods; in screening; and in registry studies.

Occupational epidemiology deals with the occurrence of work-related health hazards and the risks associated with them. A typical focus has been the study of possible causal relations between occupational exposures and observed illnesses among working populations. On the other hand, the aforementioned broader definition for occupational epidemiology allows us to study all health-related (also socially related) outcomes and their determinants in occupational settings.

Under this definition, a *determinant* may be an event, a characteristic, an exposure to a hazard, a genetic trait, a behavior, or any other definable factor that brings about change in a health condition or other defined characteristic. More simply, all factors influencing the occurrence of disease can be called the determinants of disease. In occupational epidemiology, the determinants are usually various chemical or physical exposures, workload, and various stress factors that tend to drive, or dominate, the risk in groups of workers. General determinants such as age, sex, smoking, and other lifestyle factors must also be considered because workers are also subject to the same determinants of risk as the general population.

Determinants may actually cause the disorder; in the literal sense, they may be part of the sequence of events that results in the disease, or they may contribute to an increase in the probability that the disease will occur, possibly by setting the stage for the exposure. For example, one of the most powerful determinants of pesticide toxicity is illiteracy: when workers cannot read, they are less able to follow instructions and to handle pesticides safely; therefore, excessive exposure is more likely to take place.

Determinants are very important on a population basis and, as in the case of cigarette smoking, may powerfully drive the health status of a national population. Epidemiology is a more general guide that describes how determinants work statistically in populations. However, individual cases of a disease may or may not result from these statistical determinants of disease. Individual cases have to be decided on the basis of their own circumstances. Epidemiology can provide only a general guide to what is most likely in the individual case.

In this chapter we will present a short introduction to occupational epidemiology from a practical point of view, and we will describe why and how epidemiology can be used in occupational settings.

OCCUPATIONAL EPIDEMIOLOGY

Epidemiology is one of the basic disciplines employed in studying occupational health issues. Most studies concerning occupational health problems are based on epidemiological methods. It is therefore important to understand the methods of epidemiology in order to understand where occupational health knowledge comes from. An understanding of occupational epidemiology depends on knowing what questions it asks and why it asks them, as in **Table 3.1**. Mostly these questions concern the relationship between occupational exposure and disease. The analogous questions can be presented in psychological or sociological contexts.

The first and most basic question in epidemiology is: "Does exposure increase the risk of disease?" This is a basic relationship that is characteristic of the cause of a disease or the circumstances that are likely to produce an injury. The second question, "What is the quantitative relationship between exposure and disease?" is important for many reasons. It is part of the proof that the relationship is causal, because increasing exposure to the cause normally leads to an increased frequency and, for many outcomes, increased severity of the disease it causes. Quantifying the relationship is essential to provide information for risk assessment and the development of standards or occupational exposure levels. Ideally, such studies help to identify a level of exposure that is acceptably safe and that will prevent disease. The question "Is the risk of disease increased at low levels?" has tremendous practical importance because if the disease is serious and potential exposure is unavoidable when, for example, a chemical is used in the workplace, there may need to be a ban on its use or, at the very least, different approaches to controlling exposure, such as the use of personal protective equipment. "What factors modify the relationship between exposure and disease?" is of great practical importance to understand why the disease occurs in some people but not others and what else might be possible to decrease the risk of the disease if direct exposure cannot be further reduced.

The clarification of causes and causal mechanisms is important for scientific progress but also for risk management in practical working life. Knowledge based on results from epidemiological studies is necessary for both purposes.

Occupational conditions can be improved depending on the available economic resources. For this purpose it is necessary to gather information on the consequences of avoidance of the studied occupational agent before managers of companies or society will be willing to initiate practical measures of prevention. The question "Is control of exposure effective in reducing the risk of disease?" is important as a practical matter to ensure that control efforts work and also represents a scientific confirmation that exposure is likely to be the cause of the disease.

Thus, epidemiology can be seen as an important instrument in the identification of risk factors, assessment of risk, and risk management, including preventive measures.

Finally, many occupational diseases have more than one cause and may have interacting or complicated or multiple causes. The question "Which factor or which factors together cause disease in multiple exposures?" opens the door to a better understanding of the disease and also to alternative ways of preventing it by controlling different risk factors.

A variety of behavioral or biomedical factors affect the health status of a worker both on and off the job. Many determinants of disease have similar effects as common occupational hazards, for example, both smoking and exposure to asbestos cause lung cancer. Control of lung cancer due to asbestos requires control of asbestos in the workplace. However, control of cigarette smoking requires public education and community action to support a change in individual behavior. In order to prevent disease more effectively, it is important to evaluate the etiological fraction of each potential causative factor and to design control strategies that work for each major determinant.

One of the main tasks of occupational epidemiology today is to separate out important occupational determinants from other causes in *multicausal* or *multifactoral* diseases such as low back pain, asthma, or coronary heart disease. These are disorders that are common and are not all or even primarily caused by occupational determinants. However, occupational factors contribute to the risk of these common disorders, as do many non-occupational factors. For example, generally known risk factors for coronary heart disease are high blood pressure and elevated serum cholesterol. In industrial settings, exposure to carbon disulphide or carbon monoxide is a known occupational risk factor for coronary heart disease; however, cold climate, physical load, stress, and shift work may also increase this risk.

Epidemiological methods are most challenged when diseases with a long latency time from the onset of exposure to clinical illness are studied. Occupational cancers have been given the most attention thus far. The risk of cancer caused by smoking was revealed by epidemiologists in 1950s. Presently so-called molecular epidemiology is studying the mechanisms of cancer. The methods of molecular epidemiology should make it possible that epidemiologists will not have to wait for the disease to express itself before knowing that it will occur. Based on the results of new technology, preventive measures could then be initiated much sooner. For example, it would then be possible to identify and regulate occupational carcinogens without having to wait 20 years, the typical latency period for cancer, before epidemiological studies can be done.

Models of Epidemiological Research

Occupational epidemiology is a particularly large and well-developed branch of epidemiology. The power of epidemiology lies in its ability to draw conclusions based on data that reflect the human experience. To do this requires the collection of data on people or access to data that have already been collected on people. These data have to be examined, summarized, and analyzed in a systematic, rigorous way. Epidemiology of all types and study designs requires mathematical analysis. The methods that epidemiology uses for studying populations and summarizing their characteristics and relationships are part of a branch of mathematics called *biostatistics*.

Biostatistics provides the essential tools of epidemiological analysis. The basic assumption of biostatistics is that each study is based on a sample of a much larger, complete universe of subjects. For example, a study of 100 painters is a sample of all painters. A study of 3,000 Italian automobile workers may be a sample of all automobile workers or a sample of working-age Italians, depending on the study. Measurements made, or data collected, on the sample are assumed to approximate the most common measurements (central tendency) and distribution of measurements that would be found in the total population. The diversity of measurements is expressed by a number called the *standard deviation*. However, the sample may also be different from the population and fail to reflect its characteristics for reasons of chance alone. Perhaps the sample happened by chance to be unusual. A basic principle of biostatistics is that there is always uncertainty regarding the true value when the measurements or data are summarized. A particular measurement may be very accurate or not at all accurate for an individual subject, but when the measurements for the sample are grouped together and summarized, there remains a question of statistical uncertainty as to whether they accurately reflect the characteristics of the total population. When epidemiologists summarize or calculate a value, such as average height, as a single number (called a *point value*), which is the most likely true value, they also calculate, using the standard deviation, what is called a *confidence interval*, usually providing the range of numbers that reliably would include the true value 95% of the time if the study were repeated over and over. Epidemiologists provide confidence intervals (typically abbreviated CI 95%) for derived values such as risks and ratios (which will be described below). The confidence interval is also useful in comparing two values, because if the confidence intervals do not overlap, the values can be presumed to be different at a 95% level of confidence, the level of conventional statistical significance. Biostatistics is, in a sense, the language and analytical tool of epidemiology.

Standard models of epidemiological study design are illustrated in Figure 3.1.

Occupational epidemiological studies are usually *observational*, meaning that they observe and describe the experience of the group of people being studied, but the investigator does not or cannot intervene or change the exposure or conditions under which people are working. Observational studies are often done by examining the experience of groups of people who have been exposed in the past,

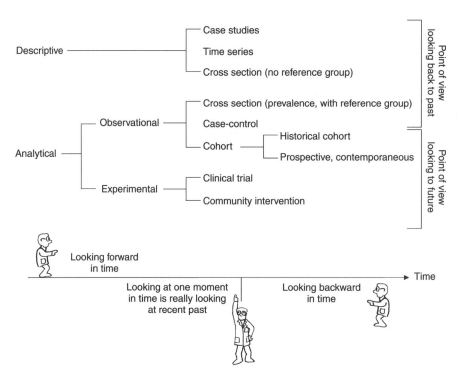

Figure 3.1 Standard models for epidemiological studies. Cohort, or prospective, studies look forward to what happens after the exposure begins, even if the study is based on information gathered in the past.

TABLE 3.1

QUESTIONS CONCERNING EPIDEMIOLOGY IN OCCUPATIONAL MEDICINE

1. Does exposure increase the risk of disease?
2. What is the quantitative relationship between exposure and disease?
3. Is the risk of disease increased at low exposure?
4. What factors modify the relationship between exposure and disease?
5. Is control of exposure effective in reducing the risk of disease?
6. Which factor or which factors together cause disease in multiple exposures?

(Adapted from Venables, K. M. 1994. "Epidemiology." In *Occupational Lung Disorders*, edited by W. R. Parkes, 3rd ed. Oxford: Butterworth-Heinemann.)

in which case they are often called *retrospective*, or by following the experience of people into the future, in which case they are called *prospective*.

The observational approach in occupational epidemiology is in contrast to experimental approaches, such as randomized clinical trials. Clinical trials are common in trials of new drugs or treatments and are similar to a laboratory experiment. In clinical trials, subjects are given the exposure (medicines or forms of treatment) on a random basis under the supervision of the investigator, and the result is a study similar to a laboratory experiment. It is not possible to do this in occupational epidemiology, because the investigator almost never has the capability, authority, or even the legal or ethical right to change the exposure experienced by subjects of the study. The exposure has occurred or will occur as a result of characteristics of the job or workplace that are beyond the control of the investigator. The observational approach enables a study to be conducted in many situations in which a randomized trial would be unethical or impractical. However, the lack of control over exposure is also the main limitation of occupational epidemiological studies. Observational studies are susceptible to more and different biases than experimental studies.

An observational study can be *descriptive* or *analytical*. Descriptive studies simply describe the patterns of what is observed. A particularly important class of descriptive studies is surveillance studies, which are conducted to see if the number of cases or rates of a disease are getting more or less frequent, indicating that the situation is getting better or worse. An analytical study seeks to identify associations with these patterns that may lead to clues about the cause and the conditions under which they occur. Analytical studies probe more deeply and are usually designed to identify causes that can be controlled in order to prevent disease.

Descriptive epidemiology is intended to get a big picture of the situation to determine the basic pattern of the disorder: how common a disease or injury may be and who in the population is affected or where the disease or injury may be occurring. Descriptive studies often form a sufficient basis for administrative decisions; for example, if respiratory symptoms and occupational allergic diseases were frequent in a bakery, it would be worthwhile to invest in ventilation to make the work environment less dusty.

Descriptive studies are of two types, *cross-sectional studies* and *time series*. A cross-sectional study design provides information on many factors at one point in time. Time series are studies that look at one number or indicator over a period of time, such as the number of cases or (when adjusted for the size of the population) the rate of a disease over several years. Time series show trends in the measurement over the period (called secular trends), and the studies are often also called *longitudinal studies*. Time series, or longitudinal studies, are particularly useful for determining whether a problem is getting better or worse over time. However, they provide no information on what is driving the trend, even when they include a comparison with other populations or places.

Descriptive *cross-sectional* studies describe the numbers of cases or rates of a disease, exposure to hazards, or other features of a population at one point in time, such as a given year or month. The observational unit can be any defined group of people, such as the population of a city, workers of a certain profession, or all workers in a company or in a particular plant. Cross-sectional studies may be used to describe who (in terms of age, sex, or other characteristics) gets an occupational disease, where it tends to occur (in which department of a plant, for example), what symptoms or problems are reported, and when the person remembers first developing the symptom or how long he or she has had it. It may be important to know how many persons in a particular population (for example, the fraction of workers in a bakery) have respiratory symptoms and allergic diseases. However, cross-sectional studies are usually limited in what they can reveal.

They do not capture information over time and so are less reliable for determining when a problem began and identifying a cause-and-effect situation. A descriptive cross-sectional study is not generally informative on the subject of causality and is often conducted without a comparison group and so cannot be considered scientific. A simple cross-sectional study design may nevertheless fill the needs for practical decision making.

The information from descriptive studies is summarized mathematically using *descriptive statistics*, such as the average (an example of a measure of central tendency that summarizes the data and shows what is the most likely value), the range (a simple measure of variability that shows how far apart the smallest and lowest values are), or the standard deviation (a more sophisticated measure of variability that shows how scattered the data are). More sophisticated studies are required to show relationships, however.

Analytical studies try to establish the presence or absence of relationships by examining the probability, compared to chance, of an association between the outcomes and significant risk factors or determinants. This is usually done by comparing the frequency of the outcome (e.g., allergies) in a group with the exposure (e.g., wheat flour) to the frequency of the outcome in a group without the exposure (e.g., workers in the bakery who package bread that is already baked or clerks in a store that sells the bread). If the outcome occurs more often when the determinant is present or present at a higher level, then this could be evidence that the determinant caused or is in some other way associated with the outcome. (For example, if allergies appeared only among those workers in the bakery who worked with flour and not among those who did not, or among clerks in the bread store, it would suggest that flour might either be a cause of the allergies or might coexist with whatever else it might be that was causing the allergies, perhaps a filling for a pastry made with wheat flour.) Because apparent associations may occur by chance alone, which is often called "coincidence" in daily life, the frequencies have to be studied with statistical methods that compare the likelihood of the number or rate arising by chance alone. These statistical methods are called *inferential statistics*. Using these methods, analytical studies can separate out those findings that are likely to have occurred just by chance from those that are more likely to be true associations.

Analytical studies come in four basic study designs: *cross-sectional, cohort, case-control,* and *experimental.* (These are described later in this chapter.) Analytical or etiologic epidemiology deals with causality: the relationship between potential causal factors and the outcome (e.g., disease) is studied by testing different hypotheses (the assumption of this causality). The observational unit consists of an individual. The concept of causality in epidemiology means that the risk factors bear a "causal" relationship. They either establish necessary conditions or set a mechanism into motion that results in the outcome.

CAUSALITY IN EPIDEMIOLOGY

A cause is a factor or determinant that contributes, alone or together with other factors, to the likelihood that an outcome will occur. In epidemiology, a cause is a specific determinant that increases the possibility of an occurrence of a disease in a population. Such causes are usually also deterministic causes, in the sense that they actually contribute to the sequence of events that results in producing the outcome. However, the epidemiological definition does not require this. It is enough, in epidemiology, that the cause contributes to an increased risk of the outcome.

Causal relationships have to be separated from other types of relationships between determinants and the risk of an outcome. It is common, even among professional epidemiologists, to make false interpretations of causality, if an epidemiological study has shown an association between a suspected (risk) factor and the incidence of disease. The associations may be only an illusion, produced by chance or by bias. An example of this type of error is demonstrated if one tosses a coin four times and each toss comes up heads. It would be an error to conclude that the coin toss will always come up heads in the future or that there was something special about this coin toss, because each flip of the coin is truly independent. The chance of four straight heads is known to occur once, on average, in 16 sequences (one sequence equals a coin tossed five times). Random error, when a result goes one way or the other due to chance only, is corrected using inferential statistics or by repeating the study in a different population. Bias is more difficult to manage.

Bias is a form of error in which the result is affected by a consistent or predominant tendency, not by random events. For example, the determinant may be related to another truly causal exposure (e.g., exposure to wheat flour may go along with baking bread but also with making cakes) that is related to the outcome (in this example, allergies), even when the first determinant is not (e.g., the allergies may actually come from ingredients that compose the filling in the cake). This is a common form of bias called *confounding*, discussed below. There are many other types of bias, which may reflect the assumptions behind the study, how the data were collected or recorded, errors in how the subjects were classified or exposures were measured, the reliability of answers to questions, etc.

Cross-sectional and most observational studies are unable to produce reliable information for causal inference, but observational studies can strongly suggest causal associations that can be further investigated using other methods.

Few diseases are caused by only one factor. Determinants of disease are not all the same in importance. Determinants of disease are considered in terms of their contribution to the risk of the outcome:

- A *necessary cause* is one that must be present for the disease to occur in the first place (e.g., one cannot get tuberculosis without the TB organism, and one cannot become allergic to wheat flour without exposure to wheat flour).
- A *sufficient cause* is one that is enough by itself alone for the disease to be initiated (e.g., exposure to asbestos and smoking both increase the risk for lung cancer, and both are sufficient causes, but not everyone exposed to either gets lung cancer during their lives).
- *Contributing causes* are determinants that increase the probability of the outcome (e.g., exposure to both smoking and asbestos increases the risk of lung cancer and exposure to both greatly, and disproportionately).

Although it is often impossible to assess which causes are necessary, sufficient, or predictable in an individual case as a cause, say, of lung cancer, it is generally clear which determinants are important on a group level. A determinant can be evaluated by calculating the *attributable risk* (usually expressed as the attributable risk fraction), which is the part of the overall risk that is explained by the determinant acting alone. The attributable risks can be calculated, and compared, for a population, but not for individuals or very small groups.

Work-related diseases are often *multifactoral*. In many cases, multifactoral diseases or health conditions are produced by causes that interact or interrelate with each other. Social factors mix with occupational ones. The causal network or chain of events can be complex or long, respectively, and thus an individual occupational factor may remain undiscovered or found at the very beginning of this chain. This effect can be seen, for example, in coronary disease, where mental (possibly occupational) stress may enhance the effect of other risk factors (e.g., by increasing smoking and elevating blood pressure).

Observational epidemiology provides only indirect evidence for causation. Proof of causation usually requires additional studies in toxicology or other forms of biomedical research. However, epidemiology can be a powerful tool that points in the direction of a causal relationship. Epidemiologists have derived criteria for evaluating epidemiological evidence to determine if an association is likely to be causal.

The most widely accepted criteria for assessing the likelihood of causation reflected in epidemiological data are those proposed by Sir Austin Bradford Hill, a British biostatistician, in 1965. Hill's criteria are presented in **Table 3.2.** The more these criteria appear to be fulfilled, the more likely the observed association is truly causal. However, Bradford Hill himself emphasized that these criteria are not absolute. When the criteria are considered in more detail, there are overlaps, discrepancies, weaknesses, and irrelevancies. For example, a weak association (Criterion 1) does not necessarily exclude causality. The exposure or the measurement of it may vary between studies. Also, a lack of consistency (Criterion 2) does not exclude causality because different methodologies or studies with varying study designs may produce different results. Specificity (Criterion 3) is not always evidence for causality because many exposures of interest may cause several diseases. In available studies, the magnitude of exposure to a truly carcinogenic chemical may not be enough to demonstrate the excess risk of an occupational cancer (Criterion 5). It is not always possible to attain experimental evidence (Criterion 8), at least in an occupational setting. On the other hand, Criterion 4, that cause must precede effect, is absolutely necessary. The criteria, for all their usefulness, do not address many common problems in occupational epidemiology. It may be difficult to assess whether a long-term effect (e.g., cancer) is really caused by the exposure or by some other factor, because a long latency period may give the subject the chance to encounter many other exposures.

In epidemiology, risk factors that are related to primary causes, but are not the risk factors of primary interest in a given study, are called *confounding factors*. *Confounding* is a situation in which the effect of two processes is not separated and leads to the confounding bias mentioned above. The confounding factor distorts

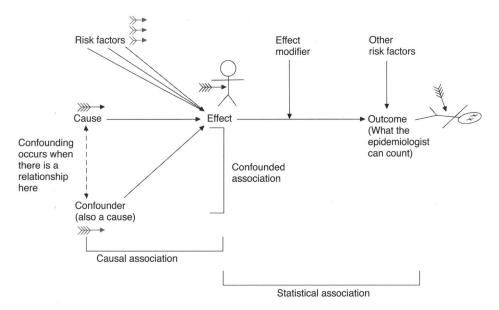

Figure 3.2 Relationships in epidemiology can be complicated. There may be two or (sometimes many) more causes for a particular effect; when causes are related to each other and to the effect, they are said to be "confounded" and may be difficult to separate statistically.

TABLE 3.2
SIR AUSTIN BRADFORD HILL'S CRITERIA FOR THE PLAUSIBILITY OF
A CAUSAL ASSOCIATION

1. Strength of association

2. Consistency among studies, by different techniques

3. Specificity of outcome

4. Exposure precedes disease outcome (temporality)

5. Dose-response relationship (epidemiologic)

6. Plausibility of a biological mechanism

7. Coherence of chain of evidence

8. Experimental association, especially dose-response (toxicologic)

9. Analogy to similar effect produced by a similar agent

(Adapted from Hill, A. B. 1965. "The Environment and Disease: Association or Causation. *Proc Roy Soc Med* 58: 295–300)

the apparent magnitude of the effect of a study factor on risk. Such a factor has to be both a true determinant of the outcome of interest (causal effect) and unequally distributed among the exposed and the unexposed. For example, smoking causes chronic bronchitis, as does occupational exposure to dusts. If a study is conducted on workers in a dusty workplace where smoking is permitted, and the prevalence of chronic bronchitis among these workers is then compared to that of workers in a clean office where smoking is prohibited, the association between dust exposure and chronic bronchitis will be overestimated because of confounding by smoking. However, if the comparison is with another dusty workplace where smoking happens to be prohibited, and if the proportion of smokers is roughly equal in the exposed and unexposed populations, smoking will not become a confounding factor.

EPIDEMIOLOGICAL STUDIES

Epidemiological studies are usually launched because a specific problem requires solution or because there has been an observation in the community that suggests a problem. Some epidemiological studies are designed to answer particular questions necessary to establish standards or to determine how big a problem there is with a particular hazard or outcome. A few epidemiological studies are performed to learn something new, to add to the knowledge base of occupational health. All of these are good reasons to do an epidemiological study. However, epidemiological studies are not easy to conduct and cost money and time. Many studies that ought to be done cannot be done because they cost too much or are too difficult. The design of epidemiological studies is always a compromise between what should be done to learn the most and what is practical given the resources available.

The first step in designing an epidemiological study is to read the literature to find out what other researchers have written on the same topic. This helps the investigator to form a mental picture of what is happening and to conceive of a prediction, or *hypothesis*, that can be tested in a well-designed study. The most common hypothesis in occupational epidemiology is that an exposure is associated with an increased risk of a disease or injury. For example, one hypothesis might be that "exposure to isocyanates causes an excess of respiratory symptoms and allergic diseases." This hypothesis can be tested by examining the frequency (the number in proportion to the number of people) of the outcome and associating this statistically with exposure to isocyanates, taking into account the level of exposure. A second hypothesis, related to the first, is that an increasing exposure to isocyanates is associated with an increased risk of respiratory symptoms and asthma, an expression of the exposure-response relationship. (In practice, these hypotheses usually follow the questions in **Table 3.1** closely.)

The design of the study is based on the hypothesis once it is formulated. The investigator proceeds, ideally, in the following order:

- selection of the type of study
- study design
- selection of a study population or sample of the population at risk
- exposure assessment, measurement, or reconstruction
- case definition of outcome (description of symptoms, allergy)
- standardized and validated methods are chosen to make the necessary measurements and to collect the data
- confounding factors are identified and decisions are made on the management of information on them in the study

- a plan to analyze the data is developed (a biostatistician is usually consulted at this point, long before the study begins)
- the study design and analysis plan need to be examined to anticipate possible sources of bias and to correct them to the extent possible

The selection of a study design depends on the study problem, the setting of the question, and available resources. One of the major decisions to be made in the study is what population to study and how to take samples if the population is too large to study in its entirety. Standardized and validated methods should always be used if they are available; a study that is based on an unreliable or untested method is usually worthless. Cigarette smoking is the most common confounding exposure; thus, when possible, investigators try to collect data on smoking, even when this is not their primary interest. At every stage of study design and implementation, the investigator has to keep in mind possible bias and sources of error and must control them to the extent possible.

A large study may require special funding, a budget, hiring personnel, and setting up special facilities or equipment. However, even small-scale studies should be carefully planned and outlined in advance in writing. Finally, the study is carried out and data is collected, put into a standardized form, and added to a database. The gathered observations are analyzed, often with the assistance of a biostatistician. The investigator must then interpret the results and figure out what they might mean. This may require going back to reanalyze data in a different way or looking for patterns that were not initially anticipated.

In conclusion, the investigator will write a scientific report, usually in the form of a paper that will be published in a scientific journal, read at a scientific meeting, or submitted to a government agency or other sponsoring organization. This paper will always include sections describing the methods that were used, the results, an interpretation of the results, and conclusions, and usually will begin with a short *abstract* (a summary) and introduction explaining why the study was done.

The most critical steps in designing an epidemiological study are discussed in more detail below.

Study Population

The steps outlined above represent the ideal situation. Often, studies can be done only on certain records, and access to desired populations, such as workers in a particular plant, may be impossible. At other times, a study is designed to answer a question that is specific to a particular population because a problem has been identified in a particular working group or plant or because a population becomes available for study and the investigator wants to learn something new. For this reason, and because understanding the study designs depends on an understanding of populations, the sequence below will start with the population.

A fundamental question in occupational epidemiology is to determine whether a defined group, or cohort, can be identified. Studies may be conducted among *dynamic populations*, in which workers are moving in and out of the workforce, or in *cohorts*, in which a distinct group of workers is identified and only those subjects are studied. For example, the workers in a given factory or the workforce in a particular city normally form a dynamic, or open, population. There would be a constant turnover in population due to people moving in and out of the neighborhood, leaving the job for another, migrating to different work assignments, and variously entering the workforce for the first time, leaving and coming back from maternity or paternity leave or illness, retiring, or dying. For some occupations and communities, this turnover can be very high. For the epidemiological investigator, this is a problem because in a dynamic population the work group consists of different individuals at different times. Studying this work group does not reveal much about the risk of exposure because too many workers in the workforce are new and too few workers who have been exposed in the past stay in the workforce.

Studies among dynamic populations are sometimes useful to identify the magnitude of current problems or, if they can be repeated, so that changes in disease prevalence can be tracked over time. Sometimes they can be compared to changes in exposure. However, the differences that are observed may be related to a change in turnover of workers, rather than a change in the workplace. A fall in prevalence of chest radiographic abnormalities in active miners might, for example, be caused by a reduction in dust exposure but may also be the result of miners being removed from underground work at the first signs of radiographic changes, in which case the miners with initial abnormalities are not included in subsequent surveys.

Cohorts are groups of workers (or other subjects) that are separately identified as individuals and share a common characteristic at a specific time or during a given period. The workers in the factory *on a certain day* would form a cohort. Cohorts are described in more detail below.

The ideal population on which to do a study is large enough to have enough statistical power to derive conclusions in the analysis of small subsets, have very low turnover, be diverse enough to have a range of characteristics in the workforce (e.g., age, sex, ethnicity, social class, and especially the prevalence of confounding exposures such as smoking), have excellent records of exposure and employment, and feature a variety of jobs or locations among which the exposure to the hazard of interest varies a great deal but where exposure is nearly constant (or at least known) in any one place. These characteristics make it much easier to link exposure to outcome, to keep bias to a minimum, and to take confounding into account. These ideal characteristics are never found in the real world. As a consequence, all studies in occupational epidemiology are imperfect and subject to interpretation because of their potential flaws. Occupational epidemiology depends on replication, analysis, and meticulous examination of all potential flaws to arrive at correct conclusions.

In reality, selecting a population to study may depend on whether the plant still exists, what records are available, whether the owner or employer allows entry into the workplace, whether there is cooperation or opposition from a union, where it is located, how much money is available, and numerous other practical considerations. It is common to do *feasibility studies*, in which a scaled-down version of the study is attempted to see if it can be done, before undertaking major epidemiological studies.

Employers are often reluctant to allow studies to be done in their facilities because they do not want to disrupt the normal activity of the workplace, lose productivity, raise concerns among employees, or gain a bad reputation (which may not be deserved) for having potential health problems. It is often even harder to gain access to comparison populations because employers may see no reason to submit to a study if they are not the ones who have a health problem among their employees.

Study Design

The most appropriate study design can be chosen from different types of analytical studies. In general, cohort studies of a prospective nature are better as an inferential research tool than case-control studies, and case-control studies are almost always better than cross-sectional studies. If the investigator wants to clarify the consequences of one exposure, a cohort study is recommended if at all possible. On the other hand, if one wants to study several risk factors of one disease (outcome), one usually chooses a case-control design because it is faster and cheaper than conducting a cohort study. A descriptive, cross-sectional study is often a first step and provides the basis for planning an analytical study in which a relationship between a suspected cause (exposure) and outcome (disease) is hypothesized. A combination of the following designs can also be used. For example, it is common to conduct a case-control study inside a cohort study to find out more about a previously unanticipated outcome that becomes recognized while the study is underway.

Cross-Sectional Studies Cross-sectional studies are performed at a single point in time (although they may be repeated) and describe patterns among the dynamic population of workers that is present at that time. They are often called *prevalence studies* because they are used to measure the frequency of characteristics.

Cross-sectional (prevalence) studies examine the frequency of disorders and characteristics in question among subjects at one point in time, usually by comparing two or more groups. They cannot capture information from subjects who are no longer there, and they cannot capture information about what will happen to the subjects in the future.

A common type of cross-sectional study is the survey. In a survey, people are counted, questioned, or information is obtained in a systematic way to determine the situation at a given time. The geographical occurrence of certain types of disease may be very revealing, for example, in a developing country with limited human resources and equipment to invest in occupational health. For example, in Vietnam in the 1990s, the Provincial Medical Centers were surveyed to assess the magnitude of silica-related disease as an occupational health problem and to assess the resources available for prevention. The survey found that over 70% of the workers exposed to silica were concentrated in five provinces, which indicated where the Ministry of Health should concentrate its efforts. The existing number of trained personnel and equipment (pumps and cyclones for dust measurement and analysis of silica content) was found to be far less than needed and justified a search for additional resources for prevention.

Cross-sectional studies are usually descriptive. They identify the frequency of characteristics in one population and usually do not try to compare that experience with another group. The usual measure that is reported is prevalence, which expresses the frequency of a disease or characteristic at one point in time, taking into account the number of cases in proportion to the number of people who are at risk. The prevalence of disease best measures the frequency of long-lasting or permanent conditions in a population at a selected point in time (e.g., the number of diabetes patients or left-handed people in a population). Prevalence is calculated only for defined populations, such as a specific community or a work group, in which the specific number of people at risk can be known.

Prevalence and incidence are usually expressed as rates (often per 10,000 people) comparing the number of cases of the disease or condition that can be identified with the number of people at risk, meaning the total number who could have developed the disease (whether they did or did not).

$$\text{Prevalence} = (\text{Number of cases})/(\text{Number at risk at a given time})$$

Prevalence is usually calculated for conditions that will last more than a few weeks or months and most often for conditions that are permanent, such as permanent disability from injury or diseases that are chronic, e.g., asthma or diabetes. Obviously, it is of no interest or use to calculate prevalence when the denominator includes persons who are not at risk. For example, it would be useless to calculate the prevalence of pregnancy in the total population, because the risk is not distributed among women of all ages and is not shared with men.

The *period prevalence* measures the frequency of cases that were present in a population over a short period of time (e.g., in a year), including current cases and any new ones. However, prevalence measures do not give a picture of how often new cases appear. For this, a different measurement is required—the incidence rate. The period prevalence rate is particularly useful for planning purposes, for example, to ensure that health care resources are allocated correctly in an annual budget.

Analytical cross-sectional studies compare the experience of the work group of interest with a comparison population (such as another unrelated plant or the general population) at one point in time. (For example, the proportion of workers in a bakery who are allergic to wheat flour may be compared with the proportion in a store that sells bread in order to determine whether exposure to raw flour prior to baking the bread is causing allergies.) However, analytical cross-sectional study designs are still considered weak. A cross-sectional study is done only at one point in time. Historical information is lost or subject to unreliable memory, and no future information is collected. A cross-sectional study cannot document that exposure to a hazard took place before the outcome occurred and so can only weakly suggest an association between a hazard and an effect. Causes must precede effects, and because cross-sectional studies cannot take the sequence of events into account, they cannot readily identify causes that are not already known or suspected.

Even with their disadvantages, it is possible to use analytical cross-sectional studies to determine connections between different factors. Causal relations may stay hidden, however. Diseases that take a long time to develop, that lead almost immediately to the worker leaving the workplace, or that are rare cannot be meaningfully studied by this methodology. Etiological factors can be studied using a cross-sectional study design only if a close time relation exists between exposure and outcome. For example, cross-sectional studies can show that on a particular day people in one building have more eye and throat irritation than in another building, because these common symptoms occur on the same day as exposure in a building with indoor air quality problems.

Cross-sectional studies do have some advantages. They may be the only feasible approach when past exposure cannot be documented and historical records are unavailable. They are relatively easy to do. Like prospective studies, they can examine many different outcomes at the same time. Descriptive cross-sectional studies are useful for many purposes. For example, ascertaining whether workers have high serum cholesterol, high blood pressure, or low levels of physical activity may be important information for planning health promotion programs for workplaces. It may be important to identify workers who are capable of performing certain types of work or to know the number of workers who have diagnosed chronic diseases (such as diabetes) in the company at a particular time and who may need special measures to protect their health.

However, cross-sectional studies, when used alone, suffer from many disadvantages. They do not accurately reflect the experience of the group over time. Such studies are relatively inefficient because they cannot identify subjects who will develop disorders in the near future and are usually unreliable in detecting subjects who have had disorders in the past but are now well. They are particularly limited in providing information on occupational disabilities and chronic disorders because workers who develop conditions that interfere with their work are likely to leave the job and will therefore be absent from the group at the time of the study (this is called *selection bias*). For this reason, prevalence estimates in cross-sectional studies of occupational groups are almost always likely to be underestimates of the risk of disability and disease.

Cross-sectional study designs are especially vulnerable to selection bias. For example, workers who become allergic to chemicals or dusts at their workplace often leave their job because of their constant, uncomfortable symptoms.

For example, in one exceptionally well-designed analytical cross-sectional study (Uitti et al. 1997), the frequency or prevalence of allergic sensitization to fur allergens was found to be surprisingly low among fur farmers. However, this study also collected information on fur farmers and subjects in a comparison group (plastic factory workers) who had left their jobs and gone to another workplace. Questionnaires sent to both groups of former workers revealed that many workers had left because of health complaints in both groups, but fur farmers changed jobs more often because of respiratory symptoms, indicating more frequent work-related allergies compared to the subjects in the comparison group.

Cross-sectional studies are particularly weak in recognizing causes, and that is why etiologic problems usually require a longitudinal design. Cross-sectional studies are, however, excellent initial steps in the development of more comprehensive studies. By themselves, cross-sectional studies are of limited usefulness, but in combination with other techniques they are immensely valuable.

In cross-sectional studies many outcomes and causes can be studied simultaneously, and they can serve as a good base to a cohort or case- control study.

Cohort Studies A cohort is a group of identified individuals who share a common exposure at a given time. Once identified, all persons in the cohort will be followed, and no new persons will be included. Unlike a dynamic population, a cohort has no turnover. The same people are followed into the future after their exposure (or other common characteristic) is established. With a cohort study, it is possible to clarify whether the frequency of a disease or the death rate will change because of the exposure. By examining what happened to the people who were exposed, it is possible to evaluate many outcomes and to identify new or previously unexpected outcomes that result from the exposure.

Usually, two or more cohorts are selected for the study. In one group, the subjects have not been exposed to the agent being studied. These subjects are often called *unexposed control subjects*. Persons in the group where exposure is measured or confirmed are the *exposed subjects*, and there may be different groups with different exposures or exposure at different levels. These people are then followed for a relatively long period of time (many years in a study of the occupational causes of cancer, chronic disease, or death). The frequency of new cases of disease or of death (the rate of death is called *mortality*) is then compared between these groups.

A cohort study can be either prospective or *historical* (sometimes called *retrospective*) or a mixture of these two.

In a prospective study, the groups are formed at the present time and then followed into the future. Exposure is documented at the beginning and often monitored and recorded over time. Potential confounding exposures (other possible determinants of disease) can be documented for later use in analysis. The study team may actively follow each member of the cohort for several years, collecting information about their health from medical records, by questionnaires, or through testing. This is time consuming and expensive but leads to the most accurate results. Large cohort studies are very valuable sources of health information, and some of the most important have continued long after the investigators who started them have retired. It is common for cohort studies that last a long time to be used to address hypotheses that were not originally part of the study or were not developed when the study was initiated. Outside of occupational epidemiology, large cohort studies of risk factors for heart disease have been the source of most of what is known about the determinants of risk for cardiovascular disease.

In a historical (or retrospective) cohort study, the cohort groups were formed in the past, and their exposure was documented in some kind of record. Ideally, exact measurements might have been taken at the time but, at least, there are records of when workers began on the job and how long they worked. Over time, the number of those who develop the disease during the follow-up period is identified, usually from records such as death certificates or cancer registries. The benefits of the retrospective cohort are that a follow-up time of many years can be achieved, and one can also study past exposures. It may, however, be problematic to obtain all the relevant details about the exposure and persons exposed.

The great advantage of a prospective study is that it is relatively free of mis-classification bias because it is possible to form the groups with reasonable accuracy and to measure the exposure at the time that it takes place. Cohort studies are more revealing in studying relationships and demonstrating that suspected causes actually occur before the effects. In this type of study, information on exposure is collected at one point in time on both the working group of interest (e.g., bakers coming onto the job for the first time) and another comparison group (e.g., new clerks). The outcome of concern (e.g., new allergies) is monitored over time, and the number of new cases is recorded. At the end of the study, the investigator looks back over, usually, several years and determines, using inferential statistics, whether the rate of new outcomes is greater in the exposed group relative to the comparison group. Cohort studies are very powerful and are generally considered to be highly reliable if done properly. They are subject to less bias than other types of studies because the information on exposure is collected at the beginning of the study.

The most important basic measurement in cohort studies is the *incidence rate*, which is an estimate of the risk of developing a disease during a specific period of time. The incidence rate measures the frequency of new cases in the cohort or in a population. The prevalence rate, by comparison, measures the frequency (number in proportion to the number at risk) of cases that were present at a specified time, whether new or old. An incidence rate may be calculated for acute (short-term) or chronic (long-term) conditions but counts only new cases. A new case is always counted when the condition was first identified, not when it is thought to have begun.

Incidence = (Number of new cases)/(Number at risk in a given time period)

Incidence usually gives the best clues to causal determinants in occupational epidemiology because the incidence rate will be higher where the causal factor is present. Incidence refers to the frequency of new cases during a specific period of time. It is expressed in person-years (such as 5 deaths/100,000 persons per year). In cohort studies each individual will be followed from the beginning of the study to the onset of the expected disease, to his or her death, or to the end of the follow-up time. Person-years sum up all these time periods for the group.

Mortality is one type of incidence measure. It indicates the number of deaths in a population. Mortality is widely used in epidemiological research because both the number and causes of deaths are registered in many countries. Usually, mortality is reported as the number of deaths during one year by age group.

The incidence is an expression of the formal concept of *risk*, which is the probability of an adverse outcome, and can interpreted as both a statistical statement of the risk that was experienced by subjects in the cohort (or members of the population) over the period of time and as the best estimate of the risk that would have been experienced by any one subject in the cohort (or member of the population), all other things being equal. Measuring risk as incidence allows the investigator to see how the frequency of new disease may have changed over time and to compare risks between groups.

The incidence rate for a particular cohort is often compared with the incidence rate in another population. In cohort studies, this comparison often takes the form of a ratio between the incidence of the disease among subjects in the exposed cohort and the incidence among subjects in the unexposed cohort, although the comparison can also be made to the general population or some other relevant comparison group. The experience of the unexposed cohort or comparison group is what the exposed cohort would have been expected to experience in the absence of exposure to the hazard. It is therefore called the *expected rate*. The experience of the exposed cohort is what was actually seen in the group that was exposed to the hazard. It is therefore called the *observed rate*. Dividing the observed by the expected rate yields a ratio that compares what was actually seen to what would have been seen had the exposure not occurred. This ratio is called the *relative risk*.

The relative risk is calculated and expressed in various ways. Articles and reports of epidemiological studies are not always careful to specify which expression is being used. The explanation below is a simplification. In practice, relative risks are almost always adjusted or standardized, meaning that they take into account the age structure of the cohorts and comparison groups.

Often, the measure of primary interest is the *rate ratio* (also called the *incidence density ratio*). This is the ratio of the incidence rate in the exposed group in relation to that of the unexposed control or comparison group. If, for example, the incidence rate is 0.03 per person-year in the exposed group and 0.01 per person-year in the control group, the rate ratio is 0.03/0.01 = 3.00. This ratio is usually simply called the relative risk in scientific papers.

Another commonly used effect measure is the *risk ratio* (*cumulative incidence ratio*). This is the ratio of the cumulative incidence (**see Box 3.5**) in the exposed group to that in the control group. If the outcome is rare, the risk ratio is almost equal to the rate ratio. This involves adding up the number of cases that were observed in the exposed group and dividing by the number of expected cases (taking into account the age structure). The most common risk ratio used in occupational epidemiology is the *standardized mortality ratio* (SMR), which is a form of risk ratio developed for studies using death certificates (**See Box 3.1**). SMRs are usually expressed as a percentage without the % sign. For example, if there were three cases of a disease found in the exposed cohort, and a calculation of the rates in the general population for the same age groups showed that only 1.7 would be expected, the relative risk would be 1.76. The SMR is expressed as O/E = 3.0/1.7 = 176.5. Although the SMR is the most common form of risk ratio, other forms are used, such as standardized incidence ratios or standardized morbidity ratios (when the outcome is not death) and proportionate mortality ratios, which is based on the fraction of deaths among the total from a particular cause when other information is lacking.

Linkage studies are a special type of cohort study and are described below.

Case-Control Studies Although cohort studies are always preferred on theoretical grounds when they are feasible, case-control studies are perfectly acceptable. The basic idea of a case-control study is the same as in a cohort design: to find out if the studied disease is caused by a specific exposure. The only difference is that the

BOX 3.1
======

Interpreting a Cohort Mortality Study

Cohort mortality studies are studies of death rates in cohorts defined by occupation or, often, chemical exposures and are conducted using death certificates. The usual measure of risk in a cohort mortality study is the standardized mortality ratio. The idea of the SMR calculation is to estimate the mortality experience of the exposed group in relation to the mortality experience of a comparison group. It can be defined as follows:

$$SMR = \frac{\text{Number of observed deaths in the exposed group}}{\text{Number of expected deaths in the exposed group}}$$

To calculate the expected deaths in the exposed group, the cause-specific death rate in the same age groups of the comparison population is needed. If
O_i = Observed deaths at age (i) in the exposed group
R_i = The death rate in the control group at age (i)
T_i = Person-years in the exposed group at age (i)

$$SMR = \frac{\Sigma\, O_i}{\Sigma\, (T_i R_i)}$$

The SMR is always standardized for age distribution, but it can also be standardized for a calendar year, smoking habits, or other known risk factors.

It is important to notice the limitations in interpreting the absolute magnitude of an SMR. SMRs of different cohorts are not directly comparable with each other because different exposed groups have different age distributions, and the expected number of deaths is highly dependent on age. Thus an SMR of 180, for example, may indicate a greater risk than an SMR of 150 in another cohort if the age distribution is similar in the cohorts. However, if the latter group is younger, the risk may actually be smaller.

information will be gathered with a different method, one that works backward rather than forward. Mathematically and theoretically, case-control studies are cohort studies in reverse but where the cohort has been sampled instead of being studied in its entirety.

Often, a case-control study design is a better practical choice than a cohort study—when results are needed quickly, when the disease to be studied is rare, when an exposure may have occurred in the past but there has been no documentation or record of it and the only way to identify exposed workers is to ask them today, and when the exposure in question is suspected of causing one very specific disease that can be identified accurately. As a general rule, case-control

> **BOX 3.2**
>
> ## Interpreting a Cohort Study Using Relative Risk
>
> A retrospective cohort investigation was conducted among Swedish bakers (2,923 subjects) to estimate the asthma incidence rate and the risk to develop asthma compared to unexposed controls. Self-administered questionnaires were used. The incidence rate (cases per 1,000 person-years) for asthma among male bakers was 3.0, referents 0.9–1.9. The relative risk of male bakers to develop asthma during baker work was also increased to 1.8 (95% CI 1.3–2.6) compared with referents. Among female bakers, no higher incidence for asthma was noted. Persons who had ever worked as bakers reported more frequently that they had changed work because of asthma (2.5%) than referents (1.1%).
>
> (Based on Brisman, S. J., and B. G. Järvholm. 1995. "Occurrence of Self-Reported Asthma among Swedish Bakers." *Scand J Work Environ Health* 21: 487–493.)

studies can be done more quickly and at less cost than cohort studies. With a case-control design, the investigator is limited to one disease or outcome but can study possible relationships with many exposures. However, these studies are harder, and usually impossible, to perform using only medical and employment records, and they are more subject to bias.

Selection of cases is the first step in a case-control study. The subsection below, on definition of outcomes, discusses the case definition of the study. In this subsection, case selection, which is also called case ascertainment, is discussed from the standpoint of sampling and validity of a case-control study.

Cases can be selected from many sources (e.g., from hospitals, from different registers) as long as the accuracy of diagnosis is reliable and consistent. If the diagnostic accuracy of a source is poor, the cases may not be valid, and this type of *misclassification bias* can easily destroy any possibility of finding a true connection between disease and exposure.

After the cases have been identified, a sample of *control subjects* (often called *referents*) is taken from the same group, community, or population. These referents do not have the disease (or at least the diagnosis) at the time that they are chosen. Sophistication in the design of case-control studies rests on how to select referents, whether or not they need to be matched on age or sex or other characteristics, and how many there should be for every case. If there are only a few cases, statistical power may be better if three or four referents are selected. Sometimes referents are *matched* with cases, i.e., selected to be the same age, gender, or social class. Excessive matching, however, may cause one to miss interesting data because there will not be enough variability in the groups to see the differences. Matching factors in the suspected causal chain, such as matching on exposure, completely defeats the purpose of the study, but it is a common inadvertent error because exposure can closely parallel other factors, such as duration of employment and age. The referents, together, form the *reference group*.

Data is then collected on the cases and referents, using identical techniques, by a research technician who often is not informed as to which subject is a case or a referent. Data may be gathered from medical or employment records, but the most common source of information is to ask the subject directly using a standardized questionnaire. The questionnaire usually includes queries about what jobs the subject held, what exposures he or she experienced and for how long, what other exposures he or she has experienced in life (such as smoking), and information on potential confounders.

The analysis of a case-control study is based on a statistic called the *odds ratio* (OR). Where the relative risk was a ratio of incidence rates, the odds ratio is a ratio of the frequency of risk factors as they are found among cases and among controls. The frequency of a characteristic (exposure to the hazard) occurring among cases with the disease is compared to the frequency of the characteristic among referents, who do not have the disease. Odds are a different way of expressing a comparison of frequencies. Odds of 1 means that the frequency of exposure to the hazard is the same among cases and referents. Odds of X means that the frequency of exposure to the hazard among the cases is X times that observed among the referents. The OR is more than 1 if cases are exposed more often than referents, and less than 1 if exposure has been more usual among controls. The data in a case-control study is often presented as a *fourfold table* (**See Box 3.3**).

An example of a typical case-control study is a Swedish study of heart disease and its possible association with shift work (Knutsson et al. 1999).

In this study, investigators identified 2,006 cases from hospitals and registers in Stockholm and in the province of Västernorrland who had suffered a first heart attack (myocardial infarction). Age- and sex-matched referents ($n = 2,642$) without any known myocardial infarction were selected from the same community or *base population*. Information about risk factors for coronary heart disease was collected with a questionnaire and by telephone interviews. Shift workers were defined as persons who, in the last five years, had worked shifts outside of the usual working hours most people spend on the job (6:00 a.m.–6:00 p.m.). Smoking was classified as smokers, non-smokers, and ex-smokers (people who had stopped smoking at least two years prior to the study). Work stress was classified using responses to the items from a structured questionnaire. Information on the level of education was also obtained. The results indicated that shift workers were more often smokers, were more often dissatisfied with their work, and had a lower educational level than those who worked only during the daytime. The odds ratios were elevated, suggesting that shift work was a risk factor for heart attack among both men and women. The total OR was 1.3, 95% confidence interval (CI 95%) 1.1–1.6 for men and for women; the OR was also 1.3, 95% CI 0.9–1.8. Among workers 45–55 years old, the OR was 1.6 (men) and 3.0 (women).

Experimental Studies Experimental epidemiological studies are rare in occupational epidemiology but can be used to assess the effects of interventions in the

Interpreting a Case-Control Study Using the Odds Ratio

An example (following the fourfold **Table 3.3** below) is a study of a possible connection between farming work and asthma. The investigators selected cases (identified asthma patients) from hospital records and chose controls from inhabitants living in the region served, called the *catchment* area, of the hospital. In this example, 500 cases and 500 referents were collected, making this a rather large case-control study. If 150 cases and 65 controls were farmers, what is the odds ratio?

In this fourfold table, sometimes called a *2 × 2 table*, the letters correspond to the following values:

TABLE 3.3

Case-control studies are usually presented as fourfold tables in the format below:	Number of workers with the disease (cases)	Number of workers without the disease (referents)	Total
Number with exposure	a	b	a + b
Number without exposure	c	d	c + d
Total	a + c	b + d	a + b + c + d

a = the number of workers who have the disease and who have been exposed to the hazard

b = the number of workers who do not have the disease but who have been exposed to the hazard

c = the number of workers who have the disease but who have not been exposed to the hazard

d = the number of workers who do not have the disease and who have not been exposed to the hazard

The *odds ratio*, abbreviated OR, is a comparison that examines the odds of exposure cases (a/c) and among referents (b/d) by constructing a ratio between them. The prevalence of exposure among cases a/(a + c) and referents b/(b + d) can also be calculated. The odds ratio is a mathematical estimate of relative risk, RR, and a cohort study and a case-control study of the same population should yield very similar results.

$$OR = \frac{a/c}{b/d} = ad/bc$$

In this example, the total number of cases is a + c = 500, and the total number of referents is b + d = 500, a = 150, b = 65, c = 350, and d = 435. Thus OR = (150 × 435)/(65 × 350) = 2.87. This is a high odds ratio suggesting a strong association between asthma and farming.

workplace. They are similar to cohort studies in concept. The population is divided into two or more groups, preferably randomized to reduce bias. Randomization is important, when possible, because it distributes known and unknown confounding factors similarly within the study groups. One or more groups will be exposed to the factor of interest or will receive an intervention (which may be intended to prevent an occupational disease or other outcome). The other group is the unexposed reference group.

The scientific community today favors experimental studies, but they are expensive and laborious to carry out. A long period of follow-up may reduce the number of participants, and the compliance also varies depending on interventions.

However, it is impossible and unethical to conduct an experiment with hazardous agents at a workplace and expose workers at random.

Treatments of musculoskeletal disorders have been the most frequent topics of experimental interventions. The following example shows how such studies are performed. The effectiveness of two competing treatments for acute low back pain was studied with a controlled trial (Malmivaara et al. 1995). The two treatments were bed rest and back extension, which is a form of stretching exercise. Patients who presented to an occupational health center with a complaint of acute, non-specific low back pain were randomly assigned to one of three treatments: bed rest for two days, back extension exercises, or nothing other than the continuation of ordinary activities as tolerated (control group). Outcomes were assessed twice, after 3 and 12 weeks. After 3 and 12 weeks, the patients in the control group had better recovery than those in either treatment group. There were significant differences, all favoring the control group, in the duration of pain, pain intensity, ability to work, disability, and number of days absent from work. Recovery was slowest among the patients assigned to bed rest. This study demonstrated very convincingly that acute low back pain (in people who do not have other diseases or signs of serious injuries) is best treated by continuing to be active, that bed rest is actually harmful, and that back-extension exercises were not effective.

Record Linkage Studies Record linkage studies are studies that can be done on existing computerized records. Most are done using a cohort study design. The large number of computerized databases in existence today makes it easy to perform different types of cohort studies when the databases are compatible or identifying information can be linked. Data sources may include national, local, and company administrative databases, disease registries, and vital statistics (death and birth certificate) databases. The key is to link one database with another by identifying the subject (by national identity number, name, birth date, or other means) in each data set and collecting the data on each subject for use in a new database that can be easily analyzed.

Typical databases on the national level are mortality statistics, cancer registry, registry for occupational diseases, registry for developmental defects, statistics collected concerning health behaviors (e.g., smoking, eating habits), and work activity classifications, etc. Local or provincial databases include hospital records, employment records, vital statistics (birth and death registration), motor vehicle driver's license registration (which shows that the subject is alive), and registration for health insurance. Because many of these records are confidential (vital statistics usually are not), the databases are strictly protected by laws and regulations designed to ensure privacy and to protect individuals from being specifically identified.

The advantages of linkage studies are that they can be done using existing data that is already collected for another purpose (such as health insurance) and, when done on a national level, can survey very large populations at a low cost. These record linkage studies are technically easy to carry out and quickly produce a lot of information, even for rare disorders and exposures. On the other hand, the accuracy of information can be poor in some databases due to errors in collecting

BOX 3.5

The Cumulative Prevalence and Incidence

Incidence is the rate of appearance of new cases during a period of time. For many diseases, it is normally expressed as the number of cases per 100,000 per year. However, there is another way of expressing this rate that is called the cumulative incidence.

The cumulative incidence is the number of new cases occurring in the population during a specified period of time, divided by the number of healthy persons in the beginning of a certain period of time. The result is a percentage. For example, if the cumulative incidence of heart attack among 55-year-old men is 20%, it is a good indicator for risk assessment and can be called a "risk" for this disease.

Cumulative prevalence is useful when the outcome may eventually include a large fraction of the subjects if exposure continues. An example of the practical use of cumulative prevalence is in the prevalence of opacities (X-ray changes) suggesting a lung disease called pneumoconiosis (Zitting et al. 1995). The extent of the X-ray changes is measured by the ILO Classification of the Pneumoconiosis, a system that involves, for the purposes of this example, a series of categories for severity, from 0/0 to 1/1 and greater. The table shows that among people who were probably exposed to asbestos, a larger fraction of workers had developed greater degrees of changes in their X-ray.

PREVALENCE (%) OF SMALL LUNG OPACITIES BY ASBESTOS EXPOSURE AMONG 3,274 FINNISH MEN AND 3,811 FINNISH WOMEN. (ILO = INTERNATIONAL LABOUR OFFICE)

ILO profusion of small lung opacities	Probably exposed		Possibly exposed		Unlikely exposed	
Men	N	%	N	%	N	%
Profusion 0/0	160	36.4	871	50.2	532	48.3
Profusion 0/1	185	42.1	598	34.5	422	38.3
Profusion 1/0	67	15.3	206	11.9	105	9.5
	27	6.2	59	3.4	42	3.8
Women						
Profusion 0/0	11	37.9	777	44.8	135	56.8
Profusion 0/1	9	31.0	474	34.1	773	32.4
Profusion 1/0	7	24.1	106	7.6	199	8.3
Profusion > 1/1	2	6.9	32	2.3	62	2.6

or entering the data. For example, the diagnostic data in health insurance databases are usually highly inaccurate (mostly because the data are entered for billing purposes before the diagnosis is confirmed). This leads to a problem with misclassification bias and a tendency for some of these studies to underestimate risks.

An example of a record linkage study was a Finnish study on the relationship between work and asthma (Karjalainen et al. 2001). In Finland, people with persistent asthma are registered for reimbursement of their medication costs from the national health insurance scheme. In this study, the authors combined data for these individuals with information on the same individuals from the population census data of 1985, 1990, and 1995 to estimate the attributable fraction of work as a determinant of adult-onset asthma. The follow-up covered the entire 25- to 59-year-old employed population of Finland from 1986–1998. Relative risk (RR) for occupational categories was estimated in comparison to those employed in administrative work. There were 49,575 asthma cases. The attributable fraction of occupation was 29% (CI 25%–33%) for men and 17% (95% CI 15%–19%) for women. Work was especially associated with asthma in agricultural, manufacturing, and service work. It is important, as a test of the validity of any study, that it be able to identify associations that are already known. In addition to identifying known occupations at a high risk of occupational asthma, e.g., food and beverage work, the analysis also identified a large number of occupations with significant excess of asthma incidence.

Definition of Outcome The aim of most occupational epidemiological studies is to describe the conditions at work and the state of health of the workers. These studies have to be performed with available techniques and measurements. In this kind of epidemiological research, definitions of exposure and outcome can be blurred a little without losing their usefulness. Cases of the disease may not be easy to diagnose, physicians may be unavailable or unsure, and the usual tests may carry some uncertainty. On the other hand, the value of a good study design is lost if the definition of the disease fails to identify most of the cases or if the definition is so loose that it includes many cases that do not actually have the disease. However, the definition does not always have to be completely accurate or inclusive for the study to be useful. For the purpose of conducting the study, the investigator develops a case definition, which is an operational set of criteria (such as a set of symptoms or test results) that are consistently associated with the disease at a high level of probability. The case definition is not the same as a diagnosis. The investigator does not usually try to include rare or unusual forms of the disease and does not usually try to include early or uncertain cases in which the relevant criteria are not yet met. Instead, the investigator tries to develop a case definition that will reliably identify most cases.

A case definition for the disease is not the same thing as a diagnosis for the disease. The disease may be defined differently in epidemiological studies than in clinical studies and even differently in different epidemiological studies because it is not possible to use the same methods of clinical diagnostics as would be used in clinical research. Instead, the investigator may have to use *indicators* that strongly suggest the diagnosis but are not completely accurate in all cases. For example, an investigator may need to use information from old medical records, from a death certificate (death certificates, in general, are accurate for some causes but inaccurate for many), from a questionnaire, or from records of what medicines a patient took instead of conducting more specific tests to confirm the diagnosis. Often, occupational diseases are defined in local legislation for purposes of compensation and may be characterized differently in different countries.

A good example of how case definition may apply is in the diagnosis of asthma. Asthma may be defined in a questionnaire as "ever has had asthma diagnosed by physician" or by a series of questions concerning shortness of breath with a standardized algorithm (a stepwise procedure for arriving at a diagnosis), or by questions combined with clinical physiological examinations (e.g., measurement of airways hyperreactivity, obstruction on spirometry), etc. (Toren 1993, Pekkanen and Pearce 1999). The highest sensitivity and most reliable results have been observed when subjects report that asthma was diagnosed by a physician.

If a questionnaire is used in the case definition, it should be *pretested*, and the results must correspond with the phenomenon in reliable examinations of "real" respondents in the same population. For example, if anxiety or depression is being studied using a questionnaire, the questionnaire and the specific questions being used to assess mood and feelings should be validated against psychological/psychiatric examinations with the best available methods in that community to see if the questionnaire accurately identifies most patients with anxiety or depression. If it does, the questionnaire is valid and can be used for a broader survey.

Examples of some indicators, as used in the epidemiology of respiratory diseases, are presented in **Table 3.5**. These examples describe the way in which functional results may represent a disease; stress or other states of human health or well-being can also be measured indirectly.

TABLE 3.5

SOME RESPONSE INDICATORS OF RESPIRATORY DISEASES USED IN OCCUPATIONAL EPIDEMIOLOGY

Indicator	Example
Mortality	Cancer
New case in the clinic	New cases of heart attack, coronary heart disease
Cancer registration	Cancer
Radiographic (X-ray) abnormality	Pneumoconiosis
Change in lung function test: e.g., decrease of FEV_1 over time	Chronic obstructive pulmonary disease
Change in FEV_1 across a work shift	Airways narrowing (possible asthma)
Decreased value in a test of gas exchange in lungs: diffusing capacity	Alveolitis, emphysema
Respiratory symptoms typical to disease: coughing up phlegm (sputum)	Chronic bronchitis
Response to special tests: e.g., hyperreactivity of bronchial airways	Asthma
Variability in peak expiratory flow	Asthma
Skin tests, immunological tests	Allergy

(Adapted from Venables, 1994. (See Table 3.1.))

It is advantageous for a study if the definition of outcome is crystallized, unequivocal, and valid. Unfortunately, this is not the case in many fields of occupational and environmental epidemiology. For example, musculoskeletal disorders are affected by injuries, poor ergonomic conditions, muscular "microtraumas," vibration, and static muscle load. Pathophysiological mechanisms are obscure, and the measures of exposure (workload) need more specific concepts. Thereafter, the risks are better understood if the development of operational measures has lead to consistent results.

Exposure Assessment Assessments of populations with differing exposures are needed in order to determine whether an exposure causes a disease and if there is an exposure (dose)-response relationship in either the epidemiological sense (the disease becomes more frequent with higher exposure) or in the toxicological sense (the disease becomes worse with higher exposure). Careful determination of the exposure-response relationship may identify a threshold below which the disease does not occur. Such thresholds are valuable for establishing standards and occupational exposure levels (see Chapter 2). It is also critically important to determine that exposure has, in fact, occurred in order to validate the study.

Many groups of workers are exposed to several chemicals or other factors at the same time, although exposure may vary during the course of their work. In occupational studies of such groups, it is desirable to assess exposures on an individual level.

Examples of exposure assessment include measurements of airborne concentrations of impurities. Biological monitoring of many agents, or their metabolites, can be conducted in humans by testing blood or urine for a class of biomarkers that indicate personal exposure. Such biological monitoring (often called *biomonitoring*) yields information on total exposures but cannot separate workplace exposures from environmental or voluntary exposures. Most workplace exposures are sufficiently higher than community exposures, so biomonitoring of workers usually accurately reflects exposure in the workplace. Other exposure measurements may include physical measurements, e.g., noise, heat, radiation, or vibration.

Sometimes the only information available concerning the jobs in the population of interest is job classification or job description. In such situations, one can approximate the exposure by using a job exposure matrix (JEM). In the simplest use of the JEM, an expert may rank the jobs of employees in a factory under study on an ordinal scale. This ranking would be made by an occupational hygienist based on his or her observations, inspection, and generally known information regarding exposure in that trade. These rankings can be validated by actual measurements where there is an opportunity to do so, but the JEM is used when measurements are not available for individual subjects (Venables 1994). "Heavy," "moderate," and "light" exposures are the most frequently used categories for classifying exposure using JEMs. For chronic occupational lung disease (Heederik and Attfield 2000), lung cancer (Kromhout et al. 1992), and asthma (Kennedy et al. 2000), matrixes have been created for the use of researchers in order to determine whether adverse respiratory effects are being caused by exposure to dusts or to other impurities in the workplace air.

Although the measurements are generally available for current exposures, sometimes the exposure of the work group occurred in the past when the levels were different. The retrospective assessment of individual exposure is difficult and is sometimes based on a simulation of conditions as they existed in the past, when this is possible. More often, exposure assessment is estimated based on extrapolation from historical trends.

Internal comparisons within studies are very useful. When workers in certain occupations have had higher exposures than workers in otherwise similar jobs, their experience can be compared within the same study and often within the same plant or company (e.g., underground miners compared to above-ground strip miners, insulators compared to sheet metal workers, and workers in old compared to new plants). In such cases, more highly exposed workers may be compared with a correspondingly less exposed population.

In many cases, information concerning job history is the only basis for exposure assessment. Depending on the aim and the outcome of a particular study, this information can be utilized in different ways. If it concerns the outcome of social, educational, or other behavioral scientific matters, the descriptive job history may give sufficient information for the comparison of different job categories. For example, early retirement occurs more frequently among construction workers than among persons with a clerical working history. Studies of disease outcomes generally require more information on total exposure. Often, duration of employment is all that is available to indicate level of exposure. However, length of employment alone is not always adequate for assessing exposure, particularly in studying cancer risk. Exposure may vary over time in the same job, especially if the worker moves into better jobs or becomes a supervisor. Exposure duration, length of employment, and latency for chronic disease also occur together during the same time period and are difficult to sort out.

Table 3.6 shows the many different types of exposure data that are used in occupational epidemiological studies (Checkoway et al. 1989).

Statistical Analysis

Statistical analysis must be planned in advance in the design of an epidemiological study. How the data will be analyzed will determine the best way to store and manage the data, what computer software is needed, and what specific data is required.

TABLE 3.6

TYPES OF EXPOSURE DATA USED IN OCCUPATIONAL EPIDEMIOLOGICAL STUDIES

Type of Data	Approximation to Dose
1. Quantified personal measurements	Best
2. Quantified job-specific data	
3. Ordinally ranked jobs or tasks	
4. Duration of employment in the industry	
5. Ever employed in the industry	Poorest

Power One of the most important attributes of a study, and one of the first things that should be examined, is statistical *power*. Power is a concept expressing the probability that a study will detect a true effect if it is there. A power of 80% means that if a disorder or outcome is present in the studied group at a given level that is higher than in the comparison group (for example, twice as frequent), the study will have an 80% chance of detecting the difference as a statistically significant finding or a 20% chance of missing it even if it is, in fact, present. A power of 0.80 is considered to be acceptable for most purposes, but the higher the power the better. A power of 0.50 means that the chance of detecting a true difference is only 50%, which means even odds or a "50-50" chance, no greater than flipping a coin. If the power of a study is low, the absence of a finding cannot be considered to be convincing evidence that an effect does not exist, because it could easily have been missed.

There are sometimes good reasons to do studies with low power. Sometimes, populations or groups of workers are small but need to be studied anyway. In other cases, a condition is rare but very important as an occupational disease.

Statistical power can be calculated by using statistical formulae. Power depends on the number of expected cases or background cases (unrelated to the exposure of interest) likely to appear in the population. It also depends on how great an effect the exposure is likely to have (*effect size*). Large studies will have greater power to detect an association, even with a relatively low effect size. Rarer disorders require a much larger population to yield the same power, unless the effect size is very high.

A sample size that is too small or that has a bias may simply miss the true effect, which is then called a *false negative*. A study that does not show a finding is often called "negative," but this is poor terminology and should be avoided. Many negative results are due to other factors than true lack of effect. A "non-positive" result is a better term that includes the possibility of false negative conclusions. A finding that suggests an effect that is not really there is called a *false positive*. False positives may arise from chance but are more likely to arise from bias and are generally less common than false negatives in epidemiological studies. This is because low power and most forms of bias (especially the most common, misclassification) produce an underestimate of risk and therefore tend to produce more false negatives.

Bias Bias is the type of error that is *systematic* and occurs regularly, consistently, or at least more often in one way or on one side than another. Random error, by comparison, occurs by chance and on any side. Random error makes it harder to see relationships because it increases the noise and obscures the relationship between determinants and outcomes. Control of random error can be adjusted for using biostatistics. Bias is more difficult because it results in unreliable data and can produce misleading results. All epidemiological studies have some degree of bias, but in the best studies the bias is minimized, anticipated, and, to the extent possible, corrected.

Biases are very important to account for in assessing the validity of study results. However, just because a study shows bias does not mean that it is invalid.

A study that is known to be biased can be analyzed or interpreted to take the bias into account. The strength and direction of the bias can be considered, and sometimes even measured, and studies with different biases can be compared.

Selection biases arise from the procedures by which the study subjects are selected from the study base. Selection bias is not a problem in cohort studies, but is of concern in case-control studies and is almost impossible to avoid in cross-sectional studies. Selection bias can occur if controls are chosen in a way that does not represent the whole population or group and is related to the outcome. For example, selection bias may occur in a study of asthma if suspected cases are chosen from among asthma patients sent to an occupational medicine clinic and are then studied to see if their asthma is occupational in origin. The subjects probably went to an occupational health clinic because they had already shown indications of occupational asthma.

Information can be biased in many ways:

- Recall bias occurs when cases (persons with a disease) recall their exposure better or more clearly than healthy referents (usually because they have been thinking about it or have already been asked the question before the study, e.g., for insurance purposes).
- Observer bias occurs if cases and referents are not interviewed in the same manner or with the same degree of accuracy. An interviewer can, for example, ask an interviewee, "What kind of exposure did you experience in your work?" Or, if the interviewer/observer is aware of the exposure of interest, he or she may lead the referent by suggesting, "I suppose you didn't experience exposure in your work."
- Information bias also occurs if somebody gives wrong information on purpose. This sometimes happens in the case of occupational diseases because workers may expect compensation or because they may have strong emotions toward their employer.

Comparison bias may occur if referents are selected from a reference group that is unusual or in which the exposure of concern is also a strong risk factor. The most common example of comparison bias occurs when an investigator draws both cases and referents from admissions to a hospital and identifies them from records. For many outcomes, hospital referents are poor comparisons because patients in the hospital are not representative of the general population. For example, if one is studying the association between smoking and lung cancer, hospital referents may lead to a strong underestimate of the odds ratio for smoking as a cause. The reason is that a disproportionate number of people who smoke are in the hospital for reasons that do not include lung cancer and will be counted as referents. Similarly, it is often misleading to use one occupational group as a comparison for another, especially if there are heavy exposures involved and differences in social class (and smoking). Studies that compare the risk of heart disease and cancer among firefighters and further compare them to police, for example, have shown quite different results than other studies that compare both to the general population. That is why a "neutral" reference group or population-based referents should always be selected.

Misclassification bias occurs when the subjects are inaccurately classified as either exposed or unexposed or as cases or referents. For example, a worker who is being interviewed for a case-control study may forget that he or she was exposed to a chemical, or the worker may think that exposure occurred when it did not. On the other hand, a person may be falsely labeled as having a disease (perhaps he or she has a similar disorder) and is counted as a case, or a person who actually has the disease but does not know it may be counted as a referent. In general, the effect of misclassification bias is to reduce the power of a study by making it less efficient. Misclassification alone usually does not change the direction of the risk if it is truly elevated, but results in an underestimate. This may lead to a false negative.

Publication bias refers to the tendency of journals to accept studies that show a finding over studies that show no finding or that are equivocal. A positive publication bias is found overwhelmingly in the scientific literature. Not only are positive findings more interesting to the reader, but due to the considerations mentioned above, it is more difficult to be certain of a so-called negative finding.

Underestimation Epidemiologists spend a great deal of energy trying to avoid or to manage positive bias, which results in false conclusions, but not errors that cause underestimation and false negatives. However, the underestimation of "real" risks because of studies with low quality and false interpretations is a serious problem in epidemiological studies.

Many errors result in an underestimation of the effect. These are summarized in **Table 3.7**. The most common problem resulting in underestimation is a lack of statistical power that may result from

- a study population that is too small
- an ineffective study design
- inaccurate indicators of exposure
- too low a level of exposure
- too short a period of exposure
- false populations or working groups
- too short a period of follow-up (latency period)
- misclassification bias

An ineffective study design might mean, for example, that a cohort study has been chosen as the type of study instead of a case-control study in a situation where the disease of interest is rare. False populations are a form of selection bias. For example, in a cohort study of the risk of lung cancer associated with a particular chemical exposure, retired workers are excluded. Because retired workers are more likely to get lung cancer than current workers who are young and are probably less exposed, and because lung cancer is unlikely to appear before retirement age, excluding them virtually guarantees that there will be an underestimate of the true risk and that no excess of cancer may be found even when the chemical is truly a lung carcinogen.

TABLE 3.7

FACTORS LEADING TO UNDERESTIMATION OF THE EFFECTS (HERNBERG, 1981)

1. Small sample size
2. Study group or "survivors" in employment
3. Exposure that has been too low or that has lasted for too short a time to give an effect
4. Follow-up time shorter than the latent interval of disease
5. Random variation in measure of exposure
6. Random variation in indicator of outcome (disease)
7. Overestimation of exposure
8. Insensitive indicator of disease
9. Comparison with general population
10. Comparison with a group who is at increased risk of disease because of other exposures
11. Confounding

The Healthy Worker Effect

The "healthy worker" effect is frequently encountered in occupational epidemiology. It occurs when the prevalence or incidence of a disease in an exposed cohort is compared with the expected values of the general population. The incidence, or risk, of disease and especially of death is almost always lower for the working population and sometimes much lower. This often leads to misinterpretation about which risks are truly elevated for working populations.

The healthy worker effect is a form of comparison bias, although it is often mistaken for selection bias. There are several reasons for it:

- People who are healthy are more likely to enter working life and become employed.
- Many employers screen employees for their health and hire only people who are fit.
- People who become ill while they are working are more likely to leave the working population because of their illness.
- People who develop minor ailments that later become more serious are more likely to leave the occupation, especially in jobs with higher demands (high physical load), and are more likely to be lost to follow-up.
- The general population includes many people who cannot work such as those in institutions, those who are chronically ill, and those with disabilities. In general, these people have a shorter life expectancy and are more likely to develop disease.

Meta-Analysis and Pooling

In order to correct for the biases inherent in many studies and to attain greater statistical power, methods have been developed to analyze studies in combination.

Using these methods, several smaller studies can be combined and studied as if they were one large study. These methods are called meta-analysis or pooling when the data from the studies can be directly combined. By summarizing the data of separate small studies, it is possible to increase statistical power and to analyze dose-response relations. It also enables better risk assessment of important problems involving low exposures (e.g., passive smoking and lung cancer, electromagnetic fields and brain tumor).

There are various methods for summarizing data: a review article, quantitative summary of published data, or meta-analysis and pooled analysis.

A review article is a scientific paper written to summarize the literature on a subject and to compare the findings of various earlier papers. A good review paper not only summarizes the findings but points out differences and possible explanations for them and what needs to be done in the future to resolve open issues. It is increasingly common for an author to provide an assessment of the quality of the published studies used in a review article. It is important that the author of the review article state how the papers were chosen and whether they represent all the papers that could be found on the topic and if not, why not. The author should state why certain articles were used and others were not and how complete they were (Weed 1997). One major problem of review articles, even when carried out carefully, is publication bias. Studies with positive results are more likely to be published than those with negative results.

Meta-analysis is a method of combining studies that are published when the original data cannot be easily pooled. It involves the re-analysis of data of many individual studies. A meta-analysis requires a clear protocol, written in advance, that describes the aim and design. It is important to report how the studies have been obtained and selected and what statistical methods are used, and it is important to declare the inclusion criteria for single studies. Meta-analysis of published data involves estimating the quantitative effect of risk factors using the same measures as in the original studies: relative risk (RR) or standardized incidence ratio (SIR). Because of publication bias, meta-analysis may tend to give an overestimation of the risk. However, because the power of the underlying studies may not be very large (which is one reason for doing meta-analysis), and meta-analysis cannot correct for bias, there may also be underestimation. Published studies may differ greatly in their methods, subjects, designs, and definitions of exposure. If the studies are very heterogeneous, the estimate will be unreliable. Strongly biased studies should not be included. There are statistical tests for heterogeneity that can be used. Meta-analysis is generally accepted as a reasonably reliable guide to the evidence but is not necessarily accepted as conclusive by many scientists.

Pooled analysis (a form of meta-analysis going back to the individual data) can solve some of the problems described above. Publication bias can be reduced if unpublished data are included in the analysis, assuming that the unpublished data are of high quality. A larger sample size can enable the study of rare or weak exposures. It is not possible to improve data quality, but some errors in the data or analysis may be partially eliminated by going back to the original data and pooling. The best result can be achieved if studies are planned in cooperation with different centers and pooling has been designed in advance. There will always be more heterogeneity in multicenter studies than in single-center studies, but researchers that plan together can establish comparability in design, data collection, and analysis of individual studies (prospectively planned pooled analysis).

Meta-analyses and review articles have been particularly important for evidence-based medicine and have been applied extensively to epidemiological experiments in treatment-randomized clinical trials.

4

EXPOSURE ASSESSMENT

Rauno Pääkkönen

Occupational hazards may be divided into chemical, physical, biological, and psychological. Psychological hazards depend on the social environment and on perceptions and are discussed in another chapter. The other three are the result of interaction between the worker and the physical or material world. A typical modern plant may include several hundred chemicals, complicated noise exposures, difficult thermal conditions, unidentified carcinogenic compounds, and strong electromagnetic fields. The task of experts in workplace *exposure assessment* is to prioritize and classify the most important hazardous agents and, within reasonable cost, to develop practical control methods to protect workers from adverse effects.

Health and safety personnel must decide on the acceptability, unacceptability, and uncertainty of exposure to the agents in question. Unacceptable exposure must be controlled and uncertain situations must be analyzed. This requires data. Chemical, physical, and biological agents in the workplace are becoming more and more complex; therefore, risk assessment and management methods are more frequent components of the world of occupational hygiene. At the workplace level, these methods should be as simple as possible but should nevertheless be efficient enough to determine all the important agents and substances of exposure.

Exposure assessment can be defined as a systematic approach to the classification of hazards and to performing a hazard analysis. Exposure assessment may be performed for several reasons and usually a combination of them:

- to ensure protection from health risks
- to carry out research so that these hazards will become better understood
- to assess the effectiveness of the technology for their control
- to evaluate a workplace that has problems
- to conduct an audit for the purposes of risk management
- to identify possible problems that are not obvious
- to document compliance with regulations and occupational exposure levels

Exposure assessment must be done at the workplace level. This assessment can be technically complicated, but, if done properly, the exposures can be determined

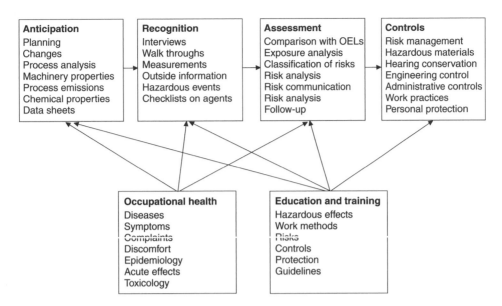

Figure 4.1 Relationship of anticipation, recognition, assessment, and controls.

and the necessary control methods can be applied. If the exposure assessment is not done, then the effectiveness of control actions to manage the problem cannot be known. In the worst-case scenario, environmental exposures may continue to cause people to become ill or their productivity at work to be reduced, despite the appearance of adequate controls.

The profession that conducts, interprets, and designs interventions based on exposure assessment is called *occupational hygiene*. (In North America, the term *industrial hygiene* is usually used.) Occupational hygienists are trained in safety, engineering, hazard control (see Chapter 5), chemistry, and epidemiology. The role of occupational hygiene is to anticipate, recognize, evaluate, and control workplace hazards (Box 4.1). Occupational health professionals rely heavily on authoritative sources of such information, such as chemical hazard profiles, material safety data sheets, safety and hygiene handbooks, and occupational exposure limits or recommended values. Most of this information can now be found on the Internet.

OUTLINE FOR EXPOSURE ASSESSMENT

Exposure precedes risk. If there is no exposure, then there is no risk. Thus, the first task of an occupational hygienist is to determine whether an exposure has occurred and, if possible, to measure it. Exposure assessment is multidisciplinary work, and many areas of science must be applied. Occupational hygienists have varying backgrounds and fields of expertise, e.g., physics, engineering, chemistry, biology, or medicine. In difficult cases, many different experts are often involved, and the necessary multidisciplinary analyses may be very complicated.

BOX 4.1

A Workplace with Multiple Hazards

In one workplace in a metal fabrication plant, steel plates are being welded. The work consists of grinding metal, inert gas welding, slag grinding, and slag hammering. There can also be some other hammering work. No stainless or acid-tolerable steel treatments are being carried out in this particular part of the plant. The workers always use hearing and eye protection, and they always have available and use gloves and protective clothing. The workers are comfortably warm but not hot and complain of a cold draft only during the wintertime.

At this workplace, noise exposure is 87 dBA. There is low-frequency vibration generated by tools (workers use vibrating tools for no more than 4 hours daily). Welding fumes (iron dust concentration 2 mg/m³) occur frequently. Ultraviolet radiation from welding is strong.

The safety or occupational hygiene officer for this plant is expected to know the OELs for every significant exposure and to have an understanding of what they mean. Information on OELs can be obtained from the Internet or health and safety books.

In this country, the OEL for noise is 90 dBA, but there is an action level requiring regular monitoring and the availability of hearing protection if the noise is above 85 dBA 8-hour TWA. It is known that at the levels usually encountered in such workplaces, the skin and the eyes of unprotected workers can be affected by ultraviolet radiation within 10 seconds, but the source (usually the arc in arc welding) seldom lasts that long and the workers use eye protection. Workers are not required to wear protective clothing. The level of welding fume exposure is not covered by a single OEL because welding fumes are mixtures. However, at their maximum, the welding fumes that reach the breathing zone of the welder do not exceed the ceiling (peak allowable) levels for the constituent gases and particles and because they are so short, on an 8-hour TWA basis, the exposures are within the relevant OELs. The ventilation system may or may not be good enough to prevent other workers from being exposed to welding fumes above the OELs because it has not been tested in three years.

What then is the result of the exposure assessment of this workplace? There is a moderate risk of hearing loss and a moderate risk of lung irritation (associated with bronchitis and worsening asthma) and possibly even cancer (associated with some types of welding). For unprotected skin and eyes, the risk of ultraviolet radiation is unacceptable. Workers who use tools for extended periods of time have a moderate risk of white finger disease as a result of exposure to vibration.

What do the workers in this workplace need? The effectiveness of existing hazard controls needs to be validated by exposure assessment. Personal protection is necessary for eyes, ears, hands, and the whole body. For accident prevention, welders generally use safety shoes. If this personal protection is accommodated, then the risk is moderate. If local ventilation and general ventilation are effective, or respiratory protection is provided, then the risk is moderate. If the daily use of tools is fewer than 4 hours a day, the risk of vibration is also moderate. If the exposure in this workplace differs from typical examples, for example, if other metal alloys are used, then the relevance of the OELs must be reassessed. If there is a question, completion of the assessment may require an expert opinion, additional measurements, or some other investigation.

Planning and the Preliminary Investigation

Chemicals can enter the body through inhalation, ingestion, or skin contact, as outlined in Chapter 2. Some agents can have several routes of exposure simultaneously. For example, solvents may be inhaled from the air and absorbed through the skin at the same time.

The exposure assessment expert will come prepared with equipment required to measure the exposures most likely to be present. The expert also reviews in advance problems that have already arisen in the workplace and is alert to possible exposures that he or she should look for.

Generally, adverse effects are greater or more frequent when exposure is greater. There can also be several types of combined effects; for example, exposure to toxic substances when combined with noise exposure can cause a greater hearing loss than noise exposure alone. In a similar way, exposure to combinations of radon, asbestos, and smoking significantly increases the risk of lung cancer compared to a single exposure. In addition to conventionally toxic chemicals (see Chapter 2), carcinogenic, mutagenic, allergic, sensitizing, and corrosive agents must be identified and, if present, monitored and evaluated.

Data on exposure can be gathered by interviewing employees, walking through factory areas, making measurements, taking biological samples, tracking the use of chemicals, etc. Occupational health personnel, labor protection officials, or safety personnel can provide suggestions as to how to identify possible exposures. Symptoms, discomfort, complaints, occupational diseases, and general information can provide indications of possible unacceptable exposures. Training and educating workers can also lead to the eventual identification of possible hazards. Figure 4.1 illustrates possibilities for exposure assessment.

Acute single events can be hazardous. One isocyanate exposure can cause asthma; similarly, one rifle shot can cause permanent hearing loss when the gun is next to the person's ear. During a visit to a workplace, these forms of intense exposure may not be seen or may not be recalled, but these types of exposures must also be accounted for if exposure analysis is to be of high quality.

Measurement

Measurements of work environment factors play a significant role in exposure analyses in the field of occupational hygiene. An occupational hygiene measurement requires technology to detect the presence and concentration of a chemical, biological agent, or physical factor and an estimate of the quantity or intensity (concentration for a chemical).

Measurement needs are specific to a particular situation: for example, in engineering, measurements are made to make sure parts fit together, and the measurement may or may not need to be very exact, depending on the technology and the mechanical requirements. In occupational hygiene, measurements usually reflect either the current exposure level or the worst-case situation. Measurements in this sense are estimates of the true dimensions of a quantity or intensity and are not expected to be exact for every situation. To estimate a quantity of the whole, or the average, one samples the whole (e.g., taking a wipe sample) or samples at one point in time or over a representative period of time. Thus, measurement in this situation always has two sources of error, the intrinsic error of the measurement technology (which is never exact) and statistical error (which arises from statistical properties when a sample is taken from the whole). In other words, the ruler may be inexact or too big for the job (causing an error in precision), and vision may be fuzzy (leading to random error in accuracy). Whether one gets the same result when measuring the same thing several times depends on both types of error but mostly on the intrinsic error of the measurement technology.

Measurement methods have been developed for many types of agents, and new technology is developing rapidly that improves exactness and reproducibility of multiple measurements of the same sample. However, it is much more difficult to reduce sampling error because that usually requires a larger or more representative sample and, depending on the circumstances, how good a sample one can get. The goal is to obtain a measurement that is as close as possible to the true value. If a measurement is very close to the true value, it is called *accurate*. If a measurement is highly reproducible, it is called *precise*. It is quite possible for a measurement to be inaccurate but very precise, for example, if a meter is not calibrated and always reads exactly five units above the true reading. This is called *measurement bias* and is compensated for by calibration and comparing measurements against known concentrations or blanks (samples in which the chemical, biological agent, or physical factor are totally absent). It is generally more difficult to be imprecise and accurate at the same time (see Figure 4.1), but it is possible for the measurement to be so affected by error that it overestimates and underestimates the true value as often and to the same degree, making the

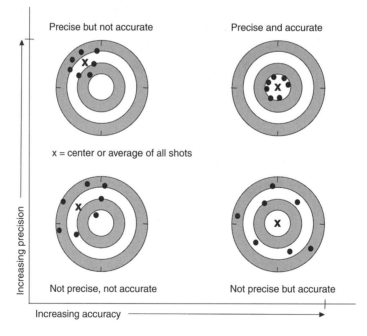

Figure 4.2 Precision describes the reproducibility of measurements, but accuracy describes how close they are to the real value; the illustration is an analogy to shooting at a target.

average value highly accurate. This is usually the case when the measurement technology is inexact but the main source of error is statistical error due to sampling, a common problem in available tests for biological agents.

Often, one is interested in the level of exposure at one point in time. One may wish to determine current levels under representative conditions, conditions of maximum exposure, or to protect workers from a hazard during upset conditions. Concentrations of chemicals and intensity of physical exposures are often measured by direct-reading meters, biological sampling, or surface wipe tests. Sampling methods provide measurements at one point in time for these devices. Direct-reading chemical instruments include explosimeters for measuring the concentration of volatile organic compounds and carboximeters for measuring carbon monoxide. A direct-reading noise meter tells the user what the level of continuous noise is at the moment, and an impulse meter tells the user how loud a single impulse noise was at its transient maximum. Biological sampling for living organisms, such as bacteria and molds, and wipe samples for chemicals on a clean surface, such as the counter of a laboratory or the inside of a cleaned tank, are taken to reflect levels at one point of time and are usually measured in a laboratory by special techniques. New technology has provided field instruments for chemical testing that can measure levels on the site to save time. Further technology is being developed for rapid identification of biological agents. Generally, these methods are forced to sacrifice accuracy to achieve precision and sensitivity, but they are useful in the field to capture actual conditions that may be changing.

However, in occupational health one is usually more interested in average values over longer sampling times. This is particularly true when one is concerned with cumulative exposure and with monitoring compliance with occupational exposure levels (OELs) (see Chapter 2). It is possible to take multiple measurements at one point in time and estimate the average, but more commonly the occupational hygienist uses different instruments, called *dose meters*. A dose is a quantity that represents the cumulative amount of the chemical, biological agent, or physical conditions to which the body is exposed over a given period, and therefore represents concentration over time.

Many types of dose meters have been developed, specifically, for noise, electromagnetic fields, and vibration. The dose meters integrate over the time of concentration or intensity, as described in equation (1). If the exposure varies or if it is intermittent, or if the calculation can be made simpler than equation (1), it is typical to calculate *time-weighted averages* (TWA) for the exposures (equation 2):

$$(1)\ E = \int c\,dt,$$
where E = exposure
$$c = \text{concentration or intensity}$$
$$dt = \text{differential time}$$

$$(2)\ TWA = (c_a t_a + c_b t_b + c_c t_c + \ldots + c_n t_n)/T,$$

where $c_a, c_b, c_c, \ldots, c_n$ = concentrations or intensities over periods of $t_a, t_b, t_c, \ldots, t_n$
T = total evaluation period (1 week, 8 hours, 15 minutes, or some other period)

Some chemicals present special technical problems; nickel, carbon monoxide, isocyanates, molds, and acids, for example, require special care and cannot be evaluated by the same standard methods employed for other metals or for other organic chemicals. Mixtures are especially difficult: e.g., the analysis of plastic degradation products, some welding fumes, and exhaust gases can be technically complicated.

Analysis

In simple cases, workplace personnel can do their own exposure assessment. As systems become more complicated, occupational safety and health personnel should be consulted because they have specific information and experience in the field. Occupational health personnel are especially qualified to evaluate health consequences. If these experts cannot decide whether or not the exposure is acceptable, then an occupational hygienist can measure exposure levels to provide more information on which decisions can be based.

However, it is common that workplace personnel or experts must decide very quickly whether the existing exposure is acceptable or not. Government occupational health agencies have set standards via legislated or regulatory limits that are called occupational exposure standards (OELs). These standards are legally enforceable and compliance is required by law. Information on legally mandated OELs can be obtained easily from the Internet, government publications, or health and safety books. The relevant OELs should be obtained, reviewed, and understood before a survey is done. (Most OELs have some technical aspects that should be understood; they are not just peak exposure limits.) Many times advisory OELs obtained from other sources are stricter than government-required standards and are thus more protective of workers' health. Whenever there is a conflict between government-required occupational exposure standards and OELs that are recommended by an international agency or other recognized authority, it is wise to try to reduce exposure to the lower of the two levels in order to achieve additional protection for the workers.

In exposure analyses, the measurements or estimates of exposure are compared with the appropriate OELs. OELs are calculated as time-weighted averages for various time periods (for example, the usual working shift of 8 hours, a longer work shift of 12 hours, a period in which a worker is performing a particular task such as 1 hour, or a period of special hazard lasting 15 minutes) or as maximum or *peak exposure* (often called *ceiling*) levels. The OEL may require recalculation if this period is different in a particular workplace situation (e.g., if the worker is working overtime). The exposure evaluation must take these factors into account, and the measurement is compared against an OEL that has been adjusted according to these factors.

In practice, workplaces mostly do their own exposure assessment even in cases in which the information available is limited. In such circumstances, the classification of risks must be done with special care, and engineering controls must be emphasized to help reduce the risk. In cases of chemical exposure, even when there are no signs of exposure, measurements must be carried out to ensure compliance with regulations and to guarantee that exposure is not being overlooked. The same precaution applies to high-level impulse noise and some radiation exposure.

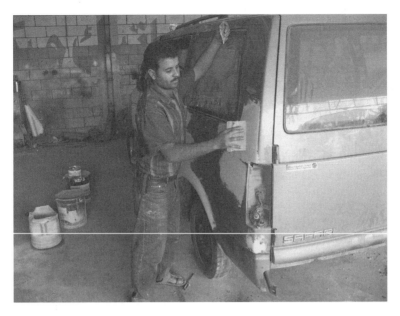

Figure 4.3 Automobile body work uses filler material consisting of fibrous glass, resin, talc, and styrene, which serves as a solvent and which evaporates. This results in exposure to styrene in a poorly ventilated area and in skin exposure, as in this garage in Saudi Arabia. (Photograph by Seifeddin Ballal, King Faisal University, Saudi Arabia.)

The effectiveness of hazard control measures should be checked by occupational hygiene measurements after the measures are installed and periodically thereafter to be sure that they are still working (see Chapter 12).

The use of chemicals that can cause dermatological problems must be carefully evaluated. Skin exposure can cause a dermatological disease, and many gaseous agents can penetrate the skin. Many factors influence the risk of skin disease, such as skin properties, duration of exposure, degree of skin contact, cleanliness of the environment, quality and use of gloves, work schedules, and so on.

Building-Related Illness Building-associated illness and symptom outbreaks are very common. They are often referred to by the general term *sick building syndrome* (Box 4.2). This section describes the evaluation of typical sick building syndrome cases. A case study is provided in Box 4.3 of a sick building study in which an explanation was eventually found. However, in most cases, no easy solution is discovered even after extensive investigation.

Building-related illness and symptom outbreaks may relate to any of several possible causes:

- "tight-building syndrome," which is a condition of poor ventilation that occurs when a building is made relatively airtight to save energy and heating costs
- poor indoor air quality, which is a common problem usually associated with poor ventilation

BOX 4.2

A Plan for Investigating Cases of Sick Building Syndrome

Office buildings frequently raise issues with respect to indoor air quality. Office buildings, schools, and workplaces in service industries not involving chemical processes are now often implicated in outbreaks of illness among employees. It is important to determine whether these problems are due to air contamination in the indoor environment or to some other cause. This has become a major challenge for occupational health professionals.

New buildings are served by complex ventilation systems for the delivery of fresh air and the removal of stale air and air recirculation within office buildings. New sources of contamination have been introduced into the marketplace, including furnishings treated with chemicals (for waterproofing and to be resistant to wear) and constructed using volatile chemicals in their glues or finishes.

A major factor contributing to the concerns with the indoor environment has been the emphasis on energy conservation in both new and old buildings. The frequency with which such outbreaks are associated with such buildings created a major problem for the construction and building management industry in the 1980s and 1990s. In the current era of concern for "green buildings," these mistakes are being repeated, and many new structures are being built with inadequate attention to occupant spaces. For example, a recently constructed, award-winning building in Maryland (USA) has been praised for its energy efficiency and intelligent monitoring systems to adjust the indoor conditions, but the spaces for maintenance and cleaning workers are unventilated.

Tightly sealed buildings that accumulate indoor air pollutants result in what is known as the tight building syndrome (TBS). The sick building syndrome, which is incorrectly used as a synonym by many people, refers to outbreaks of illness or discomfort, mostly related to respiratory symptoms and eye and throat irritation, in occupants of such buildings.

This is such a common problem that occupational hygienists have developed standard protocols for the evaluation of buildings with such problems. This box presents one such protocol used in the Canadian province of Alberta, developed in collaboration with Dr. Robert Rogers at Concordia College in Edmonton.

1. *Initial walkthrough and record review.* A simple visual inspection should be conducted of the entire building, not just the workplace where the complaints arose. This should include sources of odors (all workspaces, service areas, corridors and hallways, kitchens, lunchrooms, lounges, garages, maintenance areas (loading docks) and can be very helpful. Records of maintenance and repair of the ventilation system can be especially revealing. Consider the following:
     1.1. Is there evidence of water damage?
     1.2. Is mold growing in the building or in the ventilation system?
     1.3. Is the inside of the ductwork clean?
     1.4. Were strong chemicals used to clean the system?
     1.5. Is the system well maintained and tested every year?
     1.6. Has the system been "balanced" to provide even airflow?
2. *Personal interviews of affected workers.* Workers may be given a questionnaire asking the following:
     2.1. Did you smell an odor?

2.2. What type of odor was present?

2.3. Was it the odor that caused you to feel ill?

2.4. Where was the odor strongest and when did it appear?

2.5. What types of symptoms occurred?

3. *Air conditioning inspection and record review.* Ventilation equipment should be visually inspected. The investigation may include a description of the types of agents used during maintenance and operation, e.g., degreasing agents, solvents, and cleaning agents. Facilities adjoining ventilation intakes should also be inspected. Emphasis should be placed on

   3.1. Filters

   3.2. Humidifiers

   3.3. Outside roof area

   3.4. Inside plenum (a space, usually in the ceiling of an office building, where air is supplied or removed—it equalizes pressure and mixes air)

   3.5. Return air duct (a duct is a channel, usually made of metal, by which air is supplied or removed)

   3.6. Fresh air intake (roof area)

4. *Outdoor area inspection.* An extensive inspection of the surrounding area may be performed to determine if there are any outside sources of contamination (e.g., exhaust from neighboring buildings, leaks at nearby service stations, aerial pesticide sprayings.

5. *Ventilation testing.* Ventilation testing can be conducted utilizing a velometer for measuring air flow velocities and smoke tubes (which release small quantities of visible but harmless fumes) for determining air flow patterns. Wind directions and speeds should be determined daily. All accessible vent systems (exhaust and return systems) should be inspected.

6. *Odor test.* An olfactory (smell) test should be conducted immediately after the system is turned back on. Is there a detectable odor? Is it in the same area where an odor was reported earlier?

7. *Ventilation filter test.* The air filters located on the roof and plenum areas should be inspected and routinely replaced by new filters. The old filters should be placed in airtight plastic bags and then removed from the building entirely. Chemicals that may have accumulated on the filters may be detectable. This test is usually conducted by utilizing a direct reading instrument to detect organic gases that have accumulated in the plastic bag over 24 hours.

8. *Collection and analysis of cleaning agents.* Cleaning agents with a potential for creating odor or releasing vapors should be identified and inspected. The time when the ventilation system was last cleaned should be checked.

Certain characteristics suggest a low probability that the complaints result from indoor air contamination:

- People report the onset of symptoms within a building in a pattern that does not cluster in time or space, which would suggest a common source of exposure
- The pattern in time suggests that the new onset of symptoms goes from person to person, similar to propagating a communicable disease
- Absence of chemical contamination or evidence of poor indoor air quality
- Absence of consistent findings specific to a particular illness, response to airborne agents, or condition

- Adequate ventilation in the building
- Resolution of the problem without specific action being taken and no physical changes in the building or adjacent environment.

Of particular importance are the patterns of illness in time and space. When patterns are incompatible with a point source exposure, especially one borne by airflow patterns, one should consider the timing of the new onset of symptoms. If the incidence of new cases in various locations, called the *epidemic curve*, resembles the pattern of a transmissible agent, the outbreak is probably psychogenic.

Great care must be taken before concluding that an incident is psychogenic. It is not enough to observe that some individuals are overreacting. Anxiety and suggestibility may easily accompany true exposure incidents, so the observation of hyperventilation or the presentation of symptoms or illnesses with a psychological component among unexposed individuals is not in itself helpful in ruling out a toxic exposure. Anecdotal evidence regarding people who could not possibly have been exposed but who complain of compatible symptoms or have shown signs of anxiety does not mean that others with similar symptoms were not exposed. Human beings may demonstrate suggestibility and stress-related symptoms in any situation of urgency. However, these complaints are usually fairly stereotypical and limited to the known symptoms of hyperventilation and acute stress.

Mass psychogenic illness is a conclusion that is justified only after all alternatives have been ruled out on the basis of unequivocal documented evidence. Truly dangerous unrecognized toxic hazards must be exceedingly rare, if they ever occur, in the typical setting of a sick building syndrome in an office. Most cases are related to low-grade irritants affecting susceptible people and causing discomfort and anxiety. They are very troubling and often can be difficult to manage.

Contributed by Tee L. Guidotti

- sources of irritants in the workplace, such as the emissions from new carpets, adhesives, and new furniture or bioaerosols, such as pollen, plant debris, or mold
- specific building-associated illnesses, including hypersensitivity pneumonitis, inhalation fever, and infection, all of which are relatively rare
- asthma and allergies, with aggravation by exposure to nonspecific irritants or to allergens in the workplace (people with asthma and allergies are more susceptible to the effect of irritating chemicals as well as reactive to the substances to which they are allergic)
- psychogenic outbreaks, in which people develop symptoms due to anxiety because they truly believe that their health is affected (this is more common in schools)
- a community-acquired illness, such as influenza, that merely reflects what is happening in the community as a whole but clusters among the workers

Ventilation in buildings and the clearance of accumulated air contaminants indoors have become substantial problems in exposure assessment (Box 4.4). A major

BOX 4.3

A Building-Associated Outbreak of Non-specific Symptoms

Cases in which health symptoms are associated with a particular building are often called sick building syndrome. There are many causes, all aggravated by lack of ventilation. This is an unusual case of sick building syndrome because a very specific explanation was suggested by the evidence. Most cases of sick building syndrome are never fully explained. However, this case illustrates many important principles of ventilation.

The Incident

On a Monday morning, June 6, employees arriving for work on the 16th floor of an office building in Edmonton, Alberta, Canada, noticed a strong, foul odor as they stepped off the elevator. It was described as similar to that of burning plastic or chemical fertilizer. The odor was strongest in the east corridor and one office.

Over the course of the day, four employees complained of a headache, and some complained of nausea, eye irritation, irritability, and lethargy. The following day, five employees were absent all or part of the day, including the initial four who had complained of headache.

Over the subsequent several days, reports of an odor decreased but complaints of headache, eye irritation, and irritability persisted, peaking again on Monday, June 20, when an unusual odor was again concentrated in the east wing of the floor. June 6, 7, 10, and 20 were the worst days in terms of the frequency of complaints. The strong odor, described as similar to burning electrical wires, was highly associated with the onset of complaints. The symptoms always seemed worse on Mondays.

These symptoms were always relieved by leaving the area for several hours; they never persisted after the worker left for home. In retrospect, some workers remembered that there had been a similar odor a week earlier, but no health complaints were reported at that time. The episode ended two weeks later and did not occur again. Air sampling during that period did not indicate the presence of contaminants that could cause the symptoms recorded.

The Investigation

Operating records for the building were examined. During the previous month, only 10% of the normal volume of supply air was being directed to floors 11, 12, 13, 14, 15, and 17. The rest of the supply air was going to the 16th and 18th floors, thus creating a significant imbalance in the system. The high-volume air conditioning unit (HVAC) operates on weekdays only between 6:00 a.m. and 6:00 p.m. each day, a common practice to save energy costs. This means that air contaminants would accumulate over the weekend.

The water must be kept clean and free of algae, bacteria, and mold. Treatment chemicals were normally added on Wednesday afternoons at 5:00 p.m. The humidifier water treatment chemicals consist of an algicide, defoamer, and liquid organic chlorine, all but the last of which were common additives for such a system. The chemicals were added most recently on June 8. No chemicals were added on June 15, during the period of the odor problem.

The operation records for this period show a difference of 1 to 2 orders of magnitude between static pressures in the supply and return sides of the air-conditioning unit, which is a large difference in air flow between supply and return systems. This circumstance probably led to a relatively positive pressure on the 16th and 18th floors. Because of this there was probably inadequate entry of fresh, "make-up air" on those floors and consequently ineffective dilution of stale air in the building on those floors.

In March the original modular cellulose humidification system in the HVAC unit had suddenly collapsed. After new replacement units were installed in April, the system operated without problems until early June. According to the supplier, the humidifier units were a laminated cardboard lattice bonded with phenol-formaldehyde resin adhesive. This resin is normally used where resistance to temperature and humidity is required. The humidifier units were kept wet by pumping treated water over them as the supply air passed through the units.

The question of the actual airborne contaminants that caused the health complaints still remained. Fortunately, a piece of the humidifier material had been rescued and stored in a covered pail along with a small amount of water since the episode in June. An analysis of the water indicated 5 ppm formaldehyde (HCHO) and 9 ppm phenol, both components of the adhesive resin used in the humidifier components. However, the presence of phenol and formaldehyde in the water sample from the original humidifier material indicates that some of the phenol and formaldehyde from the adhesive became dissolved in the humidifier water. This is likely to have resulted from erosion of the resin by the water. The chlorine may have played a part in accelerating this erosion; it is not normally used in building humidifier systems.

The Reconstruction of the Incident

An explanation was eventually found. At that time of the year (June), there was little need for additional humidity and the contaminated water would not have been circulated over the phenol-formaldehyde lattice. The release of contaminants into the air would have been highest on those few occasions when the water circulation pump was operating. The smell of "burning insulation" would have occurred whenever air was moved through the rapidly degenerating lattices. This smell probably resulted from release of formaldehyde, phenol, and some unidentified nitrogen-bearing substances (from the water treatment chemicals) into the air. The latter were odorous but not particularly toxic. If the formaldehyde and phenol were present in humidifier water during June, they would certainly have been vaporized. The imbalance in the ventilation at that time would have directed all of the vapor to just two floors instead of eight. This redirection of air and the ineffective ventilation caused by poor return flow very likely led to a significant accumulation of vapors on the 16th floor. The concentrations would rise slowly over the day until the ventilation system shut down at 6:00 p.m. This cycle could have occurred each day that these substances were present in the water.

The intermittent episodes of frequent and severe complaints (June 6 and 10) occurred a few days after chemicals were added to the water. This latent period may have been required for the resin to decompose and the vapors to accumulate above the threshold concentration for irritation and other effects. Formaldehyde and phenol vapor concentrations in the air may have reflected those in the humidifier water due to the efficiency of the humidifier.

Despite the paucity of direct evidence regarding airborne contaminants, it is reasonable to conclude that the rapid deterioration of the cellulose humidifier units in early June released formaldehyde and phenol into the humidification system water of HVAC unit AS-5. The contaminants were then carried by supply air to just two floors in this building. The redirection of ventilation away from unoccupied floors and the consequent oversupply of air to the 16th and 18th floors led to an accumulation of airborne contaminants and airborne concentrations that were well above the odor thresholds of these substances. Exposure-effect data indicate that formaldehyde concentrations in the air could have reached 5 ppm. Phenol was probably present as high as 9 ppm. The additive acute effects of these substances made conditions intolerable and resulted in acute illnesses over a period of two weeks.

This left the question of why the humidifier units suddenly decayed, releasing contaminants into the water. The previous unit had lasted 11 years but ended up disintegrating almost overnight. The water treatment chemicals themselves do not appear to be implicated in the exposure. A change in the manufacturer's supplier of phenol-formaldehyde adhesive resin or an isolated batch of poor-quality resin, however, could account for the episode in June.

Formaldehyde was undoubtedly the major contaminant causing discomfort to the workers. Concentrations of formaldehyde even less than 1 ppm (the 8-hour OEL) can cause many of the symptoms observed. A second measurement conducted on the original water sample resulted in a concentration of 46 ppm and indicated that, assuming the airborne concentration of formaldehyde was directly proportional to the concentration in the humidifier water, the vapor concentration could have been even higher than 5 ppm and may have peaked at as much as 45 ppm in the case of complete equilibration between water and air. The second, higher reading was obtained after the water had been clarified, thus allowing a more accurate and reliable colorimetric analysis. This further supported the opinion that formaldehyde was the primary cause of irritation experienced on the 16th floor in June of this year.

The presence of traces of phenol and other substances with odors detectable at concentrations below the occupational exposure limit would serve to aggravate the discomfort. The unbalanced airflow in the building caused an accumulation of the air contaminants on the 16th floor, especially over the course of a weekend.

Why did the degenerating lattice occur in only one of several humidifier units in the building? The manner in which chemicals were added to the system was reviewed. Periodically, depending on the amount of water consumed, the maintenance technician would add 1/2 cup of algicide, 1/2 cup of defoamer, and 1/2 teaspoon of an organic chlorine compound. The bottles used for dispensing some of these compounds were almost identical. It would be easy to mix up the bottles and to add too much or too little of one or the other.

The algicide is a compound known as 1-(alkylamino)-3-aminopropane, and the organic chlorine compound is sodium dichloroisocyanurate dihydride (DIC). The names of these chemicals were verified with the supplier. The supplier "did not know of any special hazards associated with these compounds, especially when diluted according to directions." The algicide, an amine compound, is the likely source of nitrogenous compounds contributing to the odor. DIC is a highly reactive substance having 57% available chlorine. It is used as a bactericide in much the same way as sodium hypochlorite (household bleach) or chlorine is used in water treatment. A comprehensive data profile on DIC was obtained from "Cheminfo" files of the Canadian Centre for Occupational Health and Safety to confirm its properties.

Only 1/2 teaspoon of DIC is added to the humidifier's water trough to produce the desired chlorine concentration (around 2 ppm). It would be an easy mistake to add too much DIC given the rather primitive dispensing method used by the building technicians. If 1/2 cup was added inadvertently, not only would unwanted reactions take place with the other chemicals (giving rise to the "burning insulation" smell), but this would also cause the premature degradation of the phenol-formaldehyde bonded lattice. Unfortunately, no information appears to be available regarding the interactions of chemicals used as additives in air conditioning systems or on the action of these chemicals on the filters and other media with which they come into contact.

Under present circumstances, it is not possible to guarantee that another incident will never happen again. There is nothing to suggest that the new phenol-formaldehyde lattices will resist degradation any better than the old ones. We were not aware of any tests in the literature that have been carried out to evaluate this. Neither is there any means of assurance that the correct amounts of chemicals will always be added to the system.

Health Implications

The odor threshold of formaldehyde and phenol are approximately 0.5 ppm and 0.05 ppm, respectively. If one attributes the complaints to formaldehyde and phenol, then the exposure-effect data available indicate that their irritation effects were additive. Formaldehyde at 5 ppm causes irritation, headache, and sinus congestion. Formaldehyde has been identified as the burning smell. Phenol even at <10 ppm can cause nausea and vomiting, dizziness, and weakness. These signs and symptoms would certainly account for the subjective sense of irritability reported by many of the people involved. Phenol's odor could also have been detectable, but may have been masked by the formaldehyde. Low relative humidity (<30%) would magnify the irritant effects of formaldehyde, but no records were available in this regard.

Fortunately, the exposure to formaldehyde and some odorous air contaminants in the office was quite brief, a matter of a few days or weeks. The OEL for formaldehyde in Alberta is 1 ppm 8-hour TWA. A short exposure should not result in any long-term adverse effects. However, some people are exquisitely sensitive to formaldehyde and are bothered by it even at very low levels. Having once been exposed to the irritating effects of formaldehyde, some other individuals may become more sensitive in the short term to the smell and irritation, and this experience may be worse on subsequent occasions. What this means for the office building is that if there is a recurrence of the incident, one would probably be quickly alerted by health complaints to the need for appropriate remedial action.

The concentrations of formaldehyde achieved (and that of any other product likely to have been released) would be unlikely to cause a direct toxic effect but could easily have been sufficient to cause discomfort, nausea, and irritation. Nausea is a nonspecific human response to foul odors and is often accompanied by other signs of "vagal" activity (i.e., a reaction involving the vagus nerve, which is involved in vomiting, hiccups, and slowing of the heart rate). These nonspecific symptoms often lead to a headache, and the stress of working under such conditions adds further to the headache reaction. Thus, the illness employees experienced on June 6, was probably a direct reaction to the odors and irritation, not an unusual toxic effect.

Some people are more susceptible to the effects of irritants such as formaldehyde or sidestream cigarette smoke than others. Most of these relatively susceptible people were identifiable only by the fact that they were bothered at lower concentrations. A few people are predictably bothered at lower levels, however. These include people with allergies (especially seasonal hay fever), chronic eye inflammation, and asthma. There is no evidence that susceptibility to the irritant effects of the chemicals implies susceptibility to other, more serious health consequences.

Recommendations Made

The following recommendations were made to minimize the likelihood of recurrence:

1. The adoption of a fail-safe way to ensure that only the right amounts of chemicals were added to the system
2. Regular inspection of the phenol-formaldehyde lattices for any signs of deterioration each time chemicals were added; instruction of technicians to report immediately any unusual smells or other observations at the time of inspection
3. A system for identifying the service age of the lattice panels and replacement annually unless it can be demonstrated that no deterioration has taken place
4. That the building operators obtain reliable reports from the chemical suppliers regarding the interactions of the additive chemicals and an assurance that no harmful substances will enter the atmosphere under the conditions normally prevailing in the humidification systems
5. If there is a recurrence of the problem in the future, investigate further

Contributed by Tee L. Guidotti; Peter L. Bullock and Herb Buchwald also worked on the investigation.

BOX 4.4

Standardizing Risk Classification

An important phase in exposure assessment is the determination of risk. Exposure assessment and risk assessment are intertwined. Typically, risk assessment matrices have two axes: exposure (in terms of the likelihood of being exposed to harmful levels of a chemical) and consequences (in terms of how harmful the exposure may be).

For example, in British standard BS 8800 (Box 4.5), the consequences are classified as slightly harmful, harmful, and extremely harmful.

The degree of harmfulness is classified as follows:

- Slightly harmful equals irritation, mild disease, discomfort caused by drafts, etc.
- Harmful represents conditions such as burns, skin rashes, permanent mild diseases, hearing loss, vibration white fingers, welder's eye, frostbite, etc.
- Extremely harmful indicates work-related cancer, asthma, poisoning, and life-shortening diseases.

The probability of exposure to a level that could cause harm (which may be a function of concentration, duration, and frequency), expressed as the likelihood of harm, is classified as

- highly unlikely
- unlikely
- likely

In occupational hygiene, this classification is defined as assuming exposures of less than 50% of the OEL, 50% to 100% of the OEL, or exceeding the OEL, respectively. **Table 4.1** presents a health risk classification based on British standard BS 8800.

TABLE 4.1

A SIMPLE HEALTH RISK CLASSIFICATION FOR CHEMICAL AND PHYSICAL FACTORS BASED ON BRITISH STANDARD BS 8800

Consequences/ probability	Slightly harmful	Harmful	Extremely harmful
Examples of the harmfulness of consequences	Discomfort, irritation, mild disease, draft, small burns, reddening of the skin	Long-lasting serious effects, burns, frostbites, hearing loss, vibration white finger, electric eye, skin rashes	Constant serious effects, life-shortening diseases, poisoning, work-related cancer, asthma, drowning, loss of vision, heart attack
European Union Directives that apply	R20, 21, 22, 36, 37, 38, 66, 67	R23, 24, 25, 33, 34, 40, 43, 48, 62, 63, 64, 68	R26, 27, 28, 35, 39, 41, 42, 45, 46, 49, 60, 61
Highly unlikely less than 50% of the OEL	Trivial risk (no action)	Tolerable risk (monitoring)	Moderate risk (action needed)
Unlikely 50%–100% of the OEL	Tolerable risk (monitoring)	Moderate risk (action needed)	Substantial risk (action necessary)
Likely to exceed the OEL	Moderate risk (action needed)	Substantial risk (action necessary)	Intolerable risk (instant action)

*Refers to applicable European Union directives that define these terms. There are warning sentences for different health effects.

factor contributing to the concerns with the indoor environment has been reduced ventilation and an enclosed, sealed environment for energy conservation in new and old buildings. Gaseous chemicals that evaporate or are released (or *outgas*) from new carpets, synthetic fabrics, and adhesives used to apply paneling and other features contribute to atmospheric contamination.

Figure 4.4 demonstrates, through the idealized example of solvent released during painting a wall in a classroom, how the concentration of evaporated solvent decreases in an enclosed space logarithmically with ventilation and how it peaks again with subsequent application of paint. Single releases follow this general pattern. Continuous releases find equilibrium between release and dispersal and removal over time and maintain a more or less constant concentration in an enclosed space, depending on ventilation.

A major contributor to indoor air pollution is cigarette smoke. This includes smoke emissions from burning cigarettes and the exhaled smoke inhaled by smokers, but the former, called *sidestream smoke*, is of greatest concern. *Mainstream smoke*, as inhaled by the smoker, is filtered through the cigarette itself and is further modified by the respiratory tract of the smokers; this reduces the risk to passive smokers, although the risk to smokers remains very high. Sidestream smoke, on the other hand, has a much higher concentration of major toxic constituents, including several recognized carcinogens. Sidestream smoke is further modified by dilution with room air and possibly by chemical and odor changes

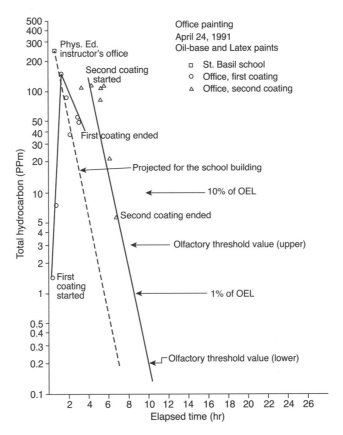

Figure 4.4 Reconstruction of the concentration of paint fume concentrations in a school building in Canada, based on measurements from sampling at given times (triangles). After each coat of pain is applied, the concentration of solvent fumes (hydrocarbon) is at its peak but rapidly (logarithmically) declines with ventilation (air turnover) in the room. Note that the scale of concentration is logarithmic, not linear. (Olfactory threshold = concentration at which a person can smell the paint; OEL = occupational exposure limit.)

over time after emission. The major health problems associated with sidestream smoke include eye and throat irritation and an increased risk of lung cancer if exposure is continuous. Individuals with asthma and other airway conditions are particularly susceptible.

In the typical "sick building" syndrome, workers in a building without a particular source of chemical emissions, usually an office building, complain of irritation of the eyes and throat and often a feeling of mental confusion. Workers with allergies are usually the first to be affected, but there may be no obvious substance in the workplace to which the worker is known to be allergic.

Sick building-associated outbreaks are very difficult to investigate. Usually, health and hygiene professionals are called in following the incident, often after odors or evidence of possible chemical contamination have dissipated or are greatly reduced. Analysis depends on the reconstruction of the episode, which is often made difficult by unreliable memories and uncertain chronology. Environmental monitoring data often do not detect evidence of a significant chemical exposure.

The first step in the investigation of a building-associated outbreak is to record the time and date of onset of reported symptoms and the precise location in the building where the affected workers spend their time. This information should pinpoint or at least point to a particular location within the building, either on the basis of a source of exposure or the flow characteristics of the building's ventilation system. A thorough occupational hygiene survey should be conducted, emphasizing any exposure that appears to be likely on the basis of the reported symptoms (which are seldom specific) or activity patterns within the building. The ventilation system should be inspected, with careful attention to the ducting, filters, and humidifiers, and a review conducted of the recent maintenance records.

The investigation of a building-associated outbreak can be as elaborate as the chemical analytical technology that is available. It is useful to divide the investigation into two phases: facility and personnel investigation and sampling and analytical strategy. The facility and personnel investigation phase emphasizes localization of the problem and identification of possible sources. The sampling and analytical strategy emphasizes characterization of the hazard level and identification of the actual exposure.

Box 4.2 also presents a general strategy for investigation of sick building incidents. Methods for the direct measurement of indoor air quality fall within the professional role of occupational hygienists. Some of the methods routinely used in the investigation of serious indoor air quality measurements include:

- visual inspection
- ventilation testing
- sampling for later laboratory analysis
- direct measurement on site
- gas chromatograph/mass spectrometer (GC/MS)

The gas chromatograph is a means of separating and quickly identifying and measuring low concentrations of chemical components of a complex mixture.

Odor plays a very important role in indoor air quality. Odors or very mild irritants may result in a disproportionate psychogenic response. Odors that are noxious, strong, or psychologically linked to unpleasant associations (such as body odor or feces) may precipitate nausea and a vasovagal reaction in susceptible individuals. Unfortunately, odors cannot be detected or quantified by conventional instruments, even GC/MS.

In many cases, outbreaks of acute illness among occupants of buildings that are not necessarily tightly sealed occur, yet no exposure can be implicated. Such incidents cause great anxiety among all parties concerned but usually end inconclusively. Many of these incidents arise as a result of psychological factors or a combination of psychological factors and low-level exposures that initiate an exaggerated response. These are called *psychogenic outbreaks*. If the pattern does not logically coincide with building ventilation characteristics, the possibility of psychogenic factors should be considered, but an outbreak should never be dismissed as psychogenic until chemical exposures and ventilation problems are ruled out.

5

MONITORING AND SURVEILLANCE

Jukka Uitti and Panu Oksa

It is the employer's duty to inform and the employee's right to know about possible chemical and physical hazards, physical and mental strain, and the risks of accidents in the workplace. Workers and employers are primarily informed about hazards through occupational hygiene and hazard assessment. The goal is to control exposure to hazards to prevent or reduce the risk of disease or injury. However, control of occupational hazards can be incomplete and uncertain.

To be sure that control is adequate, it is important to identify the effects these hazards may be having on workers and whether the risk of occupational injuries and disease is increasing or decreasing. *Monitoring and surveillance programs* seek evidence of preventable injury and disease among workers as a method of tracking occupational health progress, solving specific occupational health problems that are discovered, and providing early medical attention for cases of occupational disease.

Due to technological and economic limitations, it is often impossible to eliminate all health hazards in the workplace. Under such circumstances, the surveillance of workers' health plays a major role in worker protection.

Ideally, information from surveillance of work environments is combined with information from other sources (epidemiologic research, observations from workers' health status) in order to piece together a total picture of worker health. In practice, surveillance programs are often all that is available to determine whether the health of workers is being adequately protected.

Monitoring and surveillance programs are valuable because they provide information on the effectiveness of occupational hygiene and hazard control. In some industries, such as manufacturing, exposure to a hazard is predictable, and the effectiveness of control measures can be assessed directly. However, exposures vary considerably in many other settings and occupations that are undertaken in workplaces that are less easily controlled. Maintenance and construction work are two examples of variable work conditions that may involve notably harmful exposures and are difficult to monitor and/or control.

Many methods can be used to evaluate health effects as possible consequences of exposures to occupational health hazards. Workplace surveys and hygienic measurements can be used as direct and effective means of monitoring work conditions. When done properly and regularly, these methods provide good information on the possible health hazards of workers. However, the use of technology solely to monitor conditions in the workplace cannot completely account for all existing exposures. In a closed chemical process, technical malfunctions and failures can occur and cause exposures that are higher than normal or that are unexpected.

One obvious strategy for protecting workers' health is to examine workers regularly for early signs of disease. Monitoring workers, as individuals and as groups, for early indications of adverse health effects of workplace exposures has historically been one of the most important functions of the occupational health physician. *Periodic health examinations* are regular medical evaluations, usually conducted annually, to assess the fitness of workers for certain jobs.

The purpose of these examinations is to assess health impairments linked to exposure to harmful agents and to identify cases of occupational and work-related diseases that have been defined by legislation. When data from periodic health examinations are collected, analyzed, and reported for purposes of prevention, the effort constitutes *medical surveillance*.

The occupational health physician or nurse is often called upon to provide occupational health surveillance for workers employed in high-risk occupations (e.g., potential for exposure to lead, noise, asbestos, pesticides, known chemical carcinogens, or other chemical or physical hazards). Such surveillance programs may be conducted for a group of workers with unknown and unpredictable levels of exposure, such as employees in a certain area of a manufacturing plant, where hazardous materials are used or the workers are exposed to multiple hazards.

SURVEILLANCE AND MONITORING

When the risk of a particular disease outcome is known to be elevated in a particular industry, surveillance is one strategy to determine the group experience with that health outcome. When a particular outcome is not necessarily anticipated and the overall health experience of the group is to be observed, the more general strategy of monitoring is employed. Surveillance is useful if the conditions in question are common or specific to a particular industry, such as the case for asbestos-associated lung diseases. Surveillance programs are usually restricted to certain high-risk groups and are required by law to be provided at the employer's expense for workers exposed to specific hazards, such as asbestos, noise, and lead. Surveillance depends on the accurate identification of new cases of the disorder in question among workers at risk. On the other hand, monitoring depends on the complete ascertainment of the health outcomes experienced by a defined population. It is useful in discovering previously unrecognized health problems.

When a specific health outcome is known or suspected, the task of observing a population's health experience is simplified. Surveillance programs do not require the population to be as carefully controlled as monitoring programs do, and they are usually much less expensive. They are targeted toward specific high-risk groups, as defined by workplace assignment, known exposure history, and exposure measurement data. When a surveillance procedure is required by regulation, it is called *mandated surveillance*. The activities of health authorities, enterprises, and occupational health organizations that follow the health of workers are dependent on current legislation or on the health-care practices of each country.

Another important component of a general program set up to observe the experience of a population is *environmental monitoring*. Environmental monitoring is the periodic testing of the workplace environment for hazardous or excessive exposure conditions, and it complements medical monitoring. Another method of monitoring the work environment is by monitoring workers themselves. Exposure to hazardous chemical agents can be measured from biological samples, usually blood or urine, using tests to determine the magnitude of the exposure's effect on the body and measuring the toxic substance or its metabolite directly.

Surveillance in Occupational Health Services

Occupational health services should include surveillance of the work environment and surveillance of workers' health. International Labour Organization [ILO] Convention No. 161 and Recommendation No. 171 (1985) is the key international convention for monitoring and surveillance and provides detailed guidance on what it should include. The surveillance of the work environment should include the following:

- identification and evaluation of environmental factors that may affect workers' health
- assessment of hygienic conditions and organizational factors
- assessment of collective and personal protective equipment
- assessment, where appropriate, of exposure to hazardous agents through the use of valid and generally accepted monitoring methods
- assessment of control systems designed to eliminate or reduce exposure

It is not always possible to prevent the hazardous exposure of workers by technology. Therefore, technology should not be exclusively relied upon to prevent worker exposures. Surveillance should include all the assessments necessary to protect the health of workers (ILO 1985) including:

- health assessments before assignments to specific tasks that may involve a danger to health
- health assessment at periodic intervals during employment if there is exposure to a particular health hazard
- health assessment on the resumption of work after a prolonged absence for health reasons for the purposes of determining possible occupational causes, recommending appropriate action to protect the worker, and determining the worker's suitability for the job
- health assessment on and after the termination of assignments involving hazards that may cause or contribute to future health impairment

Occupational health professionals cannot firmly identify all health risks in advance or, for that matter, all hazards in the workplace. (The database on exposure-response relationships among humans to support standards setting is generally poor and spotty. Exposure controls are based on estimates and standards that reflect expert judgment.) However, workers in some situations may still be adversely affected despite compliance with standards or, in some cases, a standard may be found to have been inadvertently exceeded. For example, the most common occupational exposure level for noise, 90 dBA 8-hour time-weighted average, may still cause noise-induced hearing loss in as many as 15% of workers. Exposure monitoring merely defines the most likely or the worst levels of exposure (depending on the exposure assessment) that are likely to have occurred and therefore what is expected to happen at that level of exposure. That is too indirect. The exposure assessment could be wrong or inadequate for the individual worker, and the worker may or may not be susceptible to the exposure. Medical monitoring verifies the exposure status and health risk of workers. Medical monitoring is a safeguard and check on the safety of the workplace.

Types of Health Evaluations

Health examinations assess the fitness of workers to carry out their jobs and determine the occurrence of health impairment and occupational diseases. Evaluating the health status of workers is important when new workers are recruited, when new technologies are introduced, and when individual workers need follow-up because of individual health characteristics.

Evaluations for Fitness to Work These evaluations are conducted to determine whether an employee is fit to do the work required safely and to ensure that there is no health threat to the employee or other workers. These evaluations are described in detail in Chapter 17. *Fitness-to-work evaluations* are usually mandatory.

General health evaluations, or *examinations* are not mandatory. Employees may take advantage of the opportunity if they wish, and these examinations are often considered a benefit of employment. Employers may make them available to all employees or may offer them to only certain groups, determined for example by age or by the department in the company.

Often, these evaluations are given to executives and key employees of a company in order to ensure that the leadership remains uninterrupted and the interests of the company are protected. Examinations are carried out to diagnose latent disease (e.g., diabetes, hypertension), to identify serious disease as early as possible, and to provide health education and promotion. Health evaluations may also be a good way of initiating health promotion activities within the company.

Health Evaluations After Duty Involving Hazards Examinations are often performed after the termination of assignments that involve hazards that can cause health problems. The post-duty *health evaluation* establishes the health condition of the worker at the time of termination or reassignment. The worker's health is evaluated and compared with the results of previous examinations. This is done partly to ensure that the worker is still healthy and partly to protect the company against later claims that the hazard made the worker ill. The worker is also encouraged to visit his or her personal physician if periodic health examinations are needed after the cessation of exposure (for example, after substantial asbestos exposure). In some countries, such as the United States, the law requires periodic health surveillance only while a worker is employed; follow-up examinations must be conducted at the worker's expense or paid for in some other way.

Periodic Health Evaluation Programs

One might assume that occupational health problems can be effectively identified by the worker's own physician during routine care, without systematic surveillance and monitoring procedures. In the real world, this is seldom the case. Occupational illnesses are encountered only occasionally in a typical medical practice and are seldom immediately recognized for what they are. A worker's personal physician is rarely knowledgeable of the complete picture of the health experience of employees in a particular industry or plant.

A structured medical monitoring program that evaluates workers systematically can be used to identify problems due to inadequate control of exposure. Periodic health examinations should always be done in cases of suspected or known health risks, based on the best available knowledge of work conditions, and conducted by occupational health personnel.

Workers need periodic health evaluations when there are known or suspected harmful exposures in the workplace and when technical monitoring and workplace surveys have been insufficient or lacking. The general objectives of periodic health examinations are the following:

- to detect changes before clinical disease becomes apparent in order to remove workers from further exposure to prevent the disease from worsening
- to detect disorders early enough to treat them to improve the likelihood of complete recovery
- to identify new or previously unsuspected health problems
- to confirm the absence of health problems to ensure the efficacy of control measures such as technical monitoring
- to give information to the worker individually

Periodic health evaluations in hazardous work should be structured and performed systematically with appropriate tests and methods so that the data are not only reliable but also comparable to findings from other workplaces and from the same workplace at different times. Good clinical practice requires that tests and diagnostic procedures should be valid and sensitive enough to detect the initial (pre-disease) effect on the worker or the disease in the subclinical phase or at least at an early reversible or curative stage.

Examinations of an individual worker can be done by an occupational health nurse or an occupational health physician, depending on the type of tests and usual clinical practice in different countries. Occupational health nurses can competently handle routine examinations, worker information, and standard clinical tests,

Box 5.1

Example: Setting Up a Health Evaluation Program
in a Construction Company

Construction work involves several types of health risk. When the need for periodic health evaluation was assessed in a middle-sized construction company in Finland, an examination program was set up after discussions between the employer and employees' representatives. The process involved following these steps.

1. Walk-through surveys on two different construction sites were done by an occupational health physician, an occupational health nurse, and safety personnel. No hygienic measurements were done.
2. Risk assessment resulted in the conclusion that workers were exposed to noise, silica dust, and poor ergonomic work positions.
3. It was decided that all workers would be examined at three-year intervals and that the examination would include
    (a) hearing test
    (b) chest X-ray
    (c) lung function measurement (spirometry)
    (d) clinical examination and information (nurse)
    (e) clinical examination by physician (in case of symptoms or abnormal findings)
    (f) additional examinations if needed
    (g) worker feedback
    (h) feedback on work ability to employer
4. An optional set of tests for coronary heart disease and physical fitness tests in the examination (even if these were not mandatory). A questionnaire and serum cholesterol, blood pressure, and fitness tests were added to every worker's health examination, and an electrocardiogram was included for workers over 45 years of age. Both sides were willing to include this optional package because of the importance of heart disease.
5. Health examinations were carried out as planned.

The program found several workers who were at risk of serious disease. One person was suspected to have coronary heart disease. Two workers were found to have occupational hearing impairment. When the data of all the health examinations were analyzed, it was noted that carpenters as a group had impaired hearing, and the average serum cholesterol value of all the workers was higher than that of the general male population.

   After discussions between the employer, representatives of the employees, and the occupational health and safety personnel, it was decided to design a special program for preventing hearing damage in carpenters and to start a health promotion program for all the workers to prevent coronary heart disease. Both the employer and the workers considered the program a great success.

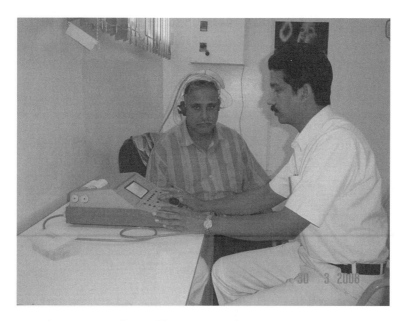

Figure 5.1 Audiometry is a form of hearing test that is performed, as shown here, as a screening test to detect noise-induced hearing loss. More elaborate versions of audiometry are used for diagnosis and evaluation (as in Figure 13.3). (Photograph courtesy of the Shuaiba Occupational Medical Centre, Ministry of Health, Kuwait.)

whereas the use of physicians is more appropriate for complicated cases, specialized tests, and evaluations that are not standardized.

A worker's periodic health evaluation should include the following basic elements, usually in sequence:

1. Tests, diagnostic procedures, and clinical examination, selected to identify the most common, serious, and characteristic health outcomes associated with the job
2. Possible additional examinations to evaluate abnormal results
3. Information on possible health hazards (and how to avoid them)
4. Feedback to the worker
5. Documentation of the worker's work ability to the employer (see Chapter 17— "Fitness to Work")

Ideally, periodic health evaluations are incorporated into a comprehensive program for worker protection. A model program in described below:

1. Occupational hygiene monitoring of the workplace and hygienic measurements
2. Risk assessment of health hazards
3. Design of periodic health examinations (identify workers at risk, content, frequency)
4. Expert advice given and discussed with the employer and the employees' representative (If health examinations are mandated by law, permission from

neither party is obligatory, but both parties need to know the situation so commitment to further preventive steps is obtained.)

5. Periodic health evaluations provided on a regular cycle (usually annually)
6. Analysis of data from health evaluations
7. Findings discussed with the employer and employees' representative
8. Occupational hygiene investigation of problem areas
9. If deficiencies found, improvements undertaken

Surveillance Programs

Surveillance programs have one or more of the following goals:

• to track trends in disease incidence across industries, over time, and between geographic areas
• to define the magnitude or relative magnitude of a problem
• to identify new hazards, risk factors, or populations subject to risk
• to target interventions
• to evaluate efforts of prevention and intervention

Table 5.1 provides a guide for designing, initiating, and operating surveillance programs (modified from Wagner 1996). Figure 5.2 describes the sources that have input into the development of a periodic health surveillance program.

Over time, the practice of surveillance has progressed from *passive surveillance*, in which the occurrence of new cases is simply recorded and reported to a central data repository (for example, disease registries) to *active surveillance*, in which occupational health professionals actively search for evidence of the disease and

TABLE 5.1

QUESTIONS TO BE ASKED WHEN INITIATING A SURVEILLANCE PROGRAM

• What is the purpose of the program?
• Who is responsible for the design, conduction, and evaluation of the program?
• What exposures are creating the health risk?
• What disease or state of health or condition is the target of the program?
• Which workers are eligible for participation?
• Is the program legally mandated or voluntary? If mandated, is legal enforcement tied to program performance?
• Is worker participation in testing voluntary or mandatory?
• Which tests are to be performed?
• What is the frequency of each test? In relation to initial exposure or cessation of exposure?
• Who performs the test and under what conditions?
• What constitutes an abnormal test result?
• What actions will be taken because of an abnormal test result?
• Are the actions mandatory or voluntary?
• How will the effectiveness of the program be assessed?

Source: Wagner 1996

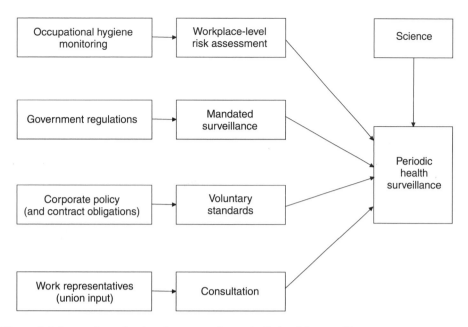

Figure 5.2 Inputs into the development of a periodic health surveillance program.

collect data on injuries, as well as compiling statistics that are used for the active analysis of data in order to generate an appropriate public health response. In passive health surveillance, ill workers are expected to consult occupational health professionals who then report the illness. However, passive surveillance systems inevitably miss some cases and almost always have problems with underreporting. Active surveillance, which is more costly but much more reliable, can take many forms, including periodic medical evaluations for all workers, medical examinations for workers exposed to specific health hazards, and screening and biological monitoring of selected groups of workers. The major components of surveillance programs are:

1. periodic identification and collection of health information
2. evaluation and interpretation of the information
3. reports and intervention for the purpose of prevention

Public institutions, managers, large companies, or occupational health services may wish to conduct surveillance programs in order to determine whether they have a hazard problem and whether the problem is under control. Sources of data for surveillance systems include workers' compensation claims, health insurance statistics, government records of worker illness and injury, hospital discharge information, disease registries, national health surveys, death certificates, and physician reporting. Simplicity, flexibility, acceptability, and timeliness characterize effective health surveillance systems. Surveillance systems should comprise sensitive indicators of the level of disease in the population at risk. Occupational health services have been urged to set up written action plans for their activities together with the client (i.e., representatives of the employer and employees). Such plans should also include procedures for the monitoring and surveillance of workers. In addition to the demands of legislation in each country, employers or public health organizations may provide some resources for their occupational health services to use in promoting the health of workers and maintaining their work ability. These comprehensive health programs are voluntary for companies and often include elements of primary and secondary prevention for common diseases such as coronary heart disease, especially in countries where these diseases are important reasons for loss of work ability, early retirement, and mortality.

Pilot projects may help determine the effectiveness and acceptability of programs before they are launched in full scale. Surveillance programs should be built around the best available testing procedure at the time of initiation. However, a test that is difficult to interpret or that varies greatly from tests applied in the past may lead to confusion and uncertainty. Therefore, the most widely applied mandated surveillance procedures are based on relatively simple and straightforward tests: blood lead for lead exposure, audiometric screening for noise exposure, and chest X-rays for asbestos exposure.

A surveillance or medical monitoring program is also a commitment to action. Abnormal findings must be acted upon, not filed away and forgotten. A medical monitoring program is not a substitute for action to control workplace exposure. Health examinations should be conducted in parallel with the surveillance of the work environment. Protecting the health of workers by controlling exposure is the primary objective, and medical surveillance and monitoring is the next essential step to protecting the worker's right to a safe workplace.

Screening Tests

The terms *screening* and *surveillance* are often used interchangeably, with confusing results. Screening is the use of medical testing for the presumptive identification of a disease in an individual, at a time before medical care would ordinarily be sought and when available intervention can favorably affect the health of the individual. Surveillance, on the other hand, involves the periodic collection, analysis, and reporting of information relevant to health for the purposes of disease prevention. In contrast to screening, surveillance is directed toward improving the health of populations and is a component of public health practice. Information generated by screening can be the raw data of a surveillance program.

Screening is the administration of a test or series of tests (questionnaires, medical examinations, laboratory tests) to individuals in order to detect organ dysfunction or disease at a point when intervention would be beneficial in disease prevention. Preferably, the screening test would identify *subclinical* disease before symptoms and signs of the disease appear. Ideally, such a test would detect an adaptation to the exposure well before subclinical impairment develops. Positive screening tests may indicate the presence of disease or the strong likelihood of disease and the need for confirmatory testing. Ultimately, the goal of medical screening should be the secondary prevention of disease (see Chapter 18).

The selection of a screening test is based on the following three variables: the *sensitivity* of the test, its *specificity*, and the *prevalence* of the disease in the community (see Table 5.2). These terms describe essential concepts that also apply to the use of diagnostic tests in the recognition of any disease.

Sensitivity is the proportion of diseased persons who are correctly identified as diseased by the screening test in the screened population. It is partly an intrinsic property of the test and partly a reflection of the diversity of the abnormality in a group of patients with the disorder. Sensitivity is an empirical measurement of the probability that a given case of the disorder will be actually identified by the test (true positive rate).

The higher the sensitivity of the test, the more likely it is that diseased persons will be identified.

Specificity is the proportion of non-diseased persons who are correctly identified by the screening test. It is generally considered an intrinsic property of the test, but may also depend on the distribution of the abnormality in a normal group of people. It is a measure of the probability that a non-diseased person, free of the disorder, will be correctly identified as disease-free by a screening test (true negative rate).

The higher the specificity of a test, the more reliably it will exclude non-diseased persons. A test with low sensitivity but high specificity will detect only a small fraction of diseased persons, but a positive test will be a reliable indication that disease is present in any person. A negative test result in the same situation will not reliably rule out the disease, however. A test with high sensitivity and low specificity will correctly identify most true cases but will also be positive for many persons

TABLE 5.2

MEASUREMENTS OF TEST PERFORMANCE

Test Outcome	True State		Total
	Disease Present	Disease Absent	
Positive	a	b	a + b
Negative	c	d	c + d
Total	a + c	b + d	a + b + c + d

a = Diseased persons detected by the test (true positives)
b = Non-diseased persons positive by the test (false positives)
c = Diseased persons not detectable by the test (false negatives)
d = Non-diseased persons negative by the test (true negatives)

$$\text{Sensitivity} = \frac{a}{a + c}$$

$$\text{Specificity} = \frac{d}{b + d}$$

$$\text{Predictive value (positive)} = \frac{a}{a + b}$$

$$\text{Predictive value (negative)} = \frac{d}{c + d}$$

who do not, in fact, have the disease. In other words, an insensitive but specific test yields many false negatives. A sensitive but non-specific test yields many false positives, so if a disease is rare in the population, the false positives may outnumber the true positives and require additional diagnostic tests to confirm the result. Tests that are both highly sensitive and highly specific are ideal. Most tests in clinical use fall short of the ideal and thus require confirmation with additional studies.

Predictive value is the probability that a person with a positive result on the test will actually have the disease; correspondingly, the predictive value of a negative test is the probability that a person with a negative result on the test will be free of the disease. The (positive) predictive value of a test depends on the sensitivity and specificity of the test, but also on the prevalence of the disorder in the population. Tests become increasingly less reliable as the prevalence of the disorder in the population decreases.

Table 5.3 summarizes the essential characteristics of any test considered for inclusion in a surveillance program. Because screening tests are applied to people who are not likely to have a serious illness, they must be safer and more tolerable than a clinical test that may suggest the need for life-saving treatment for someone who is ill.

Box 5.2 provides an example of a screening program conducted in Finland for asbestos-exposed workers.

ETHICS AND SOCIAL ISSUES

The rationale for monitoring and surveillance programs is currently under intense scrutiny. Some authorities have suggested that there is a potential conflict between individual human rights and monitoring, surveillance, and other medical evaluation programs that gather information on employees. The thrust of this argument is that abuses have occurred and are likely to occur in the future and that guidelines are needed for monitoring or evaluative medical programs. Most of these issues relate to the confidentiality of medical information and the risk of discriminating against workers with abnormal results. A consensus among occupational health professionals emerged from this issue in Canada in the 1980s, after a long debate (see Table 5.4).

TABLE 5.3

CRITERIA FOR THE SELECTION OF SCREENING TESTS FOR MONITORING AND SURVEILLANCE PROGRAMS

1. The test should be sensitive and specific.
2. The test must be simple and inexpensive.
3. The test must be very safe, to avoid causing more harm than good.
4. The test must be acceptable (i.e., not inconvenient, time-consuming, uncomfortable, or unpleasant) to the subjects and to those conducting the test.
5. The test should be capable of detecting disease at a time when intervention is likely to result in cure.

Example: Screening for Asbestos-Induced Diseases in Finland

Screening was carried out for asbestos-induced diseases in Finland in 1990 and 1992. The aim was to find workers with asbestos-related diseases in high-risk occupations. Both active and retired workers were asked to take part. The examination included a personal interview on work history and asbestos exposure and a chest radiograph. The target group comprised workers less than 70 years of age who had worked at least 10 years in construction, 1 year in a shipyard, or in the manufacture of asbestos products. A preliminary questionnaire was sent to 54,409 workers, of whom 18,943 participated in the screening. The mean age of the workers was 53 years; 95% were employed in construction. The criteria for a positive screening result were a radiographic finding clearly indicating lung fibrosis (at least ILO category 1/1) and a radiographic finding indicating mild lung fibrosis (ILO category 1/0) with uni- or bilateral pleural plaques, marked abnormalities of the visceral pleura, or bilateral pleural plaques. The positive cases totaled 4,133 (22%) and were sent for further examination. During the screening, information about the presence of asbestos in the work environment and the prevention of asbestos exposure as well as the health effects of asbestos exposure and smoking was given to the participants. The screening acted as a preliminary survey to prompt additional national follow-up of asbestos-induced diseases among the exposed workers (Koskinen et al. 1996).

TABLE 5.4

GUIDELINES FOR MONITORING AND EVALUATIVE MEDICAL PROGRAMS

1. Outcome monitoring and surveillance programs for working populations of interest are not an acceptable substitute for exposure monitoring and control.

2. Employers, health professionals, and any other parties involved in monitoring or other health evaluation programs have a moral and ethical obligation, and often a legal duty, to see that the workers under evaluation understand the purpose, degree of validity, and consequences of participation.

3. Workers have an absolute right to be informed of their individual results and the implications for their health and well-being; this information is confidential.

4. Employers have no right to information that does not pertain directly to either occupationally related disorders or to the capability of a worker to perform the job assigned.

5. Unusual or special evaluation techniques, such as a biomedical monitoring procedures under development and not yet standardized, especially if invasive, should be conducted only with the specific consent of the worker.

6. Commitment to a monitoring or surveillance program implies that the data will be gathered for a purpose and that the findings will be acted upon.

7. Data from medical monitoring and surveillance activities should not be used as the grounds for personnel actions, such as laying off or firing workers.

8. Employers should be responsible for the cost of the program because they are ultimately responsible for protecting the health of workers.

The health status of an individual worker is confidential and should not be communicated to the employer or to anyone other than the individual worker. On the other hand, the occurrence of an occupational disease is of public health significance. The insurance company must be informed, and in most countries it is mandatory to report new cases to safety authorities and to an occupational disease registry. At the workplace, new cases should be reported to the employer, the supervisors, and the occupational safety personnel. This is necessary information that will improve the work environment.

Following "good clinical practices" is one of the ethical principles for occupational health. Occupational health professionals must keep their skills at a high level and must maintain their independence, even though the employer is paying for the services. Occupational health personnel are not workers' advocates, either. Rather, they are independent consultants who are able to draw conclusions by using the facts and scientific knowledge available to them.

6

SAFETY

Tee L. Guidotti

Safety is a broad field of study, grounded on a few basic principles, with many highly specific applications in occupational health. The term safety, or *safety science*, refers to the application of technology, behavioral science, and administrative controls to prevent incidents resulting in injury, property loss and lost productivity. In recent years, the practice of safety science has largely merged with the field of loss and liability control. Safety positions in industry, but not government, now often include duties to prevent incidents that result in lost work time and damage to property as well as injuries to workers. As a result, many safety professionals work closely with insurance experts and corporate managers responsible for insurance against loss.

An eternal question about worksite safety is why it is so difficult to show progress when the problem is so apparently simple. The fact is that achieving progress in safety is difficult because changing human behavior is difficult. Change in behavior is not readily accomplished with single-point interventions; the change in behavior must be supported, reinforced, and sustained over time in an environment that does not encourage lapses to familiar old routines. In other words, safety is a profoundly social activity because changing risk-taking behavior depends on social interactions, not just individual perceptions and motivation, and on social factors such as work organization.

Behavior-based safety (BBS) is a school of thought within safety that seeks to change behavior using culture change, peer influence, positive reinforcement (rewards and encouragement rather than punishment), and open discussion. BBS has become increasingly popular in recent years because, in many developed countries, injury rates have flattened out. That is, improvement in injury rates has slowed, and not much progress is being made. This has led safety professionals to search for further ways to change workers' behavior and the realization that this is not only very difficult to do but not sufficient in itself. Most practitioners of BBS emphasize these key concepts about behavior change:

- BBS contributes significant, lasting, and sustainable results only after the workplace environment has been changed, through safety measures, design, and ergonomics.

- BBS depends on the culture of the organization: if management does not recognize and reward safe operations or make safety part of the performance review of supervisors, or takes risks with safety, BBS is much less effective.
- BBS will not work in a culture where workers are not encouraged to be open and free in discussion of safety or when they feel that they will be penalized for reporting "close calls" or "near misses."
- BBS takes time and considerable effort throughout the enterprise: it cannot reverse poor safety performance in a few months.

There has been a strong trend away from the word "accident" toward substituting the words "injury" for the outcome and "incident of injury" for the event. The argument is that "accident" implies a fatalistic view of injuries. This chapter uses the word "accident" only in a historical context, since the terms "accident causation" and "accident prevention" were heavily used in the past. The word *incident*, which has replaced it, also includes events that result in property loss.

Safety science tends to be highly specialized, and safety professionals usually focus on a particular industry and sometimes a particular type of hazard. The following is a list of common divisions of safety science:

- chemical safety (see Chapter 2), which emphasizes plant and facility safety, safe methods of storing and handling chemicals, and protection against chemical explosions
- hazardous materials management, which emphasizes handling chemicals safely and managing smaller-scale incidents, such as chemical spills
- fire science, which emphasizes prevention and suppression of fires (i.e., how to put them out), building fire safety, and industrial fire protection
- risk and liability management, which emphasizes corporate policies, insurance management, keeping track of potential safety problems, and controlling them to prevent injury and loss
- incident investigation, which often is a specialty of safety professionals in government and in insurance companies
- transportation safety, which emphasizes protecting workers, passengers, and cargo on planes, ships, trucks, buses, and other public transportation
- disaster management, which emphasizes prevention and *mitigation* (reducing the impact) of incidents on a large scale
- electrical safety, which emphasizes prevention of burns, fires, and shocks due to electricity
- occupational safety, which is a general field in which safety personnel become experts in the prevention of injuries on the job in common situations, such as handling materials and working at heights.

In addition, every major industry has its own specialized safety issues and often its own professional safety organization, such as the oil and gas industry, mining, the chemical industry, the microelectronics and semiconductor industry, the maritime (shipping and passenger) industry, and airlines, to name a few important examples. Chapter 25 presents some of these issues.

The prevention of occupational injuries through redesign of the workplace and the control of physical hazards falls mostly into the domain of two specialized occupational safety and health professions, ergonomics and safety engineering. Ergonomics is the discipline concerned with designing the workplace and tools to conform to human factors for optimum efficiency, comfort, and safety. Safety engineering, discussed below, is the field concerned with identifying and correcting physical hazards in the workplace that might cause injury. In addition, occupational hygienists are usually trained in safety, and many workers become safety officers on an informal basis in their companies, usually after long experience on the job.

Fatalities are deaths due to injuries on the job. Fatalities are always tragedies affecting all concerned and society as a whole. Often involving young workers with families, a death on the job has profound consequences for the family, the community of which the worker was a part, and coworkers. A fatality usually strains and sometimes breaks the trust between management and the workers. Fatalities are handled differently from other injuries by occupational health and safety authorities and always require investigation. A fatality often results in extended legal action and always results in psychological trauma to the family and survivors.

THINKING ABOUT SAFETY

Societies around the world have developed many different ideas about injury causation and why injuries happen, often attributing them to fate, divine intervention, or hidden human motivation. These ideas are summarized in Table 6.1.

TABLE 6.1

THEORIES OF INCIDENT CAUSATION AND PRESENT STATUS

Theories	*Critique*
Single factor theories:	
1. The "accident-prone" worker	Discredited, except insofar as a mismatch may exist between worker and task
2. Psychodynamic origin of incidents in conflicted behavior	Discredited, except in trivial sense as individual carelessness or distraction may contribute
3. Social-environmental model: goals-freedom-alertness	Lacks credibility as complete explanation but is useful in multifactoral models' concept of worker autonomy and participation
4. Domino model: factors sequentially conditioning the unsafe act	Simplistic, omits data, lacks credibility except as framework for understanding worker's role in an incident investigation
Multiple factor theories:	
1. Epidemiologic model: host-environment-agent	Useful in analysis, basis for modern conceptualization
Systems approaches:	
1. Human engineering: perception-understanding-response	Incorporated in Haddon's matrix and the basis for contemporary theory
2. Expectancy-skill-decision: emphasis on information handling, reality checks, and information receiving capacity	Useful in understanding incidents during deviations from routine or during slow pacing of work

Ergonomics and modern safety science did not begin until the late 19th century, when human factors emerged from the studies of Frederick Taylor. In this theoretical framework, occupational injuries were seen as the result of excessive demands or burdens compared to the human capacity to do the job or as errors of perception or of reaction time. This led to the idea that they could be remedied by correct design in the workplace. The problem with the human factors approach is that it often became too narrowly technical, and sometimes it became a matter of reducing the job to a very limited number of tasks that were unsatisfying and alienating to the worker. Workers often felt that they were being harassed and that changes were being made only to increase production, not to protect them. Since that time, however, human factors has matured and split into modern safety science, which emphasizes the prevention of injury, and modern ergonomics, which emphasizes better workplace design and adaptation to the worker.

Around 1960, another school of thought emerged, this time from safety engineers. This was called the "3E's" formulation and it dominated safety science for the next 20 years. This formulation included three elements:

- engineering—to eliminate, guard, or provide personal protection against the hazard
- education—to provide insight, new behavioral patterns, and training
- enforcement—including monitoring, evaluation, and accountability

This was a great advance. It kept the principles of ergonomics and human factors but brought in human elements. It had a number of drawbacks, however. One was that there was no place in this formulation for critical incidents and near misses, which are by far the majority of the incidents. The "3E's" did not guide safety officers to prioritize among hazards, treating one set of hazards much the same as another. It was too dependent on changes in behavior, which are very hard to accomplish. BBS is a return to this school of thought.

Since the 1980s, the modern approach to safety science has borrowed heavily from epidemiology and public health to look at the problem of injury as a multifactorial risk. Safety professionals who look at multiple causes may then see multiple remedies. They try to find among several sometimes unrelated trends what the single common factor is that may be easy to remedy. This approach accepts risks as being inevitable but also manageable and accommodates the idea of loss, liability, costs, and other related issues that these other systems had isolated and had not considered together. This more sophisticated approach is embodied in the formulation called *Haddon's Matrix*, described below. This matrix provides a more complete framework for identifying the elements that come together in an incident resulting in injury.

Today, modern safety science recognizes that no one knowingly exposes oneself to an unacceptable risk but that adults must often take risks to achieve objectives. An adult, with powers of reasoning and control over impulsive behavior, is able to decide when a risk is worth taking. To a large extent, the capacity to do this reflects the difference between an adult and an immature person or a child. Incidents occur as the result of predisposing elements that are in place before the incident. They occur in specific situations that bring together the worker and the hazard in the workplace, often involving unusual events (such as a new process, a worker who is new on the job, pressure to finish a job hurriedly, or when the workplace is upset by some production problem). They occur under certain conditions (such as inadequate lighting, wet surfaces, noisy workplaces where workers cannot hear warnings), and they have certain effects. They are unexpected, but in retrospect it is usually easy to see how they happened.

PRINCIPLES OF INJURY PREVENTION

Injuries usually appear to have been easy to prevent, in hindsight. Before they happen, however, they are rarely anticipated or foreseen.

The essential elements of an incident resulting in occupational injury are:

- the person susceptible to the injury
- the hazard that is capable of inducing the injury
- an environment that brings them both together in the workplace

The conjunction of these elements, under the right conditions, creates the predisposing situation for the incident. A person may decide whether or not to take a risk on the spur of the moment, may not perceive the hazard, may make an appraisal of it that is faulty in some way, may be distracted, or may make a decision that in retrospect was not reasonable. There is a very critical period just before the incident where these things come together into a particular risk-facilitating situation. Most of those will be a near miss, an incident that does not occur. Eventually, with a certain probability, those factors will come together and the incident will occur. The consequences may include injuries, damage to property, financial loss, legal liability, future costs, and increased overhead costs. However, incidents can be prevented, and when they do occur, their effects can be minimized.

THE INJURY PYRAMID

The "injury pyramid" is a graphic representation of the relative frequency of fatal, serious, minor, and near-miss incidents resulting in only property damage (Figure 6.1). Pyramids for agricultural and childhood injuries look very different from those for occupational injuries.

Figure 6.1 presents a typical injury pyramid for occupational injuries. The exact proportions are not important; it is the shape of the injury pyramid that matters. The injury pyramid for occupational injury is very wide at the base and narrow at the top, suggesting that there are very many common, minor injuries and relatively fewer fatal or severely disabling injuries. For every one fatality, there are many seriously disabling injuries. For every seriously disabling injury, there are many, approximately 10 in these data, minor injuries resulting in some degree of inconvenience and minor impairment but without permanent impairment. For every one of these minor injuries, there are several injuries in which

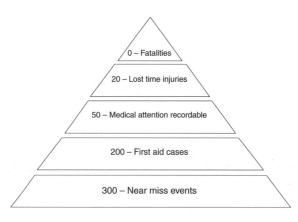

Figure 6.1 The injury pyramid for occupational injuries varies from industry to industry; this is one such pyramid reported for occupational injuries overall in a country.

there is only property damage in a workplace setting and more near misses for every incident involving property damage or worse consequences.

Considering only fatalities or serious injuries underestimates the importance and impact of injuries. However, the fatal and disabling injuries produce the greatest cost to society in terms of medical care expenses, rehabilitation, retraining costs, compensation benefits for lost wages, and psychological impact.

The injury pyramid shows that liability, legal liability for serious injury, costs in property damage, costs in compensation, costs in medical care, loss from property damage, and risk of each are all very much interrelated. By preventing injury, one may also prevent legal liability, reduce insurance premiums, reduce workers' compensation assessments, and minimize direct loss and property damage if the effort is coordinated as part of a comprehensive program.

The pyramid of occupational injury suggests two general ways to approach the prevention of injury.

One is to reduce the number of incidents so that the near misses do not happen, on the theory that the fewer near-miss incidents that occur, the fewer incidents with property damage and so forth. This can be done by engineering controls, traffic direction, training, and many other means. If one prevents incidents at the base of the pyramid, in other words, one may prevent a similar proportion of events all the way up and down the pyramid if the incidents are causally related. This approach makes use of information captured concerning near misses. This is extremely difficult because near misses are not usually reported in industry. A special effort must be made to encourage workers and supervisors to report them. If near misses are reported, they may alert supervisors to problems that can be corrected before a costly injury occurs.

Another approach is to prevent an incident in which only property damage occurs from escalating into an incident resulting in an injury by minimizing the impact of the incident. This can be done by building in safeguards, insisting on the use of personal preventive equipment, minimizing the damage resulting from an injury that occurs despite best efforts, providing the seriously injured with prompt attention, and minimizing the amount of hazardous energy that is available to cause the injury, as discussed below.

Haddon's Countermeasures and Matrix

Haddons 10 "countermeasures" for controlling energy release to prevent incidents from becoming injuries is a useful framework for thinking about the problem (Table 6.2). One may conceive of an incident as an unintended release of energy resulting in an injury. The ideal is to channel energy away from the individual and to minimize the amount of energy that can be released in an unintended way.

Haddon also developed a useful tool for analyzing incidents and situations called *Haddon's Matrix* (see Box 6.2). This tool analyzes the distribution and timing of release of the energy that caused, or could cause, the injury and the factors that aggravate or mitigate the damage once the incident occurs. The matrix divides the factors associated with an injury first by actor:

- person—the characteristics of the worker or victim who is injured
- hazard—the characteristics of the hazardous exposure, expressed in terms of potential and kinetic energy
- environment—the characteristics of the setting that brings the person together with the hazard

The matrix then considers each actor with respect to the timing of the incident:

- pre-incident—factors that were in place before the incident, factors that developed or played a role during the incident
- incident—factors operating during the incident
- post-incident—factors that followed the incident that made the consequences worse or better

TABLE 6.2

PRINCIPLES OF CONTROLLING HAZARDS INVOLVING ENERGY*

1. Prevent initial build-up or accumulation of the form of energy
2. Reduce amount of energy collected in one place
3. Prevent release of energy
4. Modify rate of spatial distribution of energy release from its source
5. Separate in time and space the energy released from the susceptible structure
6. Separate energy being released from the susceptible structure by interposition of a material barrier
7. Modify contact surface, subsurface, or basic structure that can be affected by the energy released and that in turn may convey energy to the person potentially exposed
8. Strengthen living or nonliving structure that might be damaged by the energy transfer
9. Move rapidly to detect and evaluate damage and to counter its continuation and extension
10. Prepare for all measures needed during the emergency period after the damaging energy exchange and before the final stabilization of the process

*Energy may be thermal, electrical, mechanical, electromagnetic, or any other type.

Pre-incident factors may be longstanding conditions or those that developed just before the incident occurred. In theory, these are the critical factors that could have been modified to prevent the injury or to mitigate its effect. In a multifactoral model of occupational injury prevention, these are the factors most under the control of an employer.

Pre-incident factors for the person might include, for example, level of training and experience, performance skill, understanding of the hazard, judgment, literacy, mental alertness, distraction or stress, and whether the worker was already impaired from a previous injury or illness. For motor vehicle incidents, the pre-incident personal factors might involve whether the worker was driving, how skillful a driver he (assuming the driver is a man) was, whether he had been drinking, how tired he was, whether he had been taking medicines that made him drowsy, and whether he was used to heavy traffic.

Pre-incident factors for a hazard might include whether there was adequate separation or a barrier between the hazard and the worker, disruptions due to maintenance or unusual conditions, whether safeguards were in place at dangerous locations, how easy a piece of machinery was to operate, how fast a vehicle was moving, the geometry of a workplace and the worker's location in it, the design of a piece of equipment (and whether the machine could, for example, catch or pinch a worker's hand), or temperature. For motor vehicle incidents, the pre-incident hazard factors might include the condition of the vehicle.

Pre-incident factors for the environment of the workplace might include other activities around the location that might have distracted the worker, the layout of the workplace, whether there was unrestricted access to the worker's location, the

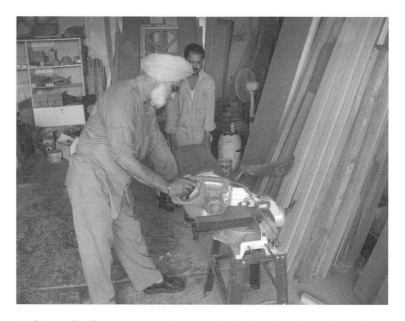

Figure 6.2 This worker has not properly secured the board he is sawing. (Photograph by Seifeddin Ballal, King Faisal University, Saudi Arabia.)

presence or absence of signs and visual clues that the worker could read and interpret, whether the workplace was in compliance with safety laws of the jurisdiction, and the safety policies of the employer. For motor vehicle incidents, the pre-incident environmental factors may include the condition of roads, whether signs were adequate and easy to read, the condition of road traffic, whether the speed limit was enforced, and how steep a hill or road embankment might have been.

Likewise, the factors during the incident can be characterized for each actor. However, the time frame is very different. Incidents resulting in injury generally take place quickly, and so there is much less time available to prevent injury and to mitigate its effects. Incident-related personal factors might include how susceptible a worker was to injury (e.g., if he or she was recovering from a previous injury), where he or she was located relative to the release of energy (e.g., where in the car during a crash), what the worker was wearing, and how quickly he or she was able to react. Incident-related hazard factors might include the amount of kinetic energy released (e.g., how fast the vehicle was going, how large the vehicle was) and whether the energy release was contained or absorbed (e.g., absorbed by the metal of the vehicle folding rather than collapsing or released if the gasoline tank exploded). Incident-related environmental factors might include the absence of an escape route (e.g., to get out of the way in order to avoid a collision), the presence of an object (e.g., if the vehicle hit a tree), the presence of other people nearby, and the presence or absence of barriers (e.g., traffic barriers) that could contain the energy. Anticipation of incident-related factors is difficult because all possible incidents can never be imagined. However, realistic scenarios

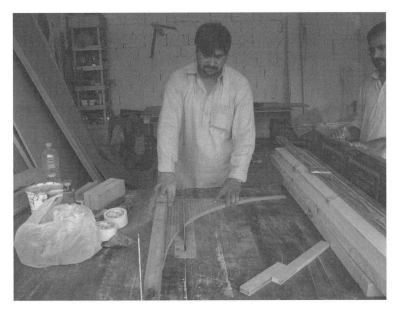

Figure 6.3 This worker is hand-feeding a piece of wood into a table saw with fingers, without a guard to protect his hand or eye protection. (Photograph by Seifeddin Ballal, King Faisal University, Saudi Arabia.)

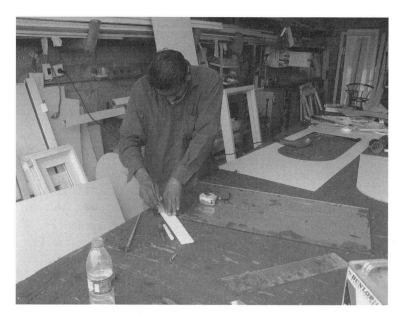

Figure 6.4 This worker is cutting glass with no protection for hands or eyes. (Photograph by Seifeddin Ballal, King Faisal University, Saudi Arabia.)

can be used to identify the most likely incidents that could happen, and there are engineering methods that can be used to predict the incidents most likely to cause damage and injury.

Post-incident factors are also more subject to planning and anticipation than incident-related factors. They are important in the response and mitigation of the results of the incident, which is called *consequence management.* Post-incident personal factors might include the extent of the worker's injury, how it is treated, how well the worker deals with it psychologically, how much rehabilitation treatment is required, and how prepared and motivated the worker is to retrain if he or she is partially disabled. Post-incident hazard factors might include secondary hazards that result from the incident (e.g., cuts from broken glass). Post-incident environmental factors might include the speed with which help arrives, the quality of emergency response and medical services, the availability of counseling and rehabilitation services, and whether other jobs are available for a worker who is disabled by the injury.

Box 6.1 gives an example of the application of Haddon's Matrix to an incident in the oil and gas industry.

Work Organization

Investigators at the Finnish Institute of Occupational Medicine identified a number of behavioral factors related to work organization that play a major role in predisposing toward a higher risk of accidents. The strength of these studies is that data were collected directly on injuries rather than depending on reports

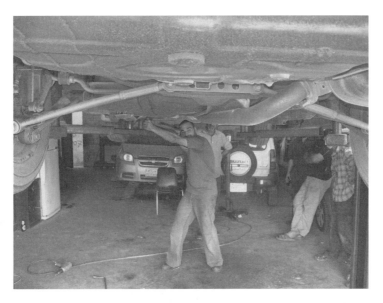

Figure 6.5 These workers are doing repairs under a car in a body shop under unsafe conditions: the frame holding up the car is not as secure as a hydraulic lift. (Photograph by Seifeddin Ballal, King Faisal University, Saudi Arabia.)

Box 6.1

Haddon's Matrix Applied to an Occupational Injury

A 33-year-old, healthy worker in an oilfield is assigned to repair a pipeline compressor that does not seem to be generating enough pressure. The pipeline runs from a sour gas collecting station (where natural gas containing sulfur is collected from several wells) to a desulfurization plant and treatment plant about 100 km away, where the dangerous sulfur-containing gas hydrogen sulfide is removed and the natural gas is then shipped by pipeline to world markets. The compressor is located in a small building with metal walls and a concrete floor in an isolated, rural area in very cold weather (−30°). The worker arrives after a long drive with a companion in a truck that carries tools and has "self-contained breathing apparatus" (SCBA) personal respiratory protection for both of them. He enters the shed wearing his hard-hat and is immediately overcome with the rotten-egg smell of hydrogen sulfide and within moments loses consciousness and falls to the ground. His companion, who was standing outside, realizes what has happened, runs back to the truck, puts on the SCBA equipment, and runs back to the shed, where he pulls his coworker out. The worker is still breathing and within a few minutes regains consciousness. They return to the truck, where it is warm, and call their company to alert them that there is a gas leak. The coworker takes the worker to hospital, where he is examined, found to be in good health, free of head injury (a concern because of the fall), and released. The affected worker does not remember smelling hydrogen sulfide before entering the shed or during the incident, but the coworker recalls smelling it during the rescue. At high concentrations, hydrogen sulfide paralyzes the sense of smell.

The compressor station is repaired the next day by a team of workers wearing SCBA and watching each other for signs of hydrogen sulfide toxicity. They observe that the alarm that was supposed to warn of increased hydrogen sulfide concentrations was malfunctioning.

This is a familiar event in many industries: a *confined space incident*. In this case, toxic hydrogen sulfide collected in the shed from a leak. The worker suffered what is commonly called a *knockdown*, which is loss of consciousness. Fortunately, this incident was not fatal, but it easily could have been. Confined space incidents are often tragic because the gas accumulates to dangerous levels, exposure is high, and rescue is often difficult because of tight spaces. Too often, coworkers will rush to save the affected worker before putting on personal protection themselves. All too often, the result is two or more casualties instead of a rescue. These workers were well trained, however. The second worker recognized the situation and took the necessary steps to protect himself both for personal safety and so that he could carry out the rescue successfully.

Haddon's Matrix for this incident is presented below.

TABLE 6.3

Timing/ Factor	Person	Hazard	Environment
Pre-incident	Worker: • was healthy • was well trained to recognize hazard (but did not in this case) • was wearing hardhat • apparently could not smell the odor of hydrogen sulfide initially (possibly because of cold effect on nose)	Pipeline or compressor leak: • releasing hydrogen sulfide • at high concentrations	Incident occurred: • in a confined space • remote location • accessible by truck • alarm failure • coworker was also well trained
Incident	Worker: • was overcome by hydrogen sulfide • sense of smell probably paralyzed on entering shed • was unconscious • fell down but protected by hardhat • was removed from exposure after a short time	Toxic gas exposure: • present throughout incident • exposure level sufficient to paralyze sense of smell • possibly exposure was reduced when door was open	Circumstances: • coworker was present • SCBA readily available on truck • Floor of shed was concrete • Truck was warm
Post-incident	Worker: • was revived in open air • was able to get into truck to avoid cold	Hazard: • dealt with the next day by crew which was better prepared	Circumstances: • Long distance to get help • Medical care too late to be helpful but not necessary in this case

Box 6.2

Occupational Injuries in an Economy Dependent on High-Risk Industries

Interpreting injury rates is not easy. Many trends that affect injury rates occur simultaneously during the same time period, and disentangling them can be difficult. The absolute number of injuries is of interest in terms of the overall problem of injury in the workplace, but the rate of injury is used to set priorities for industry-specific programs. The injury rate identifies industries at greatest risk given the size and activity of their workforce. Using rates, industries can be classified as high or low risk.

The general patterns of injury in the workplace are illustrated by the experience in Alberta, a province of Canada, from 1988 to 1993. Lost-time claims are insurance claims (under the workers' compensation system) for injuries that result in more than three days off work for the injured workers.

The economy of the province is dominated by industries that have parts, or subsectors, that present a high risk for injury, such as forest products, which require logging (tree-cutting); underground and surface mining (the latter primarily for the oil sands, a fossil fuel resource); and oil and gas (which consists of upstream, involving exploration and development of new production, and downstream, involving refining and distribution). The patterns observed in Alberta in any one year were typical of those encountered elsewhere (Table 6.4).

Breaking out injury rates by subsectors within a given industry presents a different picture. For example, meatpacking stands out as having much greater, essentially double, risk of injury compared to other manufacturing subsectors (Table 6.5). Oil and gas, which is the main economic driver of the province, concentrates its risk in exploration, drilling, and servicing oil wells and pumps in the field, which employ relatively few people; otherwise it is low in risk overall (Table 6.6). Construction, which was the second-most hazardous industry sector, demonstrates a very high risk in certain trades where there is a physical hazard, such as falling off a roof. It is clear that injury rates for hazardous areas of an industry tend to be buried or averaged out in the lower risk of the industry sector as a whole, so that aggregate data can be misleading.

During this period there were improvements in injury rates throughout North America, but the improvement in Alberta over the five years is remarkable. During this period there was much attention given to safety because Alberta was perceived as having excessively high injury rates. Several interventions occurred at once: the Workers' Compensation Board provided a financial incentive program for employers to reduce injury rates, several Alberta industry associations organized "safety associations" to disseminate information on safety, and highly visible demonstration projects in community injury prevention were launched in Edmonton, Red Deer, and Fort McMurray.

There are many theories as to why injury rates fell so rapidly during this period. They include the following:

- Industry-specific programs. Major employers, particularly large hospitals (which had experienced a high injury rate), instituted programs to reduce the injuries in their facilities.
- Industry safety associations. The safety associations were valuable in disseminating information within their sectors, especially in sectors such as construction

that are difficult for outsiders to influence. However, they sometimes took credit for unrealistically rapid improvement in injury rates in their sectors, without waiting to see if these improvements could be sustained.

- Financial incentives. The Workers' Compensation Board of Alberta created a rebate program for employers with favorable injury trends, but in the absence of an independent means of verifying the injury reports, this also created an incentive to underreport injuries.
- Cultural trend toward risk aversion. Injury rates fell for all residents and communities across the province during this period, not for occupational injuries alone. In the past, safety may not have been as much a societal value as it is today, and that risk-taking behavior may have been more widely tolerated as a cultural norm.
- Recessionary restructuring of employment. The province went through a recession in the early 1990s due to the reduced price of oil. Historically, injury rates tend to fall when jobs are scarce and employees are being laid off. They rise when jobs are plentiful but labor is scarce and inexperienced workers are hired.
- Incentives to underreport injuries. The extent to which at least part of the reduction is spurious cannot be known for certain. During this same period, the Government of Alberta strongly favored "individual responsibility" or partnership programs to encourage employers to comply with regulations voluntarily and to reduce both the number of inspections and sanctions for poor compliance. One piece of evidence suggesting that the private sector as a whole began to underreport injuries is that injury rates in public administration, where reporting was not influenced by these policy changes, did not change much during the period.

from the employer or statistical summaries, reducing the likelihood of bias, underreporting, or withholding information.

The investigators found that the factors that were most often associated with serious incidents were related to time pressure. Beating timetables and saving time on production were the most prominent factors. Another, more general factor was "incautiousness," meaning an unconscious disregard for consequences in an effort

TABLE 6.4

INJURY RATES BY INDUSTRY SECTOR IN ALBERTA (CANADA), 1988–1993, LOST-TIME CLAIM RATE (PER 100 PERSON-YEARS)

	1988	1993	% Change
Forestry	14.9	6.7	−55
Construction	10.9	6.0	−45
Manufacturing	9.6	5.7	−59
Transportation/Utilities	6.0	4.4	−27
Trade	4.4	3.7	−16
Public Administration	3.8	3.7	−3
Oil, Gas, Mines	3.5	1.9	−46
Service	3.4	2.8	−17

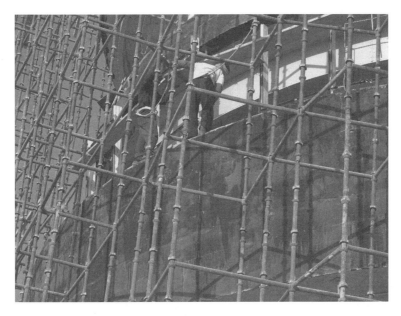

Figure 6.6 This worker is working on open scaffolding without a hardhat but is using basic fall protection (see the rope leading under his T-shirt). (Photograph by Seifeddin Ballal, King Faisal University, Saudi Arabia.)

to get the work done expediently. Other factors played a role: wage system (piecework favored risk-taking and a higher injury rate compared to hourly wage), "professional pride" (possibly including "showing off" behavior), influence of coworkers, influence of foremen, and responding to demands by customers.

As expected, the highest rates of serious injury were observed in the construction industry, in which rates were about five times the sector's representation in the total workforce. Manufacturing and transportation were also relatively elevated, approximately double their proportion of the workforce.

There is an inverse correlation between the size of the company and the risk of serious accidents, even for the smallest enterprises (< 10 workers) in industrial settings. Even in sectors as different as manufacturing, construction, and transportation, lacerations and other injuries related to moving machinery are overrepresented in small and large enterprises.

Employees of subcontractors are at special risk. On an industrial scale, these are employees of companies hired to perform tasks on contract, such as maintaining factories, constructing new facilities, and performing special duties, such as removing waste. On a smaller scale, these may be individuals or small enterprises that do a particular job or that fill in a temporary labor need for a period. A disproportionate number of incidents occur among employees of subcontractors in the construction industry compared with regular employees. The elevated risk of subcontractors exposes the worker to an unfamiliar worksite, which outweighs experience in the job as a predictor of individual risk. As well, there may be less satisfactory worker education, enforcement of occupational health and safety, and training in good work practices when an employer turns the job over to a subcontractor.

Group behavior cannot be changed effectively by addressing a collection of single persons acting in isolation, influenced by interventions designed to reach them as individuals. The message of safety must be reinforced by a supportive environment, the availability of safe tools and equipment, and allowance for individual adaptation and comfort. There must be a well-defined policy that the employer not only enforces in the workplace but visibly follows throughout the organization, including the executive offices. Effective safety programs take into account the interaction between people and the social environment, including how work is organized.

Worker Education and Attitudes Workers sometimes treat serious or unusual hazards in their work with an attitude that seems casual or even foolhardy. There are several likely reasons for this. Workers may not have been adequately educated or may not understand the hazard. When one is working with a particularly frightening or unknown hazard, some degree of denial is inevitable. One cannot work effectively (or even safely) when one is distracted or preoccupied by fear of a hazard. An overreaction is to deny so strongly that one's attitude becomes overly casual. This tendency is often reinforced, particularly in groups of young men, by peer pressure to demonstrate "macho" (aggressively masculine) or fearless behavior. Today, younger workers are often better educated and more risk-conscious than older workers.

When workers understand the reason for safety procedures, they are more likely to cooperate, and safety procedures will be more effective. These programs must be sustained and constantly reinforced. Even well-designed training programs will have only transient effects on worker behavior unless there is a process that reinforces the adoption of new values.

Programming Safety

Injury prevention is primarily risk management. If one manages injuries, one also potentially manages risk, loss, and costs. There are several levels of injury prevention management. Safety engineering uses a set of tools that follows certain general principles of controlling hazards. Safety should be managed like any other company function, and education in injury frequency and sources in loss prevention should be treated as business outcomes to be planned, evaluated, and managed. Accountability should be instilled throughout the management structure, with each manager accountable to his or her supervisor and safety performance evaluation that is taken into account in personnel ratings. Safety is a function of loss prevention and is managed similarly: locate and define the operational errors that would permit an incident to occur and correct them.

A good safety program should be reasonable in cost. If it is not, management will not be able to sustain it from year to year. Something that is expensive and out of line with the budget or that the employer cannot afford for one year is not going to work. An injury control program has to be reasonable in cost to work effectively.

Available tools to solve a safety problem may be drawn from safety engineering, state-of-the-art ergonomics, behavioral engineering, training, and plant design.

Whatever tools are used, there must be a framework to use them effectively if injuries are to be prevented. An effective safety program must supply strategies and tactics that put those tools where they are needed and ensure maximum benefit. This means injury and incident investigation, a monitoring system, risk analysis techniques, worker participation, goal setting, defining objectives in injury reduction, incentives, and recognition for safe workers.

Safety approaches and tools should be integrated into a program so that tools, strategies and tactics are part of a coherent system or program that can be used to ensure an ongoing practical sustainable program for injury reduction. These programs should be based on a reasonable injury causation model and should be appropriate to the population of workers in the workplace. If workers have trouble speaking and reading English, the manager should have a better way to reach them than printed materials. Safety measures should be integrated into a comprehensive package so that they are mutually reinforcing, backed by company policy, specific to the hazards in that workplace, clear and explicit, and aimed toward realistic, obtainable objectives that everyone understands. Supervisors should be able to evaluate progress.

Certain situations present a high risk of injury, but they can be anticipated and controlled. They include:

- Unusual or non-routine work that results in a departure from normal, familiar procedures. Thus, it is advisable to supervise safety especially closely during maintenance and repair operations and during unusual conditions.
- Presence in the workplace of sources of energy of great intensity or magnitude that can result in uncontrolled release. It is therefore advisable to reduce energy consumption to the minimum required for the job and to avoid accumulating large quantities of reactive chemicals on site, if this can be avoided.
- Non-productive or unusually slow periods in which machinery is shut down or operations are paced unusually slowly. Slow conditions result in distraction and inattention.
- New hiring and a rapid increase in the workforce. The influx of new workers who are inexperienced is associated with increased injury rates, which is why injury rates tend to increase during an economic expansion.

TOOLS FOR SAFETY PROGRAMS

Safety professionals have many tools they can use in integrated safety programs. These include, but are not limited to:

- *Safety audits.* Safety audits are systematic inspections in which the workplace is carefully examined for hazards and policies and procedures are reviewed. They are very effective in identifying problems that can be corrected before there is an injury.
- *Materials handling.* One of the most common situations associated with injury is in handling materials, such as boxes or bulk materials. The risk can be reduced by moving materials on pallets or in containers and using lifting appliances (such as cranes or elevators) and appropriate rigging if ropes or cables are used.

- *Transport equipment.* The selection of appropriate equipment for moving materials, such as forklifts, and training in how to operate the equipment safely is also important for preventing injuries.
- *Illumination.* A well-lit workplace with a diffuse light source is generally safer than a dim workplace. Glare or excessive shadow tends to make the workplace less safe despite higher levels of illumination.
- *Safeguards.* Machinery with exposed cutting or rotating parts or *pinch points* (places where machine parts could snag and crush a hand or other body part) should have guards installed.
- *Lockout.* Machinery should be equipped with switches and guards that allow workers to cut off the power when serviced, with locks to ensure that the power is not inadvertently restarted.
- *Risk analysis procedures.* Engineers have developed many techniques for analyzing operations to determine where problems are likely to arise. Some of these methods are very sophisticated and require computer modeling, including fault tree analysis, hazard operability studies, and human error analysis.
- *Maintenance.* Many safety problems are the result of improper or inadequate maintenance. Broken machinery is often dangerous, and inadequate housekeeping often leads to a fire hazard.
- *New plant design.* New plants are more easily designed for safety than older plants. It is much easier to ensure safety in the design of a new plant than it is to modify, or *retrofit,* an old plant to make it safe after it is built. In general, a well-designed plant is a safer plant.
- *Safety policies.* A critical aspect of instituting successful injury prevention, loss control, and risk modification programs appears to be the communication of a consistent, clear, and enforceable message within the organization that safe work practices are the norm and unsafe practices will not be tolerated. Thus, incidents can be regarded as symptoms of something wrong with management that led to the tolerance or creation of the contributing factors that resulted in the incidents.
- *Educational programs.* Education and training programs must be reinforced with repeated training and workplace changes in order to be effective. Posting signs and making slogans are not effective alone. They are soon ignored by workers, who get used to them. The most effective training and educational programs are those that are focused on the particular job, are repeated (with variations) periodically, and involve the worker in solving the problem.
- *Awards programs.* Awards programs are controversial. Many authorities believe that they create an incentive to conceal injuries and unsafe conditions. They also place emphasis on the worker rather than on the responsibility of the employer to provide a safe working environment.
- *Joint labor-management health and safety committees.* These committees should have regular meetings to review problems and should have the authority to correct unsafe working conditions.
- *Provision of consultation services.* Whether within large organizations or in the community, assistance is needed for supervisors, managers, and workers in solving safety-related problems without penalizing them for asking for help.

- *Encouragement of shared services and resources.* This is particularly important for small businesses.
- *The "buddy system."* It is standard practice in hazardous situations, as in confined space operations, to have workers paired with coworkers who can call for help or render assistance if there is trouble.

Some common situations present special problems that all safety professionals must know. These include, but are by no means limited to, the following:

- *Fall prevention.* Workers who work on scaffolding or at height are at risk of falling. Guardrails, catwalks, and fall restraining devices (typically, a harness worn by the worker that is attached to a cable to prevent a serious fall) are effective in preventing fall-related injuries.
- *Trenching.* Digging trenches, or pits, is a particularly dangerous part of construction, especially in sandy or wet soil. The sides of the trench can collapse, burying the worker. The sides of deep trenches should be reinforced, or shored up, by a wooden frame to ensure that the trench does not collapse.
- *Road safety.* Motor vehicle incidents are a leading cause of occupational injury.
- *Confined spaces.* Closed or restricted spaces, such as inside tanks or other small, enclosed utility closets or sealed rooms, are dangerous for many reasons. Toxic gases may accumulate if there is a source. They are difficult to ventilate. Oxygen levels can drop below that required to sustain life. Rescue may be difficult in tight spaces. Entry into confined spaces must be controlled and the atmosphere checked for safety before entry (see Box 6.1).

INJURY STATISTICS

Adequate data collection and analysis is essential to effective injury prevention. The most important sources of data on occupational injury on a national level are usually:

- fatalities and fatality investigation reports
- workers' compensation data
- inspection records for occupational health agencies
- trauma and other medical care registries

At the level of an individual workplace, the sources of data usually available include the following:

- first aid or medical treatment logs
- reports of injury to insurance
- claims for disability
- safety inspections

Injury Prevention in Namibia

Many observers believe that small and medium-sized enterprises do not devote enough time and effort to the elimination of hazards associated with the major industrial operations. This appears to be as true in Namibia as elsewhere. The problem of preventing injuries is further compounded by the fact that data regarding the type and causes of these accidents are incomplete. The absence of reliable statistics is a substantial obstacle to government and private-sector experts who are trying to develop preventive strategies.

It is known that a high percentage of these accidents arise from workers falling to a lower level. As a result, there is a clear need for adequate training and education on the dangers associated with their work environment, promotion of personal safety devices, identification of hazards (prospective and retrospective), and evaluation of results.

The government can play a crucial role in ensuring that relevant measures are taken to promote health and prevent diseases caused by workplace hazards as well as improve the overall health and well-being of Namibian workers. This would also mean development of codes and regulations locally as well as with international experts, and initiating joint programs with other communities aimed at solving common problems.

Amwedo, A. 2000. "Accident Prevention in Namibia." *African Newsletter on Occupational Health and Safety* 10(2):4–8.

Fatalities are usually reported reliably. They are often mentioned in news reports, are alarming to other workers and to the community, are often investigated (this is required by law in many places), and are difficult to conceal. Serious injuries, especially if they are permanently disabling, are reported fairly reliably where there are insurance schemes that require such information. In many countries, the division between serious and minor injuries is determined for statistical purposes by whether the worker has lost time from work. The severity of lost-time injuries can be measured either by the length of time off work, when the worker returns to work (see Chapter 17—"Fitness to Work"), or by the resulting disability if the injury results in permanent impairment. Minor injuries are not reliably reported, and many minor injuries are either not brought to the attention of the employer or, in some cases, intentionally left out of injury reports.

There are many problems with the accuracy of injury data and the limitations of reporting. Employers who want to conceal the number of injuries their workers have experienced sometimes underreport minor injuries and may keep workers on the job, doing something else, even though they are injured. Some employers, in violation of ILO covenants and national legislation, terminate workers who have injuries. Incidents resulting only in property damage frequently go unreported unless there is an insurance claim, and near misses are rarely reported at all. In fact, there are usually disincentives that discourage employees from mentioning near misses at all because they are often afraid of reprimands or being fired, especially if a mistake was involved.

In understanding injuries and the pattern of injuries, it is important to understand the calculations used in analysis. It is difficult at first glance to interpret injury rates. There are two key rates (injuries per year or other unit of time). The first is the number of injuries that occur in a given industrial sector, usually recorded as lost time claims. These are claims for lost time injury reported to the competent authority, such as the occupational health and safety regulatory agency or the workers' compensation board. The number of cases indicates the contribution to the overall problem. These figures miss the many minor injuries that do not result in loss of time, however, and are not accurate in reflecting incidence for diseases or for injuries with a chronic or cumulative component. They are reasonably accurate for most injuries, however, and provide a basis for year-to-year comparisons. The absolute number of injuries is of some interest in terms of the contribution of a particular industry to the overall problem, but the rates (the number per employees per year) are most useful in setting priorities because they identify industries or occupations at highest risk. The second key rate is the rate of injuries reported per 100 person-years of employment, which adjusts for the workforce in that sector. The rate allows comparisons between industry sectors and of safety performance among companies in a sector (Tables 6.5 and 6.6).

Using rates, one can classify various industries into high and low risk compared to the average rate of injuries for all industries or for all enterprises in terms of claim rates. High-risk industries would be those whose experiences fall above the average, low risk would fall below the average. Over time there has usually been a fair degree of stability in the lost time claim experience for the various major industrial sectors. Forestry usually leads in injury rates; construction, manufacturing, transport, and utilities also rank among the highest risk.

There is much more to the picture than the overall experience of industries as a whole. These rates are aggregate numbers. They are the sum of the experience of a number of smaller trades, industries, and industrial operations within each

TABLE 6.5

INJURY RATES FOR THE MANUFACTURING SECTOR IN ALBERTA (CANADA), 1988–1993, LOST-TIME CLAIM RATE (PER 100 PERSON-YEARS)

	1988	1993	% Change
Meat/Poultry Packing	28.2	10.7	−62
Metal Products	15.8	8.9	−44
Wood and Building Products	11.6	6.8	−41
Food and Beverage	10.2	8.5	−17
Non-metallic Mineral	5.0	5.3	+ 6*
Printing/Publishing	2.9	2.5	−13
Petrochemicals	2.2	1.8	−18

*1992 rate: 4.2

TABLE 6.6

INJURY RATES FOR THE INDUSTRIAL SECTOR OF OIL, GAS, AND MINES IN ALBERTA (CANADA), 1988–1993, LOST-TIME CLAIM RATE (PER 100 PERSON-YEARS)

	1988	1993	% change
Oil, Gas Exploration	18.8	9.8	–48
Drilling	12.5	5.2	–58
Servicing	12.1	4.1	–66
Other Oilfield	5.9	3.7	–37
Coal, Mining	2.7	2.1	–22
Oil Sands	1.4	1.2	–14
Gas Plant, Oil Wells	0.5	0.4	–20

large industrial sector. Breaking these results down by components of the industry can yield very interesting insights.

Comparisons are frequently made between large industry and small industry. The conventional wisdom in occupational health and safety circles is that small enterprises usually have higher injury rates than larger enterprises because they lack the resources to control and monitor hazards. It is generally true that smaller employers have higher-risk injuries than larger employers. However, smaller industries are the norm in many high-risk industries: servicing oil wells, cutting timber, and performing small-scale construction. Injury rates, therefore, reflect the pattern of employer size in high-risk industries as much as the relative merits of health and safety control in small versus large industries. (Box 6.2 provides examples of occupational injury statistics.)

Construction

One clearly high-risk industry is construction. It is easy to see why construction would be a high-risk industry. It involves many trades and operations that have inherently high risk. The risk profiles of the various trades within the construction industry are fairly consistently elevated (Table 6.7). This represents an industry in which the injury rates are a general problem.

Employment in the industry varies with the economic cycle, and in recent years employment has been high in the sector. Injury rates are particularly high among minority workers in the construction sector and where language is a barrier. For example, occupational injuries in the United States are particularly elevated among Hispanic construction workers and in the less skilled trades that attract recent immigrants. The nature of fatal injuries (e.g., falls) and their concentration in population groups with low skill levels and language barriers suggests that they are relatively easily preventable. Hispanic construction workers treated at an emergency room in Washington, DC, were at greater risk for injury and for greater severity of injury, probably because employment in this group is concentrated in less-skilled trades. The impact of the injury, in terms of lost employment, wages, and disability, was also disproportionately greater, probably

TABLE 6.7

INJURY RATES FOR THE CONSTRUCTION TRADES IN ALBERTA (CANADA), 1988–1993, LOST-TIME CLAIM RATE (PER 100 PERSON-YEARS)

	1988	1993	% Change
Roofing	20.9	12.4	–41
Sheet Metal	20.1	–	–
Drywall	19.3	9.7	–50
Concrete	14.5	9.4	–35
Plumbing	9.7	7.2	–26
Painting	8.1	6.2	–23
Electrical	7.6	4.4	–42

reflecting greater injury severity and limited prospects for employment in skilled trades. Injuries in the construction industry trades vary greatly from year to year within particular trades, as would be expected due to chance variation in small numbers.

Studies in depth on one large construction site in downtown Washington, DC, confirmed that Hispanic workers had a higher rate of injuries of sufficient severity to require ambulance and trauma care services. Because the data specific to trades were gathered over only six months, trends over time are not known. The occupations and trades at highest risk were laborers, carpenters, and electricians. Most of the injuries involved a sharp object (26%, usually a piece of metal, a cutting tool, a power tool, or a nail or screw), striking an object (20%, many), or falls (17%, mostly from ladders or scaffolding or slips, trips/stumbles). Falls contributed half of all admissions to hospitals and indicated much greater severity for the typical case. In keeping with these patterns, most were lacerations (37%, presumably including penetrating injuries), sprains/strains/acute pain (22%), contusions or abrasions (15%), and eye injuries (11%). Trades at greatest risk for the most serious common type of injury (falls from height) were painters, glaziers (who install windows), drywall workers, and insulators.

The problem is really one of technology transfer and commitment rather than innovation. Like all sectors in mature industries, the construction sector is characterized by relatively few thought leaders who innovate and monitor trends and a larger group of technical experts who receive and disseminate innovation and new ideas. In other sectors, this dissemination group consists of consultants, designers, and engineers, but for most construction work this level of technical sophistication is not necessary and is not supported because it is costly. Building methods certainly do change but not as rapidly as methods in other sectors and not without extensive trial and demonstration to ensure that buildings using new technology will remain as acceptable to the owner as buildings using conventional methods. In the construction sector, therefore, this dissemination group is very small, relatively conservative, and fragmented. One conspicuous leader in dissemination in the United States is the Center for the Protection of Workers' Rights, a worker-oriented organization dedicated to occupational health and safety training and research. Thus the organization of the sector is not conducive to rapid dissemination of occupational health and safety innovation and ideas. Individual contractors are very much focused on their current work, and the market does not readily accept early adoption. On the labor side, small scale and fragmentation is reflected in the trades and the personal autonomy of craftspeople, who usually see occupational safety as a personal rather than collective responsibility and commitment.

Laborers are another story. The hazards they face are largely unchanged over the years because they reflect traditional methods of material handling and assembly. Laborers are especially transient in this most transient of workplaces and have little in the way of assets or training to protect themselves.

7

ERGONOMICS

Veikko Louhevaara and Nina Nevala

Ergonomics, as applied to occupational health, is a scientific and practical discipline examining and changing interactions between humans and physical elements of a workplace and work system (Figure 7.1). The ultimate mission of ergonomics is to promote the health, safety, and well-being of individuals, both during work and leisure time, and to increase productivity. Individuals use various tools in their work, and the objective of ergonomics is to achieve the best possible match between the tool and its users. Additionally, work activities often require handling materials and products. Thus, another objective of ergonomics is to achieve the greatest efficiencies and safety in materials handling. As life becomes more competitive due to globalization and free market forces, it is more important than ever for business, in particular, to minimize errors and to maximize success with respect to human abilities, needs, and limitations related to the use of new technology.

Ergonomics is a scientific and practical discipline, examining and developing interactions between humans and other mechanical elements of a system. An ergonomist (a practitioner of ergonomics) must have a core competence in the full scope of the discipline, including physical, psychosocial, cognitive, organizational, and environmental factors.

Ergonomics has many benefits. A properly designed workplace may achieve the following very practical goals:

- greater efficiency
- more productivity
- fewer acute injuries
- fewer musculoskeletal problems among workers
- less fatigue among workers
- less spoilage of work and higher-quality products or levels of service
- more satisfied workers

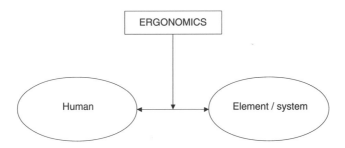

Figure 7.1 Ergonomics seeks to match human capabilities with the requirements of the work element (such as a tool, workstation, furniture) or production system at work.

ERGONOMICS AS A SCIENCE

At institutions such as the Finnish Institute of Occupational Health and the University of Eastern Finland, ergonomics is defined as a multidisciplinary field of science, based on physiology, psychology, sociology, and technical science applications. The field studies human capacities, needs, and limitations in the interaction of technical and organizational work systems. Ergonomics aims to integrate elements of work and the environment by using job design and redesign measures.

The earliest steps toward a science of ergonomics were taken in the Stone Age (Drills 1963) as stone tools were progressively shaped over centuries to be easier to use and to fit the hand better. Ergonomics was recognized in ancient Greece.

While the concept of ergonomics has changed, due to continuous and accelerating changes in society and working life, the mission and basic principles of modern ergonomics are still consistent with those first formulated by Wojciech Jastrzebowski, who founded the modern science of ergonomics in 1857, who said: "By [the] term Ergonomics we mean the Science of Work. Useful work is divided into physical, aesthetic, rational and moral work. Examples of these kinds of work are as follows: the breaking of stones, the playing with stones, the investigation of natural properties or the removal of stones from the roads so that they not give rise to untidiness or suffering for people."

Ergonomics was advanced in America by Frederick W. Taylor, who conducted "time and motion" studies to increase work efficiency and to increase the productivity—and earnings—of laborers. Ergonomics became widely recognized as a science during and after World War II, when military applications required research to produce more efficient and reliable equipment.

According to the definition used by the International Ergonomics Association (IEA), modern ergonomics is the scientific discipline concerned with understanding the interaction between humans and other elements of a system (Figure 7.1) and the profession that applies theoretical principles, data, and methods of design to optimize human well-being and overall system performance (Figure 7.2).

The fundamental principles of ergonomics can be found in several sciences, such as biology (anatomy, *biomechanics*, and physiology), psychology, sociology, and technology (Figure 7.3). Practical ergonomics requires a background in

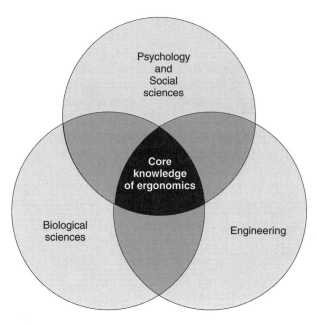

Figure 7.2 The core knowledge of ergonomics comes from psychology and the social sciences, the biological sciences, and engineering.

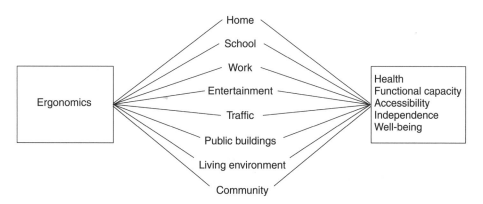

Figure 7.3 The principles of ergonomics can be applied in any setting to achieve a healthier, more efficient way of living and to ensure that people with impairments have opportunity, access, and independence.

biomechanics, the science of how the body moves from a mechanical point of view, and *anthropometry*, the method of measurement of various parts of the body.

Applied ergonomics takes into consideration the following aspects of work:

- Physical (power). Ergonomics is concerned with human anatomical, anthropometrical, physiological, and biomechanical characteristics as they relate to physical activity or work.

- Cognitive function (information handling in the brain). Ergonomics is concerned with mental processes, such as perception, memory, reasoning, and motor response, as they affect interactions among humans and elements of work-related or other systems.
- Work organization. Ergonomics is concerned with the optimization of socio-technical, work-related, or other systems, including their organizational structures, policies, and processes (IEA 2000).
- Economic and social context. Ergonomics is concerned with how business cycles and relationships between employers and workers affect the work.

APPROACHING THE PROBLEM CORRECTLY

In ergonomics, the usual problem to be solved involves a single workplace, task, or piece of equipment, and the most common object is micro-level human-machine integration. The worker has to operate the equipment, monitor its operation, interpret readings or signals, adjust it, and sit, stand, or assume whatever other position is required to do so. In designing the *human-machine interface*, where the worker and the equipment meet, the main purpose is to develop a technical system that suits human capabilities and needs. When the machine is not flexible or designed for the human, the worker may have to adjust himself or herself to the machine's dimensions and technical features: the machine may be running the worker rather than the worker running the machine.

Common approaches to solving the single workplace task include changes to make the machine or workplace more easily adjustable; to design it to fit the reach, height, or other relevant dimension of the worker; to make meters and gauges easier to read; to reduce the force required to move a lever or operate a tool; to make the fit of a tool in the hand more comfortable; to lower how high the worker must lift materials; and to reduce the number of steps or movements the worker must make to complete the work. Every problem must be examined individually, but there are general principles that guide the solution of these problems.

However, many problems in ergonomics go beyond single workplace tasks. They may involve how a series of tasks are organized, the design of the entire workplace, how work moves through a factory, and how monitoring systems keep track of worker productivity. Some of the most challenging problems in ergonomics have to do with how work is organized and how workers fit into the big picture.

The main goal of ergonomics is to develop a comprehensive, workplace-wide (or "macro-level") system that promotes the health and well-being of individuals and allows them to work efficiently and safely. When the field of ergonomics is merely considered as a micro-level discipline, and the context is missing or limited, there is no comprehensive understanding of the system. The ergonomist, who is described below, may fix the individual problem related to the task, but overall productivity may still fall short because the overall situation has not been corrected.

Developing an ergonomic solution for a single workplace is not worthwhile when there is no overall logistic system for work processes. Therefore, ergonomics needs theoretical macro-level frameworks and paradigms for outlining and analyzing complex systems such as organizations, work processes, and environments (Figure 7.4).

In macro-level ergonomics, broader societal or even global factors must be considered because they directly or indirectly affect comprehensive human-system integration. For instance, with ergonomics measures, it is possible to promote health of employees and maintain their productivity. Ergonomics, however, cannot be of much help if business is suffering, and the number of personnel is being reduced due to an economic crisis. Ergonomics should be considered as a philosophy and meta-method for understanding complex interactions between human and various physical systems.

The practitioners of ergonomics are called *ergonomists*. The training of ergonomists varies; some are trained on the job and others have doctoral degrees from universities. Either as members of a team or individually, they contribute to the planning, design, and evaluation of tasks, jobs, products, organizations, environments, and systems in order to make them compatible with people's needs, abilities, and limitations. Practical ergonomists must have a competence over the full scope of the discipline, taking into account physical, cognitive, social, organizational, and environmental and other relevant factors. A sufficient background is required in these core competencies to practice as an ergonomist:

- behavioral sciences
- physical and biological sciences
- engineering
- ability to evaluate the adequacy of applied ergonomics research and generalize the conclusions to operational settings

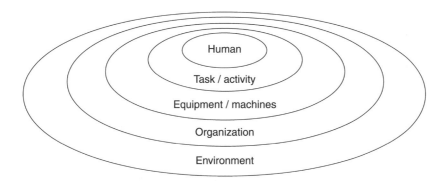

Figure 7.4 Ergonomics works on the scale of tools, machines, workplaces, and the built environment but is always centered on human capabilities.

- ability to carry out and evaluate various kinds of traditional ergonomics analyses
- ability to perform and evaluate classic human-machine integration
- ability to apply knowledge of human performance capabilities and limitations under varying environmental conditions
- sufficient knowledge of computer modeling, simulation, and design methodology to appreciate their utility in systems development
- ability to apply knowledge of education and training methodology to the evaluation of training programs
- ability to assist in the development and evaluation of job aids and related hardware that allow persons with disabilities to do the job
- ability to apply the organizational behavior and motivational principles of work group dynamics, job enrichment, and redesign
- specialized expertise in at least one area of human-system integration technology

The competency demands of an ergonomist are continuously changing due to the rapid development of society and working life. For instance, new information technology requires special knowledge in cognitive ergonomics in order to avoid

---

BOX 7.1

Ergonomics in a Research Laboratory

Biotechnology is a rapidly growing industry that requires laboratory technicians to use pipettes. Ergonomists describe the pipette as a thumb-actuated, in-line hand tool. Laboratory workers often suffer from upper limb disorders, and using a pipette for more than 300 hours a year is associated with an increased risk of hand and shoulder disorders. The aim of this study was to test the ergonomics and usability of two mechanical and one electronic pipette by analyzing upper limb musculoskeletal strain and assessing the features of usability.

The subjects were 11 healthy female laboratory employees (ages 30–49 years) from eight laboratories. The subjects were right-handed, and they were accustomed to using the three models of the pipettes at their normal work.

This was a comparative cross-sectional study. The measurements of each subject were carried out during one day in a simulated work situation in the ergonomics laboratory. The measurements of three one-channel pipettes were done during a seven-minute pipetting task: tip taking, liquid dosage from a test tube into an Eppendorf tube, and finally tip ejection.

Ergonomics and usability were tested with the measurements of wrist angles, muscular activity, perceived musculoskeletal strain, and perceived usability features. Wrist extension/flexion and ulnar/radial deviation were measured using a two-channel electronic goniometer attached to the wrists of the subject with skin adhesive tape.

Output from the goniometers was sampled with a portable device, ME3000P, at a frequency of 200 Hz, averaged at a time constant of 0.1 seconds, and stored on a computer for analysis with ME3000P software.

The surface muscular activity (electromyography = EMG) was recorded from four muscles of the right body side (m. trapezius pars descendes, m. flexor digitorum sublimis, m. flexor pollicis longus, and m. flexor pollicis brevis) with a portable ME3000P device. The EMG was recorded using the averaged mode, a time interval of 0.1 seconds, and a bipolar setting of disposable surface electrodes. The maximal muscle activity was registered bilaterally during a maximal voluntary contraction (MVC), and the mean muscular activity at work was standardized as the percentage of the MVC (% MVC).

Visual analogue scales were used to analyze musculoskeletal strain and perceived features of the pipettes. The subjects rated their strain and perceived features on a modified visual analogue scale, the result of each scale being reported in millimeters (range: 0 to 100 mm with end points of 0 = no strain to 100 = very straining; 0 = very bad to 100 = very good). Variance analysis and t-tests were used to test differences between the pipettes.

Mean muscle activity (% MVC) of flexor digitorum sublimis and flexor pollicis longus muscles was lower when the subjects used the electronic pipette compared to the mechanical pipettes. Mean extension of the right wrist was 32° when the subjects used the mechanical pipettes and 37° when they used the electronic pipette (p < 0.01). Electronic pipettes caused less strain on the thumb area than manual pipettes. The location and height of the dispensing button were perceived to be better in the electronic pipette than in the manual pipettes.

The ergonomics and usability of the pipettes were tested in a situation that represented the most typical use of the pipettes. Physiological measurements have seldom been used when testing for the usability of products. However, new usability testing methods are needed to provide valid and reliable data on how well people use products and how they like using them. The validity of the electric goniometers and the visual analogue scale lines and the reproducibility of the EMG measurements were known to be good.

Musculoskeletal strain of the right shoulder and upper limbs were lower; perceived strain of the right thumb was lower; and the perceived features of usability were better when the subjects used the electronic pipette compared to the use of the manual pipettes. However, the extension of the wrist was larger when the electronic pipette was used. In conclusion, the use of both electronic and manual pipettes during everyday pipetting tasks will reduce upper limb strain, especially in the thumb area. The posture of the wrist should be taken into account when the design of the electronic pipette is developed.

(Adapted from Nevala-Puranen, N. and M. Lintula 2001. "Ergonomics and usability of Finnpipettes." Proceedings of NES 2001. *Promotion of Health through Ergonomic Working and Living Conditions. Outcomes and methods of research and practice. Publication 7.* University of Tampere, School of Public Health, Tampere, Finland.)

sensorial strain, a term used for stressful sensory and cognitive overload, in excess of the mind's ability to process the information.

PARTICIPATORY ERGONOMICS

To prevent work-related diseases and work disability, progressive ergonomists combine ergonomics with organizationally and individually oriented measures for the promotion of health, work ability, competence, and well-being directed at improving the productivity and quality of work (Figure 7.5). This necessarily involves the participation of workers themselves in the design of their workplace, and this is called *participatory ergonomics*.

In working life, worker participation and commitment are needed to develop and implement ergonomic measures, thus this participation and commitment can be considered a true value of ergonomics. Participatory ergonomics is evaluated and developed within the workplace in collaboration with employees, supervisors, and occupational health and safety practitioners. This type of participatory approach requires a comprehensive theoretical understanding of the job in question. It is important to develop (i.e., design or redesign) the whole work process, instead of making some small, partial improvements. The design process can be

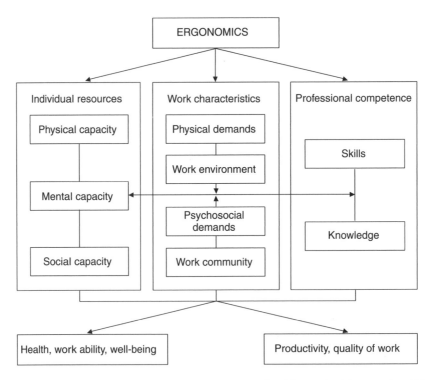

Figure 7.5 Ergonomics is a key measure for promoting health, work ability, and well-being in the working life.

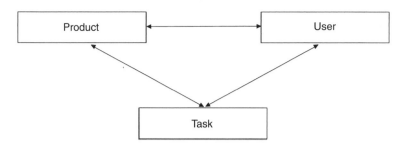

Figure 7.6 Ergonomics brings together the product, the user, and the task in the design of an efficient and easy-to-use system.

described as a systematic learning process carried out in teams. The teams must consider the job's background and the current problems involved in the work tasks and generate practical measures for systematically improving the ergonomics of the tasks and work environment. Thus, ergonomics should decrease the technical or organizational obstacles necessary to carry out productive and qualified work (Louhevaara 1999).

The drawback of participatory ergonomics is that it can be demanding and slow because it requires consultation, discussion, and a group process. However, participatory ergonomics ultimately strengthens the motivation and commitment of employees to institute and to accept ergonomic measures and improvements. Participatory ergonomics interventions are effective and practical methods to reduce workload and strain at worksites.

ERGONOMICS AND USABILITY

The objective of ergonomics is to achieve the best possible match between the product and its users in the context of the task to be performed (Figure 7.6). The following criteria for successful matches have been proposed: functional efficiency, ease of use, comfort of use, health and safety, and quality of working life. Usability is defined as the extent to which a product can be used by specified users to achieve specified goals with effectiveness, efficiency, and satisfaction in a specified context, for example, in terms of the International Standards Organization (standard number SFS-EN ISO 9241-11). Good usability is most often based on user-centered design of the product. User-centered design should be based upon the physical and mental characteristics of the human users. User-centered design means not only designing *for* users, but also designing *with* users. The terms "design for all" and "universal design" are used to describe design approaches aimed at designing products and services that meet the needs and circumstances of the widest possible range of users, including disabled and aging people.

Usability testing refers to any technique through which users interact systematically with a product or system under controlled conditions in order to perform

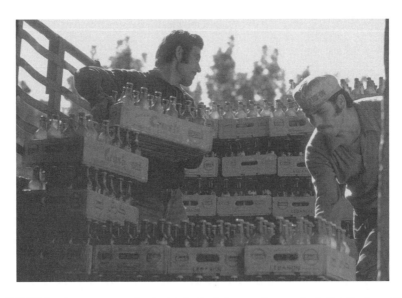

Figure 7.7 Lifting heavy cases of soft drinks in Lebanon for product distribution. Note the strain on the worker's lower back (right) and the awkward movement required to raise the cases above chest height (left) (Photograph by Nick Wheeler, courtesy of Saudi Aramco World/SAWDIA.).

BOX 7.2

Participatory Ergonomics

The participatory approach was applied in carrying out ergonomic interventions at work sites. The jobs consisted of professional cleaning, home care work, vehicle inspection, and metal work. All jobs encompassed physically demanding tasks. Professional cleaning and home care work were typical service jobs held by female workers with low occupational status. Vehicle inspection was also a service occupation, but technically oriented. The inspectors were men with a medium level of technical education. The auxiliary jobs of metal employees comprised simple manual materials-handling tasks in an industrial environment. The purpose of the participatory ergonomic interventions was to reduce acute load and strain at work. Technical and organizational redesign measures were used that optimized the load and strain on the musculoskeletal and cardio respiratory system, taking into account each employee's individual characteristics.

The employees were both men and women aged 19 to 62 years. The interventions lasted for 11–12 months for the cleaners and home care assistants and 3–4 months for the metal workers and vehicle inspectors. In each intervention, ergonomic measures were linked with other organizational or individual actions related to the promotion of health, work ability, and well-being. The redesigns of the ergonomic processes were completed by applying teamwork supplemented with practical training of new work techniques. This was done in collaboration with all relevant personnel groups.

The results of this intervention were evaluated by taking similar ergonomic measurements on the new work processes and by a survey of workers and management. Follow-up studies found the following:

- Harmful static postural load on the musculoskeletal system reduced
- Cardiac strain decreased measured by working heart rate
- Necessary occupational knowledge and skills increased
- Better possibilities for regulating work rate
- Rushing work activities decreased
- Satisfaction, appreciation, and interest toward work increased

The results and experiences suggest that the key prerequisites for feasible and successful ergonomics interventions included the following:

- Unreserved support of top management
- Close collaboration with occupational health and safety practitioners
- Interventions were carried out in normal work units, using teamwork and practical training systems
- Process and redesign measures considered the actual needs of the employees
- Quick feedback from the worksite assessments enhanced the motivation and commitment of the employees

The investigators concluded that participatory ergonomics is an efficient and feasible method for reducing work load and increasing well-being at work. In addition, it often produces innovative and consistent improvements at workplaces.

a goal-oriented task in an applied scenario. According to the standard (SFS-EN ISO 9241-11), product developers can develop appropriate measures of efficiency, effectiveness, and/or satisfaction. Both objective and subjective data collection methods have been used in assessments of usability. Usability can be evaluated by means of any technique through which users interact systematically with a product or system and perform a goal-oriented task under controlled conditions.

8

PHYSICAL HAZARDS

Tee L. Guidotti

Physical hazards have in common the release of energy in various forms. This release may be sudden and uncontrolled, as in an explosion or mechanical safety hazard, or sustained and more or less under control, as in conditions of work that expose the worker to excessive noise or heat. A sudden, uncontrolled release of energy usually involves the physician only insofar as the treatment of trauma is required. Prevention of injuries due to the sudden release of energy is discussed in general terms in Chapter 6 and the injuries themselves in Chapter 14. This chapter will address the health implications of pure energy sources and of physical conditions of work, with an emphasis on exposure over the long term to physical hazards.

IONIZING RADIATION

This section addresses occupational health concerns specifically associated with *ionizing radiation*. Ionizing radiation is radiation carrying sufficient energy to dislodge electrons on impact from their otherwise stable orbital cloud in an atom. This results in the production of charged ions or free radicals inside the cell. These altered atoms and molecules are highly reactive and therefore potentially toxic to the cell. Non-ionizing radiation is discussed below.

Although ionizing radiation is a typical occupational hazard in its principles of control and safety, the technical nature of ionizing radiation hazards together with the history of radiation use has led to the development of a professional occupational health specialization, the *radiation safety officer*.

Ionizing radiation occurs in two types: electromagnetic radiation and particle radiation. Electromagnetic radiation is a beam of energy carried by photons, infinitesimally small particles that behave as waves. Ionizing electromagnetic radiation is observed in the form of X-ray or gamma radiation of about 100 nm or shorter. Ionizing electromagnetic radiation is therefore of a shorter wavelength (and therefore higher frequency) than the non-ionizing electromagnetic radiation described below and thus carries much more energy than electromagnetic radiation at longer wavelengths. This is why it can ionize atoms and molecules in cells.

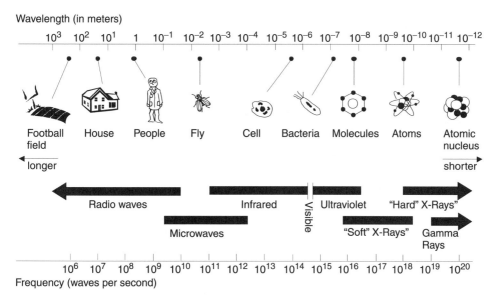

Figure 8.1 The electromagnetic spectrum, showing objects that are of the same magnitude in size as the wavelength of the radiation.

Particulate radiation consists of atomic fragments or particles, observed in the form of alpha or beta radiation, or neutrons.

- *Alpha particles* consist of two protons and two neutrons (the stripped nucleus of a helium atom) and are heavy and slow. Although they carry much energy, they do not penetrate materials effectively: they can be stopped by a piece of paper or by human skin. For this reason, alpha particles are mostly a concern when they are released inside the body by ingested or inhaled radioactive atoms (radionuclides).
- *Beta particles* are electrons stripped from their atoms. They are light, fast, and penetrate thin plastic but not lead.
- *Neutrons* are relatively heavy, carry much energy, and are deeply penetrating. They are a practical concern only in nuclear fission technology because they are not produced by any nonnuclear process.

Sources of radiation on Earth include natural *radionuclides* (isotopes in which spontaneous decay results in emission of a particle and X-ray), outer space (cosmic radiation), medical and industrial X-ray technology, and nuclear fission and fusion. Approximately 82% of the radiation dose received by most people is of natural origin, over half of which results from a common natural radionuclide, *radon* (Rn), and the remainder in roughly equal amounts from cosmic radiation, terrestrial sources in rocks and soil, and internal sources in the body; manmade sources are mainly medical applications. Occupational exposures are concentrated in a relatively few but expanding number of industries, including health care, energy production, mining, metal products and fabrication, and defense. Cigarette smoke contains radionuclides in small quantities (mostly polonium, ^{210}Po) that deposit in the lung.

The hazards of the nuclear energy industry and of research and technological development in fusion and high-energy physics are a highly specialized area of concern usually handled by health physicists and specially qualified radiation health officers. A detailed discussion of these industries is beyond the scope of this book.

Exposure to radiation may be "whole body" or limited to a particular body part. Whole-body radiation might occur due to an exposure to an unshielded source in an uncontrolled incident. Limited or segmental radiation may come from an external source when a worker passes in front of the beam or if the shielding is faulty. Limited radiation may also arise from an internal source such as inhaled radionuclides that may either remain in the lung or migrate to bone. Alpha emitters that accumulate in lung or bone, such as plutonium (Pu) and radon (Rn) daughters, are of particular concern in this regard because they emit radiation of high energy that, although it does not penetrate far, damages vulnerable cells in the unprotected tissue and can cause cancer.

In occupational health, the most important measurements of ionizing radiation are the gray (Gy), the sievert (Sv), and the working level (WL). The gray is a standard measurement of absorbed dose, indicating the deposition of energy in the material absorbing the radiation (10,000 erg/g). The sievert is a measurement of the absorbed dose adjusted by the effect of the type of radiation in tissue and is therefore important in dosimetry or estimating health risks. The sievert is the SI (metric) replacement for the rem: 1 Sv = 100 rem. Working level is an administrative unit used in uranium and other underground, hard-rock mining and some other settings in which radon and radionuclides are present. It is a quantity of radiation from exposure to radionuclides in any combination that results in a certain total quantity of alpha particle emission energy (130,000 MeV). Standards and guidelines for work underground were based on the cumulative length of time a miner was exposed at this level, usually expressed in "working level months" (WLM). It had some utility in defining the maximum time a miner was allowed to spend underground in a particular mine, and it has been used in epidemiological studies to quantify exposure; however, it is not very useful otherwise.

Instruments used to take workplace measurements in occupational health surveys take many forms but are usually based on ionization of air; ionization and production of current in a detector tube (the familiar Geiger counter); scintillation counting, which identifies interactions with a liquid; electron entrapment and release from thermal heating; and interactions with photographic film emulsions. Special techniques are used in high-energy physics and the nuclear industry.

Measurement of the personal exposure of individual workers to radiation is universal in health care and in industries in which a radiation hazard exists. Film badges (which show the effect of ionizing radiation on photographic film), thermoluminescent dosimeters (which detect ionization), and pocket ionizing chamber dosimeters (which are based on electrostatic repulsion resulting from ionization) are most often used for assessing individual worker exposure.

Radiation sickness is a syndrome that results from intense whole-body radiation. It may occur after external beam irradiation or internal absorption of a radionuclide. It is usually fatal at exposures above several Gy. Widespread cellular injury results in progressive multisystem disease, beginning with those tissues in which cell turnover is most rapid. Because cell replacement is inhibited by the radiation-induced genetic damage, radiation sickness is characterized first by loss of function in organs that require rapid cell turnover: failure to produce blood cells or new hair and failure to repair skin and intestinal lesions. This results in failure of the immune system, leading to infections, ulcers, hair loss, and loss of blood from bleeding into the damaged gastrointestinal tract. Radiation also affects the brain and can result in brain damage. People can recover from moderate exposure to radiation but are at risk for dementia, cancer (particularly acute leukemia), cataracts, and infertility.

Limited or segmental external radiation, as from a beam of particles or X-rays at high intensity, may produce skin redness at the site of exposure, tissue death, and variable risk of cancer with high exposure. Specific effects of local irradiation may include thyroid cancer with irradiation of the neck (relatively rare), brain swelling and dementia with heavy irradiation to the head, and birth defects, particularly neurological, with irradiation at relatively low levels during pregnancy.

Incidents in which radionuclides are absorbed into the body are rare. Radionuclides may enter the body by inhalation (most common), ingestion, or by implantation when there is a penetrating wound or an explosion. The effect of a radionuclide inside the body depends on where the radionuclide goes in the body. ^{131}I is heavily concentrated in the thyroid and is strongly associated with an increased risk of thyroid cancer; immediate administration of stable iodine blocks uptake of ^{131}I and so is standard treatment when someone is exposed to this isotope. Alpha emitters, such as ^{239}Pu and Ra isotopes, Rn and its "daughters," and ^{210}Po, are most likely to be inhaled, and once in the lung cause heavy exposure to alpha particles in a small, circumscribed area of tissue immediately around the particle. This results in an elevated risk of lung cancer. ^{238}Pu and other Pu isotopes are also concentrated in bone, where they may be associated with the risk of bone cancers. These are mostly problems in the nuclear industry. The alpha-emitting isotopes most likely to be of significance in occupational health outside the nuclear industry are radon and its daughters. ^{32}P, used in some nuclear medicine applications, is distributed widely in the body, exchanging freely with intracellular phosphorus.

Certain radionuclides present particular shielding problems. ^{32}P, for example, is a beta-emitter. The beta particles are released at an energy level that produces X-rays passing through lead and must therefore be shielded with thick plastic.

Some radionuclides also have toxicity unrelated to their radiation hazard. Uranium, for example, is toxic to the kidney.

ELECTROMAGNETIC FIELDS (EMF)

Magnetic fields are generated by current-carrying electrical conductors and are present in all electrical appliances, power lines, and even current running to ground in steel beams and plumbing. Magnetism is a fundamental force in physics and is linked to electrical current in conducting materials, in a direction perpendicular to the movement across field strength lines. Magnetic fields of strengths greater than the background field of Earth are everywhere in urban life.

Magnetic field strength is measured in gauss (G) and is independent of electrical fields; both fall off rapidly with distance from the source (following the "inverse square rule" that strength declines as the square of the distance from the source).

Some studies have suggested that EMF strength associated with power lines may be associated with an increased cancer risk, particularly for childhood leukemia. As a result, this issue has been intensively studied, with several very large studies. The evidence is highly inconsistent, and the better and more powerful studies generally do not show an association. Very large studies conducted in Sweden, France, and Canada have not confirmed the risk. Magnetic field strength may be confounded as a risk factor with other risk factors that are associated with housing type. The International Agency for Research on Cancer has concluded that limited evidence exists for an association between exposure to electromagnetic fields and leukemia in childhood. At present, the idea that exposure to magnetic fields is associated with adverse health effects remains speculative.

Recently there has been similar speculation that mobile phones, which operate at 900 MHz at much lower power levels than most appliances, may be associated with brain tumors. The initial evidence for this was a suggested preponderance of tumors on the side of the head that corresponded to users' handedness in holding the phone. Again, there has been much research, but the evidence for an association has been inconsistent and not persuasive.

Adult cancers have been extensively investigated in studies of electrical workers and radio transmission operators and have a possible association with brain cancer and, more weakly, adult leukemias have been suggested but not confirmed.

At present, the health implications of exposure to magnetic fields remain unproven. The risk of cancer associated with EMF exposure does not appear to be great even if it exists, and the available evidence to date is not persuasive that it does.

NON-IONIZING RADIATION

Non-ionizing radiation consists of electromagnetic waves radiating from the source at energies too low to ionize atoms in matter; unlike ionizing radiation, no particles are involved (other than photons, the basic unit of electromagnetic energy). Figure 8.1 illustrates the electromagnetic spectrum; non-ionizing radiation starts at about 350 nm. The electromagnetic spectrum below about 100 nm can be divided into several spectral ranges, described by wavelength or frequency. The longer the wavelength, the higher the frequency and the less energy the wave carries: Ultraviolet light (for health purposes, 100–400 nm), visible light (400–700 nm), infrared (700 nm–300 μm), microwave (0.1 cm–10 m), and "long" radio frequency waves (>10 m). They are discussed here in order of their place on the electromagnetic spectrum.

Ultraviolet Radiation

Ultraviolet radiation (UV) is a common and serious occupational hazard in outdoor work and certain occupations such as welding, in which radiation is produced by open electrical arcs. There are many components to the UV spectrum, but only three are significant with regard to health. UVA (400–320 nm) is often called "near UV," or "black light." It is relatively low in energy and weak in causing sunburn. UVB (280–320 nm) carries more energy and is more potent than UVA in producing sunburn . UVC (280–100 nm) kills bacteria and is destructive to other cells but is readily absorbed by air and by ozone in the stratosphere.

Exposure to UV is a hazard of outdoor work, regardless of temperature or climate. Exposure to UV is associated most characteristically with sunburn in light-skinned people, skin cancer, and eye problems, including cataracts. UV generated during welding can cause eye inflammation, which is called "welder's flash" and is quite painful, although it goes away after a few days.

Control measures in the workplace include painting walls and other surfaces with nonreflective paints (containing titanium dioxide or zinc oxide), hanging UV-impermeable plastic curtains between workstations, and segregating activities such as welding into enclosed booths. Personal protection can be achieved by protective work clothes and by viewing the welding arc through helmets or hand shields with filter lenses.

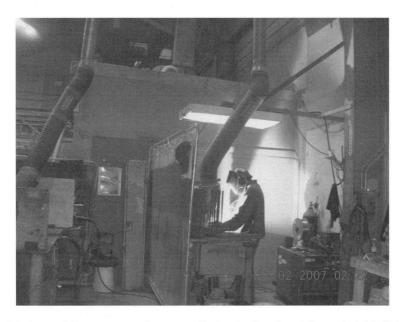

Figure 8.2 Arc welding generates intense radiation in the ultraviolet and visible light parts of the electromagnetic spectrum. The welder's helmet has built-in eye protection against ultraviolet radiation, and the yellow curtain centered in the picture filters out ultraviolet radiation to prevent others in the shop from being exposed. Note also the moveable area ventilation system. (Photograph by Julietta Rodríguez Guzmán, Universidad El Bosque, Colombia.)

Light in the Visible Spectrum

Illumination is a fundamental requirement of almost all work. The adequacy of illumination is a limiting factor for accuracy and safety. Inadequate lighting is associated with headaches and fatigue, as considerable effort must be exerted to keep details of work in focus, but there is no long-term damage to the eye itself from squinting or eyestrain. As the worker ages, accommodation becomes more difficult, and increased light levels are required to see and resolve small or distant objects. It also becomes more difficult to adapt to changes in illumination, such as when entering a dark room from the sunny outside and in seeing through glare. Although these changes make illumination particularly important for older workers, the productivity and comfort of younger workers also suffers when illumination is inadequate. Illumination levels should be adequate to meet the needs of work, regardless of the standard. The smallest detail of work should be easily resolved visually, there should be sharp contrast between the objects worked on and the background, and sources of glare should be identified and removed.

When the waves of light coming from a source are lined up and ordered so that they form a narrow, high-energy beam, this is called *coherent light*. Coherent light, in the form of laser beams, carries much more energy over a much longer distance than diffuse visible light. This makes coherent light useful in applications such as surgery, materials cutting, measurement instruments, and signal transmission. Laser light presents a serious hazard to the eye and may cause burns on skin and other tissue. When focused by the lens on the retina (the structure at the back of the eyeball that senses light and converts it to a nerve cell impulse), a laser beam can cause severe injury and permanent destruction, resulting in partial blindness. Safeguards should be present on all lasers that are not completely contained so that lasers cannot be inadvertently pointed toward someone. Enclosures for the beam should be constructed of nonreflective, fireproof materials. Reflecting surfaces must be removed from the area or covered because a reflected laser beam carries almost as much energy as the original beam. Training in the safe use of lasers is mandatory whenever they are used.

Infrared

Infrared radiation is produced by all objects in proportion to their temperature. The radiation carries heat away from the object. Radiation heat loss is a major cooling mechanism for the human body, for example. Infrared radiation intense enough to present a burn hazard is produced by objects that are significantly hotter than the human body. In occupational health, exposure to infrared radiation may be a problem in any occupation or industry in which hot processes play a role, including foundries and steel mills, glassblowing works, heating and dehydrating operations, and welding operations.

Absorption of the infrared radiation results in heating. In the human body, the tissues most sensitive to heat are the skin and eye. Infrared does not penetrate well, and it is usually these superficial structures that are affected by infrared itself.

Exposure to infrared may result in skin changes, cataracts, and potentially severe eye injury. In situations where there is heating of the total body, heat stress may be a significant hazard. Exposure to infrared also may also result in thermal burns.

Microwave

The term *microwave* refers to radiofrequency radiation on the spectrum below infrared in frequency but above conventional radio and television transmission. These frequencies include the so-called "extremely high frequencies" (EHF, 30–300 GHz, wavelength in millimeters), "super high frequency" (3–30 GHz, wavelengths in centimeters), and "ultra high frequency" (0.3–3 GHz, wavelength in tenths of meters). UHF is familiar as an ancillary spectrum used for television transmission; "very high frequency" (VHF, 30–300 MHZ) is the standard television transmission range and is present on the electromagnetic spectrum just under the microwave channels.

Microwave transmissions are used for radar, communications beacons, heat-sealing, cooking, diathermy, and plywood bonding, among other applications. The microwave beam can be highly focused and reflected. Microwaves on the order of one centimeter in wavelength have the property of directly imparting their energy to molecules of water and other small molecules, thus increasing molecular movement and directly causing heat. This is the way that microwave ovens work. Radiofrequency radiation in this range, as in the case of microwave ovens, may disturb the function of cardiac pacemakers and so presents a hazard to people who have them.

Although microwaves do not appear to be common or important causes of injury to workers, the possible effects of microwaves on human health are very controversial.

Noise

Noise is the most widespread and common occupational hazard. It is an important cause of deafness, which is then called *noise-induced hearing loss*. Noise-induced hearing loss is usually partial deafness, tends to occur later in life, and interferes with communication and daily life. Noise consists of individual sounds that are waves of air pressure. These pressure waves propagate from the source of the sound in all directions.

The loudness of a sound reflects the magnitude of pressure of the sound wave propagated in air. The loudness of sound is measured in "bels" (B), named after Alexander Graham Bell, who also invented the telephone. The bel scale is exponential; 4B is 10 times louder than 3B and 100 times louder than 2B. A bel is an inconvenient unit to use for most purposes, so it is customarily divided into tenths, or "decibels"; a 40 dB noise is equal to 4B and is 10 times louder than a 30 dB (3B) noise. Because the scale is exponential, but divided into tenths, the logarithm of doubling is about 3 dB; a 43 dB noise is about twice as loud as a 40 dB noise. (Table 8.1)

The pitch, or musical quality, of a sound is called its tone. Tone is the frequency of a sound and is measured in Hertz (Hz), which corresponds to the number of cycles or waves in one second. Most sound in real life is mixed, consisting of different tones, overtones (in musical terms, sounds that are an octave above or below), and harmonics. A pure tone consists of a single frequency. Although pure tones rarely exist in real life, the human ear hears all sounds as the sum of their individual pure tones and is tuned to these pure tones.

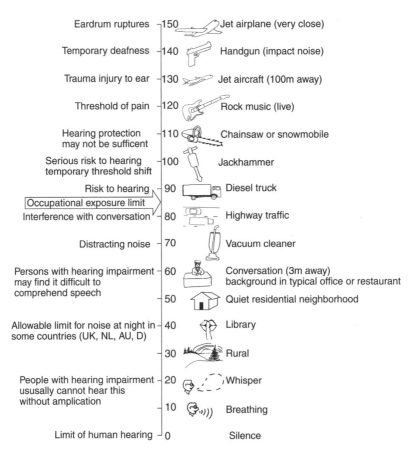

Eardrum ruptures	150	Jet airplane (very close)
Temporary deafness	140	Handgun (impact noise)
Trauma injury to ear	130	Jet aircraft (100m away)
Threshold of pain	120	Rock music (live)
Hearing protection may not be suffcient	110	Chainsaw or snowmobile
Serious risk to hearing temporary threshold shift	100	Jackhammer
Risk to hearing	90	Diesel truck
Occupational exposure limit		
Interference with conversation	80	Highway traffic
Distracting noise	70	Vacuum cleaner
Persons with hearing impairment may find it difficult to comprehend speech	60	Conversation (3m away) background in typical office or restaurant
	50	Quiet residential neighborhood
Allowable limit for noise at night in some countries (UK, NL, AU, D)	40	Library
	30	Rural
People with hearing impairment ususally cannot hear this without amplication	20	Whisper
	10	Breathing
Limit of human hearing	0	Silence

Figure 8.3 Noise levels produced by various sources, showing effects on hearing and the human body.

Human beings hear differently at different frequencies. A pure tone at 1000 Hz sounds louder than a pure tone carrying the same energy at 250 Hz. In order to accurately adjust for how the hearing mechanism and the brain respond to different frequencies, physical measurements of sound using the decibel measurement are modified by electronically varying the sensitivity of the measurement device to the frequency components of the noise, using a formula called the "A-scale."

In addition to tone and loudness, sounds also may be *continuous* or *impulse*. A continuous noise may vary in tone and loudness but continues for at least a few seconds without interruption. The effect of continuous noise on the ear is primarily related to its loudness and tone. Impulse noise is of very short duration, sometimes less than a second, and carries high energy in a single or small number of waves. Impulse noise, which might be generated by a hammer, a crash, a gunshot, or an explosion, is usually of mixed frequencies, and its effect on the ear depends on the energy it carries, which is perceived as loudness. When impulse noise is very sudden and very loud, it is called a *blast wave*, and the injury it causes is traumatic, the result of the physical pounding that the ear receives when the blast wave hits it and the energy is transmitted through the ear.

Devices that measure continuous sound are called *sound level meters* (SLM) and read automatically in "dBA," decibels weighted by the A-scale. (There are other scales with other applications.) Devices that measure sudden, direct noises are called *impulse meters*. Those that measure the total exposure to noise over a given time are called *noise dosimeters*. (A dosimeter is any device that measures total dose rather than the exposure at one point in time.) The noise dosimeter is used to determine what the average noise exposure is over a period of time, usually 8 hours to correspond with a normal work shift. The sound level is averaged by measuring the loudness over time and averaging over the total period of time; in practice, this is equivalent to weighting the loudness by the length of time it lasted. For this reason, the average sound level is called a *time-weighted average* (TWA).

Table 8.1 also gives examples of dBA readings that one might encounter in common situations. In practice, SLM readings are usually made in the workplace by safety officers, occupational hygienists, audiologists, or acoustical engineers and in the community by noise control officers representing local government. Exposure to noise in the workplace occurs in jobs in many industries and depends on the process being performed, the acoustics of the workplace, the controls on the machines or noise sources, the distance between the source and the worker, and what type of personal hearing protection the worker may be using. Exposure in the community is usually less intense but may be increased for residents of communities near major airports, highways, or industrial plants or for individuals who indulge in motorcycle riding, shooting firearms, or listening to music at high volume.

Noise-induced hearing loss can be prevented by avoiding exposure to excessive noise. This requires a program of both noise control and monitoring workers for early detection of hearing loss (Table 8.2). Noise control is a highly technical specialization that may involve acoustical engineering, plant design, engineering controls, and containment or isolation of noise sources. However, most problems involving excessive noise can be handled effectively and inexpensively using basic principles.

Occupational noise exposure standards in many countries, including the U.S. and Canada, require employers to measure the noise level in the workplace if the noise is loud enough to interfere with easy speech communication or to cause discomfort. The permissible exposure level or occupational exposure level in North American jurisdictions is 90 dBA (8-hour TWA). If the eight-hour time-weighted average (TWA) is 85 dBA or greater, then the employer must institute a hearing conservation program.

Hearing conservation programs should include regular monitoring of the workplace, baseline and annual audiograms for all exposed workers, in-service and pre-service worker education regarding hearing conservation, systematic record keeping and worker notification when problems are detected, and the provision of hearing protection to all exposed workers. Many programs in industry also include referral of affected employees to specialists, administrative controls to limit the duration of assignments in noisy areas, and noise control measures. Noise-induced hearing loss is discussed in detail in Chapter 17.

TABLE 8.1

THE DECIBEL SCALE

Relative loudness	Bel	Decibel	Example
10^{11}	11	110	Chainsaw
10^{10}	10	100	Jet flying overhead at 300 m
10^9	9	90	Motorcycle or diesel truck at 10 m
10^8	8	80	Many occupational settings in manufacturing
10^7	7	70	Television set in same room
10^6	6	60	Office with air conditioner
10^5	5	50	Office with no background noise
10^4	4	40	Quiet home
10^3	3	30	Barely perceptible background noise
10^2	2	20	Limit of most acute human hearing
10^1	1	10	Perceived as complete quiet
10^0	0	0	Occurs only in acoustically insulated spaces

The weakest part of most industrial hearing conservation programs is personal protection. To be effective, a variety of effective hearing protection devices must be made easily accessible to all exposed workers, who also must be trained in their proper use and motivated to wear them. Hearing protection devices vary considerably in their effectiveness and are rated by their ability to attenuate sound. A device that is overly impermeable to sound for a given job could be a safety hazard if it interferes with communication. In practice, this seldom occurs, and workers usually have no problems understanding speech once they become accustomed to the device. Individuals vary considerably in their ability to tolerate various models of earmuffs and plugs, and a selection must be available for workers to choose what they prefer. Workers must be instructed in their correct use: nondisposable earplugs must be kept scrupulously clean, deformable-type disposable plugs should never be inserted with dirty fingers, and earmuffs should be seated properly on the head. If the devices are uncomfortable, inconvenient, inaccessible, or

TABLE 8.2

ESSENTIAL COMPONENTS OF HEARING CONSERVATION PROGRAMS

Noise monitoring in the workplace

Acoustical noise abatement

Training of employees

Annual audiometric evaluations

Employee notification and referral

Personal hearing protection

Systematic record keeping

look funny, some workers will simply not use them or will remove them as soon as they are unsupervised. Rolled cotton earplugs are often used but are completely ineffective due to their poor sound-absorbing characteristics.

Pressure

Pressure levels in the atmosphere are called barometric pressure. Normal barometric pressure is determined by the thickness of the atmosphere and weather conditions and is measured in units of bars or atmospheres (one atmosphere is the normal barometric pressure at sea level). Conditions in the workplace may subject the worker to much greater or lesser pressure levels. Barometric pressures substantially

---

Box 8.1

Noise-Induced Hearing Loss at an Old Factory in Korea

Many enterprises in Soth Korea, as in other countries, have unsatisfactory hearing conservation programs. Permanent hearing threshold shifts, that is, noise-induced hearing loss, have been documented among employees. The problem is mostly occurring at older factories in workplaces using old production equipment. The employers are under great pressure to keep costs low because of competition from China. At the time of this study, wages for Korean workers were 10 times higher than wages for Chinese workers. The Korean companies are losing their market due to competition from Chinese companies. They are therefore reluctant to make further investment to improve the environment of the workplace.

For instance, one company in Korea produces bronze pipes with equipment that is 50 years old. The production processes of extracting and dropping the pipes are very noisy. Noise surveys have measured a maximum noise level of 102 dBA. The equipment itself produces noise as high as 95 dBA. The noise level in the factory has been found to be 92 dBA 8-hour time weighted average (TWA), clearly above the Korean and international occupational exposure levels. However, the dominant type of noise of the workplace is not the steady state noise averaged in these measurements. It is transient, or impact, noise, which has been measured as having a very high sound pressure level of 102 dBA at the worker's location.

There is a particular problem in one group of workers. Noise-induced hearing loss is even more frequent among the technicians who are fixing the equipment than among workers who are operating the equipment. The technicians have not been trained well in wearing the hearing protection device, though they are spending many hours checking and fixing the old equipment and are exposed to high levels of noise.

The best way to reduce the noise level of the factory is by replacing the old equipment with new equipment. Another necessary intervention is to modernize the production line through automation or to modify the production process using quieter tools. However, workers are provided only with personal hearing protection, without a complete hearing conservation program, which should include noise monitoring, audiometric (hearing) tests, and noise control.

Any intervention imposes additional costs the employer. The managers of many enterprises do not wish to invest more money in their operations because there is no proportional benefit to the employer from a big investment.

The Korean occupational health authority has intervened in the case of the pipe manufacturer. The authority is enforcing the requirement that the employer comply with the Korean regulation for daily noise exposure of 90 dBA 8-hour TWA.

The employer and the managers of the enterprise were concerned at first that they could not comply with the regulation without investing much time and money to improve the environment of the workplace. As it happened, the working hours were decreasing at the workplace because of reduced job orders. Thus, the workplace did eventually meet the regulation for continuous noise through reduced production activity.

However, this was not enough. The problem with impact noise continued. Although the workplace could meet the regulation, the remaining impact noise level was harmful enough by itself to change the hearing threshold of the workers, in the absence of an appropriate hearing conservation program with the hearing protection devices.

A comprehensive hearing conservation program is needed. One key individual in the workplace should be responsible for education, coordination, and management of the hearing conservation. So far, this has not been happened.

Contributed by Chang-Myung Lee, Professor, University of Ulsan, Korea

---

above or below one atmosphere are part of the conditions of work in special environments. The absolute pressure is usually less important than the changes that are experienced by the worker. The direct adverse effects of these pressure changes are called *barotraumas* and are of particular interest in aerospace and undersea medicine. There are also a number of problems that result from the dissolving of gases into and release out of body fluids. The literature in both is highly specialized and technical and is firmly grounded in physiological principles. In occupational health generally, problems associated with pressure changes are relatively uncommon except as they relate to commercial air travel or shallow diving.

Hyperbaric Effects Hyperbaric pressure is pressure above normal atmospheric levels. It is a particular problem in diving and in work in caissons, in which air pressure is pumped up above one atmosphere in order to allow workers to work underwater.

Compression occurs when a diver descends underwater or a worker in a caisson is subject to elevated pressure. Health problems associated with compression are relatively uncommon at depths where industrial activity is likely to take place; decompression effects are more commonly severe coming back up from those depths. The body normally adapts to increased external pressure relatively rapidly. Gases such as oxygen and nitrogen in air dissolve into tissues of the body quickly and can cause toxic effects. Air in spaces in the body is compressed. Problems with compression-induced barotrauma arise when there is no free communication from an enclosed space to the outside through which to equilibrate pressure. The increased external pressure pushes against a relative negative pressure inside the enclosed space, causing ear trauma. *Nitrogen narcosis* is a condition that occurs during deep dives while breathing air that contains 78% nitrogen, instead of a helium atmosphere specially designed for deep diving. Normally, nitrogen gas is inert and causes no toxicity. Under pressure, however, it causes central nervous system toxicity when dissolved in the blood, resulting in euphoria (feeling drunk), hallucinations, and unsafe behavior.

Decompression Decompression is a more common problem in diving. When a diver returns to surface too quickly or when workers who are in compressed chambers, such as caissons, are depressurized too quickly, nitrogen and other gases in the blood that dissolved under pressure come back out again and form bubbles. This is *decompression sickness*, also known as "the bends." The bubbles may accumulate and block blood vessels, causing a stroke or spinal cord injury. Treatment is by repressurization, either by immediate return to depth or in a hyperbaric chamber on the surface. Guidelines for the safe rate of ascent for divers are well known to professional divers.

High Altitude Rapid ascent to high altitude (7000 to 9000 m or more) without time to adjust can cause *high altitude sickness*, a potentially life-threatening condition. This tends to be a problem among mountain climbers rather than workers. Few industrial activities are carried out at elevations this high.

Temperature Extremes

The human body regulates its own temperature very closely to keep it close to an average 37° C (as measured in the mouth). Problems arise when temperature variations exceed the ability of the body to adapt or mechanisms of adaptation, such sweating, are impaired. The body can gradually, over several days, adapt or get used to elevated temperatures. This process is called *acclimation* and makes the body more efficient in losing heat and, up to a limit, more resistant to the effects of higher temperatures. There is no such protective mechanism against lower temperatures, however.

There are fewer ways to warm up the human body than there are to cool it. The principal physiological mechanism to increase heat production is shivering. The major mechanism to reduce loss of heat from the skin is by constricting blood vessels, called vasoconstriction. Neither mechanism is particularly effective or can be kept up over long periods of time. As a consequence, human beings are highly dependent on clothing, heating technology, wind screening, and increasing exercise levels. The primary risk of generalized cooling is hypothermia, which is rarely an occupational health problem even in extreme Arctic or alpine environments. Frostbite occurs when exposed body parts freeze, often the ears, nose, toes, and fingers. It usually occurs because clothing does not adequately cover and insulate the face or hands or becomes wet from perspiration. Severe frostbite occurs when a body part is frozen all the way through and is a medical emergency.

Heat stress is not limited to tropical climates or jobs involving proximity to a heat source. It can also occur as the result of excessive heat retention due to the combination of heavy clothing and strenuous exercise or in combinations of heat and humidity that interfere with evaporative cooling.

Heat stroke is the most serious disorder related to heat stress. Heat stroke starts with nausea, vomiting, hyperthermia (core temperature often above 39° C), headaches, and dizziness. The victim shows signs of mental confusion and may have a seizure. Heat stroke is a medical emergency requiring immediate treatment in a hospital.

Heat fatigue is a condition of temporary weakness, fatigue, and muscle cramps caused by salt depletion, often aggravated by dehydration. Taking salt tablets may provide too much salt replacement for workers and is not recommended. *Heat exhaustion* also results from salt depletion and starts with dizziness, headache, weakness, fainting, cold and clammy skin, sweating, vomiting, blurred vision, and an upset stomach. Both conditions respond quickly to rehydration, cooling, and rest. *Heat syncope* is loss of consciousness associated with a drop in blood pressure that briefly reduces supply to the brain. The person feels dizzy and falls down but quickly recovers when the head is lower than the heart, restoring blood pressure to the brain. Heat syncope often occurs when a person has been standing for a long time without moving because blood pools in the legs. *Miliaria rubra*, or "prickly heat," is a skin rash.

Prevention of Heat Stress Heat stress can be prevented by shade, cooling, drinking plenty of fluids, eating a diet with sufficient salt (much better than salt tablets), and acclimatizing the worker. Acclimatization requires a period of adjustment to the

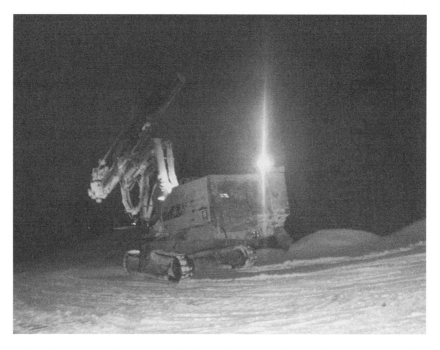

Figure 8.4 Construction in northern Québec often takes place under extremely cold conditions. (Photograph by Julietta Rodríguez Guzmán, Universidad El Bosque, Colombia.)

temperature, limiting the level and duration of activity until the worker is adapted. Clothing worn in hot workplaces should not constrict any part of the body or prevent air movement against the skin. Heavy exercise should be limited to short intervals in hot environments, and frequent rest breaks may be necessary.

Alcohol contributes to serious heat stress by causing dehydration and relaxing blood vessels, allowing blood to pool. Drugs for heart disease often increase the risk for heat stress-related disorders.

Vibration

Whole-body vibration occurs when the entire body is shaken, particularly at frequencies that shake the trunk disproportionately. Low frequency, whole-body vibration is the most characteristic and unusual exposure of vehicle drivers and heavy equipment operators. This kind of vibration appears to be associated primarily with gastrointestinal disorders and back pain.

Segmental vibration affects a particular body part, usually the arm and hand when using handheld power tools, including chainsaws, riveting guns, pneumatic drills, grinders, air hammers, chippers, and cutting devices for concrete. The most characteristic effect of prolonged exposure to vibration at the hand is *vibration vasculitis*, or "white finger disease," in which blood vessels constrict, initially in response to the vibration and later in response to cold or spontaneously.

9

CHEMICAL HAZARDS

René Mendes

The general principles of toxicology and chemical safety are outlined in Chapter 2. This chapter describes chemicals that are commonly found in the workplace and their characteristic hazards and toxicity.

ASBESTOS

Chemical Formula: Si_xO_y, fibers consisting of silicone and oxygen, variably of magnesium, calcium, iron, and sodium.

Asbestos has been known since antiquity and was always regarded as a valuable natural substance. The name derives from the Greek adjective *asbestos* meaning "unchangeable," "non-perishable," "non-combustible."

Asbestos is the name used for various types of minerals that naturally form fibers. It is not a single mineral. The individual minerals have different chemical compositions, although all are silicates, based on silicon and oxygen, and also exist in forms that do not form fibers. The term *asbestos* covers the fibrous forms of six naturally occurring minerals that can be grouped on the basis of their mineralogical properties into two families: serpentines, which includes chrysotile (white asbestos), and amphiboles, of which there are five types. Of these, crocidolite (blue asbestos) and amosite (brown asbestos) are the most widely used in industry.

Asbestos was once used widely in the production of industrial and household products because of its useful properties, including fire retardation, electrical and thermal insulation, chemical and thermal stability, and high tensile strength. Asbestos products have also been built into a multitude of different devices: ovens, kilns, cooking and heating stoves, boilers, irons and ironing boards, work surfaces, plumbing fixtures/sanitary fittings, refrigerators, water heaters, motors and alternators, vehicles (brake linings, clutch assemblies, gaskets), railway equipment, ships, aircraft, electrical equipment, and components used in civil engineering (sewage systems, water distribution, road surfacing) and buildings (roof tiles, elevator doors, fire dampers, seals, partitions, etc.). Table 9.1 lists common uses for asbestos and materials that can replace it.

World production reached its highest level in 1975 at over 5 million tonnes. It is still around 2 million tonnes a year now, most of the asbestos produced (more

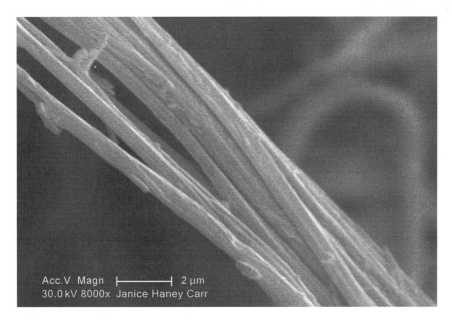

Figure 9.1 Chrysotile asbestos, at a magnification of 8,000x. (Photograph by Janice Haney Carr, Public Health Image Library, U.S. Centers for Disease Control and Prevention.)

than 90%) being chrysotile. The leading producers are Russia (39%), China (16%), Kazakhstan (15%), Canada (9%), Brazil (9%), and Zimbabwe (7%). Table 9.1 lists many of the uses of asbestos.

Today, however, asbestos is recognized as a health hazard if inhaled. Exposure to asbestos causes a range of diseases, such as lung cancer, mesothelioma, and asbestosis (fibrosis of the lungs), as well as changes in the pleura (lining of the chest wall), including plaques (local areas of thickening), diffuse thickening, and effusions. There is also evidence that it causes laryngeal and possibly some other cancers.

The International Labour Organization (ILO) estimates that over the last several decades 100,000 deaths globally have been due to asbestos exposure, and the World Health Organization (WHO) states that 90,000 people die each year globally because of occupational asbestos exposure. The burden of asbestos-related diseases is still rising, even in countries that have banned the use of asbestos in the early 1990s. Because of the long latency periods attached to the diseases, stopping the use of asbestos now will not result in a decrease in the number of asbestos-related deaths until after a number of decades. Currently, about 125 million people in the world are exposed to asbestos at the workplace.

Asbestos as a Hazard

Over 90% of asbestos fiber produced today is chrysotile, which is used in asbestos-cement construction materials: asbestos-cement flat and corrugated sheet, asbestos-cement pipe, and asbestos-cement water storage tanks. Other products still being manufactured with asbestos content include vehicle brake and clutch

TABLE 9.1

SOME ALTERNATIVES TO ASBESTOS-CONTAINING PRODUCTS

Asbestos Product	Substitute Products
Asbestos-cement corrugated roofing	Fiber-cement roofing using synthetic fibers (polyvinyl alcohol, polypropylene) and vegetable/cellulose fibers (softwood kraft pulp, bamboo, sisal, coir, rattan shavings, tobacco stalks, etc.); with optional silica fume, fly ash, or rice husk ash
	Microconcrete (Parry) tiles; galvanized metal sheets; clay tiles; vegetable fibers in asphalt; slate; coated metal tiles (Harveytile); aluminum roof tiles (Dekra Tile); extruded uPVC roofing sheets; recycled polypropylene and high-density polyethylene and crushed stone (Worldroof); plastic-coated aluminum; plastic-coated galvanized steel
Asbestos-cement flat sheet (ceilings, facades, partitions)	Fiber-cement using vegetable/cellulose fibers (see above), wastepaper, optionally synthetic fibers; gypsum ceiling boards (BHP Gypsum); polystyrene ceilings, cornices, and partitions; façade applications in polystyrene structural walls (coated with plaster); aluminum cladding (Alucabond); brick; galvanized frame with plaster-board or calcium silicate board facing; softwood frame with plasterboard or calcium silicate board facing
Asbestos-cement pipe	*High pressure:* Cast iron and ductile iron pipe; high-density polyethylene pipe; polyvinyl chloride pipe; steel-reinforced concrete pipe (large sizes); glass-reinforced polyester pipe
	Low pressure: Cellulose-cement pipe; cellulose/PVA fiber-cement pipe; clay pipe; glass-reinforced polyester pipe; steel-reinforced concrete pipe (large-diameter drainage)
Asbestos-cement water storage tanks	Cellulose-cement; polyethylene; fiberglass; steel; galvanized iron; PVA-cellulose fiber-cement
Asbestos-cement rainwater gutters; open drains (mining industry)	Galvanized iron; aluminum; hand-molded cellulose-cement; PVC

Source: World Bank Group 2009

pads, roofing, and gaskets. Though today asbestos is hardly used in construction materials other than asbestos-cement products, it is still found in older buildings in the form of friable surfacing materials, thermal system insulation, non-friable flooring materials, and other applications. The maintenance and removal of these materials warrant special attention.

Asbestos also occurs as a contaminant in some deposits of stone, talc, vermiculite, iron ore, and other minerals. This can create health hazards for workers and residents at the site of excavation and in some cases in the manufacture and use of consumer products the materials are used to make.

Asbestos creates a chain of exposure, from the time it is mined until it returns to the earth at landfill or unauthorized disposal site. At each link in this chain, there is both occupational and community exposure. Workers in the mines are exposed to the fibers while extracting the ore; their families breathe fibers brought

BOX 9.1

A Brazilian Perspective

It is well known that Brazil holds a major position and visibility in the international scenario of asbestos mining and exportation. Currently 100% of asbestos fibers are chrysotile ("white asbestos"), a serpentine fiber extracted from just one mine (Canabrava), by one company (Sama/Eternit), close to Minaçu, State of Goiás, in the middle of Brazil, close to Brasilia, the country's capital. Geological and commercial assessments and forecasts estimate productive reserves ranging from 40 to 60 years.

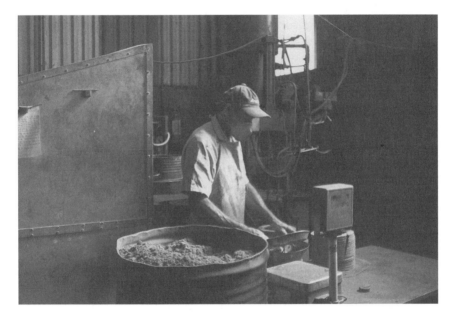

Figure 9.3 Dry asbestos being mixed with phenolic resin to make brake linings in a workplace in Brazil in 2005. Dust is visible on the table, scale, and on the worker's hands. The dust mask worn by the worker is completely inadequate to protect him. After these unsafe working conditions were documented, the company first developed a containment method to prevent exposure of workers and then replaced asbestos entirely, without financial loss. Asbestos is no longer used. (Photograph by Fernanda Giannasi, Ministry of Labor, Brazil.)

In fact, Brazil is ranked in fifth among major producers of chrysotile, with an annual production around 273,000 tons. Around 63% (171,000 tons) is exported to the international market, mainly to India, Thailand, Indonesia, Malaysia, United Arab Emirates, Mexico, Bolivia, Sri Lanka, Iran, Nigeria, Colombia, Ecuador, China, Mozambique, Vietnam, and Syria. In spite of the movement to ban asbestos all over the world, Brazilian exports are increasing, and this trend is inversely proportional to the decreasing trend of internal consumption, thanks to step-by-step progress in banning asbestos in Brazil.

home on work clothes; workers in the mills and factories process the fiber and manufacture products with it; and their families are also secondarily exposed. Communities around the mines, mills, and factories are contaminated with their wastes; children play on tailings piles and in contaminated schoolyards; transportation of fiber and products contaminates roads and rights-of-way. Tradesmen who install, repair, and remove asbestos-containing materials are exposed in the course of their work, as are bystanders in the absence of proper controls. Disposal of asbestos wastes from any step in this sequence not only exposes the workers handling the wastes but also local residents when fibers become airborne because the source, usually insulation, is uncovered and disturbed. Finally, in the absence of measures to remove asbestos-containing materials from the waste stream and dispose of them properly, exposure is often repeated when discarded material is scavenged and reused.

Production of chrysotile-containing shipboard and building insulation, roofing and, particularly, flooring felts, and other flooring materials, such as vinyl asbestos tiles, has declined considerably, with some of them disappearing from the marketplace. Friable chrysotile or amphibole-containing materials in building construction have been phased out in many countries, but there are large quantities of these materials still in place in buildings, which will continue to give rise to exposure to both chrysotile and the amphiboles during maintenance, removal, or demolition. Chrysotile has been used in hundreds (or even thousands) of products that have entered global commerce. These existing products may also give rise to exposure.

According to WHO, uncontrolled mixed exposure to chrysotile and amphiboles in the past has caused considerable disease and mortality in Europe and North America. Studies in European countries have clearly indicated that a larger proportion of mesotheliomas occurs in the construction trades than in production. Far more chrysotile than other types of asbestos was used in most construction applications.

In some industrialized countries, the manufacture and use of all forms of asbestos (including chrysotile) and its derivatives is now prohibited, or at least their use is extremely limited or restricted. Table 9.2 lists countries that have banned asbestos as of the time of this writing (2010). But people are still exposed, and will continue to be exposed for many years to come, both at work and in the home, because asbestos-containing materials are still in place in existing structures. Those at risk are predominantly specialists working in demolition, asbestos removal, and maintenance (in other words, those concerned with all types of construction finished and fittings).

In most countries, however, asbestos is not banned. Unfortunately, some countries have maintained or even increased their production or use of chrysotile in recent years. World production of asbestos in the period 2000–2005 has been relatively stable, at between 2,050,000 and 2,400,000 metric tonnes per annum.

So high-risk exposures to asbestos fiber dust continue, putting a lot of people at huge risk. And in many of these countries, not only adults but also adolescents and even children are already heavily exposed in a range of working environments, increasing their risk of developing an asbestos-related illness and of developing it earlier.

TABLE 9.2

COUNTRIES THAT HAVE BANNED THE USE OF ASBESTOS

1. Argentina	16. Greece	31. Poland
2. Australia	17. Honduras	32. Portugal
3. Austria	18. Hungary	33. Republic of Korea
4. Belgium	19. Iceland	34. Romania
5. Bulgaria	20. Ireland	35. Saudi Arabia
6. Chile	21. Italy	36. Seychelles
7. Cyprus	22. Japan	37. Slovakia
8. Czech Republic	23. Jordan	38. Slovenia
9. Denmark	24. Kuwait	39. South Africa
10. Egypt	25. Latvia	40. Spain
11. Estonia	26. Lithuania	41. Sweden
12. Finland	27. Luxembourg	42. Switzerland
13. France	28. Malta	43. United Kingdom
14. Gabon	29. Netherlands	44. Uruguay
15. Germany	30. Norway	

(Source: World Bank Group, May 2009)

Mechanisms of Action

Asbestos fibers break down into fibrils and are inhaled in the form of very fine dust that penetrates deep into the lungs. The longer and thinner these fibers are, the harder it if for the body to eliminate them. Many persist for a long time in the lung (Figure 9.2). The body's defense mechanisms cannot cope, and the physico-chemical properties of the fibers trapped within the respiratory system mean that they cannot be broken down and destroyed. They then very gradually cause inflammation and then fibrosis of the lung tissue (asbestosis) or the membrane—the pleura—that covers the lungs and may cause a variety of pleural conditions. On contact with the lining of the bronchi the fibers can interfere with cell division and, after a lengthy latency period, cause cancerous changes leading to a lung tumor. The risk is exacerbated if there is simultaneous exposure to other carcinogenic agents. Certain fibers may migrate outside the pleural cavity, where they evoke localized fibrosis (pleural plaques) or cancer of the pleura (mesothelioma).

The most dangerous fibers are those that are long (more than 5 μm) and thin (less than 3 μm), with a length-to-diameter ratio greater than 3:1. However, whilst the likelihood of developing an illness depends very largely on the size and nature of the asbestos fibers, and thus varies according to the type of asbestos concerned, the fact is that all types of asbestos are carcinogenic.

There is considerable uncertainty about the mechanisms responsible for the more rapid removal of chrysotile fibers from the lung than in the case of amphibole asbestos fibers. It is uncertain whether the more effective removal of chrysotile fibers is due to more rapid fiber dissolution or to more rapid clearance of shorter fibers as a result of breakage. Another explanation may be movement and dispersion in the watery atmosphere in the lung.

An important question in the evaluation of the possible risks associated with the ingestion of asbestos fibers is whether fibers can migrate from the lumen into

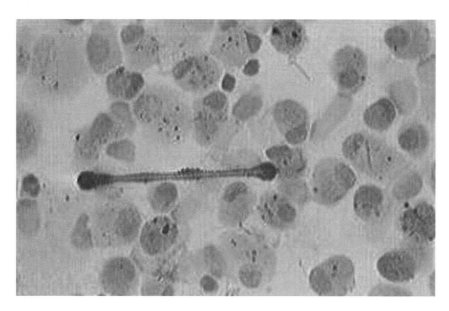

Figure 9.2 An "asbestos body" is a fiber of asbestos that has remained in the lung for a long time and has been coated by cells with protein and iron deposits. Asbestos bodies are much more visible in the lung than uncoated asbestos fibers. (Photograph courtesy of David Koh and Gregory Chan, National University of Singapore.)

and through the walls of the gastrointestinal tract to be distributed within the body and subsequently cleared. The current understanding is that:

- It is not possible to conclude with certainty that asbestos fibers, mainly chryso-tile, do not cross the gastrointestinal wall. However, available evidence indicates that, if penetration does occur, it is extremely limited.
- There is no available information on bioaccumulation/retention of ingested asbestos fibers. Simulated gastric juice has been shown to alter the physical and chemical properties of chrysotile fibers.
- There is no difference in the level of urinary chrysotile between subjects drinking water with high compared to those drinking water with much lower natural chrysotile contamination.

Asbestos-related Diseases

Asbestosis Asbestosis is a pneumoconiosis produced by inhalation of asbestos fibers. It is a chronic disease with slow onset that usually requires several years of exposure, depending on the intensity of exposure. Clinically, it is characterized by diffuse interstitial pulmonary fibrosis, often accompanied by thickening and some-times calcification of the pleura. Shortness of breath on exertion is the most common presenting symptom. A chronic dry cough is common, but the cough may be productive, especially among smokers. Finger clubbing may appear in advanced cases.

In most cases, the first and often the only physical sign are crackles, also known as "rales" (with a "Velcro®" quality), usually detected near the end of a full inspiration. Chest X-rays reveal small, irregular opacities commonly distributed in the middle and lower lung fields. With disease progression, all lung zones may be affected, and honeycombing, especially in the lower zones, is not unusual. Late manifestations can include an irregular diaphragm and cardiac border, which is associated with pleural plaques and diffuse pleural thickening.

In diffuse interstitial fibrosis, particularly cases of low levels of profusion, other etiologies should be considered. These include interstitial pneumonitis leading to idiopathic pulmonary fibrosis; interstitial lung disease associated with connective tissue disorders; and lipoid pneumonia, all of which can present with irregular opacities in the lower lung fields. If rounded opacities are prevalent, the possibility of exposure to silica or coal dust should be considered.

Lung function tests can help to quantify the level of pulmonary dysfunction and extent of impairment. In advanced asbestosis, vital capacity, functional residual capacity, and total lung capacity are reduced. Diffusing capacity is also decreased, and in more advanced cases, resting arterial oxygen tension may be reduced. Obstructive defects may occur, even in the absence of smoking. Currently, the most common abnormality seen in patients with asbestosis is a mixed restrictive and obstructive pattern in lung function. This is consistent with pathological observations that show peribronchiolar fibrosis early in the course of asbestosis, with distortion of the airways in some advanced cases.

Diagnosis usually requires a history of sufficient exposure to asbestos, established by an accurate occupational history, by the presence of pleural thickening or plaques, or by asbestos bodies in sputum or bronchoalveolar lavage, and by sufficient latency (usually 15 or more years), combined with some or all of the following features: "rales" or crackles; positive chest X-ray or high-resolution CT (most sensitive) findings for fibrosis (which may only appear later in the course of disease); reduced lung function (vital capacity, total lung capacity, diffusion capacity, or arterial oxygen tension reduction with exercise); and shortness of breath on effort.

There is no specific treatment, apart from alleviation of the symptoms. Patients with asbestosis are at higher risk than others of developing lung cancer, and that risk is significantly higher if they smoke. Workers with asbestosis should be removed from further exposure as the risk that parenchymal scarring will progress appears to increase with cumulative asbestos exposure.

Studies of workers exposed to chrysotile asbestos in different sectors have broadly demonstrated exposure-response relationships for chrysotile-induced asbestosis, insofar as increasing levels of exposure have produced increases in the incidence and severity of the disease. However, there are difficulties in defining this relationship due to factors such as uncertainties in diagnosis and the possibility of disease progression on cessation of exposure.

Lung Cancer Asbestos (actinolite, amosite, anthophylliyte, chrysotile, crocidolite, and tremolite) has been classified by the WHO International Agency for Research on Cancer (IARC) as being carcinogenic to humans. Exposure to chrysotile, amosite, and anthophyllite asbestos and to mixtures containing crocidolite results in an increased risk of lung cancer.

Despite reduced use, lung cancer is a major asbestos-related disease, accounting for about 20% of all deaths in asbestos-exposed cohorts, and up to 7% of all lung cancer is attributable to asbestos exposure.

In fact, high and protracted exposure to asbestos fibers increases the risk of developing bronchopulmonary cancer, even where there is no asbestosis. There is clearly a dose-effect relationship here, but the threshold for cancer induction cannot be identified. Exposure to other carcinogens, especially tobacco smoke, exacerbates the risk. At the same level of exposure, the risk to smokers is 10 times that of non-smokers. Latency periods between exposure to asbestos and the onset of pathological symptoms are on average 15–20 years, and may be as long as 30 years. The disease and its progression have no specificity compared with other cancers of the lung. The same applies to the options for treating it, which vary depending on the nature of the tumor, its stage, and its site. Whilst the prognosis is still often very poor, lung cancer can be cured, especially if it is diagnosed early.

Exposure-response relationships for lung cancer have been estimated for chrysotile mining and milling operations and for production of chrysotile asbestos textiles, asbestos-cement products, and asbestos friction products. Risks increased with increasing exposure. The slopes of the linear dose-response relationships (expressed as the increase in the lung cancer relative risk per unit of cumulative exposure (fiber/ml-years)) were all positive (although some not significantly) but varied widely. Textiles produce the highest risk. Risks for production of cement products, friction materials (slopes 0.0005–0.0006), and chrysotile mining are lower. The relative risks of lung cancer in the textile manufacturing sector in relation to estimated cumulative exposure are, therefore, some 10 to 30 times greater than those observed in chrysotile mining. The reasons for this variation in risk are not clear.

Malignant Mesothelioma Malignant mesothelioma is a cancer with unique features of etiology, diagnosis, management, and prevention. This tumor is uncommon, accounting for only a small fraction of deaths caused by cancer, but it and other asbestos-related diseases have been of great interest to occupational health physicians, public health professionals, biomedical researchers, and personal injury attorneys.

The first case reports of mesothelioma associated with asbestos were published in the 1940s, but the problem received scant attention until 1960, when diffuse pleural mesotheliomas were associated with asbestos exposure in the Cape Province of South Africa.

There has been a dramatic epidemic increase in incidence throughout the world during the past 40 years. The total global burden of asbestos-related mesothelioma in the 20th and 21st centuries has been estimated by the ILO at 2 million cases, with most cases yet to occur.

The ILO and WHO have estimated incidence in North America, Western Europe, Japan, Australia, and New Zealand at 10,000 cases per year, and a greater number of cases per year elsewhere in the world. Incidence in the United States is estimated at 3,000 cases per year. More than 90% of cases are pleural; less than 10%, peritoneal. Incidence in males is 5 to 6 times that of females. Incidence is increasing in both sexes and is predicted to reach a maximum in 2020 in Western Europe, in 2010 in Australia, and much later in Japan, Eastern Europe, and developing countries. Incidence may be leveling out or decreasing in the United States and Scandinavian countries, which restricted asbestos exposure earlier than other countries.

Malignant mesothelioma most commonly occurs in the pleura, less commonly in the peritoneum, and much more rarely in the pericardium and other lining tissues. Nearly all cases are related to asbestos exposure. The clinical presentation of the pleural tumor is often a pleural effusion (in 95% of patients), chest pain, and dyspnea (in 40% to 70% of patients). The peritoneal tumor commonly presents with ascites or bowel obstruction.

A detailed history of occupational and environmental asbestos exposure is vital to diagnosis. Mesothelioma is a disease of long latency, generally 20 to 50 years from first exposure to the time of diagnosis. A history of asbestos exposure can be obtained in approximately 90% of cases. Accounting for about 5% of cases is non-occupational exposure to bystanders, in domestic or hobby situations, or environmental exposure near a mine, factory, or natural or human-made surface deposits of asbestos.

Epidemiologic data show that exposure to asbestos can result in mesothelioma, without a clear dose-response relationship. Also, although both chrysotile and amphiboles can apparently cause cancer, there is some evidence that amphiboles are more likely to produce mesothelioma and lung cancer.

Chest radiography and tomography demonstrates pleural opacity. Tissue diagnosis can be made on pleural or peritoneal fluid cytology or pleural biopsy obtained via needle biopsy, thoracoscopy, or thoracotomy. Peritoneoscopy or laparotomy may be required to obtain tissue in peritoneal mesothelioma.

Despite active research into new treatments, mesothelioma is nearly always fatal, with no effective curative therapy available. Thus, mortality equals incidence. Median survival from initial diagnosis is generally about six months. Peritoneal tumors have a worse prognosis than pleural tumors.

Other Pleural Conditions Asbestos fibers migrate very readily from the lung to the pleura, where they cause a range of lesions: pleural plaques, pleurisy, diffuse pleural fibrosis. Pleural plaques are areas of fibrosis, with pleural thickening and, sometimes, calcifications. Unlike asbestosis, these benign pleural plaques do not in general cause problems. They are usually identified on a chest X-ray. Regarded as a "marker" of asbestos exposure, they are not a predictor of mesothelioma.

International Recommendations on Prevention of Asbestos-related Diseases

Bearing in mind that there is no evidence for a threshold for the carcinogenic effect of asbestos and that increased cancer risks have been observed in populations exposed to very low levels, the most efficient way to eliminate asbestos-related diseases is to stop using all types of asbestos. Continued use of asbestos cement in the construction industry is a particular concern because the workforce is large, it is difficult to control exposure, and in-place materials have the potential

Asbestos in India

"Rapidly industrializing India is described by the International Monetary Fund as a young, disciplined, and vibrant economy with a projected growth of 6.7% for 2005. The total workforce of 397 million has only 7% of workers employed in the organized sector with construction, where asbestos exposure is prevalent, employing 4.4%. The domestic production of asbestos declined from 20,111 tons in 1998–1999 to 14,340 tons in 2002–2003. The imports from Russia and Canada increased from 61,474 tons in 1997–1998 to 97,884 tons in 2001–2002. The production of asbestos cement products went up from 0.68 million tons in 1993–1994 to 1.38 million tons in 2002–2003. The asbestos industry has been delicensed since March 2003. The number of asbestos-based units stood at 32, with the western state of Maharashtra having the largest number. According to official figures, the industry employs 8,000 workers. The occupational exposure standard is still 2 fibers/mL, worse still, mesothelioma is not recognized as an occupational disease. The latest cancer registry data have no information on mesothelioma. The health and safety legislation does not cover 93% of workers in the unorganized sector where asbestos exposures are extremely high. Workers remain uninformed and untrained in dealing with asbestos exposure. Enforcement agencies are not fully conscious of the risks of asbestos exposure. Industrial hygiene assessment is seldom carried out and pathologists do not receive training in identifying mesothelioma histopathologically [under the microscope]. The lack of political will and powerful influence of the asbestos industry are pushing India toward a disaster of unimaginable proportion."

Quoted from: Joshi. T. K., U. B. Bhuva, and P. Katoch. 2006. "Asbestos Ban in India: Challenges Ahead." *Ann New York Acad Sci* 1076: 292–308.

to deteriorate and pose a risk to those carrying out alterations, maintenance, and demolition. In its various applications, asbestos can be replaced by some fiber materials and by other products that pose less or no risk to health.

Materials containing asbestos should be encapsulated and, in general, it is not recommended to carry out work that is likely to disturb asbestos fibers. If necessary, such work should be carried out only under strict preventive measures to avoid exposure to asbestos, such as encapsulation, wet processes, local exhaust ventilation with filtration, and regular cleaning. It also requires the use of personal protective equipment—special respirators, safety goggles, protective gloves and clothing—and the provision of special facilities for their decontamination.

WHO has announced that, in collaboration with ILO and with other intergovernmental organizations and civil society, they will work with countries toward elimination of asbestos-related diseases in the following strategic directions:

- recognizing that the most efficient way to eliminate asbestos-related diseases is to stop the use of all types of asbestos

- providing information about solutions for replacing asbestos with safer substitutes and developing economic and technological mechanisms to stimulate its replacement
- taking measures to prevent exposure to asbestos in place and during asbestos removal (abatement)
- improving early diagnosis, treatment, social and medical rehabilitation of asbestos-related diseases and by establishing registries of people with past and/or current exposures to asbestos

---

Box 9.3

The ILO/WHO Model National Program for the Elimination of Asbestos-related Diseases

In 2006, the International Labour Organization declared that "… the elimination of the future use of asbestos and the identification and proper management of asbestos currently in place are the most effective means to protect workers from asbestos exposure and to prevent future asbestos-related diseases and deaths …" The World Health Organization and the ILO have jointly launched the "ILO/WHO Model National Program for the Elimination of Asbestos-related Diseases," which includes the strategic actions outlined below:

National level

Action at the national level should create a political, regulatory, and social environment and appropriate institutional framework conducive to elimination of asbestos-related diseases. Such action would include:

a) political commitment to the elimination of asbestos-related diseases, e.g., prepare a national report on elimination of asbestos-related diseases to be presented to the government or the parliament, including information about past and current use, estimates of health, economic and social consequences of continuing use of chrysotile asbestos, and proposals for a package of measures to be taken to phase out its use and to prevent/contain the epidemic of asbestos-related diseases

b) ratification of international legal instruments (ILO conventions No. 162 and 139, Basel and Rotterdam conventions) and development of specific laws and regulations to prevent exposure to the different forms of asbestos, to phase out their use, and to ensure the prevention of asbestos-related diseases

c) introduction of fiscal mechanisms to reduce the use of chrysotile asbestos, e.g., import and excise duties, loans for conversion to non-asbestos technologies, establishment of a national fund for elimination of asbestos-related diseases with contribution from duty holders, insurance and compensation boards, governmental subsidy, etc.

d) updating and enforcement of occupational exposure limits for various forms of asbestos, e.g., align national occupational exposure limits to those listed in the IPCS Chemical Safety Card for Chrysotile; establishment of resources for determining the mineralogical form of asbestos and for measuring and monitoring its concentration in the air; introduction of practical tools for assessment and management of the risk from potential exposure; and creation of a national reference laboratory

e) provision of an effective system of inspection and enforcement of technical standards and safety measures through strengthening the authority of the enforcement agencies in the areas of labor, building maintenance, construction, environment, public health, accreditation, and standardization; provision of guidelines for enterprises and economic undertakings for management of asbestos-related health risks, etc.

f) organization of early detection, notification, registration, reporting, and compensation of asbestos-related diseases through improving diagnostic capacities for early detection of asbestosis and non-malignant asbestos-related disorders, clinical and pathological diagnosis of mesothelioma; establishing the causal relationship between lung and laryngeal cancer with exposure to asbestos; inclusion of all asbestos-related diseases in the national list of occupational diseases and development of diagnostic and exposure criteria for their recognition; establishing a fund for compensation of victims of asbestos-related diseases

g) provision of governmental advisory services to industry, trade, and other economic undertakings, workers and their organizations, and building owners on the use of safer substitutes for asbestos, application of preventive measures, and raising awareness about the risks related to the use of asbestos

h) enhancement of international collaboration to stimulate the transfer of know-how on alternatives to asbestos and best practices for prevention of asbestos-related diseases

Regional (provincial) level

Local authorities should be involved in the efforts for elimination of asbestos-related diseases. Local authorities are usually responsible for issuing building licenses and monitoring the housing stock, landfills, etc. In addition, municipalities may employ workers for building maintenance, reparation, and demolition works that may involve exposure to asbestos. Local authorities may be able to take the following actions:

a) introduce requirements for the use of safer substitutes for asbestos products and/ or prohibit and enforce the prohibition of the production and use of chrysotile asbestos and asbestos-containing products

b) ensure that work involving potential exposure to the various forms of asbestos, e.g., demolition of structures containing asbestos, reparation, and removal of asbestos from structures in which it is liable to become airborne, are carried out only by certified employers or contractors

c) take measures to dispose properly of asbestos-containing waste wetted, transported covered, buried at special landfills, and impregnated with agents that form a crust resistant to erosion

d) increase awareness among the general public of the hazards of demolition, removal, and reparations of friable asbestos insulation in buildings and disseminate information about the risks related to the presence of undisturbed asbestos in buildings

e) organize medical surveillance of municipal workers who might be exposed to asbestos in their work

Enterprise level

Actions at this level should aim to reduce and eliminate the risks of exposure to asbestos. Enterprises can take the action in the following directions:

a) replace chrysotile asbestos with safer substitutes and prevent potential exposure to any other type of asbestos already in place
b) promote the elimination of the use of chrysotile asbestos among contractors and suppliers
c) monitor the work environment for contamination with various forms of asbestos
d) ensure compliance with exposure limits and technical standards for working with asbestos
e) establish engineering measures for control of the exposure to asbestos at the source
f) provide special training for workers involved in activities with potential exposure to asbestos
g) provide appropriate personal protective equipment
h) ensure registration and medical surveillance of workers exposed to asbestos

Detailed guidance on actions to be taken at the enterprise level can be found in the ILO Code of Practice on Safety in the Use of Asbestos (1984) and in the practical guide on best practice to prevent or minimize asbestos risks in work that involves (or may involve) asbestos: for the employer, the workers, and the labor inspector, developed by Senior Labor Inspectors Committee of the European Union (European Union 2006).

Source: International Labor Office. 2007. *ILO/WHO Outline for the Development of National Programmes for Elimination of Asbestos-Related Diseases.* Available at http://www.ilo.org/wcmsp5/groups/public/—ed_protect/—protrav/—safework/documents/publication/wcms_108555.pdf

CHEMICAL ASPHYXIANTS

Carbon Monoxide

Chemical Formula: CO; Chemical Abstracts Service Number (CAS): 630-08-0

Uses and Potential Sources of Occupational Exposure Carbon monoxide is ubiquitous in our environment, as it is a product of incomplete combustion. Common non-occupational sources include space heaters, furnaces, and internal combustion engines. It is also a product of tobacco smoke. Occupational exposure to carbon monoxide is common where combustion occurs, e.g., blast furnace operations and emissions from automobile exhaust. Automotive garage workers, traffic policemen, tunnel workers, and firefighters are at particular risk. Carbon monoxide is also a metabolite of dichloromethane (methylene chloride), a solvent and paint stripper in common industrial and home use.

Adverse Health Effects Approximately 80% to 90% of the absorbed amount of carbon monoxide binds with hemoglobin, forming carboxyhemoglobin (HbCO). HbCO causes oxygen to detach from adjacent hemoglobin, thus reducing the oxygen-carrying capacity of the blood. The affinity of hemoglobin for carbon monoxide is 200 to 250 times that for oxygen. HbCO shifts the oxyhemoglobin dissociation curve to the left, thus interfering with the delivery of oxygen to tissues. Carbon monoxide also binds reversibly to other heme proteins, such as myoglobin, cytochrome oxidase, cytochrome P-450, and hydroperoxidases. However, its most important effects are on hemoglobin.

The combination of decreased oxygen-carrying capacity of the blood, impaired release of oxygen to tissues, and interference with intracellular oxidation processes results in tissue hypoxia that is proportional to the HbCO saturation and oxygen demand. The brain, cardiovascular system, exercising skeletal muscle, and the developing fetus are the tissues most sensitive to this hypoxia. Thus, toxic effects are of concern in neurobehavioral function, cardiovascular exercise capacity, and fetal development. Carbon monoxide does not appear to have large and consistent behavioral effects on healthy, young volunteers with HbCO levels below 10%. However, exposure to carbon monoxide resulting in prolonged HbCO level of 5 to 10% may affect the performance of tasks requiring a high degree of vigilance, such as flying an aircraft or monitoring a control panel. Moreover, carbon monoxide exposure can reduce the capacity to perform strenuous physical activity at HbCO levels above 2.5%. People with coronary artery disease are particularly sensitive to carbon monoxide. Decreased exercise time to onset of angina or ischemia was observed at HbCO levels as low as 3% and increased ventricular arrhythmias at HbCO levels of 6%. Carbon monoxide exposure during pregnancy may result in low birth weight and possibly diminish the mental ability of children.

Carboxyhemoglobin (HbCO) in blood or expired air, determined by spectrophotometric methods, is by far the most common index for carbon monoxide exposure.

Hydrogen Sulfide

Chemical Formula: H_2S; CAS: 7783-06-4

Uses and Potential Sources of Occupational Exposure Hydrogen sulfide is a byproduct of many industrial processes, especially in proximity to oil wells and in areas where petroleum products are processed, stored, or used. It is also produced during the decay of organic matter and is naturally occurring in coal, natural gas, oil, volcanic gases, manure pits and sewage tanks, and in natural sulfur springs.

Adverse Health Effects Hydrogen sulfide is a highly toxic gas. At extremely high concentrations, it may exert a direct paralyzing effect on the respiratory center. Hydrogen sulfide is also known to inhibit cytochrome oxidase, resulting in altered oxidative metabolism; it can also disrupt critical disulfide bonds in essential cellular proteins. Exposure to high concentrations can result in unconsciousness and respiratory paralysis. A five-minute exposure to a concentration of 1,000 ppm can be lethal to humans. Prolonged exposure to concentrations between 250 and 500 ppm can cause respiratory irritation, congestion of the lungs, and bronchial pneumonia. Low concentrations are irritating to the eyes. Conjunctivitis may result from exposure to 20 to 30 ppm.

Hydrogen Cyanide (Hydrocyanic Acid, Prussic Acid)

Chemical Formula: HCN; CAS: 74-90-8

Uses and Potential Sources of Occupational Exposure Hydrogen cyanide is used to produce methyl methacrylate, acrylates, cyanuric chloride, triazines, sodium cyanide, dyes, rodenticides, and some pesticides. It occurs in beet sugar residues and coke oven gas as well as in the roots of certain plants, such as sorghum, cassava, and peach tree. Firefighters may be exposed to HCN in fires. Materials such as polyurethane foam, silk, wool, polyacrylonitrile, and nylon fibers burn to produce HCN.

Adverse Health Effects HCN is a dangerous, acute poison. The cyanide ion exerts an inhibitory action on certain metabolic enzyme systems, most notably cytochrome oxidase, the enzyme involved in the ultimate transfer of electrons to molecular oxygen. Because cytochrome oxidase is present in practically all cells that function under aerobic conditions, and because the cyanide ion diffuses easily to all parts of the body, cyanide quickly halts practically all cellular respiration. Lethal effects due to inhalation of its vapor depend on its concentration in air and time of exposure. Inhalation of 270 ppm of HCN in air can be fatal to humans instantly, while 135 ppm can cause death after 30 minutes. Exposure to high concentrations can cause asphyxia and injure the central nervous system, cardiovascular system, liver, and kidneys. HCN is extremely toxic via ingestion, skin absorption, and ocular routes. Swallowing 50 mg can be fatal to humans. The symptoms of HCN poisoning at lethal dosage are labored breathing, shortness of breath, paralysis, unconsciousness, convulsions, and respiratory failure. At lower concentrations, toxic effects are headache, nausea, and vomiting.

SOLVENTS

Solvents are substances (usually liquids) capable of dissolving one or more substances (solutes) with the formation of a uniformly dispersed mixture (solution) at the molecular or ionic size level. Industrial solvents are of major toxicological concern, as many are irritant or toxic to humans, especially to workers who are repeatedly exposed to a given solvent or its fumes. Organic solvents are compounds or mixtures used as solvents; they include aliphatic and aromatic hydrocarbons, alcohols, aldehydes, ketones, chlorinated hydrocarbons, and carbon disulfide. The vapors of organic solvents may be toxic. Exposure can occur by contact with the liquid or, in most cases, with the fumes or vapors. Contact may cause skin irritation, defatting, or dermatoses, especially after long-term exposure. Occupational exposure to solvent vapors is usually by inhalation, although skin absorption may also occur. Most organic solvent vapors have an anesthetic effect on the central nervous system; some are nephrotoxic and/or hepatotoxic; and some can damage the blood-forming system.

CHLORINATED HYDROCARBONS

Trichloroethylene

Chemical Formula: C_2HCl_3; CAS: 79-01-6

Uses and Potential Sources of Occupational Eexposure
Metal degreasing; extraction solvent for oils, fats, waxes; solvent dyeing; dry cleaning; refrigerant and heat exchange liquid; fumigant; cleaning and drying

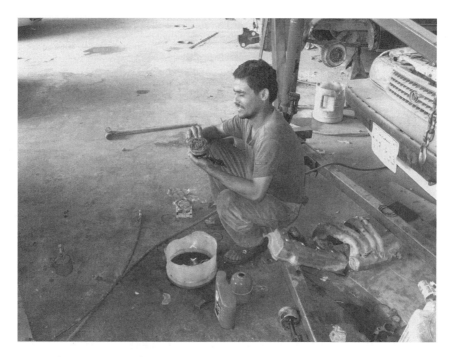

Figure 9.4 Cleaning automobile parts exposes this worker to solvents through skin absorption and through inhalation. (Photograph by Seifeddin Ballal, King Faisal University, Saudi Arabia.)

electronic parts; diluent in paints and adhesives; textile processing; chemical intermediate; aerospace operations (flushing liquid oxygen).

Adverse Health Effects The toxic effects manifested in workers from inhaling trichloroethylene vapors are headache, dizziness, drowsiness, fatigue, and visual disturbances. A 2-hour exposure to a 1,000-ppm concentration affects visual perception. Higher concentrations can produce narcotic effects. Heavy exposures may cause death due to respiratory failure or cardiac arrest. Although trichloroethylene exhibits low toxicity, its metabolite trichloroethanol, and oxidative degradation products, such as phosgene and chlorine, can cause severe health hazards. So far, this solvent exhibits evidence of carcinogenicity only in laboratory animals (International Agency for Research on Cancer [IARC] Classification Group 3). The biological monitoring of occupational exposure may use trichloroacetic acid (TCA) and/or trichloroethanol (TCE) concentration in urine.

Tetrachloroethylene (Perchloroethylene)

Chemical Formula: C_2Cl_4; CAS: 127-18-4

Uses and Potential Sources of Occupational Exposure Dry-cleaning solvents, vapor-degreasing solvents, drying agent for metals and certain other solids, vermifuge, heat-transfer medium, manufacture of fluorocarbons.

Adverse Health Effects Exposure to tetrachloroethylene can produce headache, dizziness, drowsiness, lack of coordination, irritation of eyes, nose, and throat, and flushing of neck and face. Exposure to high concentrations can produce narcotic effects. The primary target organs are the central nervous system, mucous membranes, eyes, and skin. The kidneys, liver, and lungs are affected to a lesser extent. Symptoms of central nervous system depression are manifested in humans from repeated exposure to 200 ppm for 7 hours/day. Chronic exposure has caused peripheral neuropathy. Skin contact with the liquid may cause defatting and dermatitis of the skin. Evidence of carcinogenicity of this compound has been noted in test animals subjected to inhalation or oral administration. It causes tumors in the blood, liver, and kidneys in rats and mice. Although the IARC has determined that evidence for carcinogenicity to humans is inadequate, the U.S. National Institute of Occupational Safety and Health recommends that this substance be handled as a potential human carcinogen.

AROMATIC HYDROCARBONS

Benzene

Chemical Formula: C_6H_6; CAS 71-43-2

Uses and Potential Sources of Occupational Exposure Manufacturing of ethylbenzene (for styrene monomer); dodecylbenzene (for detergents); cyclohexane (for nylon); phenol; nitrobenzene (for aniline); maleic anhydride; chlorobenzene; diphenyl; benzene hexachloride; benzene-sulfonic acid; as a solvent.

Adverse Health Effects At high concentrations, benzene has a narcotic effect on the central nervous system. Inhalation of 7,500 ppm for 30 minutes to 1 hour may cause loss of consciousness and death from respiratory failure. Levels of 3,000 ppm may cause euphoria and excitation followed by fatigue, dizziness, and nausea. Acute effects include light-headedness, headache, excitement, unsteady gait, confusion, euphoria, nausea, vertigo, and drowsiness. If exposure continues, respiratory paralysis and death, sometimes with convulsions, may occur. The chronic effects of benzene exposure depend on the level of exposure, and symptoms are typically vague.

Chronic benzene intoxication creates a disturbance in the hematopoietic (blood-forming) system that may affect every cell type. The most frequently reported adverse health effect of benzene is bone marrow depression leading to aplastic anemia, a condition in which the bone marrow stops making blood cells. At high levels of exposure, a high incidence of both bone marrow depression and aplastic anemia would be seen, and some damage would also be seen at lower doses. Benzene is a well-established human carcinogen. Epidemiological studies of benzene-exposed workers have demonstrated a causal relationship between benzene exposure and the development of acute myelogenous leukemia, the most common form of leukemia in adults. Benzene exposure may be associated with other forms of cancer, but this remains to be proven. A task group established by the WHO and the International Program on Chemical Safety (IPCS) concluded some years ago that "a time-weighted average of 3.2 mg/m³ (1 ppm) over a 40-year working career has not been statistically associated with any increase in deaths from leukemia. However, because benzene is a human carcinogen, exposures should be limited to the lowest level technically feasible. Increases in exposure level to over 32 mg/m^3 (10 ppm) should be avoided. Benzene and benzene-containing products such as gasoline should never be used for cleaning purposes."

Toluene (Methylbenzene; Phenylmethane)

Chemical Formula: $C_6H_5CH_3$; CAS: 108-88-3

Uses and Potential Sources of Occupational Exposure Aviation gasoline and high-octane blending stock; benzene, phenol, and caprolactam; solvent for paints and coatings, gums, resins, most oils, rubber, vinyl organosols; diluent and thinner in nitrocellulose lacquers; adhesive solvent in plastic toys and model airplanes; chemicals (benzoic acid, benzyl and benzoyl derivatives, saccharin, medicines, dyes, perfumes); source of toluene-di-isocyanates (polyurethane resins); explosives (TNT); toluene sulfonates (detergents); scintillation counters.

Adverse Health Effects The acute toxicity of toluene is similar to that of benzene. The exposure routes are inhalation, ingestion, and absorption through the skin, and the organs affected from its exposure are the central nervous system, liver, kidneys, and skin. At high concentrations, it is a narcotic. In humans, acute exposure can produce excitement, euphoria, hallucinations, distorted perceptions, confusion, headache, and dizziness. Such effects may be perceptible at an exposure level of 200 ppm in air. Higher concentrations can produce depression, drowsiness, and stupor. Inhalation of 10,000 ppm may cause death to humans from respiratory failure. Chronic exposure may cause some accumulation of toluene in fatty tissues, which may be eliminated over time. The chronic effects of toluene can be severe because the neurotoxicity of toluene causes brain damage in people who are heavily exposed. Toluene, unlike benzene, is not known to cause bone marrow depression or anemia. Toluene is metabolized to benzoic acid and finally to hippuric acid and benzoyl-glucoronide. The latter two are excreted in urine along with small amounts of cresols, formed by direct hydroxylation of toluene. Hippuric acid—the major metabolite of toluene—can be used for biological monitoring.

Xylene (Dimethylbenzene)

Chemical Formula: $C_6H_4(CH_3)_2$; CAS: 133-20-7

Uses and Potential Sources of Occupational Exposure Xylene is among the most commonly used solvents and is also a material for organic synthesis in industry. It is a constituent of unleaded automobile gasoline. Its uses include aviation gasoline, protective coatings, solvent for alkyl resins, lacquers, enamels, and rubber cements, and synthesis of organic chemicals. *m*-xylene (CAS: 108-38-3): solvent; intermediate for dyes and organic synthesis, especially isophthalic acid; insecticides; aviation fuel. *o*-xylene (CAS 95-47-60): manufacture of phthalic anhydride, vitamin and pharmaceutical syntheses, dyes, insecticides, and motor fuels.

p-xylene: synthesis of terephthalic acid for polyester resins and fibers ("Dacron," "Mylar," "Terylene"); vitamin and pharmaceutical syntheses; insecticides.

Adverse Health Effects The toxicity profile of the three xylene isomers is similar to that of toluene, namely, the most important occupationally related effect is suppression of the function of the central nervous system, as evidenced in various subjective symptoms.

Carbon Disulfide

Chemical Formula: CS_2; CAS: 75-15-0

Uses and Potential Sources of Occupational Exposure Carbon disulfide is a widely used industrial solvent. Its principal use is in the production of rayon and cellulose. It is used as an intermediate in the production of carbon tetrachloride and some pesticides and as a solvent in the rubber industry.

Adverse Health Effects Carbon disulfide is absorbed via the lungs and skin. Pulmonary absorption is the most significant. Pulmonary retention at the start of exposure is about 80% and declines steadily, reaching a plateau within 2 hours of approximately 40% of the inhaled concentration. Carbon disulfide is a potent neurotoxin. Peripheral neuropathies, cranial nerve dysfunction, and neuropsychiatric changes characterize the neurologic illness associated with excessive carbon disulfide exposures. These neuropsychiatric symptoms may be irreversible. Chronic long-term exposure may result in central nervous system involvement, decreased glucose tolerance, reduced serum thyroxine (thyroid hormone) levels, ocular injury, central and peripheral neuropathies, increased triglycerides and low density lipoproteins, and parkinsonism. Increases in the incidence of atherosclerosis, coronary artery disease, hypertensive disease, personality changes, and suicide rates have been reported from epidemiological studies. Xylene is also irritating to mucous membranes and thus causes eye and throat irritation.

METALS

Arsenic

Chemical Formula: As; CAS: 7440-38-2

Uses and Potential Sources of Occupational Exposure (Metallic Form) Alloying additive for metals, especially lead and copper as shot or other ammunition, battery grids, cable sheaths, and boiler tubes. High-purity (semiconductor) grade: used to make gallium arsenide for dipoles and other electronic devices, doping agent in germanium and silicon solid state products, special solders, medicine. The principal occupational hazards of arsenic exposure arise in the preparation of herbicides and pesticides and in industrial processes in which arsenic trioxide is a by-product. Exposure to arsenic is also possible when it occurs as a by-product in the smelting of certain metals, which liberates the oxidized form. Unlike most industries, in which the use of arsenic is on the decline, the electronics industry has been increasing its use of arsenic, particularly in the form of gallium arsenide, which is used in the production of semiconductors.

Adverse Health Effects All arsenic compounds are toxic; the toxicity varies with the oxidation state and solubility of the metal. Thus, the trivalent inorganic compounds of arsenic, such as arsenic trichloride, arsenic trioxide, and arsine are highly toxic—more poisonous than the metal and its pentavalent salts. The organic arsenic compound Lewisite is a severe blistering agent that can penetrate the skin and cause damage at the point of exposure. Lewisite was used as a poison gas in World War I. Less soluble arsenic sulfide exhibits a lower acute toxicity. Arsenic is absorbed into the body through the gastrointestinal route and by inhalation. The acute symptoms include fever, gastrointestinal disturbances, irritation of the respiratory tract, ulceration of the nasal septum, and dermatitis. Chronic exposure can produce pigmentation of the skin, peripheral neuropathy (often painful disorders of the nerves outside the central nervous system), and degeneration of the liver and kidneys. The toxic effects of arsenic are attributed to its binding properties with sulfur. It forms complexes with coenzymes. This inhibits the production of adenosine triphosphate (ATP), which is essential for energy in body metabolism. Arsenic is carcinogenic to humans and is associated with lung, skin, and bladder cancers. Ingestion by an oral route has caused an increased incidence of tumors in the liver, blood, and lungs.

Beryllium

Chemical Formula: Be; CAS 7440-41-7

Uses and Potential Sources of Occupational Exposure Structural material in space technology; moderator and reflector of neutrons in nuclear reactors; source of neutrons when bombarded with alpha particles; special windows for X-ray tubes; in gyroscopes, computer parts, inertial guidance systems; additive in solid propellant rocket fuels; beryllium-copper alloys, which are commonly used in aerospace and high-performance brakes for planes and trains.

Adverse Health Effects The main target organs for beryllium-related health effects are the skin and lungs. When workers are exposed to beryllium or its compounds, a small percentage of them will develop granulomatous lung disease, known as chronic beryllium disease. In the beryllium extraction industry, a large percentage of workers may develop contact dermatitis and/or beryllium skin ulcers in relation to exposure to the soluble salt. Historically, workers who extracted beryllium ore were described as experiencing chemical inflammation (nasopharyngitis, tracheobronchitis, and/or pneumonitis) with subacute onset, which resolved with the cessation of exposure to beryllium salts, always within one year of symptom onset. X-ray evaluation of these patients shows diffuse pulmonary fibrosis, bilateral haziness, varying degrees of emphysema, and microscopic granulomatous (tight local scarring) lesions in the lungs; these lesions sometimes are also seen on the skin of face and in other organs, such as the liver and spleen. In contrast, chronic beryllium disease may develop after workers have left the beryllium industry, sometimes with a latency of several decades from first exposure; it is irreversible and sometimes fatal. The diagnosis of beryllium disease requires evidence of lymphocyte proliferation to beryllium in blood or lavage lymphocytes. This specific characteristic differentiates the disease from other granulomatous diseases, such as sarcoidosis and hypersensitivity pneumonitis. Beryllium has been classified as a potential human carcinogen by the IARC and is known to be associated with lung cancer in animal studies.

Cadmium

Chemical Formula: Cd; CAS 744-43-9

Uses and Potential Sources of Occupational Exposure Cadmium is widely dispersed in the environment. In non-occupationally exposed persons, food and tobacco consumption represent the main sources of exposure to cadmium. In industries where workers are highly exposed to fumes and dust, cadmium is widely found. Occupations with potential exposure to cadmium and cadmium compounds include the following: a) high risk—alloy makers, battery workers, pigment workers, plastic workers, smelters and refiners, welders; and b) moderate/low risk—brazing workers, coating workers, diamond workers, electroplaters, electrical contact workers, enameling workers, engravers, glass workers, laser workers, metalizers, paint workers, semiconductor and superconductor workers, solder workers, transistor makers, etc. Workers may be exposed to cadmium in these occupations via inhalation of the finely ground particulates (e.g., pigment dusts) or via cadmium oxide fumes generated during heating or welding of cadmium-containing materials.

Adverse Health Effects Cadmium may cause acute and long-term effects. In humans, the principal acute manifestations are gastrointestinal disturbances following ingestion and chemical pneumonitis following inhalation of cadmium oxide. Cadmium fumes, when inhaled in sufficient concentrations, are toxic to the epithelial and endothelial cells of alveoli and cause acute pulmonary edema. In humans, the principal toxic effects resulting from long-term exposure to cadmium are renal dysfunction and lung impairment. Long-term inhalation exposure to cadmium dust or fumes in the cadmium industry has been shown to produce emphysematous lung changes. The kidney is the organ where the first signs of adverse effects are seen following long-term cadmium exposure. Some effects are irreversible. The possible role of occupational cadmium exposure for the development of cancer has been re-evaluated by IARC recently. Given sufficient evidence of the carcinogenicity of cadmium and cadmium compounds in humans (prostate cancer), cadmium and its compounds have been classified in Group 1: carcinogenic to humans.

Chromium

Chemical Formula: Cr; CAS: 7440-47-3

Uses and Potential Sources of Occupational Exposure Alloying and plating element on metal and plastic substrates for corrosion resistance, chromium-containing and stainless steels, protective coating for automotive and equipment accessories, nuclear and high-temperature research, constituent of inorganic pigments.

Several million workers worldwide are exposed to airborne fumes, mists, and dusts containing chromium or its compounds. Highest exposures to chromium VI may occur during chromate production, welding, chrome pigment manufacture, chrome plating, and spray painting; highest exposures to other forms of chromium occur during mining, ferrochromium and steel production, and welding, cutting, and grinding of chromium alloys. Chromium can exist in formal oxidation states of II to VI. The most stable oxidation states are 0, II, III, and VI. Chromium VI and III are the most common valence types in the workplace.

Adverse Health Effects Absorption of chromium compounds occurs mainly through inhalation. Chromium may reach the respiratory tract in the form of vapors, mists, fumes, or dusts, where it may be present in the hexavalent, trivalent, or elemental state. The absorption is dependent on the valence and solubility of the particular chromium species. Chromium transported by blood is distributed to tissues and organs that have a different retention capacity. The highest levels of chromium are found in the liver, kidneys, spleen, and lungs. Metallic chromium does not seem to have harmful health effects. Chromium VI compounds may cause adverse effects to the skin, the respiratory tract, and, to a lesser degree, the kidneys in humans, whereas chromium III is less toxic. Hexavalent (VI) chromium compounds seem to be more potent skin allergens, but trivalent (III) compounds may also cause eczema. Occupational exposure to the hexavalent salts can produce skin ulceration, dermatitis, perforation of the nasal septa, and kidney damage. According to IARC, there is sufficient evidence in humans to show the carcinogenicity of chromium VI compounds as encountered in the chromate production, chrome pigment production, and chromium plating industries. Lung cancer and nasal cancer have been reported frequently. There is inadequate evidence in humans to prove the carcinogenicity of metallic chromium and of chromium III compounds.

Lead

Chemical Formula: Pb; CAS: 7439-92-1

Uses and Potential Sources of Occupational Exposure People have always been exposed to lead, as it is ubiquitous in the environment; common sources include air, dust, food, and water. However, the Industrial Revolution introduced much more lead into the environment due to mining, smelting, and its use in industrial processes. The major source of exposure for children, historically, has been lead paint used in houses, leaded gasoline used in motor vehicles, and, occasionally, exposure from nearby smelting. The major source in air pollution has been leaded gasoline, which has led to a ban on leaded gasoline in many countries. It was estimated some years ago that 90% of atmospheric lead comes from automobile exhaust. Industrial emissions are also important sources in specific localities.

In many countries, a major reduction of lead in gasoline has resulted in a reduction of air lead levels in urban areas and is probably the most important contributing factor for lowering environmental lead exposure. Most studies have shown a decline in blood lead levels following a reduction of lead in gasoline. In terms of occupational exposure, the hazards from lead exist in a wide range of industrial settings. Estimates are that between 100 to 200 different occupation and job titles are considered to be associated with a potential risk of lead exposure. High-risk occupations include blasting or scraping of lead-painted metal, brass foundry work, flame welding and cutting of lead-painted metal, indoor shooting ranges, battery storage and manufacture, and lead smelting. Moderate to low-risk occupations include antique restoration, car repair, lead mining, lead soldering, and porcelain manufacture.

Adverse Health Effects Pulmonary deposition of lead particles suspended in air varies as a function of particle size distribution and respiratory rate. Particles with an aerodynamic diameter above 5 µm are mainly deposited in the upper airways, cleared by mucociliary mechanisms, and swallowed. Some of this lead is then absorbed from the gastrointestinal tract. Particles with a diameter below 1µm are deposited to a large extent directly in the alveolar region of the lung. Lead deposited in the deep lung is completely absorbed. Studies of the gastrointestinal absorption of stable lead in adults estimate an average absorption of about 10%. Once absorbed, lead is found in all tissues, but eventually more than 90% of the body burden is accumulated or redistributed into bone, where it remains with a half-life of many years. Lead is excreted primarily through the urine.

Lead poisoning is in most cases a chronic disease. The toxic effects of lead on humans can be diagnosed by observing the broad spectrum of laboratory and clinical manifestations, ranging from subtle subclinical biochemical abnormalities to severe clinical emergencies. In the beginning, inhibition of enzymes and other biochemical effects occur. At the intermediate stage, the effects of various enzyme inhibitions can be measured, such as inhibition of enzymes in the biosynthetic pathway of heme (the chemical unit that carries oxygen in hemoglobin and gives blood a red color) or accumulation of enzyme substrates. Clinically, the most significant adverse effects occur in the neurologic, hematologic, gastrointestinal, cardiovascular, renal, and reproductive systems. Wide variation exists in individual susceptibility to lead poisoning with a corresponding range in the spectrum of clinical findings. Symptoms sometimes appear in adults with blood lead concentrations as low as 25 µg/dL. More commonly, however, overt symptoms emerge in patients whose peak blood lead concentration has exceeded 40 to 60 µg/dL. Subacute or chronic intoxication is more common than acute poisoning.

Early symptoms are often subtle, non-specific, and subclinical, involving the nervous system (fatigue, irritability, sleep disturbance, headache, difficulty concentrating, decreased libido); the gastrointestinal system (abdominal cramps, anorexia, nausea, constipation, diarrhea); or musculoskeletal system (arthralgia, myalgia). A high level of intoxication may result in delirium, coma, and seizures associated with lead encephalopathy, an inflammation of the brain that is potentially life-threatening.

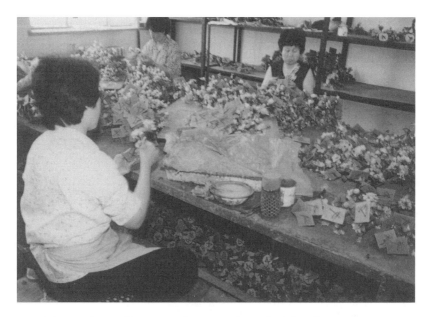

Figure 9.5 A factory (township enterprise) manufacturing glass flower arrangements, outside Beijing, in 1990. The glass contains high levels of lead, and the production of the glass leaves and flower petals exposed workers to high levels of lead; these workers are in the assembly area. (Photograph by Tee L. Guidotti, University of Alberta.)

Manganese

Chemical Formula: Mn; CAS: 7439-96-5

Uses and Potential Sources of Occupational Exposure Ferroalloys (steel manufacture), nonferrous alloys (improved corrosion resistance and hardness), high-purity salt for various chemical uses, purifying and scavenging agent in metal production, manufacture of aluminum by the so-called "Toth process."

Adverse Health Effects Finely ground dust and fumes have been linked to acute respiratory problems, including pneumonitis and increased susceptibility to infection. The literature contains numerous reports of pneumonia linked to industrial operations involving manganese (manganese ores, dusts, and fumes of manganese oxides). Methylcyclopentadienyl manganese tricarbonyl (often called MMT) and manganese cyclopentadienyl tricarbonyl, both organic manganese compounds used as fuel additives, are sometimes irritants to the skin, eyes, and upper airways.

The most prominent feature associated with chronic manganese overexposure is a neurological disorder called *manganism*, a constellation of signs and symptoms caused by a selective disruption of the dopaminergic neurons (essentially palladium, caudate nucleus, and putamen cells). Manganism, an illness similar to Parkinson's disease, is associated with exposure of several months or years to manganese or manganese compounds. It appears in several stages. Initially, an individual who is overexposed to manganese develops apathy, weakness, somnolence, a low monotonous voice, muscular twitching, stiffness in the leg muscles, and cramps. Diminished libido, slowed movements, insomnia, back pain, headache, clumsy movement, increased sweating and salivation, personality changes, instability, restlessness, a tendency to cry or laugh at inappropriate moments, and difficulty speaking, talking, and walking also develop. As manganism advances, additional symptoms of a more neurological nature develop, including a stolid, expressionless, mask-like face; muscular twitching or tremor of the hands; difficulty walking; a unique gait (because the individual tries to keep as wide a base as possible); inability to maintain balance; increased speech difficulties; memory loss; difficulty with fine movements such as writing; and urinary bladder disturbances. Walking becomes slower and spastic as the illness progresses. Recovery is rare, and dysfunction generally persists or progresses after cessation of exposure. L-dopa may improve the mental aberrations, but not the underlying neurological abnormalities.

Mercury

Chemical Formula: Hg; CAS: 7439-97-6

Uses and Potential Sources of Occupational Exposure Mercury occurs in a number of physical and chemical forms in three oxidation states: Hg0 (elemental or metallic mercury), Hg^+ (mercurous or monovalent mercury), and Hg^{2+} (mercuric or divalent mercury). Mercuric mercury also forms a number of organometallic compounds. Exposure to mercury vapor is the most common form of occupational exposure to mercury, occurring in various industries. The main route of absorption is via the respiratory tract. Mercury is used in dental amalgams, catalyst, electrical apparatus, cathodes for production of chlorine and caustic soda, instruments (thermometers, barometers, etc.), mercury vapor lamps, extractive metallurgy, mirror coating, arc lamps, boilers, and coolant and neutron absorbers in nuclear plants.

Adverse Health Effects Inhalation represents the main route of uptake of metallic mercury. About 80% of inhaled metallic mercury vapor is absorbed by the body, and about 20% is retained. Following absorption, red cell uptake, and physical dissolution of mercury vapor, mercury is rapidly transported to all parts of the body. Mercury vapor penetrates the brain and can cross the placenta. The principal sites of deposition of mercury are the kidneys and the brain after exposure to mercury vapor; the majority of mercuric mercury ends up in the kidneys. The biological half-life of mercury is approximately 2 months in the kidneys, but is much longer in the central nervous system.

Following intense exposure to elemental mercury vapor, lung damage (bronchial irritation, erosive bronchitis, diffuse interstitial pneumonitis) occurs, as do gastrointestinal and renal tubular necrosis after ingestion of mercuric mercury. Long-term exposure to elemental mercury can affect the central nervous system and kidneys; chronic exposure to mercuric mercury causes renal tubular damage. Immunologically based kidney damage (glomerulonephritis) can occur. The characteristic tremor may begin in the fingers, eyelids, lips, or tongue. Slight tremor has usually been accompanied by severe behavioral and personality changes, memory loss, increased excitability, and, in severe cases, delirium and hallucinations. This constellation of symptoms is called *mercurial erethism*. Renal manifestations of mercury exposure range from proteinuria (protein detectable in urine) at low exposures through the nephritic syndrome. Subclinical effects on the kidney have been detected through the measurement of urinary excretion of low and high molecular weight proteins and renal tubular enzymes (N-acetyl-β-D-glucosaminidase [NAG], β-galactosidase [GAL]).

Biological monitoring indices include the following: mercury in blood (indicator of recent exposure); mercury in urine (tends to reflect cumulative exposure over previous 2 to 4 months); and mercury in hair and nails (unreliable, no standardized technique available).

Nickel

Chemical Formula: Ni; CAS 7440-02-0

Uses and Potential Sources of Occupational Exposure Alloys (low-alloy steels, stainless steel, copper and brass, permanent magnets, electrical resistance alloys); electroplated protective coatings; electroformed coatings; alkaline storage battery; fuel cell electrodes; catalyst for methanation (adding carbons) of fuel gases; and hydrogenation of vegetable oils.

Adverse Health Effects Metallic nickel and certain nickel compounds cause sensitization dermatitis, known as "nickel itch," a chronic form of eczema. Nickel refining has been associated with an increased risk of nasal and lung cancer. Nickel refinery flue dust, nickel subsulfide (Ni_3S_2), and nickel oxide (NiO) produce localized tumors in experimental animals when injected intramuscularly. IARC has classified nickel and its compounds as carcinogenic to humans. Subsequently, this has been reviewed and the current consensus is that nickel cardinogenicity is species-specific (i.e., depends on the chemical form of nickel). Nickel subsulfide is clearly carcinogenic and inhalation can produce lung and sinus cancer in humans with a latency period of about 25 years. Inhalation of nickel metal dust probably does not initiate cancer.

PESTICIDES

Pesticides are any compound or formulation of chemicals used to destroy plant and animal pests or to inhibit their activity. Different pesticides are used to control different pests, and thus are referred to as insecticides (to control insects), herbicides (to control unwanted plants), molluscicides (to control snails), miticides (to control mites), rodenticides (to control rats), etc. Virtually all are toxic to humans at some level. Some, such as parathion (an important and widely used insecticide), are very toxic to human beings and have caused many deaths from poisoning. Others, such as malathion (an insecticide) and diazinon (an insecticide used on the ground), have low toxicity at levels of exposure typically encountered on the job.

The circumstances of work are usually important in cases of pesticide toxicity. Acute pesticide poisoning often occurs when workers do not use or are not provided with protective clothing and when they are not trained or cannot understand the language in which the instructions are written. Many pesticides are readily absorbed through the skin; therefore, dangerous levels of exposure may result during the mixing of pesticides for use and/or when handling concentrated pesticides in preparation for use.

Organochlorine Compounds

Organochlorine compounds or chlorinated hydrocarbons are halogenated compounds in which one or more hydrogen atoms have been replaced by chlorine atoms. They are broad-spectrum poisons and are toxic to nearly all animals, including many vertebrates. Organochlorine compounds were widely used in agriculture and malaria-control programs for decades, beginning in the mid-1940s. Their use declined in the 1960s, and today they have been nearly completely banned in most countries. This ban was instituted in response to evidence that these pesticides have a high potential for biomagnification in food chains. Evidence that many species, especially birds, were accumulating DDT in their bodies and that it was affecting their survival led to a widespread ban on DDT in most developed countries in the 1970s.

Organochlorine insecticides were heavily used and are still used in many countries for malaria control because of their low cost and high efficacy (Harbison

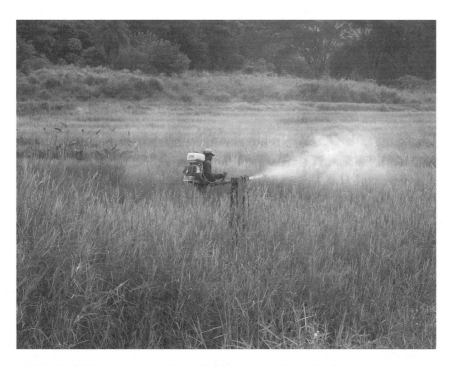

Figure 9.6 Pesticide sprayer treating a field in Costa Rica. The foggy appearance in the photograph is from the cloud of the spray that is enveloping the worker, causing high exposure by inhalation in addition to skin exposure. (Photograph courtesy of Dr. Patricia Monge, Central American Institute for Studies on Toxic Substances, National University of Costa Rica.)

1998). The amount of DDT or other organochlorine pesticides required to control mosquitoes is much less than the amount used to control insects on crops.

Among the most widely known chlorinated hydrocarbons are the cyclo-dienes such as aldrin, chlordane, dieldrin, endrin, heptachlor, and toxaphene; hexachlorocyclohexanes (HCH) such as lindane; and chlorinated ethane compounds such as dichlorodiphenyltrichloroethane (DDT) and methoxychlor (Lewis 1998).

About 100 are used or have been used as insecticides that degrade slowly in the environment and accumulate at higher levels in the food chain. They are lipophilic and accumulate in depot fat (stored fat, as in adipose tissue). The acute effects most commonly associated with overexposure to organochlorine insecticides result from central nervous system stimulation. Many of them are known to be carcinogenic (e.g., DDT), hepatotoxic (e.g., dieldrin, chlordecone), nephrotoxic, neurotoxic (e.g., chlordecone), or may produce reproductive adverse effects (e.g., chlordecone).

Organophosphorus Insecticides

Organophosphorus (OP) insecticides have replaced organochlorine insecticides for many uses. Because some organochlorine insecticides are suspected of being potential carcinogens, regulatory actions have been taken to restrict their use and sale all over the world. OP insecticides, mostly malathion, have been widely used in WHO mosquito eradication programs (non-agricultural purposes).

OP pesticides are anticholinesterase agents or acetylcholinesterase inhibitors (i.e., substances that inhibit or inactivate acetylcholinesterase, thereby preventing the hydrolysis of acetylcholine). Their action leads to an accumulation of endogenous acetylcholine with a resultant hyperactivity of cholinergic neurons, which can be lethal. Symptoms of acute poisoning can include irritability, tremors, and convulsions, with death usually from respiratory failure. A number of OP chemicals may induce delayed neurotoxicity, characterized by sensory and motor axon degeneration in distal regions of the peripheral nerves and spinal tracts. The axonal degeneration is delayed for 1 to 3 weeks after exposure.

The most representative examples of OP insecticides are parathion (CAS: 56-38-2), methyl parathion (CAS: 298-00-0), malathion (CAS: 121-75-5), and diazinon (CAS: 333-41-5). All OP insecticides provoke similar acute effects of overexposure. Parathion is the most potent inhibitor of acetylcholinesterase, if compared with other OP pesticides (the lethal oral dose ranges from 10 to 100 mg.) Malathion is currently registered in the United States as an active ingredient in more than 80 formulations. Malathion is of low to moderate toxicity relative to other OP insecticides. Diazinon (CAS: 333-41-5) is an active ingredient in more than 190 commercial formulations. Non-agricultural uses of diazinon include flea and tick collars for pets; lawn and garden insecticides; ant, roach, and spider sprays; and wasp, hornet, and fireant control.

Carbamate Insecticides

Carbamate ester derivatives are used as insecticides. Thiocarbamic acid derivatives are used as fungicides, and many others are used as herbicides. Carbamates have an anticholinesterase effect on mammals similar to that of the OP pesticides. However, acetylcholinesterase inhibition by carbamates is reversible, and spontaneous recovery is more likely. Although carbamate insecticides are of relatively low toxicity to humans, it is important to note that the lowest dose reported to produce an adverse effect is closer to a lethal dose for carbamates than for OP compounds. Humans may be exposed to carbamate insecticides through inhalation, ingestion, or dermal routes.

Carbaryl (CAS: 63-25-2) is a typical example of a carbamate insecticide and is one of the most commonly used insecticides for non-agricultural purposes. It is currently an active ingredient in more than 145 formulations. It has a relatively low toxicity in humans. Acute overexposure to carbaryl can cause acetylcholinesterase inhibition and associated signs and symptoms. Exposure may occur via inhalation, ingestion, or dermal contact. Atropine is the antidote of choice in severe cases of overexposure.

Herbicides

Herbicides comprise any substance or formulation intended for use as a plant regulator, defoliant, or desiccant. A chemical agent (an herbicide) is used to kill or seriously inhibit the growth of noxious or otherwise undesirable plants. Herbicides are classified as contact or systemic, selective or non-selective, and pre-emergent (killing weeds before they sprout) or post-emergent (killing weeds after they sprout). Many herbicides are also toxic to animals and to humans.

Triazines are some of the most commonly used herbicides in many countries. They are selective herbicides characterized by a low oral toxicity. However, triazines are relatively persistent in most environmental conditions, and this has led to concern over large-scale exposure of the general public to low levels of these compounds through drinking water. Atrazine (CAS: 1912-24-9), simazine (CAS: 122-34-9), and cyanazine (CAS: 21725-46-2) are the best-known triazine herbicides.

Among the quaternary nitrogen compounds, paraquat (CAS: 1910-42-5) is the most toxic and has been responsible for thousands of fatalities all over the world. Individuals employed in the manufacture of paraquat may be exposed to dust, vapor, or aerosol or to all three. One of the most striking aspects of paraquat toxicity is the delayed onset of acute effects. Depending on the amount consumed, patients may survive a few hours to several weeks. A second remarkable aspect of paraquat toxicity is its pulmonary toxicity. Pulmonary fibrosis is the most common effect of acute exposure and follows exposure by any route. Dermal exposure may cause pulmonary fibrosis in addition to severe burns. Ingestion is a common route of accidental or intentional acute exposure. Consumption of as little as 10 to 15 ml of a 20% solution has been proven fatal. Paraquat is most often ingested with suicidal intent. Once consumed, it directly attacks the gastrointestinal tract. This injury may include mucous membrane erosion in the mouth, bleeding ulcers, and tissue erosion in the esophagus and stomach. Gastric erosion in paraquat intoxication indicates a poor prognosis. Severe acute exposure to paraquat may also lead to renal failure. Patients who reach this level of toxicity have an extremely poor prognosis.

Other groups of toxic herbicides include the chlorophenoxy herbicides: dichlorophenoxyacetic acid or 2,4-D (CAS: 94-75-7); 2,4,5-trichlorophenoxyacetic acid or 2,2,5-T (CAS: 93-76-5); and 5-chloro-2-methylphenoxyacetic acid or MCPA (CAS: 94-74-6). The debate as to the health effects of exposure to these herbicides has been as intense as it has been lengthy. To complicate matters, it is rare to find a group of persons exposed to a single chlorophenoxy herbicide to the exclusion of others. The common contaminant 2,3,7,8-tetrachlorodibenzo-p-dioxin (TCDD) has been incriminated and is in the center of most toxicological and health concerns.

Other types of herbicides have been developed, including common products such as glyphosate, which is a common broad-spectrum herbicide used for broadleaf plants and has relatively low toxicity. The toxicity of the other herbicides varies greatly.

Fumigants

A fumigant is smoke, gas, or vapor used (usually in enclosed spaces) to control pests such as rodents or insects. It is an irritant that is usually lethal. Substances commonly used as fumigants are acrylonitrile, carbon tetrachloride, ethylene oxide, hydrogen cyanide, and methyl bromide. Fumigants, which are used industrially in enclosed spaces under controlled conditions, are highly toxic.

10

BIOLOGICAL HAZARDS AT WORK

Gregory Chan Chung Tsing and David Koh

INTRODUCTION

Biological hazards refer to microbial agents present in the work environment, including bacteria, viruses, fungi, and parasites, that can cause occupational disease. These diseases fall into two general but overlapping categories—occupational infections and occupational allergies and related immune disorders.

These disorders are considered occupational because they result directly from exposure at work. There is little or no difference between occupational and non-occupational diseases that are caused by the same microorganism. The pathogenesis, clinical features, diagnosis, and treatment are the same. If biological hazards at work are controlled, the risk of occupational infections and immune disorders, such as allergies, can be significantly minimized.

Microbial agents are found in natural or man-made environments, in animals, and in humans. They may be transmitted by direct contact with infected bodily fluids or secretions or indirectly via air, food, water, or other vectors. Entry into the human body can occur through inhalation and ingestion or through broken skin and conjunctivae. Whether clinical infection or hypersensitivity occurs and how severe it becomes depends on the virulence of the microbial agent, the degree of exposure, and the level of immunity of the worker.

OCCUPATIONAL INFECTIONS

Infections are diseases in which the microorganism enters the body, establishes itself, and grows or replicates. The disease process can be the result of the infection itself (e.g., an abscess or a pneumonia), the result of the release of toxins by the microorganism (e.g., in anthrax or tetanus), the result of damage done by the microorganism (e.g., in hepatitis), or the result of the body's reaction against the microorganism (e.g., the response to the tuberculosis organism is worse than

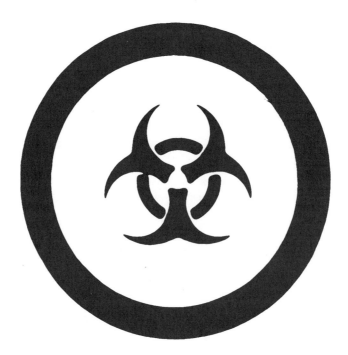

Figure 10.1 This international symbol warns against a biological hazard in transport or in workplaces where it may be present.

the damage caused by the bacillus itself). Many infections are similar in their early symptoms because the body's normal immune response to the microorganism triggers the initial signs and symptoms. That is why infections usually involve fever, fatigue, an increase in white blood cells, and signs of inflammation. These are the result of the body's normal immune response, which is typically to kill the microorganism, wall off the infection, and protect the body through the release of chemical substances (cytokines) that prepare the body to overcome the infection.

Some infectious agents are *transmissible*, i.e., they can be transmitted from person to person. The risk of exposure depends on how endemic the disease is in the local population and varies by season, weather, diurnal variation, and individual behavioral practices. Examples include tuberculosis and hepatitis B and C. For these infections, workers most at risk are those who come into intimate contact with patients, such as medical care workers. Other infectious agents are not transmissible, and exposure to the organism occurs in the course of work. Workers at risk for these infections include those who work with animals and animal products (e.g., abattoir workers, wool workers, animal breeders, veterinarians, laboratory workers who work with animals) or who work with biological materials (e.g., gardeners, laboratory workers, and pathologists).

Some workers may transmit diseases to the public or to other workers who eat food they have handled. For example, food handlers who do not use proper precautions for personal hygiene (hand washing) can transmit serious illnesses such as hepatitis B to customers if they are infected themselves. Food that is improperly prepared can infect customers or can cause *food poisoning*, which is the result of contaminating microorganisms that produce toxins. Large outbreaks of food poisoning can occur among workers who share food or who eat at a company canteen or food service if regular safety inspections and proper food preparation procedures are not enforced. These outbreaks usually consist of localized epidemics of diarrhea. Outbreaks of vector-borne disease, such as malaria and dengue, may occur among workers who live and work in environments where the risk is high.

A global mortality survey by the World Health Organization in 1995 estimated that 17 million of the 52 million deaths from all causes were due to infections, and the majority of these cases originate in developing countries. Chief among them in terms of numbers chronically affected is malaria, a worldwide disease that exists in several forms, some of which are lethal, and is caused by a parasite transmitted by the bite of a mosquito. However, more industrialized countries still have to grapple with infectious diseases. New infections, such as Severe Acute Respiratory Syndrome (SARS), are emerging, and some infections that were considered to be under control are re-emerging (such as resistant forms of tuberculosis and malaria) due to factors such as international travel, shifts in the genetic structure of infectious agents, and antibiotic resistance. These new and returning infections are called *emerging infections*. Table 10.1 below highlights the range of possible occupational infections and how to prevent them.

As noted earlier, occupational disease due to biological hazards can be prevented if the hazards are identified and controlled. Some biological hazards

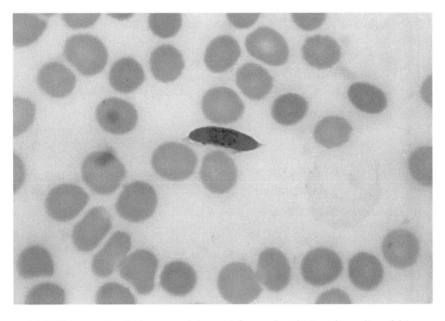

Figure 10.2 The parasite that causes the worst form of malaria: *Plasmodium falciparum*, in the bloodstream, in the macrogametocyte stage of its development. (Photograph courtesy of the U.S. Centers for Disease Control and Prevention, Public Health Image Library.)

TABLE 10.1

EXAMPLES OF OCCUPATIONAL INFECTIONS

Disease and Agent	Exposure	Target Organ	Preventive Measures
Bacteria			
Anthrax *Bacillus anthracis*	Wool or hide handlers, butchers, agricultural workers, veterinarians, researchers	Skin, lung	Immunization, personal hygiene
Brucellosis *Brucella abortus, B. suis, B. canis, B. melitensis*	Abattoir workers, veterinarians, hunters	Systemic	Personal hygiene, vaccination of livestock, serologic surveillance of affected animals
Leptospirosis *Leptospira icterhaemorrhagiae, L. interrogans*	Abattoir workers, sewer workers, agricultural workers, fishermen, military	Liver, kidney, systemic	Personal hygiene, protective clothing, vaccination of livestock, doxycycline chemoprophylaxis
Meliodosis *B. pseudomallei*	Agricultural workers, military	Skin, systemic	Personal hygiene
Tetanus *Clostridium tetani*	Construction workers, agricultural workers, animal handlers	Nervous system	Immunization
Tuberculosis *Mycobacterium tuberculosis*	Health-care workers, laboratory workers	Lung, systemic	Immunization, post-exposure surveillance and chemoprophylaxis
Viruses			
Hepatitis A Hepatitis A virus	Sewer workers, travelers to endemic areas	Liver	Immunization, personal and food hygiene
Hepatitis B Hepatitis B virus	Health-care workers, sex workers	Liver	Personal hygiene, universal precautions, immunizations
Hepatitis C Hepatitis C virus	Health-care workers, sex workers, intravenous drug users	Liver	Personal hygiene, universal precautions, immunizations
Japanese Encephalitis Japanese Encephalitis virus	Travelers to endemic areas, military	Nervous system	Immunization, personal protective measures
Dengue	Construction workers	(One form causes hemorrhagic fever, bleeding and high fever)	Mosquito suppression by removal of standing water, personal protection

(Continued)

TABLE 10.1 (Contd.)

Disease and Agent	Exposure	Target Organ	Preventive Measures
Nipah virus	Abattoir workers	Nervous system	Personal hygiene
Rabies Rabies virus	Laboratory workers, veterinarians, wild-animal handlers, travelers to endemic areas	Nervous system	Immunization, post-exposure prophylaxis with vaccine and immunoglobulins, avoidance of stray animals
AIDS HIV virus	Health-care workers, sex workers, intravenous drug users	Immune system	Universal precautions, post-exposure surveillance and prophylaxis
SARS SARS virus	Health-care workers	Respiratory system	Personal hygiene, universal precautions, respirators
Fungal			
Candidiasis *Candida albicans*	Dishwashers, cannery workers	Skin	Personal hygiene, keeping skin dry
Dermatophytoses *Trichophytom spp,* *Microsporium spp,* *Epidermophyton* *spp*	Animal handlers, athletes, military	Skin	Personal hygiene, keeping skin dry
Parasite			
Malaria *Plasmodium* *falciparum,* *P. malaria,* *P. vivax, P. ovale*	Agricultural workers, business travelers to endemic areas, construction and other workers entering high-risk areas	Blood, liver, brain, kidneys, systemic	Mosquito suppression, protective barriers, e.g., long sleeves, mosquito nets, chemoprophylaxis
Toxoplasmosis *Toxoplasma gondii*	Veterinarians, laboratory workers, cat handlers	Reticuloendothelial system, eye, developing fetus	Personal hygiene

can be detected early before clinical disease by screening methods (such as a combination of tuberculin skin prick tests/QuantiFERON ® serological tests, and chest X-rays for latent tuberculosis) that can identify workers who have encountered the organism and may have been infected. However, there is no screening test for many occupational infections. In those cases, detection and surveillance depend on early recognition of symptoms in a single or multiple cases and early diagnosis.

The principal strategy for avoiding occupational infections is *primary prevention*. This means taking measures so that the causative organism does not infect the worker in the first place. This can be done in many ways depending on the setting: by good hygiene, proper waste-handling methods, cooking food thoroughly, using biological cabinets for research procedures, and using protective equipment or immunization. Most of these measures require workers to understand and to cooperate, which means that workers must be educated and trained in prevention strategies.

Immunization is the primary strategy for avoiding infection when exposure to the agent is inevitable, unpredictable, or cannot be prevented otherwise. Vaccines are available for many infectious agents, such as hepatitis, or neutralizing toxoids against the toxins they produce, such as tetanus. A few diseases may actually be treated as well as prevented by vaccination; for example, rabies is effectively treated by a course of vaccine after an animal bite has occurred, and immunization promptly after anthrax infection can prevent the disease. However, this is unusual. Unfortunately, there is no vaccine at present for some diseases, including malaria and HIV/AIDS.

Some infections are widespread in the general population and affect workers but are not necessarily work-related. Malaria, for example, may be an important cause of disability and may greatly interfere with a worker's ability to do the job, but unless the worker was infected as a result of work-related travel to an area where malaria is *endemic* (already prevalent), or in circumstances where exposure is related to outdoor work (such as construction or field work where the risk of infection is high), it would not normally be considered an occupational infection. Some infections can be transmitted on the job. Tuberculosis is prevalent in many populations, and infection may be work-related when groups of workers are brought together on the job and an infected worker transmits the disease to others.

One of the biggest challenges facing occupational health today is the management of infection with HIV, the agent that causes AIDS. HIV/AIDS is rarely work-related in the sense that it is transmitted at work, although this is possible, but it is often indirectly related to work. HIV, and therefore AIDS, is spread mostly by sexual intercourse and by contaminated needles and syringes. In many countries, large numbers of people are infected, and workers may spread the infection through travel (such as has occurred along the routes used by truck drivers) and migration paths, particularly when migrant workers leave their homes and live in camps or dormitories for long periods of time, away from their families and tempted by prostitution and sometimes drugs.

HEALTH-CARE WORKERS AND BLOOD-BORNE INFECTIONS

There are certain categories of workers who have an increased risk of occupational infections, e.g., travelers and agricultural workers. One group at particular risk of microbial exposure are health-care workers, who may be exposed to blood-borne infections such as the hepatitis B virus (HBV), hepatitis C virus (HCV), and human immunodeficiency virus (HIV) transmitted within health-care settings, usually from patients. In the United States, for example, the Centers for Disease Prevention and Control estimates that 800 health-care workers are infected with HBV annually and has documented at least 54 cases of occupationally acquired HIV infection. Such infections are, however, uncommon and can be transmitted only by an injection that breaks the skin or through contact with an open wound, non-intact skin, or mucous membranes with blood or body fluids. In fact, the risk of transmission of HIV infection in a health-care setting is much lower than that for the transmission of HBV and HCV, with seroconversion rates following a needle-stick or cut exposure at 0.3% for HIV compared to 6% to 30% for HBV.

To reduce risk of blood-borne infections in the health-care setting, "universal precautions" should apply. All blood, body fluids, and tissues should be assumed to be potentially infected with blood-borne infections. The measures include:

- proper hand washing
- careful handling and disposal of sharp instruments
- personal protection and appropriate use of protective equipment
- use of disposable equipment, where applicable
- sterilization and disinfection
- disposal of bio-hazardous waste
- management of soiled/contaminated laundry

Injuries with "sharps" (needles, scalpel blades, and other sharp objects) are common among health-care workers. They carry a risk of infection, especially if the worker has been stuck by a needle contaminated with the blood of a hepatitis-infected or HIV-positive patient. Hepatitis B vaccination is recommended for all health-care workers, and post-exposure prophylaxis for possible HIV exposure should be made available by the employer. Unfortunately, it is often the case that it is not known whether the patient is infected with HIV or hepatitis virus, and a test sometimes cannot be done. In such cases, a decision to give prophylactic medication must be made based on the patient's risk of having the infection.

AGRICULTURAL WORKERS AND ZOONOTIC INFECTIONS

All animals harbor diseases, some of which can affect the workers who handle infected animals. Diseases that humans can catch from animals are called *zoonoses* (*zoonosis* is the singular form). There are two levels of control in the prevention of zoonoses in agriculture workers:

- controlling the disease in the animal by vaccinating against zoonotic pathogens (where possible), ensuring good standards of hygiene in animal shelters, avoiding food or water contamination, and through regular medical checks by veterinarians

- protecting the worker by means of vaccination, chemoprophylaxis, use of personal protective equipment (e.g., when examining animals and handling animal births), personal hygiene, universal precautions, and other safe working practices when handling blood or body fluids

MICROBIAL ALLERGIES

Immune disorders are diseases that are primarily caused by an abnormal immunological response. In such cases, the microorganism is not causing an infection but is merely present in the body. Certain chemicals or parts of the microorganism act as an *antigen*, a chemical substance that the body recognizes as foreign. In response, the body mounts an exaggerated, sometimes severe, immune response. The most common form of immune disorder is *allergy*. Allergies are disorders in which the body responds to the antigen in a particular way, producing cells that are primed to remember the antigen and to react to it the next time the body encounters the antigen. Common manifestations of occupational allergies include asthma, skin rashes, inflammation of mucous membranes such as rhinitis (hay fever is a rhinitis associated with plant pollens).

Asthma is a condition characterized by episodes of obstruction to the flow of air when exhaling, due to constriction and inflammation of the airways. The person with asthma feels short of breath because he or she cannot get air out of the lungs quickly and therefore may not move air fast enough to meet the body's needs. Inhalation becomes difficult as well because air is trapped in the lungs. As a result of the obstruction, many people with asthma make a noise when they

TABLE 10.2

MICROBIAL ALLERGIES

Disease Condition	Causative Organism
Extrinsic allergic alveolitis	
Bagassosis	*Thermoactinomyces sacchari*
Cheese washer's lung	*Penicillium spp.*
Dry rot lung	*Serpula lacrimans*
Farmer's lung	*Micropolyspora faeniae*
	Thermoactinomyces vulgaris
Malt worker's lung	*Aspergillus clavatus*
Mushroom worker's lung	*Micropolyspora faeniae*
	Thermoactinomyces vulgaris
Potato riddler's lung	Spores and dusts from potatoes
Sewage sludge disease	Dust of dried sewage sludge
Baker's asthma	Flour containing spores of *Aspergillus sp., Alternaria sp.*
Humidifier fever	Microorganisms in humidification systems of buildings
Occupational asthma	Varieties of fungi, actinomycetes, and *Bacillus subtilis*

breathe out called "wheezing." Most occupational asthma is caused by an allergy to some inhaled antigen in the workplace, often a biological agent. Irritation due to chemicals also causes occupational asthma.

Another immune disorder associated with microorganisms is *extrinsic allergic alveolitis* (also called hypersensitivity pneumonitis), in which an inhaled antigen results in persistent inflammation in the lung. Over time, this inflammation can result in scar tissue, or *fibrosis*, in the lung and result in serious lung disease.

Occupational microbial allergies mainly affect the respiratory tract and result from the inhalation of bacteria, spores of fungi, and actinomycetes. Table 10.2 below shows the various types of occupational microbial allergies and their causes.

CONTROLLING BIOLOGICAL HAZARDS

Controlling biological hazards usually calls for one or more of the following measures:

- Assessment of health threats at the workplace. For this, it is necessary to know the diseases endemic to the area of work and the specific health hazards pertaining to the nature of the work.
- Environmental control measures, including good sanitation, vector control, and other public health measures at the workplace to remove potential disease reservoirs, vectors, and vehicles of transmission.
- Immunization, e.g., for anthrax, HBV, cholera, and diphtheria. Use of a vaccination should be weighed against the efficacy, costs, and adverse effects of the vaccine. Post-exposure vaccination can be considered in certain diseases (e.g., rabies and anthrax) but is not as reliable as primary prevention.
- Chemoprophylaxis. *Prophylactic* (preventive) medication to prevent infection such as for malaria, leptospirosis, and typhus, is an alternative when a vaccine is not available. It does not prevent infection but may reduce the severity of clinical outcome. Post-exposure prophylaxis can also be considered in some cases (e.g., HIV and HBV) when appropriate medication is available.
- Surveillance and screening. Early disease detection contributes to successful treatment of disease and enables precautionary measures to break disease transmission, including isolation of infectious disease cases. Identification of the implicated organism can take various forms including positive cultures, serology, immunofluorescence, and genetic material (e.g., polymerase chain reaction).
- Outbreak response. When outbreaks occur, prompt investigation to determine the source, control of the source, prompt and effective treatment, and, if necessary, isolation of the affected workers is essential.
- Fitness to work. Pre-employment and periodic examinations are required to determine whether the worker has any existing health condition that may worsen the effects of an infection or increase susceptibility of contracting one. For instance, immunosuppressed or pregnant individuals may not be allowed

hazardous biological exposures. Workers who are infectious may pose a risk to coworkers, the public they serve, their families, or others.

- Safe workplace practices and use of personal protective equipment should be backed by education of the workers on health risks and good hygiene measures.

11

STRESS AND PSYCHOLOGICAL FACTORS

Tsutomu Hoshuyama

Every person in modern urban life is under some degree of stress as he or she fulfills multiple roles as citizen, parent, manager, worker, and individual. Job-related stress is a problematic issue that is not as simple as it may initially seem. It has many causes, probably many effects, and many possible solutions. The effects of psychological stress in the workplace on human health are complex, difficult to quantify, and subject to modification by social support and individual host factors.

Stress in this context may be considered to be a physiological response induced by the psychological reaction to an imbalance between demand and capacity (or expectation) and comfort level. The body's response to this demand is non-specific. The physiological pattern of the body's response to stress is the same as the preparation to flee or to attack a threat. In the absence of a manageable threat, however, the stress response becomes maladaptive, causing stress-related symptoms rather than preparing the body for short-term exertion.

The influence of stress seems to be more strongly felt by individuals with existing health conditions or who are experiencing complicated life situations. There is a tendency to think of stress as one might think of other occupational hazards—by assuming that exposure to a stressor results in an increased risk of a predictable outcome or a cluster of outcomes that can be monitored, such as injuries or occupational diseases. However, stress is very different from other occupational hazards. There is no one specific outcome associated with stress, as illustrated by Table 11.1. Stress often magnifies the effects of other conditions and the perception of the discomfort and disability associated with many outcomes, especially chronic pain and illness severity. Mood, sleep, and other behavioral patterns are altered by stress; it may even affect immune function. Stress also reduces one's ability to cope with other hazards and stressors in daily life and work because of distraction and worry.

Stress at work is intimately mingled with stress in one's personal life: just as the troubled and distressed worker brings some job stress home, the worker brings some degree of life stress to the job from home. Background levels of stress coexist at home and in the worker's personal life. However, the important role that work plays in most individuals' lives increases the potentially constructive impact that industry can have in helping workers change their lifestyles to cope better with stress. If the home life is tense, then the worker may be less able to cope with work-related stress than would normally be the case.

Stress is paradoxical and feeds on itself; people can be neurotically stressed by worrying about the presence of stress in their life. There is also "positive stress," in which stress perceived as experienced for a purpose is followed by a sense of release. Excitement, a sense of commitment, teamwork under pressure, achievement, and successful response to a disaster can all be exhilarating, energizing, and constructive. Positive stress is a highly individualized perception, however. It is not *imposed* on an unwilling worker by demands of management. It does not carry on indefinitely but ends with a sense of accomplishment. It is associated with clear goals that the worker can identify with, not the personal goals of a supervisor. It calls for team building and camaraderie, not divisiveness and not standing by waiting for something to happen. Positive stress implies a goal worthy of the worker's efforts.

Personal competence and the ability to cope with social realities are markers of mental health status. Personal competence conveys a sense of mastery and control and particularly the capabilities for coping with life situations and stressful events. Individuals, for the most part, deal with stress by resolving the source, avoiding it, or ignoring it, but can sometimes need help to resolve their response to stress. Social support is very important and can be provided by social networks or helping networks: family and spouse, neighbors, friends, and coworkers. Those with few sources of social support are more vulnerable to stress than those who have the problem-solving and supportive resources of a personal helping network.

Combinations of factors within and outside the work situation interact and contribute to disease, so the relationship between job stress and illness is complex. This makes it difficult to study. Most of the research that links stress to illness has not been done in occupational settings. However, a growing body of knowledge is documenting the effects of occupational stress on the etiology and development of physical and mental disease. Employers need to be aware of work-induced stresses that may affect their employees and their operations. The ideal situation is an organizational atmosphere in which the worker feels free to express concerns and to ask for help.

One of the most common situations associated with stress in occupational settings is excessive demand for increased production. Working overtime or for long hours can be sustained for short periods, after which fatigue, frustration, and ultimately stress-related symptoms set in. However, there are many other causes of job-related stress, as summarized in Table 11.2.

The pioneering work of Karasek from 1981 has demonstrated that stress is strongly associated with two job characteristics: a high volume or pace of work and lack of control over the job and workplace. A highly demanding job that comes with authority to make decisions and to structure one's own work may not be as stressful as a lower-demand job in which the worker has no control. That is why many investigators believe that the frustration associated with boredom, inactivity, and a sense of wasting time can be as stressful as overload, time pressure, and interpersonal conflict, particularly for those whose self-esteem is heavily bound to their work.

However, stress occurs at all levels of employment. Managers at all levels are evaluated by those on a higher level; similarly, the chief executive officer is evaluated by a board of directors. To minimize levels of stress, interpersonal relationships on all levels should be tolerable, but need not necessarily be perfect.

Another theory of stress is the "effort-reward model" developed by Johannes Siegrist, who proposed that stress occurs when the effort a worker is putting into

TABLE 11.1

CONDITIONS WITH A STRONG ASSOCIATION WITH STRESS

Headache	Depression
Low back pain	Insomnia or hypersomnolence
Gastrointestinal symptoms	Irritability symptoms
Spastic colon	Alcohol abuse
Duodenal ulcer	Distraction, irritability
Chest pain	Eating disorders
Labile hypertension	Sexual dysfunction
Autonomic effects*	Violence
Emotional lability	
Panic attacks	Post-traumatic stress syndrome

* Symptoms associated with the autonomic nervous system, such as clammy skin or sweating palms

TABLE 11.2

FACTORS CONTRIBUTING TO STRESS IN THE WORKPLACE

Isolation	Overload
Stagnation	"Career arrest"
Lack of challenge	Shift work
Personality clashes	Public disapproval
Absence of personal identification with work	Paced work, speedup
Role conflicts	Ambiguous or contradictory directives
Unfair evaluations or labor practices	Lack of recognition for performance
Lack of job security	Discrimination due to prejudice
Unpleasant working environment	Inefficient working environment (as perceived by worker)
Disagreement with management policy	Employment in a job substantially below abilities
High responsibility/low authority	Concealment of alternative behavior or lifestyles (perceived as "deviant" by the majority)

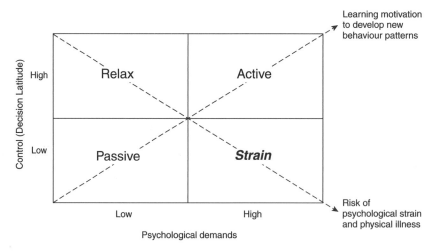

Figure 11.1 The Karasek model of "demand-control" is a powerful tool for analyzing workplace stress and has been shown to correlate with the risk of cardiovascular disease.

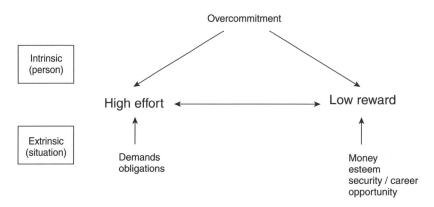

Figure 11.2 The Siegrist model of "effort-reward" adds an additional dimension to the analysis of stress in the workplace and tends to be associated with motivation, engagement with work, and the risk of "burnout."

the job is not recognized or compensated with an appropriate reward. The reward does not necessarily have to be money or material compensation. The reward may be favorable attention, a feeling of contributing something of value, personal satisfaction, a feeling of solidarity with a group or larger cause, social standing, or other intangible benefits.

A special type of occupational stress is associated with participation in or observation of a disaster, such as an industrial accident or near miss. This form of psychological trauma and the post-traumatic stress syndrome is common and is associated with experiences, such as being witness to a serious incident or having had a serious occupational injury, that are outside the normal experience of life. This is a special problem and will not be discussed in this chapter.

STRESS REDUCTION

Measures for reducing stress in the workplace may be introduced at the group level through changing work organization, or at the individual level through intervention designed to reduce personal stress. Personal stress reduction programs are also often included in health promotion programs and employee assistance programs. Table 11.3 outlines several general approaches to stress management in the workplace. These are general approaches and should be adapted as needed to a particular situation in the workplace. Different people have different stresses and different reactions to these stresses, as well as very different lifestyles and needs. Therefore, the best solutions are what is appropriate for each individual.

Maintenance of a positive worker attitude is critical to effective teamwork. Management can induce stress by changing working conditions and negatively impacting a person's attitude toward his or her work and job. A worker can be pulled from a team, given repetitive work, denied due recognition, or compelled to meet extremely difficult and apparently arbitrary production demands. The manager who does not allow or encourage feedback from staff may be doing harm to the employer by excluding useful suggestions on production issues or problem solving. In many cases, managers with such attitudes are unable to tell when employee morale is deteriorating until it is reflected in performance and is more difficult to turn around.

Work is a social environment and provides a worker with many rewards. Most workers enjoy their work and deal with it on a daily basis with motivation and interest. One of the most rewarding aspects of work is a sense of belonging to a community with a shared purpose. The worker who does not enjoy a feeling of participation may develop resentment that his or her work is not valued or feel a sense of diminished self-esteem because he or she has little to contribute.

If the work environment is a significant contributor to stress, management may consider changes in work organization that improve the quality of working life. These may involve increased worker participation in the decision-making process about particular jobs, plans, or operational decisions. A higher level of participation at the workplace may increase satisfaction, stimulate interest, and result in higher productivity. Some other approaches that might be tried include changing reporting structures, changing the division of labor, changing control and monitoring procedures, increasing control by the individual worker over the process or job he or she performs, and changing the social interactions among workers. If there are power struggles in the workplace, encouraging leaderless or self-organized work teams may help to reduce perceived competition and personal alienation. Managers can share problems with their subordinates as a group rather than attempt to conceal them. Often, workers have well thought-out solutions to workplace problems but feel constrained from offering them to management.

Information flow in both directions is critical to maintaining responsive relationships between workers and their superiors. Communication must be fluid between the worker and those not only above, but on the same level and below the worker. Not being able to talk with someone in the workplace, especially to one's supervisor, about problems is itself stressful. Behavioral approaches to the management of psychological and physical responses to stress have been developed in the past decade. Relaxation techniques, assertiveness training, guided imagery, meditation, biofeedback, and physical exercise are useful as prevention as well as in treatment. Table 11.3 summarizes some of the stress management techniques that can be used in individual cases.

Supervisors can be made aware of the signs of stress, which may include changes in attitude, changes in work quality, absence from work, or reports of domestic troubles. Management, when requesting an increase in production with no increase in staffing or resources, should be aware of the potential for increasing stress and ideally should seek the means to mitigate it and to provide adequate resources. If an individual worker is identified as abusing alcohol or drugs or is affected by a mental health or dependency problem, he or she can be referred for help in an employee assistance program. If there is a physical health problem as a result of stress, the worker should be evaluated by a physician who is an expert in that particular specialty before the assumption is made that the problem is due entirely to stress. The occupational implications of any impairment should be evaluated by applying the fitness-to-work process (see Chapter 17).

Methods of job enrichment may also be used to increase job satisfaction. Job enrichment is the redesign of work to include tasks and activities that promote the psychological involvement of the worker in the work itself. This may include rearranging tasks and processes, adding new ones, increasing feedback on results and performance, increasing work variety, and increasing the level of contact with other workers.

TABLE 11.3

APPROACHES TO MANAGING STRESS IN AFFECTED INDIVIDUALS

- Identify and control particular stressor
  - Awareness
  - Modifications in work environment
  - Speak to supervisor
- Union grievance
- Change jobs (if no alternative)
- Behavior modification ("stress inoculation")
- Social support and self-help networks
- Individual psychotherapy
- Time out
- Holiday
- Days off

(Continued)

TABLE 11.3 (Contd.)

- Unstructured break during day
- Recreation or enjoyable activities on own time
- Schedule different work patterns
- Relaxation techniques
- Autogenics (autosuggestion)
- Self-hypnosis or hypnosis
- Meditation
- Progressive relaxation
- Biofeedback
- Deep breathing
- Stretching
- Control of substance use
- Short-term use of tranquilizers and hypnotics
  - (risk of dependency—used primarily to break pathological behavioral cycles)
- Control stimulant intake: coffee, tea, cola drinks
- Control depressant intake: alcoholic beverages, prescription drugs
- Lifestyle interventions
- Diversion or rewarding avocation or sport
- Regular exercise, improved fitness
- Avoid hassles of daily life (to extent possible)
- Regular bedtime
- Cognitive coping interventions
- Positive attitude—visualization techniques, self-talk, rehearsal
- "Minimizing" coping style (reduce perceived seriousness)
- Decreased sense of vulnerability
- Improved coping skills

TABLE 11.4

APPROACHES TO REDUCING STRESS IN THE WORKPLACE

- Conduct a "stress audit" to identify perceived sources of stress among workers and managers
- Stress management training sessions for workers and supervisors
- Supervisor training to control sources of stress
- Employee assistance programs
- Health promotion programs
- Management restructuring and policies designed to reduce ambiguity, insecurity, and confusion over goals
- Restructuring of the workplace for improved efficiency, worker convenience, and comfort
- Encourage participation of workers in planning their tasks and workplaces
- Change work organization to provide greater variety of tasks, skills training, and social interaction
- Share information on group goals and performance with workers

Although some authors have attempted to relate shift work to significant clinical disease, the evidence that shift work is a major, as opposed to contributing, risk factor for disease is weak. Although an association with risk of cancer has recently been noted by the International Agency for Research on Cancer (IARC), the most prominent effects of shift work are likely to be psychological and social. It is known, however, that a few people like shift work, some strongly dislike it, yet most workers have learned to live with it. The popularity of shift work has increased over the last 30 years. This increase appears to be due to two major factors. In manufacturing that factor is production efficiency, and in service occupations the factor is increased access to meet demand.

In manufacturing, shift work exists primarily for the efficiency of production, and the limiting factor in heavy manufacturing is usually how long the plant can operate during the day. Technological advances, energy costs, and more efficient usage of heavy machinery have resulted in a preference for continuous production in order to reduce costs of equipment maintenance and shut-down. It is often more profitable to run a plant "round the clock" in order to raise the level of annual operating hours and, therefore, profit. Productivity during some shifts may be low with respect to workers, but equipment productivity is more critical in these industries. Machines work longer hours than their human counterparts. Shift work not only saves capital but reduces operating costs as well. Shift work is also instituted to allow production at times of reduced cost, avoiding peak load electrical rates and decreasing traffic congestion.

A second factor, of more importance in service occupations, is the need to provide certain services on a 24-hour basis. This has long been the pattern for medical care and public services, such as fire and police protection and utility services. With increasing emphasis on personal convenience, retail, food, and transportation services are increasingly available throughout the day and night, requiring staffing by shifts. Sometimes, this leads to additional problems, such as violence or the risk of robbery, which may be increased at night and at times when there may be only one or a few employees present and the workplace has cash on site (e.g., a fast-food restaurant). Such events, and the knowledge or fear that they may occur, are very stressful for staff. Some customer-service occupations that operate at night, such as convenience stores, may hire young adults, and stress may increase when there is a threat they are not experienced enough to handle.

In 2008, the International Agency for Research on Cancer (IARC) concluded that night-shift work may be associated with an elevated risk of cancer, presumably due to hormonal changes. IARC classified night-shift work as a "probable" human carcinogen, based on animal and epidemiological studies.

Despite the constant performance characteristics of plant equipment and the ongoing demands of society, human performance and the reliability to meet these demands cannot remain constant. Significant reductions in performance occur on a night shift, as measured by reaction time, accuracy of perception, and error rate. The nadir of performance appears to occur between 3:00 and 6:00 a.m., corresponding to the lowest point in the diurnal variation of body temperature, and is further reduced by the number of days spent on the night shift in a particular week.

Jobs requiring repetition, mental acuity, and vigilance regarding signs or observing details do not lend themselves as readily to satisfactory shift work as physical labor. Visual perception and response times are prolonged at night and if the worker is fatigued and sleep deprived. Unfortunately, jobs requiring these higher-level skills include many occupations that are assigned by shifts, such as nursing and transportation workers, including airline pilots.

Circadian rhythms are cycles that human beings experience throughout the day. Workers on a permanent night shift or a rotating shift appear to be negatively affected mainly by the disruption of circadian rhythms and reduced contact with their family and the community. Physiologically, the body has many different circadian rhythms, including those that affect body temperature, pulse, breathing rate, blood pressure, urine production, and brain activity. These rhythms are usually well synchronized by external events, such as light/dark cycles and the alarm clock, but can be artificially altered by long periods of isolation from external stimuli. Permanent night shift workers show less extreme swings and desynchronization in their circadian rhythms. The periodicity of the human circadian rhythm is approximately 25 hours; it is reset daily by routine and visual cues, including daylight. Therefore, it is easier for individuals to postpone sleep than to advance the time of sleeping or rising earlier. Shift rotations of day-evening-night, either having a day off or working a double shift on the day of transition, are therefore better tolerated in general than day-night-evening. It takes approximately 15 days to adjust fully to a new shift, approximately one day for each hour of change in going to sleep. More rapid schedules of rotation, while acceptable to many workers, do not permit synchronization to stabilize at any point and are disliked by most workers.

The *diurnal* (day-night) cycle of body temperature appears to be one of the cycles most sensitive to change. Studies have shown a correlation between body temperature and performance, as judged by vigilance (alertness to hazards), accidents, and manual dexterity. The optimum time to work is when the body temperature is high, that is, during the day. When these cycles are changed, e.g., by a transcontinental flight, the change in the pattern of body temperature seems to determine fluctuations in levels of performance, rather than the actual time of day. Night workers typically get less sleep than day workers, and what sleep they do get is often of poor quality. Rapid eye movement (REM) sleep, which occurs more frequently after a person has been asleep for more than five or six hours, is a biological necessity. Night workers who sleep at odd hours may use hypnotics to aid in falling asleep, and their REM sleep may be disturbed by the medication. With inadequate REM sleep, chronic fatigue may develop.

Permanent shift workers may be different from other workers in matters of job preference, personality, or social ties, so there may be a selection factor confounding studies of the health effects of shift work. Management of certain chronic illnesses, such as insulin-dependent diabetes and epilepsy, is certainly made more difficult by shift schedules and sleep deprivation, respectively. Night-shift workers tend to use sleeping pills more often than day workers, and there may be other differences in use of medication and alcohol.

There are some obvious advantages and disadvantages to the various shift schedules. Steady day shifts have the most advantages as well as fewer disadvantages.

A day-shift schedule fits best into the family's schedule as well as social schedules. The disadvantages, which are relatively minor, include the worker's inability to tend to outside personal business during the day and the necessity to rise early in the morning.

Steady afternoon shifts also have significant advantages. Often the worker arrives home at an hour when he or she can enjoy uninterrupted quiet time with a spouse or companion. The worker often has enough free time during the day to take care of outside business. The worker is able to sleep during normal hours and to sleep late in the morning. However, this shift has major disadvantages for workers with families and significant relationships. One will not have much time to see young children because they are asleep when one comes home and at school when one wakes in the morning. The major disadvantage of this shift for most people is that it interferes greatly with social activities.

While the steady night shift is often thought to produce the most detrimental health effects, there are benefits available for the worker who can make the adjustment. This shift may actually interfere less with family and social obligations than the afternoon shift. As with the afternoon shift, working at night allows for useful free time during the day. Night workers seldom work fewer hours, but usually get paid more and often do not have to work as hard. The major disadvantage is having to sleep during the day. A night worker's demand for sleep in the daytime, if children are active and the home is noisy, can be a source of friction within a family. However, most permanent night workers, once conditioned, appear not to have major adjustment problems.

The rotating shift is the most commonly used form of shift work for a number of reasons. Permanent afternoon workers would express dissatisfaction finding themselves permanently cut off from family and social activities on workdays. Therefore, shift rotation is used to spread the inconvenience around. The pay differentials commonly offered to night workers are not usually enough to compensate for the human costs of working nights on a permanent schedule. Shift work in general interferes with family life in many other ways, making it difficult to have meals with the family, provide child care, and run errands. The amount of difficulty experienced is a function of the amount of disruption to the family's schedule.

One solution is to adjust the timing of the shift to minimize worker effects. The amount of time between cycles of rotation could be lengthened to allow for adjustment of circadian rhythms. Similarly, increasing the frequency of vacations could allow for more free time between work periods. Minimizing the number of hours worked on a night shift could be beneficial, and the deficit could be made up on the other shifts. The shifts logically should be adjusted to circadian rhythms relating to body temperature. The dawn shift would run from 4:00 a.m. to noon, sunset shift from noon until 8:00 p.m., and the night shift from 8:00 p.m. to 4:00 a.m., thus allowing the night worker to get more sleep.

With employers utilizing a rotating shift, the opportunity to work a fixed shift is often not available. Employers that take into consideration personal preferences for shifts may allow those preferring the night shift to work it permanently. Certain personality types who may lead solitary lives may enjoy working at night. Younger workers, "evening" people, extroverted personalities, and those with high amplitude circadian rhythms appear to adjust more easily to shift work. Maintaining some consistency in daily routine, such as the time of a major meal with family, can help mitigate the effects of shift work.

As shift work becomes more the norm, the activities and services of a community could be changed to gear activities to shift workers. In some communities dominated by a single employer requiring shift work, it is not unusual for businesses to adjust their hours.

Box 11.1

Case Study of Deadly Stress—Health Impact of Stressful and Intensive Work in Japan: Karoshi and Karo Jisatsu

The average number of working hours in Japan was reportedly higher than in any other industrialized country between the mid-1970s and the beginning of the 1990s. While this extreme commitment to work resulted in rapid increases in the Japanese market share, it also led to death from overwork. This phenomenon, called *karoshi*, has been a cause of social concern domestically and, increasingly, internationally. Karoshi is defined as fatal incidence and associated work-related disability due to cardiovascular events such as strokes, myocardial infarction, or acute cardiac failure, which could occur from the aggravation of hypertensive or arteriosclerotic diseases, triggered by heavy workload. The term *karoshi* is used for legal purposes, such as occupational disease compensation in Japan. More recently, a further syndrome has been added: *karo jisatsu*, or suicide due to overwork.

Why did Japanese workers work such long hours? According to sociological studies, this tendency developed due to the structure of the working-time system and the sociocultural background of labor. Contributing factors included the lifetime employment system, the consequently weaker influence of unions, the lack of a two-day-per-week rest system, the concept of loyalty to the company, and the collectivist mentality of Japanese workers. The employer's assessment of workers relates to their attendance rate, also promoting long working hours and unpaid overtime.

There is, however, insufficient evidence to conclude that working long hours alone adversely affects health. Some articles indicate the adverse effect of overwork on mental health and cardiovascular disorders, but the evidence is not conclusive. A case-control study on sudden unexpected death among Japanese workers found no significant correlation with the mean number of working hours during the four weeks before death (Hoshuyama et al. 1993). A second case-control study by Sokejima and Kagamimori (1998) found a U-shaped relationship between previous mean working hours and the risk of acute myocardial infarction among Japanese workers. This means that people who worked short hours and very long hours were most at risk, and people who worked a moderate amount were least at risk.

Recently, a Japanese government expert committee on the issue of workers' compensation published a report stating that the criteria for a decision that a worker had died of karoshi should be enlarged to consider the quantity of non-scheduled work in addition to regular working hours (*overtime* or overwork), up to six months before the death from the current one month). This may be in response to the increasing number of complaints about negative decisions regarding karoshi. Adverse health effects of long working hours may also depend on not only the quantity but also the quality of work. In fact, in karo jisatsu, a recent phenomenon occurring among Japanese workers, 10% of cases may be due as much to physical as psychological exhaustion in the current economic slump and record unemployment. Only an epidemiological intervention study, while difficult to conduct, may be able to scientifically resolve the causal factors in karoshi and karo jisatsu.

In the meantime, work patterns are changing in Japan. In the 1990s, the lifetime employment system diminished, and the five-day workweek was introduced. The currently amended Labor Standards Law regulates legal working hours to 40 per week. Some young workers prefer to do part-time work rather than permanent work. Thus, some of the factors associated with karoshi are changing.

BURNOUT

Job burnout can be defined as a debilitating psychological condition, characterized by a sense of disappointment, lack of fulfillment, and anxiety brought about by unrelieved work stress that may result in

- depleted energy reserves
- lowered resistance to illness
- increased dissatisfaction and pessimism
- increased absence due to illness

There is still considerable controversy over whether stress on the job affects immune function and renders a person more likely to develop clinical illness, such as respiratory tract infections. However, most would agree that workers under great stress are less able to cope with illness. The fatigue, mental state, possible self-medication, and sleep disturbances may make workers more susceptible to injury, substance abuse, and depression, as well as a wide range of psychosomatic disorders. It was once believed that the major risk factor in job burnout was the high degree, frequency, and intensity of intrinsic stressors in highly pressured occupations such as corporate executives, emergency responders, physicians, nurses, firefighters, police, social workers, and clergy. Occupations with few or no obvious sources of stress were considered to be at low risk. In recent years, however, it has been shown that workers in many jobs traditionally thought to have few or no sources of stress also experience job burnout.

Job burnout may begin gradually and varies from individual to individual. The worker may become bored or dispirited with the job, may become lackadaisical toward job responsibilities, may begin to procrastinate, and may fail to perform at a level compatible with past standards or his or her potential. These patterns soon become noticeable to superiors. When the decrement in performance is brought to the worker's attention, the worker may become even more frustrated. As the worker becomes increasingly dissatisfied with the job, he or she may begin looking for any excuse to call in sick, and absence episodes may increase. Workers may develop psychosomatic illnesses or may experience exaggerated symptoms from real complaints that under normal conditions would be rather minor, especially chronic pain. Sleep disorders are common, and workers may become depressed.

When the worker becomes frustrated with the job, there may also be acting out behavior directed at those who are closest, such as spouses and children. Instead of confronting the problem at work, the worker may bring feelings home and complain to the partner or spouse and take out frustrations on the family. This increases tension at home and may put family relationships in jeopardy.

The pace of work is not, within limits, the determining factor in job burnout. Workers who receive too few stimuli often feel that their job is monotonous and that they are not truly accomplishing anything. Most investigators now believe that a certain amount of controlled stress in a job is not unhealthy. Stimulation allows workers the opportunity to feel a sense of accomplishment and satisfaction and to feel better about themselves and their job. Feelings of depression are often more common among workers doing jobs of low complexity and less common among workers in highly complex jobs. One study showed that among workers experiencing a sharply reduced workload, assembly-line workers reported only slight dissatisfaction when they had too little to do, administrators had significantly more dissatisfaction, and police officers none. This response was correlated with the intrinsic interest reported in their work: administrators saw themselves as challenged by problems and indispensable to their employers, while assembly-line workers saw themselves as replaceable and present only to perform routine functions. Police, of course, deal with potentially hazardous situations and, for these workers, satisfaction may be the absence of problems.

One associated factor in job burnout is what has been termed the "honeymoon effect," a lack of fulfillment from the job that usually, but not always, affects those who are just beginning a new career after a prolonged period of training or education. The newly hired workers may begin very enthusiastically in the job but soon may feel disappointed because they are relegated to unchallenging duties day in and day out, or their ideas may be disregarded by their employers. They begin to feel that the time spent in preparing for their career was wasted; hence, they lose their enthusiasm and soon feel that they are in a rut.

Deskilling is another factor in burnout. With the increasing use of computers, mechanization of production, and unitizing and deskilling of work processes, many employers have created standardized, interchangeable jobs. These standardized jobs give the worker little opportunity for personal input and lack sufficient variety for the worker to increase his or her level of skill in a particular workplace. This leads to frustration and boredom in the absence of new challenges or accomplishments. When workers have been doing the same thing for many years and see nothing in their future except more of the same, they may feel trapped because they are unable to increase their status. They may adopt a "don't care" attitude in defense, which often leads to job burnout.

Another factor involved with job burnout is working hours. Many jobs, especially the professions or those that have a peak load of demand (such as waiters or bus drivers), do not accommodate a structured 40-hour workweek.

Individual personality characteristics appear to play some role in setting the stage for burnout. Individual life situations are also important factors in determining risk.

Individuals who are working below their educational status or skill level appear to be at increased risk of job burnout. They are usually of high intelligence, not easily satisfied, and are demanding of themselves and others. Often they are stuck in jobs below their appropriate level because of personality traits, or they may not be able to find more suitable work because of the state of the economy. These individuals are very ambitious and wish to make a good impression, but they may have difficulty expressing their ideas and suggestions to their employers and soon feel frustrated. Thus, they may develop a low self image and may feel there is nothing better they can do and that they are trapped in the job. These more susceptible individuals seem to be most vulnerable for job burnout when they are either starting a new job or have been in a single position for a long time.

"Workaholics" are typically individuals who have no social fulfillment outside their work. They become engrossed in their jobs as a means of retaining self-esteem. Burnout comes not from fatigue but from depression, after the inevitable realization that one is unfulfilled or after a career setback. Many ambitious people, in an effort to get ahead, put in considerable time over the usual hours and may become totally engrossed in the job. When the job becomes their only meaningful activity in life, the least setback may induce depression and feelings of inadequacy.

Workers who are in jobs for which they are ill-suited, either because they chose their careers unwisely or because a job was the best or the only one available at the time, often feel dissatisfied even if they are successful at the job. These people may continually feel that there is something missing in their lives, and unless they realize their predicament, they become more and more dissatisfied and may experience burnout.

Women with both careers and families are a special group at risk. They are actually working two jobs, one at home and the other in the plant or office, and have double the level of responsibility and work, yet only receive a single paycheck. They must fulfill the needs of others in both home and workplace, while trying to fulfill their own individual needs. Some cannot maintain this balancing act.

More individuals from disadvantaged minority groups are assuming leadership roles in business. Not only does this bring increased stress associated with a position of higher authority, but these individuals now find that they often must communicate on many levels, maintaining relations with their peers and friends and at the same time becoming accepted by members of the majority who are their subordinates. They may experience anxiety associated with the fear of failure in the new position, sometimes rooted in old thought patterns of accommodation to discrimination and the fear that they will not be able to succeed in higher positions.

While recognition and early intervention are important in the reduction of job burnout, the key to managing job burnout, like any other occupational disorder, is prevention. Ideally, rotating workers through different jobs from time to time will prevent monotony and make for a more broadly skilled employee, who will ultimately be more valuable to the employer. (However, this is often precluded by contract or union rules or is not otherwise feasible.) Seminars and workshops on stress awareness can be developed as part of a health prevention program. Promoting workers to higher-level positions from within, instead of filling higher positions with people from outside the company, instills optimism and a feeling that a job well done will be rewarded.

Personal communications with employees is difficult for some managers but is an important and effective tool in improving worker morale. Acknowledging, in person and in writing, appreciation of the work an individual has done makes the worker more satisfied with what has been accomplished and more eager to continue.

Employee input and suggestions, offered in good faith, should be received seriously and acted on, if possible. Allowing the worker a chance to participate in the employer's growth by contributing ideas and suggestions makes the worker part of the team. This promotes loyalty and makes for a stronger employee-employer relationship.

If relatively modest steps do not help with the problem, further steps may need to be taken. A discussion or, if necessary, a confrontation with the supervisor may be unavoidable. If so, a friendly third person, ideally a professional counselor, can help mediate and make the confrontation less personal or stressful. Rotating jobs or asking for a leave of absence may help. After taking time off, a worker may return with a more positive outlook toward the job. The worker may need a complete change of position or a new job in a new workplace. The younger the worker is, generally, the more one can do about burnout, but even mature workers may benefit from such interventions.

ADDICTIVE BEHAVIOR

Workers may abuse alcohol or drugs as a means of coping with stress, a process called *self-medication*. Others may have a problem with addiction unrelated to their work. Some turn to gambling or other forms of addictive behavior that temporarily make them feel better and relieves their feelings of stress. Some are surrounded by people using alcohol, such as bartenders, in settings where excessive alcohol use is tolerated, and others may have opportunities to gain access to drugs that are not open to most people.

At first, the habit may seem to reduce stress, but ultimately it may interfere with work by causing the worker to become unreliable or negatively affect his or her work performance. People caught in such addictive behavior are at risk for losing their jobs. The stress of job insecurity may make them even more reliant on their addiction.

Employee assistance programs (EAPs) are services sponsored by employers to help workers cope with these problems. EAPs, where they are available, may provide support and the interventions needed to resolve the problems. Discussing the problem with a counselor often helps to clarify matters. Talking over problems at work may give new insights on how to handle these issues and a renewed outlook on the job situation. However, EAPs must operate under conditions of strict confidentiality and privacy.

Workers with obvious addictive behaviors cause a great deal of stress for others in their workplace. They may be unreliable, act in a threatening or violent manner, or even act dangerously on the job. This is a particular problem in occupations that are responsible for the safety of others, such as airline pilots or truck drivers. Many countries require screening for alcohol or drug abuse and prohibit workers in such occupations from consuming alcohol for a certain period before, and certainly during, their work shift.

12

HAZARD CONTROL

Erkki Kähkönen

Hazards take many forms: chemicals, unsafe equipment, microorganisms, extreme heat or cold, noise, vibration, toxic liquids, poor lighting, radiation, and more. Effective control of hazards in the workplace can be achieved by a variety of interventions, including engineering controls, administrative arrangements, safe work practices, preventive maintenance, and the use of personal protective equipment.

Occupational hygiene is the field of occupational health that involves the recognition, evaluation, and control of hazards found in the workplace. The occupational hygienist is a specialist in recognizing the existence of hazards in the work environment, evaluating the risks arising from these hazards, and, where necessary, eliminating or controlling risks to acceptable levels. Preventive measures are becoming more important at workplaces in order to minimize hazardous exposures. Many measures that prevent worker injury or exposure also reduce loss from inefficient work processes, spoilage, and contamination.

The control of workplace hazards is illustrated in this chapter by the reduction of noise and vibration and by the control of exposure to silica dust. Noise is the most common occupational hazard, found in every industry, and control of noise is one of the most common problems in hazard control. Silica is a common occupational hazard and illustrates ventilation and respiratory controls.

BASIC APPROACHES

There are four basic approaches to controlling occupational hazards. Engineering controls are generally considered most effective because, properly maintained, they do not require cooperation or special effort from the worker. Preventive maintenance is essential to ensuring that engineering controls work, avoiding breakdowns that cause dangerous conditions, and reducing the accumulation of hazardous chemicals or waste. Personal protective equipment (PPE) is necessary when hazards cannot be effectively controlled by engineering, but PPE is considered less reliable because it requires regular and voluntary use. Its effectiveness depends on worker training in how to use PPE properly, voluntary compliance, proper fit of the equipment to the person, adherence to a routine, and maintenance

Box 12.1

Controlling Silicosis in Singapore

Silicosis is the characteristic lung disease caused by inhaling silica dust particles. It is the oldest occupational disease known and was first described in ancient times, yet it remains the most common occupational lung disease in the world. It is a particular problem in mining, sandblasting, foundry and metal casting, and ceramics.

As Singapore launched its industrialization program in the 1960s, the importance of protecting workers from occupational health hazards was foreseen. The government established the Industrial Health Unit in 1970, now known as the Department of Industrial Health (DIH), Ministry of Labour. One of the top priorities of the Industrial Health Unit was the silicosis problem in Singapore.

The statistics on all notified and confirmed occupational diseases are kept by the DIH. Silicosis was made a notifiable industrial disease under the Factories Act of 1970. It was the leading occupational disease in the early 1970s and was the leading occupational respiratory disease in the 1970s and 1980s (see Figure 12.1). At the end of 1995, there were 362 cases of confirmed silicosis, of which 78% came from granite quarries (Table 12.1).

TABLE 12.1

SILICOSIS BY INDUSTRY 1970–1995

Industry	No. of Cases (%)
Granite Quarries	282 (77.9)
Rubber Factories	43 (11.9)
Kaolin Quarries	11 (3.0)
Foundries	10 (2.8)
Brickworks	6 (1.7)
Others	10 (2.8)
Total	362 (100)

The risk of silicosis was particularly great in granite quarries in the 1970s. There were 25 granite quarries employing about 1,200 workers in 1970. Quarry operations involve drilling, blasting, and stone breaking at the quarry face; the granite rocks are then loaded and transferred to the crushing plant for crushing and screening. Dust monitoring carried out in 1968 and 1971 revealed very high dust levels.

A radiological survey of 1,188 granite quarry workers in 1965 revealed that 8% had silicosis. A follow-up survey in 1971 of 1,230 quarry workers showed that 15% had silicosis.

The government took a serious view of the situation and engaged a World Health Organization (WHO) consultant in industrial hygiene in 1972 to study the dust control problems in granite quarries. The consultant concluded that there was a serious dust hazard in the quarries and recommended the following:

1. Quarry operators must be required to take action to reduce dust levels.
2. Each quarry must submit a plan of action.
3. Regulations should be developed for dust control in quarries.
4. Quarry operators must establish a dust monitoring program.

All the recommendations were implemented by the government.

Following the WHO Study, the Singapore Institute of Standards and Industrial Research (SISIR), in cooperation with the Granite Quarry Owners and Employers Association of Singapore, carried out a survey in 1972 covering 21 quarries. The report published in 1973 (Leow 1973) found that only one of the quarries had an effective dust control system and that 50% of the larger quarries had very serious dust emissions. The major sources of dust emissions came from the drilling operations, the crushing units, the screen units, and the transfer and loading points. In both the WHO and SISIR reports, local exhaust ventilation together with wet method were recommended as an effective means of dust control in quarries.

Control measures were encouraged and supported by legislation. The Sand and Granite Quarries Regulations were enacted in 1971. Licensees of any quarry were required to install dust extraction systems, provide dust masks, and arrange for annual chest X-ray examinations for quarry workers. Silicosis was made a compensable occupational disease under the Workmen's Compensation Act in 1972. The Abrasive Blasting Regulations enacted in 1974 prohibited the use of sand as an abrasive for blasting. Thereafter, there were very few cases of silicosis among sandblasters in Singapore.

To focus attention on the problem and to create awareness among both workers and management, the Ministry of Labour launched a campaign against silicosis in 1973 that included a mobile exhibition and media coverage. Quarry owners were called upon to take preventive measures to protect the health of their workers.

Between 1972 and 1973, the government formally requested all 25 granite quarries to install local dust exhaust systems (Tan 1979). Despite the expected technical and financial problems, the number of quarries that installed such systems increased from 12 in 1974 to 21 in 1976. SISIR was responsible for the design of most of the dust control systems. By 1979, all granite quarries had installed dust control systems.

Regular monitoring of dust exposure is essential to assess occupational exposure and to evaluate the effectiveness of the dust control measures. There was a significant decline in dust levels particularly after the implementation of dust control measures in 1973 (Table 12.2).

In a study of 201 quarry workers from five granite quarries in 1988, the prevalence of respirator usage was about 60% to 70% among the drillers and crusher attendants, who were the more exposed group of workers (Chia 1989).

Pre-employment and annual chest X-rays have been a legal requirement for granite quarry workers since 1972 and for all silica-exposed workers in factories since 1985. Chest X-ray screening is useful in the early detection of silicosis, and as a result a large number of silicosis cases were detected in 1973.

There was a sharp decline in the number of new cases of silicosis after 1975 and a further decline after 1990. In the 1990s, occupational asthma has replaced silicosis

TABLE 12.2

RESPIRABLE DUST LEVELS (8 HR TWA) OF CRUSHER WORKERS AT GRANITE QUARRIES

Year	No. of Samples	Mean (mg/m^3)	% > 1 mg/m^3
1973	116	3.1	85.3
1976	141	1.3	42.5
1977	296	1.3	48.6
1978	291	1.1	50.1
1985	270	1.3	55.2
1986	217	1.0	34.6
1987	114	0.8	25.4

as the most common occupational respiratory disease (Lee et al. 1996). Only one case of silicosis was confirmed in 1995 and three cases in 1994. These workers had been working in granite quarries for many years.

A radiological survey of 219 currently employed workers from six operating granite quarries in 1990 showed that the prevalence of silicosis among drilling and crushing workers was 12.5% vs. 0.8% among maintenance and transportation workers (Ng et al. 1992). Among those first exposed to granite dust in 1979 or later, no cases of silicosis were noted. This may suggest that the reduction in dust levels since 1979 may have been successful in preventing silicosis among active quarry workers over 10 years.

In recent years, the government has stopped renewing the licenses of many quarries; therefore, the number of quarries has declined from 25 in 1970 to 3 in 1995.

Silicosis was a significant problem among granite quarry workers in Singapore in its early years of industrialization. The government recognized the problem and sought the assistance of experts to study the problem and to recommend solutions. Legislation was introduced in 1972, and dust control measures were enforced. At the same time, public education was carried out. Dust levels fell significantly after 1973, and this was followed by a decline in the number of silicosis cases. Today, silicosis is no longer a significant disease in Singapore. However, cases of occupational asthma have increased, reflecting changes in technology and the economy that have accompanied Singapore's development.

Prepared by: Dr Lee Hock Siang, Singapore

of the equipment. Administrative controls, such as limiting the time a worker is allowed to work in a given area, are considered the least effective when used alone, although they are critical in supporting other approaches.

Engineering Controls

Engineering controls focus on managing the source of the hazard, unlike other types of controls that generally focus on the employee exposed to the hazards.

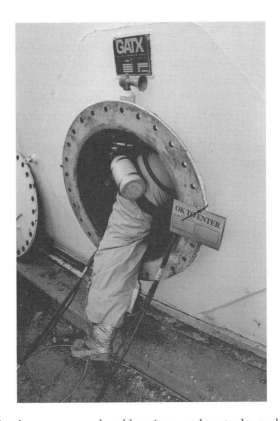

Figure 12.1 Confined spaces are enclosed locations, such as tanks, sealed rooms, reaction vessels, and pipelines. They are also created when processes are contained, which is one form of *engineering control* to prevent exposure, but sometimes have to be entered for maintenance or repair. They are especially hazardous because entry and exit may be difficult in an emergency, the air may be contaminated, fumes may build up to create a fire or explosion hazard, and oxygen levels may be too low to support life. This worker is entering a tank to repair damage after an earthquake in California. He is carrying self-contained breathing apparatus (SCBA, the metal tank visible next to his leg), which is a *supplied air respiratory personal protection* device providing about 25 minutes of air, enough time to escape in an emergency. The tank has been checked carefully for oxygen level and to ensure that there are no toxic or flammable gases present, as shown by the permit tied to the flange (an example of *administrative controls*). Workers who enter confined spaces are required to work with a coworker (a "buddy," not seen in the photograph) who stays outside and carefully monitors the situation and who will call for help in case of emergency, another example of *administrative controls*. Note that the worker's boots are taped to his pants in order to keep dust and chemicals out, another example of *personal protection*. (Photograph by © Earl Dotter, all rights reserved.)

The first and foremost strategy is to control the hazard at its source. Engineering controls minimize employee exposure by either reducing or removing the hazard at the source or by isolating the workers from the hazards. Engineering controls include eliminating toxic materials from the work process and replacing them with less hazardous ones, enclosing work processes or confining work operations, and installing general and local ventilation systems. The advantage of engineering controls is that they work whether or not the worker actively cooperates, they are usually reliable if properly designed, and they reduce the risk of unexpected incidents that result in exposure. However, engineering controls often depend on proper maintenance and have to be monitored to be sure that they are working efficiently. They can sometimes be expensive, and when they slow down production, they may be removed or bypassed by workers in a hurry.

Engineering controls include, but are certainly not limited to, the following:

- Isolation. The hazard may be located away from workers so that there is a safe distance separating them; e.g., a kiln in a ceramics factory may be located away from the main plant.
- Containment. The hazard may be fully enclosed. Most large chemical plants and all oil refineries completely contain the production process.
- Substitution. Hazardous materials may be replaced by less hazardous materials in the workplace; e.g., trichloroethane, a solvent, has replaced the more toxic trichloroethylene as a degreasing agent by industry.
- Process controls. Modern controls for monitoring and controlling the production process can reduce the risk of incidents. Chemical plants today usually control their processes very closely, but in the past there have been many incidents where chemical reactions got out of control, resulting in explosions, leaks, and production of more hazardous chemicals.
- Ventilation. The most important form of engineering control (see below).

Preventive Maintenance

Maintenance of equipment and the workplace is the best way to assure that the system will continue to give the health protection it was meant to provide. When machinery breaks down and the workplace becomes dirty, conditions can become dangerous. The frequency of the maintenance will vary for the different components of the system and the maintenance method used. Preventive maintenance is generally done at regular intervals, more frequently than the expected time between failures. The advantage of this schedule is that most of the maintenance can be planned. The disadvantage is that maintenance is not always done before a breakdown occurs. "On-condition maintenance" or "predictive maintenance" means that the breakdown of a machine is predicted with performance measures or measurements of characteristics such as vibration, because a developing fault such as a worn part or a broken ball bearing often raises the vibration level in a machine. "Run-to-breakdown maintenance," in which machines are intentionally allowed to break down, is mainly used when many machines operate in parallel, the breakdown of one machine does not affect the overall operation, and the machine is inexpensive and easy to replace.

Safe Work Practices

The design of safe work practices is based on the analysis of the hazards in work tasks. Written procedures are needed, the training of workers is important, and it is necessary that the workers understand the safety procedures and follow them.

Safe work practices also include housekeeping, good personal hygiene, hazard warning signs, and training to ensure that the work is done correctly. This may be easier to implement if the employees are actually involved in the safety analysis, thus the procedures will then be perceived as fair and be understood by all. Good work practices must be enforced to be effective; the employer should penalize workers who do not follow instructions and supervisors who do not correct this behavior.

Housekeeping and Hygiene Order and cleanliness, or industrial housekeeping, are important for safety, control of exposure to hazards, product quality, and company image. The cooperative development of standards, employee participation, modern motivation principles, teamwork, quantified measurement and evaluation, and positive feedback are the cornerstones of effective housekeeping programs. Good housekeeping includes adequate washing and eating facilities away from hazardous areas. The hands and face should be washed before eating outside dusty areas. A shower and change into clean clothes before leaving the work site is strongly recommended for any work involving chemical hazards or dusts. Dusty clothes easily contaminate clean areas at work and can lead to the exposure of family members if the worker wears dirty clothes home.

Administrative Controls

Administrative controls are measures that depend on the behavior of workers or the way that work is organized, instead of managing the hazard directly. They include organizational rules, staff rotation, standards, and training. Such controls are normally used in conjunction with others that more directly prevent or control exposure to the hazard. Administrative controls include controlling the employees' exposure by scheduling production and workers' tasks, or both, in ways that minimize exposure. For example, the employer might schedule operations with the highest exposure potential at times when only a few employees are present. Sometimes administrative approaches that rely on record keeping, such as staff rotation, can be defeated by workers or supervisors who make false records. Administrative controls are generally considered to be the weakest approach to managing hazards.

Personal Protection

When exposure to hazards cannot be eliminated completely from normal operations or maintenance work, and when safe work practices and other administrative controls cannot provide sufficient additional protection, a supplementary method of control is the use of protective equipment. Personal protective equipment, such as appropriate respiratory equipment, gloves, safety goggles, helmets, safety shoes, and protective clothing may also be required. In order to be effective, personal protective equipment must be individually selected, properly fitted, and periodically refitted; it must be conscientiously and properly worn, regularly maintained, and replaced whenever necessary. The employees must know why and how to use it and how to maintain it.

Ventilation is the most important method of reducing exposure to airborne contaminants. It also serves other purposes, such as preventing the accumulation of flammable or explosive concentrations of gases, vapors, or dust at workplaces. In addition, special ventilation is needed to control fire and explosion hazards.

For some particularly hazardous contaminants, such as asbestos, ordinary ventilation alone is not enough, and special arrangements should be made to keep the environment clean. The control of personal exposure to levels below the occupational exposure limits can be achieved in a number of ways, e.g., substituting the hazardous substance with a less harmful one, altering the process, enclosing the process totally, removing the contaminant as soon as it is generated, and providing personal protection.

Ventilation systems may be designed to move air through the workplace or to remove an airborne contaminant at the source before it reaches the worker's *breathing zone*, the space in front of the worker's nose and mouth.

A key concept in ventilation is *balance*. Air, like water, always flows from higher, relatively positive pressure (often called blowing) to lower, relatively negative pressure (often called suction). Also like water, air follows the path of least resistance: when a constant flow of air encounters resistance, pressure goes up and can force the air in a different direction, if there is another pathway. In addition, the flow of air can be broken up by obstacles or turbulence. When airflow is smooth and going where it should go, the ventilation system is in balance. Systems that are out of balance may show unexpected patterns of air movement. For example, a clogged filter may present so much resistance to airflow that the contaminated air stops moving. Where exhaust ducts come together and one contains more air pressure than the other, contaminated air may be pushed out into the workplace rather than exhausted away from it.

Although air behaves in many respects like water when it flows, there is one important difference. Unlike water, when air is compressed, the volume is reduced and it heats up. When pressure is released, the volume of air increases and it cools down. This is the basic physical principle behind refrigeration.

Worksite Ventilation

The three main methods of ventilation that control airborne contamination in a workplace are general ventilation, dilution ventilation, and displacement ventilation. The overall heating and cooling air system in a building is often referred to as the general ventilation system. General ventilation is primarily used to maintain comfortable conditions for those working or living in the building. Air conditioning is used to control the temperature, humidity, and heat load and to ensure fresh air circulation without drafts. General ventilation is generally not strong enough to provide effective dilution for air contaminants in a workplace. Sometimes, poorly designed or positioned general ventilation systems cause problems in the workplace, e.g., when the air intake is located near an exhaust vent or in an area where motor vehicles have their engines running.

Dilution ventilation is used in contaminant control systems. Incoming air diffuses throughout the workroom. It passes partly through the zone of contaminant release and dilutes the contaminant to a lower concentration. The dilution effect continues as the material moves further from the process until the exhaust fan removes the contaminated air. The air volume needed to dilute the contaminant to a safe limit may be large if the amount of contaminant released is sizeable. Dilution ventilation does not provide any control at the source of the contaminant, so the work processes should be arranged so that the air moves from cleaner to dirtier areas.

Effective dilution can be achieved from natural ventilation as well as from mechanical systems that use fans. Even moderate winds can move large volumes of air through open doors and windows. This method is useful in warm countries where industrial plants are often open to the outdoors. In such cases, the ventilation rate may depend greatly on weather. Air movement due to temperature differences between the exterior and interior of a building may provide useful ventilation in colder countries. Hot processes heat the surrounding air, and the rising column of warm air will carry contaminants upward.

In a cold climate, it is expensive to heat *make-up air*, which replaces the air that is removed from the building, to workroom temperature. On large premises, the use of heat recovery systems may be economically feasible. If the incoming air is heated, and warm air rises upward, it is possible that fresh air will never reach the breathing zone. The workers must be located far enough from the contaminant source because it may be difficult to control the employees' exposure near the contaminant source. Only low-toxicity materials should be considered for control by dilution ventilation, and the rate of contaminant release should be reasonably constant. Peak concentrations are difficult to control by using dilution ventilation.

Displacement ventilation is a technology was developed in Scandinavia and is applicable to cold climates. In spaces with displacement ventilation, the air is supplied at low velocity from large outlets directly into the occupied zone. The outlets are located near floor level. The supply air, at a temperature of 2 to 4° C below room air temperature, spreads near the floor in a comparatively thin layer and subsequently rises to the ceiling as it warms, displacing the contaminated room air. The amount of dilution airflow depends on the rate of contaminants released, their toxicity, the acceptable airborne concentration, and the relative efficiency of the total air volume flowing through the area. These data are difficult to obtain.

Local Exhaust Ventilation

Local exhaust ventilation systems capture contaminants at their source before they are dispersed into the workroom. A typical system consists of ducts, one or more hoods, an air cleaner, and a fan. The advantages of local exhaust systems include better control of worker exposure and lower airflow requirements, which reduce energy costs for premises that are heated or cooled. The collection efficiency is always less than 100% due to workers' movements, drafts, and other air disturbances, and so local exhaust alone is not sufficient.

For local exhaust systems to work properly, the whole ventilation system must be in *balance* so that negative pressures pull the airborne contaminant away from the worker, and air currents or positive pressures in other places do not push the

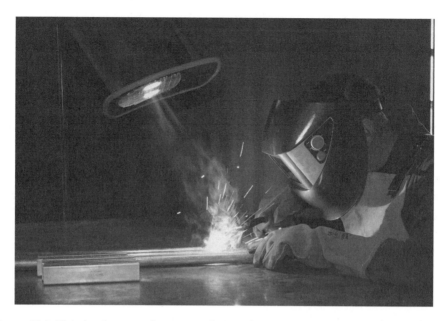

Figure 12.2 This local area exhaust ventilation duct system is designed specifically for welding operations. There is another example of this type of exhaust ventilation in Figure 8.2, the Kemper Exhaust Hood. (Photograph courtesy of the manufacturer, © Kemper America.)

contaminant back into the workers' breathing zone. Additional dilution ventilation is always needed in the workplace as a whole, but may not be sufficient alone where there is an intense source of emissions.

The hoods are the most important part of the local exhaust system. A hood, enclosure, or other inlet collects and contains the contaminant close to its source. The hood should be located so that contaminants are never drawn through the workers' breathing zone.

There are three major types of hoods:

- *Enclosures* surround the contaminant sources as completely as possible. The contaminants are kept inside the enclosure by air flowing in through openings in the enclosure. For example, fume cupboards are partial enclosures fitted with a vertically sliding front, which can be adjusted to vary the height of the opening. Negative pressure in the hood pulls the contaminant up into the exhaust and away from the worker, whose head is located outside the hood.
- *Receiving hoods* are positioned so that they catch the contaminants generated by a production process. For example, a furnace emits a hot stream of air or a grinder throws a stream of material tangentially from the point of contact. The hood is placed so that it intercepts the stream and negative pressure pulls it away from the worker and out the exhaust.
- *Capturing hoods* capture contaminants in the workroom air. Airflow into the hood is calculated to generate sufficient capture velocity in the air space directly in front of the hood. The capture velocity needed depends on the amount and

motion of contaminants and contaminated air. Tables have been published showing the capture velocity in a many situations.

There is an important physical limitation to hood design. Hoods draw air from only a short distance away from the hood opening and therefore cannot control contaminants released at some distance. Air is drawn into the fan inlet duct from the space immediately around the duct opening, a space in the shape of a sphere. The power of the negative air pressure falls off as the inverse cube of the distance from the inlet duct. This means that the farther away from the intake of the duct, the less strongly air is drawn into the system. That is why systems are ineffective beyond a short distance.

Many people believe that particles and vapors that are heavier than air tend to settle to the workroom floor and therefore can be collected by a hood located near the floor. While it is true that larger particulates tend to settle and move downward toward the floor, they cannot be controlled this way effectively. A concentration of 1,000 ppm means 1,000 parts contaminants in 999,000 parts air. The resulting density of the aerosol in the air mass is close to that of the air itself and is moved around by random air currents until it disperses throughout the room. Also, if the vapors are warm, they may move upward toward the ceiling or into the worker's breathing zone, even if they are denser than air at room temperature.

Ducts convey the contaminants away from the source. Ducts should be designed so that the air velocity in the duct, the *duct velocity*, is high enough to keep the particles suspended in the air stream. Duct diameters, the number and type of bends and elbows, as well as hoods affect the resistance to airflow in the duct network. When air passes through a narrower duct, when the duct changes direction, when there are objects in the duct (such as valves or baffles), and when the surface of the duct is uneven, resistance to airflow increases. This increases the energy cost of moving the air and may result in unbalanced flow. On the other hand, when air moves from a narrow to a large duct diameter, flow slows down, the air may stop moving, and particles may fall out. Ductwork systems should be as simple and straight as possible, and the number of changes in direction and the number of junctions should be kept to a minimum in order to avoid excessive resistance to flow.

Flexible ducting is often used where hoods are attached to moving parts of machinery. However, flexible ducting tends to wear out quickly, and flow resistance is high. Suitable materials for ductwork are galvanized sheet steel, sheet aluminum, or PVC and polypropylene, depending on the temperature, particle size, and properties of the contaminants. One must be careful in retrofitting a duct system because the addition of new openings changes airflow and resistance patterns and changes the balance in the system.

Fans generate suction that draws contaminated air in through the hoods. Fans have some built-in flexibility because their flow rates increase with higher fan speed. Fans also require maintenance and sometimes fail. In selecting a fan for a particular application, the following factors are important: air flow, total flow resistance of the system (static pressure), operating temperature, noise, type of contaminants, rotating speed, and power consumption. Data on fan performance are listed in fan rating tables in manufacturers' catalogs.

Air Cleaning Devices

Air cleaners are packaged units that are purchased and installed in local exhaust systems. Many national and international standards and recommendations require air-cleaning devices in ventilation systems to regulate the amount of hazardous air pollutants that can be discharged from certain industrial operations.

Air cleaning devices may be grouped into three basic types—air filters, particulate dust and fume collectors, and devices to remove mists, gases, and vapors. An air cleaner often represents the point of greatest resistance to the flow of air in the system.

Air filters are mainly used for cleaning air in ventilation and air-conditioning systems. Filters of woven or felted fabric are most common, although paper and woven metal are also used. The contaminant is physically trapped on the surface of the filter medium. A common reusable filter unit for an industrial exhaust system is the baghouse. Much of the collected dust can be released by a vibrating shaking device or by blowing high-pressure jets of air back through the filter. A high efficiency particulate air (HEPA) filter is a special disposable filter used mainly for particularly hazardous particulates.

Particulate collectors are designed to extract large quantities of dust and fumes from an air stream. These collectors include cyclones, fabric filters, wet collectors, and electrostatic precipitators. Electrostatic precipitators charge particles with an electrical current and trap them by electrostatic attraction. Some materials do not charge easily and thus tend to pass through these devices. However, collection efficiency is high for small particles. Cyclones create a circular motion to the exhaust gas that causes particulates to move to the outer part of the air stream, where they impact the cyclone walls and drop into the collection hopper. The cleaned air passes through a central outlet at the top of the chamber. Cyclones may also be operated as wet collectors if a water spray is installed to wet the particles at the inlet. Wet scrubbers contact particles with water or another liquid. The highly turbulent conditions break down the water into small droplets that form around the dust particles, and the droplets are then collected.

The major removal techniques for gases and vapors are absorption, adsorption, and combustion. Absorption is a diffusion process in which the contaminant moves from the exhaust gas to a liquid that is released in a fine stream in a spray chamber. Water is the most popular absorber. Adsorption is a process in which a gas or vapor adheres to the surface of a porous solid material. No chemical reaction is involved. The most common adsorbents are activated carbon, silica gel, and hydrated silicate. Thermal oxidation devices use direct and catalytic oxidation to convert organic compounds into innocuous substances (such as carbon and water vapor) in a chemical reaction.

Ventilation System Evaluation and Maintenance

Maintenance and inspection include lubricating the fan, motor, and drive; checking the fan belt for proper tension; inspecting the air cleaner internal mechanisms for visible damage; inspecting fan wheels and housing for wear and dust buildup; checking dust systems for partially plugged ducts; and cleaning the ducts. The mechanical and electrical system components should also be checked for proper operation and condition. Maintenance should be performed following the designer's and manufacturer's instructions.

Unfortunately, more attention is often given to the mechanical part of the ventilation system and to reducing costs of heating and cooling than to the effectiveness of the ventilation system in protecting workers' health. It is important to ask who is responsible for the maintenance of ventilation systems and for regular testing to be done by people who are not normally responsible for the system maintenance.

Evaluating Ventilation Systems A new ventilation system should be thoroughly tested upon installation to see that it meets design specifications and to assure that the airflow through each hood is correct and the system is properly balanced. In addition to maintenance, there may be statutory requirements that must be met in its operation. Common tests include smoke tube tracer studies, velocity at the hood opening, hood static pressure, duct velocity measurements, system static pressure, and fan tests.

Smoke tubes are a very useful tool in evaluating ventilation systems. The smoke tube contains chemicals that produce visible fumes. The smoke follows the air currents, and its velocity shows how the air flows into the hood. The smoke tube helps to identify the correct hood location, the capture distance for hoods, the turbulence around openings, the effect of cross drafts on hood performance, slight air currents and their direction, leaks in pipelines or joints, distribution of substances in vapor form, etc. Smoke tubes are particularly useful for training purposes, to show how ventilation hoods function and what factors affect hood performance.

Hood velocity measurements are needed to calculate average air velocity and volumetric airflow through a hood opening or duct with a known area. A rotating vane anemometer (a device for measuring wind speed) is used in large openings, such as doorways and large ventilated booths, but it cannot be used for small areas where the instruments fill a large proportion of the openings. Hot wire anemometers are used to measure capture velocities and air flows in ducts. By using anemometer hoods, which are calibrated for direct reading of volumetric flow, it is easy to measure volume flows at duct input and output vents. The most accurate way to measure airflows in ducts is the use of a pitot tube. The pitot tube is used to measure air velocity at a number of points across the duct cross-section. The pressure differences given by the pitot tube are measured using a manometer. By the same manometer, it is possible to perform a hood static pressure test as well as a system static pressure test. The result given by the static pressure measurements can be compared with the values given by the equipment designer or the values recorded when the system was operating properly.

Control of Particles

Particles are a common type of occupational hazard. The general term for particles suspended in air is *aerosol*. Aerosols consisting of liquid droplets suspended in air

An Innovative Policy for Controlling Silica Exposure

One of the most dramatic examples of silica dust control has taken place in China at the Anshan Iron and Steel Group, an initiative led by Chen Guohua, who played a major role in occupational health in China in the 1970's and 1980's. In the past, silica dust levels in the foundry and metal casting parts of the complex were very high, and there was high exposure among maintenance workers. Over 45 years, despite difficulties, the occupational health professionals in Anshan were able to get dust levels down to international standards of exposure, preventing thousands of cases of silicosis. One of the keys to their success was adoption of a policy called the "Three Simultaneities." This policy dictated that three critical tasks needed to be done at the same time and on an ongoing basis: design, construction, and operation of the dust control system, always in step and coordinated together with the main production facilities.

may form *droplet nuclei* as the liquid evaporates. Solid particles suspended in air are called *dust*. Dusts are a very common problem in hazard control and merit special attention. In this section, additional measures to control dust will be described, using silica as an example.

Small dust particles, below 10 µm, remain airborne for a long time and can penetrate into the deep lung. There, they may cause serious lung disease (see Chapter 16). High dust levels also irritate the throat and eyes and reduce visibility in the workplace. The hazards associated with dust depend on its composition and size. Various categories can be classified, but individual particles may belong to more than one category:

- *Fibrogenic dusts* are dusts that cause inflammation and scarring in the lung. The most common dust-related hazards are from silica and asbestos, each of which can cause its own serious lung disease (silicosis and asbestosis, respectively). These dusts, and others that are formed from natural minerals, are often called *mineral dusts*.
- *Toxic dusts* consist of or carry toxic chemicals. Lead, for example, is often carried into the lungs via particles, which then slowly dissolve and release the lead into the body.
- *Biological dusts* include mold spores, pollen, grain dust, wood dust, and other particles of biological origin. These dusts often cause allergies and, depending on their origin, may carry bacteria or other infectious hazards.
- *Droplet nuclei* are dried-out droplets of a liquid that may contain a chemical or infectious agent. Droplet nuclei from a person who coughs, for example, may carry tuberculosis or other diseases if the person is infected. Droplet nuclei from ocean spray forms tiny salt particles in the air.

- *Particulate air pollution* is the type of particle found in urban air pollution. The health effects of particulate air pollution, acting on the large population of cities, make this form of pollution a major public health hazard.
- *Nuisance dust* is the common name for dusts that consist of substances that are not very toxic. Examples include paper dust, house dust, plastic dust, and titanium dust (from white paint powder). At high concentrations, however, these dusts are still irritating to the mucous membranes of the eye and throat, and they may overload the body's immune and defense systems in the lungs.

Ventilation is a mainstay for particle control. All the measures described in the previous section apply to dust control. Droplet control is more often controlled at the source by preventing it from being generated in the first place.

To eliminate or significantly reduce employee exposure, any dirty operation can be isolated by enclosing it. Sandblasting cabinets and machines are examples of totally closed processes. Sandblasting on a small scale, e.g., for metal parts, can be done in enclosed chambers. This may involve building an enclosure around a dusty work process. An enclosure should be properly ventilated to eliminate the buildup of contaminants and as airtight as possible. Small vision ports are needed to allow inspection of certain aspects of the process.

Changes in the manufacturing process, such as the introduction of water to control silica dust levels, can be used to reduce worker exposure. When most dusts are wet, they stick together and do not become suspended in air. Wetting down is one of the simplest methods for dust control. Its effectiveness depends on the proper wetting of the dust, which may require the addition of a wetting agent to the water. Great reductions in dust concentrations have been achieved by forcing water through the drill bits used in rock drilling operations and wet sawing to protect adjacent workers from exposure. Castings can sometimes be cleaned with water instead of by sandblasting. Furthermore, if the molding sand is kept moist, the dust concentration in air will be considerably lower.

Personal protective devices must be used when there are no other ways to avoid or eliminate risks arising from the work. Respirators should not be the only method of control. National and international standards set forth guidelines for the selection of proper personal protective equipment. The anthropometric and ergonomic properties, as well as the comfort of use, are of vital importance. Common issues include (1) the service life of filters, which can be shortened by high temperature and relative humidity; (2) the purity of the air, which must be ensured when compressed air devices are used; and (3) in hot and humid countries, a full or half-face mask is inconvenient to use because of sweating. The great variety of devices and the complexity of some devices require that the users and the persons who are responsible for cleaning and maintenance of the devices be given proper training.

There are a number of technical methods for controlling and reducing workers' exposure to dust. In a foundry, for example, the risk of silicosis has been eliminated by combining several technical measures: dry sand is not conveyed on open conveyor belts; efficient general and local ventilation has been installed; sand preparation and sandblasting are done in a totally closed system; and central vacuum cleaners, not compressed air, are used for cleaning. Preventive measures

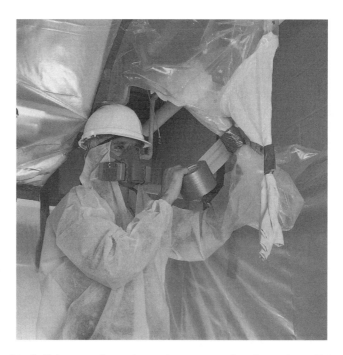

Figure 12.3 This half-face mask respirator is an example of an *air purifying* device. The cartridges on either side of the mask contain different filters or absorbing agents and are chosen for the specific hazard. The worker using the respirator is preparing a workplace for asbestos abatement by sealing it off with plastic sheeting, and he is also wearing protective clothing, safety glasses, and a hard hat. (Photograph courtesy of the manufacturer, © 3M Corporation, all rights reserved.)

must be built into the companies' management and quality assurance system and should be seen as an investment for the future that will bring dividends in the form of healthier employees and better products.

Substitution may also be possible to prevent generating the dust in the first place. Sandblasting is an industrial process that is difficult to control because it is often performed outdoors (e.g., to renovate buildings) or in confined spaces (e.g., to remove corrosion from pipes). Ordinary sand is almost entirely quartz, a crystalline form of silica. When sand is used in sandblasting, small particles break off to form respirable dust. When these small particles are inhaled they can cause silicosis, a serious lung disease. Many countries, mostly in Europe, have restricted or banned the use of quartz sand.

There are many substitutes for hazardous quartz sand, such as glass beads, cast iron, steel grit, aluminum oxide, and zirconium oxide. These media are more expensive, but they are recyclable and they have some other benefits, such as increasing the quality of the final products. Glass beads do not remove material or metal, and the cleaned surface is smooth and has a matte finish, which reduces glare. Studies show that a glass-bead finished stainless steel surface inhibits the growth of bacteria. This is particularly important for components used in the medical or food industry, where the hygiene and cleanliness of the products are

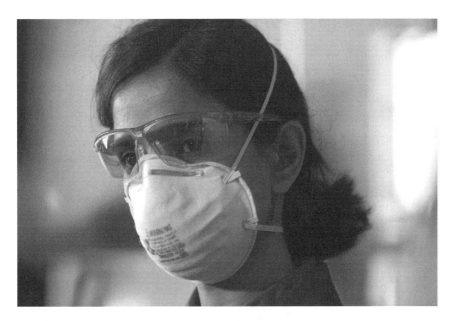

Figure 12.4 This N95 respirator is disposable and is widely used in hospital and medical services for the protection of health-care staff and patients, but it is also used in dusty workplaces. The name N indicates that it is not for use with oily aerosols (which penetrate the fabric of the mask), and the designation 95 indicates that it reduces exposure to airborne particles < 0.3 μm in diameter by at least 95%, although actual performance is usually much better than that. (Photograph courtesy of the manufacturer, © 3M Corporation, all rights reserved.)

of paramount importance. In addition, glass-bead blasting is a quicker and less labor-intensive process than conventional methods. Ferrous abrasives can include steel grit, which is sharp-edged, and steel or iron shot, which are spherical products. Iron and steel abrasives are not hazardous in themselves. Aluminum oxide is very hard, sharp-edged, and an effective cutting and cleaning medium that renders an excellent surface for painting. In foundries, silica sand is difficult to substitute. Olivine sand (the granular form of olivine, a mineral which consists of silica, iron, and magnesium) is perhaps the only economical alternative. Zircon or chromite sands are expensive, and they are used only in special cases. Solid carbon dioxide has been developed for abrasive blasting and may be used much more in the future.

NOISE AND VIBRATION CONTROL

Noise is a universal problem in work life and is the most widespread hazard in the workplace. Noise is a form of energy. In the workplace, noise is usually the sum of many sounds all mixed together. Sound consists of a pressure wave that moves through air. A continuous sound wave has a *frequency* (heard as a tone and measured as the number of cycles in one second) and *amplitude* (heard as loudness, measured in units of *decibels*). As the wave moves outward from the source, it loses

BOX 12.3

Unexpected Problems with Personal Protective Equipment in a Developing Country

For many generations, workers have been collecting salt and other chemicals from groundwater and seawater in the arid costal plains of Tamil Nadu, India. Seawater is channeled at high tide into shallow, wide pits called "pans," where the water is allowed to evaporate. Traditionally, the saltpans were scraped regularly with hand tools to break up the mineral crust, and work was done by men.

The principal hazards of this work are chemical exposure to the salt, heat, and ultraviolet radiation (see Chapter 8). The concentrated seawater becomes brine, a solution of salt that dries out the skin and causes severe skin irritation. Therefore, the workers must wear heavy rubber boots to protect their feet and legs. The ambient temperature in the summer months is 44 to 47° C, which presents a serious risk of heat stroke even to heat-adapted workers. The workers must drink huge amounts of water. The work is out in the open, with no shelter available, resulting in heavy UV exposure, both directly from the intense sunlight and from reflected radiation off the water-filled pans. Eye protection is also required.

UV radiation is associated with skin damage, skin cancer, and cataracts. Cataracts occur when the lens of the eye, which is normally clear, becomes cloudy and vision is lost; blindness may occur. This is often overlooked or unrecognized because cataracts also occur with aging and with diseases such as diabetes. However, they occur earlier, more severely, and in a different place in the eye when they are caused by intense UV exposure. Many other occupations involving water, such as fishing, share an increased risk of cataracts associated with intense UV exposure.

UV radiation also causes pterygium, a scar-like growth on the eyeball that is very common and in rare cases can grow over the lens. UV radiation may also cause damage to the retina, which is the structure in the eye that perceives light.

In order to protect the workers from cataracts, the company issued wrap-around sunglasses to protect the eyes from UV exposure. Although intended primarily to reduce the risk of cataracts, this item of personal protective equipment (PPE) would also decrease the incidence of pterygium and reduce the risk of retinal injury. However, the workers sold the eyeglasses they were given, giving up protection for the money.

Why did this happen? There are several reasons. The workers were very poor, and the small amount of money they made from selling the eyeglasses went to support their families. The money was spent on living expenses or dowries to ensure that their children were able to marry in what they considered to be a proper manner. Because sunglasses are a popular fashion item and are relatively expensive in stores, it was easy for them to get a good price for their PPE on the street.

The tragic result will be that some of these workers will lose their vision due to the lack of PPE. Why did they do it?

These people recognized the costs and benefits. They were very resourceful about getting a price for their sunglasses. They cared enough about their lives and the lives of their families to try to make more money. They may or may not have understood that the purpose of the eyeglasses was to protect their vision. They may have felt that a relatively small benefit today (the money) was worth taking a big future risk (loss of their sight) that will happen to only some workers. Each worker who sold his glasses was betting that loss of vision would not happen to him. Because the workers who do this job are impoverished and live in communities where life expectancy is not long, they may have felt that they would not live long enough to get cataracts. Because they are poorly educated and literacy rates are low, some of them may not have valued their vision as much as people who can read, although most people consider sight their most important sense.

Poverty, lack of education, and responsibility to family often interfere with hazard control. Sometimes workers act in ways that seem irrational to occupational health professionals, but there may be valid reasons that can be understood only from the workers' point of view.

Contributed by Craig Karpilow, M.D.

power proportional to the square of the distance away from the source. Noise that measures 10 decibels can barely be heard by someone with excellent hearing. Noise that measures 80 decibels is loud. Noise that measures 85 decibels interferes with comprehension of speech when spoken in a normal voice between two people with normal hearing who are standing about arm's length away from one another. Noise that measures 95 decibels interferes with speech between two people standing next to each other, often results in temporary reduction in the ability to hear after the noise stops, and can permanently impair hearing over time. Noise that measures 120 decibels can damage hearing immediately and is very painful.

The consequences of exposure to noise can be quite serious. Loss of hearing can occur from the trauma to the ear of sudden, very loud *impact noise*. Loss of hearing can also result from prolonged exposure to loud *continuous noise*. The effect of noise adds up over time: the cumulative exposure to continuous noise is what impairs hearing. Noise also interferes with communication and makes it difficult for workers to hear instructions or a warning.

Noise is mostly generated by mechanical or other physical forces such as hammering, out-of-balance equipment, rubbing parts, friction between two sliding surfaces, transformer hum, hydraulic noise, and aerodynamic noise. Once a source of noise has been identified and measured, an intervention can be designed to control it.

The key to noise control is finding a means that is both effective and economical. Today, there are new software tools to calculate the reflections of sound and sound pressure levels. Computer-aided acoustical modeling has long been used for the design of auditoriums and concert halls, where the sound distribution in a large listener area is to be optimized. Modern software allows the modeling of more complicated work spaces and estimation of the effect of making changes. The advantage of acoustical modeling is that different alternatives can be simulated and evaluated at low cost. Different calculation methods have been developed, such as ray tracing, diffuse field theory, and image-source method.

Whenever possible, noise should be controlled at its source. Properly modified tools can reduce impact noise. The engineering control of noise may include replacing or changing the location of equipment, modifying the machine (such as placing it on a rubber mat), installing acoustical tile in the room, and using barriers and enclosures. Unfortunately, most of these modifications of machines are so complicated that only the manufacturers can do them. Manufacturers of heavy equipment usually disclose the noise level a machine generates. In the long run, it is generally more economical to buy a quiet machine than to try to modify noisy machines.

Because the sound level drops as one moves away from a noise source, noisy machines should be located as far from each other and from workers as possible. Indoors, the effect of echo or reverberation bouncing off of walls and hard surfaces may limit the reduction obtained by relocating machines. Acoustical tiles and other noise-absorbing materials may reduce reverberations and therefore reduce noise levels in the workplace.

Carefully designed insulation cuts down the vibration of a part of a machine and also reduces airborne noise. Enclosures and barriers wrapped around a noisy machine can effectively reduce noise near workers. Enclosures should be as tight as possible, and ceiling and wall reflections of sound should be attenuated when partial enclosures are used. Sometimes machine operators can be isolated from their machines in sound-resistant booths or control rooms. If partial walls or enclosures are removed, they must be replaced before the equipment is put back in service.

Administrative controls have been a traditional approach to controlling noise exposure. The employer rotates workers or modifies the work schedules to limit the individual employee's exposure to noise. Those who work in noisy areas rotate with those who work in quieter areas on a regular basis. However, problems often arise because of different labor skills and wages as well as from worker resistance to changing jobs. Furthermore, rotating workers means that in the long run more people are exposed to high-level noise.

Safe work practices include the instruction, training, and selection of quiet work methods. For example, the hammering of metal sheets is noisy compared to the bending of sheets, and the use of compressed air for cleaning machines is noisier than vacuum cleaning.

Good maintenance also plays a part in reducing noise levels. Almost without exception, all machinery and equipment runs more quietly when in good condition and properly adjusted than when in poor condition. The difference may be as much as 10 to 20 dB. Some sources of noise are steam leaks, worn gears, slapping belts, insufficiently lubricated parts, unbalanced rotating parts, etc. If the noise level of a machine rises, either the maintenance interval should be shortened or the condition of the machines checked and all defective components replaced. Workers should report all unexpected or unusual machine noises to a supervisor.

Hearing protection should be used when the noise level exceeds safe limits and it is not possible to reduce noise by technical improvements. Hearing protection is the first line of defense against noise in environments where engineering and other controls have not reduced employee exposure to safe levels. Hearing protectors can prevent significant hearing loss, but only if they are used properly. Ear protectors are of four types: plugs, muffs, helmets, and electronic noise suppression devices. The most popular hearing protection devices are earplugs that are inserted into the ear canal to provide a seal against the canal walls. Earmuffs enclose the entire external ear inside rigid cups. The inside of the muff cup is lined with acoustic foam, and the perimeter of the cup is fitted with a cushion against the head and around the ear, held in place by the headband. Helmets are made to cover most of the bony parts of the head in order to reduce bone conductivity of noise as well as airborne noise. Hearing protectors must be tested in accordance with relevant standards, and they must fulfill the requirements of the standards. Electronic noise suppression devices detect the incoming noise, determine the waveform, and generate the opposite waveform, called antinoise. The antinoise cancels the noise, so it does not reach the worker. Electronic noise suppression devices are currently expensive.

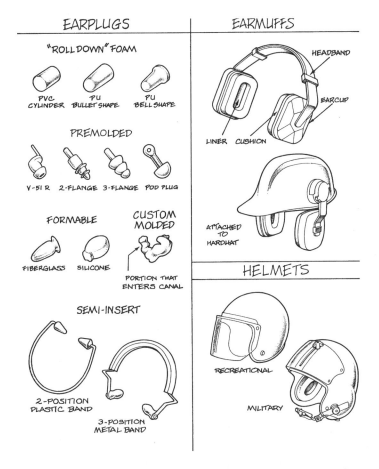

Figure 12.5 Devices used for hearing protection in the workplace. Best results are obtained when there is a selection of equipment and workers can choose which is best for the situation and is most comfortable to wear.(Reproduced courtesy of the American Industrial Hygiene Association.)

The best hazard control measures in the world do not work unless they are used and used properly. It is not enough to engineer hazard controls on equipment and to hand out personal protection. Workers need to be trained in their maintenance and proper use and to understand why they are necessary.

It is common for workers to circumvent safety measures in order to speed production, especially if they are paid by piecework or are facing a deadline. Often workers do not understand why a safety procedure is in place and consider it to be an impediment to their work. Some workers do not like the looks of safety equipment and simply don't want to wear them. Some workers feel immune to hazards and do not take them seriously; these workers tend to be young. Some workers feel that they are used to certain types of equipment and that they have the skills or experience to work safely despite the hazards; these workers tend to be older. It is almost always the case that poorly trained workers will keep their personal protection on when a boss or a visitor is around and will then take it off when they leave.

Compliance with hazard control is as important as the presence of controls in the first place. There are many ways that employers can improve compliance as part of a comprehensive safety program, some of which may be required by regulations in some jurisdictions (see Chapter 8). Here are a few steps that have been proposed:

- Train workers in how to maintain engineering control, how to use personal protective equipment, and why they are important.
- Educate workers on the hazards in the workplace and how they can affect health; safety hazards are usually more obvious.
- Monitor compliance at all times and keep a record when workers are not complying. Do not rely on audits and walk-throughs because problems are likely to be temporarily hidden or minimized.
- Hold supervisors responsible for compliance and maintenance of hazard controls and make it part of their performance review, affecting their wage increases and job security.
- Inspect ventilation, engineering controls, and stocks of personal protective equipment at irregular times and without warning. Determine whether ventilation equipment is turned off when it should not be. Determine if hazard controls and safety devices (such as machine guards) are circumvented, evaded, or removed. Observe if personal protective equipment is clean, up to date, and in plentiful supply.
- Provide a variety of personal protective equipment (such as hearing protection) whenever possible so that workers can choose the devices that fit best and are most comfortable.
- Ensure that the pace of work is not rushed to the point that workers feel forced to cut corners or work unsafely.
- Create an award in the workplace for best safety proposal. Do not give an award for lowest injury rate because that encourages underreporting.

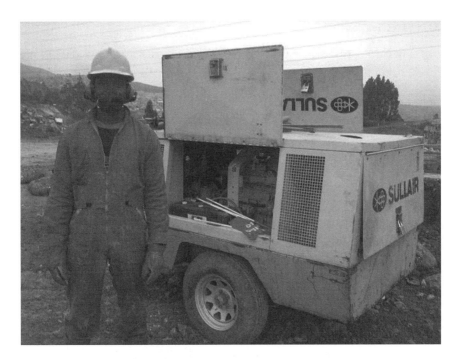

Figure 12.6 This construction worker next to a noisy air compressor looks like he is wearing appropriate personal protective equipment for his job, but he is not. Can you tell what is wrong? Note that he is wearing gloves, protective clothing, a hard hat (also called a helmet in some companies), hearing protection muffs, and an N95 respirator for protection against dust. [Answer: He is not wearing eye protection and he is not wearing his N95 respirator properly, because the headbands are around his neck, making the N95 respirator useless. (Photograph by Julietta Rodríguez Guzmán, Universidad El Bosque, Colombia.)

- Reward workers for reporting hazardous conditions and defects in safety equipment.
- Insist that all visitors, including company bosses, always wear personal protection all the time they are in a workplace with hazards. Workers will not take these measures seriously if their managers do not.
- Include maintenance of hazard controls and proper use of safety equipment as an emphasis in all behavior-based safety programs.
- Encourage workers to tell one another when they observe unsafe work practices or when a coworker is not complying with safe work practices. The tone should be constructive and friendly, not accusatory or insulting.

13

CLINICAL EVALUATION OF OCCUPATIONAL DISORDERS

Gregory Chan Chung Tsing and David Koh

"… to the questions recommended by Hippocrates, (the doctor) should add one more—What is your occupation?"

—Bernardino Ramazzini, 1633–1714

Some people believe that hazardous exposures and the risk of ill health are all part of work, a risk a worker takes to keep a job. Most people reject this belief and feel that workers should not have to sacrifice their health to make a living. However, it is an indisputable fact that all occupational diseases are preventable. Therefore, the goal should be to eliminate them.

Hippocrates, the ancient, great Greek physician, advised the physician to ask the patient's name, age, and residence in addition to asking about the patient's symptoms. Centuries afterward (in 1700), the great Italian physician Ramazzini, the Father of Occupational Medicine, added the patient's occupation to the list. Although scholars and practicing clinicians occasionally noticed specific occupational diseases in their community, occupation was first appreciated as an important general factor in disease causation by Ramazzini. In his book *De Morbis Artificum Diatriba (Diseases of Workers)*, he observed the effect of working conditions on the health of 54 categories of workers, including miners, chemists, cleaners of latrines, tanners, cheese makers, midwives, nurses, and learned men. When occupation was ignored, he said, incorrect diagnosis could occur or inadequate treatment be provided, resulting in delayed recovery and even deterioration of the patient's medical condition.

Occupational exposures contribute to the risk of many diseases. Unfortunately, work-related illness is recognized in only a small proportion of cases. Some experts believe that the relationship between work and occupation may be recognized in as few as 10% of patients with chronic illness because neither employers nor workers are aware of the relationship. At the same time, doctors and health-care professionals, who may be aware of the existence of occupational causal relationships, sometimes do not have sufficient information to make an accurate assessment.

An accurate diagnosis may result in the removal or reduction of hazardous exposures; institution of appropriate, early treatment; and facilitating quicker recovery. In addition, other control measures may be considered, including medical surveillance in workers with similar exposure, workplace modifications to keep exposure within permissible limits, and sometimes, reassessment of what are presently established safety limits.

HEALTH AND WORK

The equation below shows a two-way (bi-directional) relationship between health and work.

$$Health \leftrightarrow Work$$

Though it appears simple, the association is not always obvious. The worker may perceive the negative impact the job has on his or her health, whereas the employer will likely place greater emphasis on how the worker's health and associated disability (if any) will affect total work output. Obviously, the different perceptions are dependent on the interest of the individual parties.

$$Work \rightarrow Health$$

Basic Terminology

In order to discuss the effect of work on the health of the worker, it is important to understand certain basic terms.

- The *work environment* refers to the area within which the employee works. It will contain various environmental exposures, some of which have the potential for adverse health effects on the worker. These could be the raw materials used or the by-products generated, including loud noise and heat from machinery.
- The *work process* differs somewhat from the work environment. It relates specifically to the tasks being performed and knowledge of the workers' tools and machinery. It allows the physician to perceive potential difficulties encountered by the worker with an occupational disorder.
- Varying *adverse occupational health outcomes* occur with hazard exposure. On one hand, workplace factors can be a direct causal agent of *occupational diseases*. At the other end of the spectrum are *general diseases*, where the association with workplace factors is weak and unclear. *Work-related diseases*, conceptualized by the World Health Organization (WHO) Expert Committee on Occupational Health, make up the middle of this spectrum, where there is a possible causal role for workplace factors, in addition to other non-occupational factors. These factors may accelerate or exacerbate existing disease.

The worker is exposed to various workplace hazards. Toxic materials enter the body via three routes:

- through inhalation and pulmonary absorption
- percutaneous through the skin
- ingestion and absorption via the gastrointestinal system

How much of the exposure is absorbed into the body depends on the interaction between the hazardous agents, the work process, and the work environment. The presence of a hazardous substance by itself does not necessarily imply that the worker is at risk, if there are effective control measures. Tables 13.1 and 13.2 list some common workplace exposures and the risks associated with them.

Case Study 3

A 55-year-old bus driver was discharged from the hospital after a mild left-sided stroke with residual weakness of the left arm and leg (hemiplegia). Nobody asked about his occupation or thought about whether he could handle it. He was allowed to return to his job, jeopardizing his safety and that of his passengers because he was not in control of the vehicle.

Health→Work

It is also true that health can have an impact on work. In a fitness-to-work examination, a job match between health (measured by functional capability) of the worker and the particulars of specific work demands and work environment is required. A poor match between the health of the worker and the work could result in adverse outcomes:

- suboptimal work performance where worker productivity and product quality may be compromised
- stress-related outcomes, such as those discussed in Chapter 11
- situations in which the worker poses a safety risk to himself or herself, fellow workers, or even the community
- an injury or disability that increases the risk of a second injury or disability; for example, if a worker who is recovering from a broken arm is unable to climb a ladder safely

However, poor health alone does not necessarily imply decreased productivity to the company. It depends on the work and the situation. In the case of someone with chronic disease, workplace modification and accommodation can often reduce the discrepancy between compromised health and work demands.

Age is not, by itself, a reason for poor health or disability. The aging worker, who may not be able to do as well at strenuous tasks, may be very productive and safe in many jobs, with excellent general work effectiveness. Older workers tend to have a lower turnover rates and have specific strengths (e.g., a greater dedication to work, better routine skills, and more stable character, due to experience and age-related intellectual and personality development) that make them suitable for certain demanding jobs.

Objectives of Clinical Assessments

There are specific objectives for different types of clinical assessments. This chapter focuses on the clinical evaluation of occupational disorders, i.e., the diagnosis and management of an occupational illness. The following sections provide an overview of the other types of clinical evaluations, and they will be discussed in

TABLE 13.1

EXAMPLES OF OCCUPATIONAL HEALTH HAZARDS AND THEIR CLINICAL EFFECTS

Hazardous Factor	*Examples of Adverse Health Outcome*
Physical factors, including • Noise • Heat • Radiation • Vibration • Cold stress	Disorders include • Noise-induced hearing loss • Heat stress • Radiation injuries • Hand-arm vibration syndrome • Cold injuries, e.g., frostbite
Chemical hazards, including • Solvents • Inorganic dusts/powders • Organic dusts • Metals, metal fumes • Dyes/stains • Plastic and polymers • Irritants/gases/aerosols	Wide variety of diseases, including occupational lung diseases, occupational skin diseases, occupational disorders of the nervous system, cancers, acute toxicity, chemical hepatitis
Mechanical risk factors, including • Dangerous operations • Inadequately guarded equipment • Working at heights without restraints • Sudden or jerky movements	Injuries, including • Crush injuries, soft-tissue injuries (muscle strains and sprains) • Lacerations (cuts), pinch injuries, avulsion (body part is pulled off or out of position) • Falls, head trauma • Dislocation, avulsion
Heavy or repetitive physical work, including • Repetitive movements of a weak body part • Lifting excessive weight • Repeated heavy lifting	Musculoskeletal disorders, including • Repetitive strain injuries • Hernia • Low back pain (many causes) • Osteoarthritis (degenerative disease of joints)
Ergonomic factors, including • Inappropriate workstation design • Prolonged hours • Abnormal shifts • Inadequate lighting • Distraction • Awkward posture	Multiple outcomes, including • Lowered productivity, quality of work, and morale • Repetitive strain injury • Depression (many causes) • Squinting • Injury • Neck pain and back pain
Biological factors, including Bacteria, protozoa, fungus, viruses	Infections, allergies, malignancies
Psychological strain, including • Unreasonable work expectations • Excessively paced work • No control over work • Poor interpersonal relationships at work • Fear of losing job	Stress-related disorders, including: Psychic stress, work dissatisfaction, burnout, depression, heart disease (many causes)

TABLE 13.2

SOME OCCUPATIONS AND POTENTIALLY HAZARDOUS EXPOSURES ASSOCIATED WITH THEM

Occupational Group	Some Associated Workplace Exposures
Agricultural industry	• Biological substances • Pesticides • Organic dusts • Heat • UV light
Biotechnology and chemical industry	• Solvents • Irritant aerosols/gases • Acids/alkalis • Metals and fumes • Biological substances
Building and construction industry	• Noise • Heat • Physical work • Asphalt/tar • Welding emissions
Carpentry and lumber industry	• Wood dust • Noise • Heat • Dangerous equipment • Physical work • Pesticides
Ceramic industry	• Silica • Heat • Physical work
Electronics	• Irritant gases/aerosols • Solvents • Fiberglass
Foundry work	• Noise • Heat • Physical work
Health care	• Biological substances • X-ray radiation • Anesthetic gases
Metal works	• Metal and metal fumes • Noise • Heat • Physical work
Mining	• Coal dust • Silica • Noise • Heat • Physical work

(Continued)

TABLE 13.2 (Contd.)

Occupational Group	Some Associated Workplace Exposures
Petrochemical industry	• Benzene • Petroleum distillates • Heat • Hydrogen sulfide
Printing/Lithography	• Dyes and stains • Solvents
Sandblasting	• Silica • Heat • Noise
Spray painting	• Solvents • Metals • Irritant gases/aerosols
Textile industry	• Solvents • Metals • Irritant gases/aerosols
Welding	• Welding emissions • Heat

their respective chapters. They are not assessments done in isolation and are often done during the management of occupational disorders as well.

Fitness to Work These evaluations are done to match the worker's abilities to the demands of the job. They comprise pre-employment (when done as part of application for a job), pre-placement (when done to ensure capacity to do the job after the decision to hire is made), and periodic examinations (which are conducted at intervals during employment). They are also performed after an injury or illness to determine fitness to resume a particular line of work. The assessment of fitness to work is discussed in detail in Chapter 17. Fitness to work is often called "fitness for duty", a term some authorities prefer because it implies capacity to do a particular job rather than to hold a job or to be employed in general. This distinction, like the difference between preplacement and preemployment, is important under employment law in many countries, such as the United States and the United Kingdom.

Disability Evaluations Such evaluations aim to determine eligibility and quantify the extent of functional impairment or total disability. This allows the appropriate amount of compensation to be awarded. Disability evaluations are often called "impairment assessments", a term that is preferred by many authorities because it avoids confusion with the term "disability determination". The role of the health professional is to determine impairment and work capacity. Disability is an administrative decision that depends on how a given impairment interferes with a worker's employability in a given labor market or work capacity for their usual occupation. Disability determinations are made by the organization that is providing compensation, usually insurance companies or government agencies.

These organizations take into account the demand for a particular occupation, the worker's capacity to do it or a similar job, and the earnings that may be lost.

Monitoring and Surveillance In occupational health, these terms have specific but closely related meanings. Monitoring is a general strategy of watching for disease and disability in a population of workers. Surveillance is a strategy of searching for evidence of hazardous exposures or particular occupational diseases or injuries in a working population in which these outcomes are expected or possible. Both involve evaluating individual workers in order to detect disease, injury, or causes of disability, and both are also interpreted using epidemiological methods to determine patterns in the population. Because the concepts are very similar, the terms are often used interchangeably. Strictly speaking, however, monitoring is a process of following the general health of individual workers and by so doing learning the experience of the population, whereas surveillance is a process of looking for a particular exposure or outcome. An important goal of both strategies is to detect disease as early as possible so that the individual worker has a better chance of cure or control of the condition and so that hazards in the workplace will be recognized and controlled. (See Chapter 5.)

Occupational Health Monitoring This is a program to identify the onset and prevalence of various medical disorders as a means of identifying adverse workplace exposures and unusual diseases. Monitoring programs, sometimes called medical monitoring, are usually conducted by obtaining information from workers, by an examination by a physician, and by conducting general tests to detect disease early. A monitoring program is normally scaled to the level of what is feasible for the company. A national monitoring system may draw on different sources of information to track occupational injuries and diseases. The system in the United Kingdom, for example, supplements disease reports with surveys of clinicians.

Biomonitoring is a particular type of monitoring in which tests are performed that indicate the level of exposure to a particular chemical or other hazard among workers who are not necessarily ill.

Medical Surveillance

Sometimes referred to as biological surveillance, medical surveillance assesses whether excessive exposure and occupational diseases still occur despite the implementation of control measures. The evaluations are called periodic health evaluations. They often include an examination by a physician and special tests. The tests that are performed depend on the hazards present in the workplace. Clinical testing of various physiological parameters, such as lung function, determine if there are changes over time that could indicate newly developing disease. Tests may also involve taking biological samples from the exposed workers, usually blood or urine, to detect exposure levels and early manifestations of disease.

Sentinel Events A sentinel event is a recognized case of a disorder that is associated with an exposure that may be present in the population or workplace. A sentinel case suggests that there are other cases that may have been overlooked.

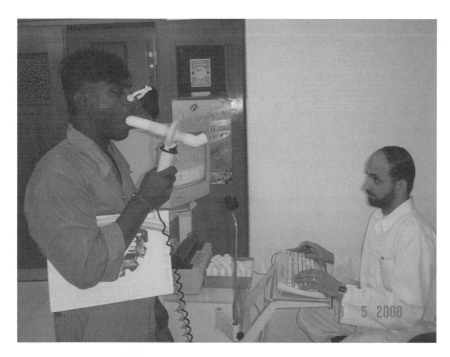

Figure 13.1 Pulmonary function testing is performed using a device called a "spirometer" that measures flow rates during breathing and the capacity of the lungs. Spirometry is a simple but extremely useful and reliable test of lung function. Spirometry alone is sufficient for screening purposes, but additional studies are usually performed for diagnosis of lung disease. (Photograph courtesy of Shuiaba Occupational Medical Centre, Ministry of Health, Kuwait.)

For example, a worker may come down with an illness that is likely to be the result of a hazardous exposure, such as asthma in a workplace where a common cause of asthma, such as an isocyanate, is present. This case is a sentinel event. Further investigation may reveal other cases that have not been reported or that are mild and have not been recognized. If so, this provides evidence that there is a hazard in the workplace that is not adequately controlled. The usefulness of sentinel events varies with the latency period or the time required for the disease to develop. If the latency period is long, as in the case of most occupational cancers, the value of a sentinel event for prevention is reduced because exposure may have occurred in the past and the workplace may no longer even exist.

Outbreak Investigation of an Occupational Disorder An outbreak is an event in which more than one worker shows signs of illness that may be due to an occupational hazard. An outbreak investigation is a specialized evaluation to actively identify other related cases and whether there is evidence for excessive exposure to a hazard. The information is used in determining the extent and source of the problem so that appropriate preventive measures can be put into place.

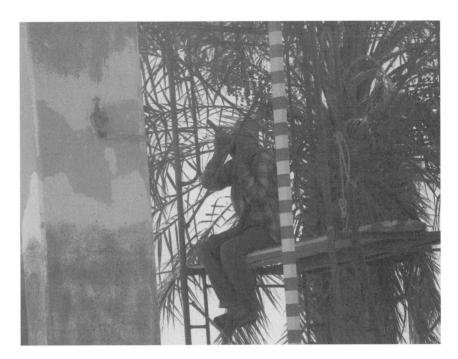

Figure 13.2 The detection of a case of occupational disease may be a "sentinel event" that identifies hazardous working conditions. This worker is sandblasting a building using silica sand, using only the cloth of his *shumag* (head cover) for protection, which is completely inadequate. He will develop silicosis, a serious lung disease. Once it is diagnosed in this worker, the risk may be recognized and other workers doing similar work may be better protected, but it will be too late for this worker and his family: because of his exposure, he will probably become disabled or die from the disease, even though it is easily and completely preventable. (Photograph by Seifeddin Ballal, King Faisal University, Saudi Arabia.)

OCCUPATIONAL HEALTH RESEARCH

Primarily epidemiological in nature, occupational health research provides evidence to support effective prevention in the workplace and the recognition and treatment of occupational disorders in occupational medicine.

BOX 13.4

Case Study 4

Mr. X, a welder in a shipyard, frequently sees the company doctor for respiratory tract infections. It appears that exposure to dust and fumes at work may be the underlying cause. However, he does not get better when he is away from work. He has asthma and is a heavy smoker. It is difficult to ascertain which exposure is the cause of Mr. X's respiratory problems. Even after excluding workplace factors, his smoking habits and home conditions need to be considered.

Clinical Evaluation of Occupational Disorders

A problem-oriented approach is required for an accurate, systematic assessment of occupational disorders and for effective utilization of limited health and safety resources in the workplace. The approach can be broadly divided into three parts with areas of overlap (see Table 13.3).

1. diagnosis
2. establishing work-relatedness of disease
3. treatment of the clinical disease
4. managing occupational issues arising from the clinical disease

TABLE 13.3

CLINICAL EVALUATION OF OCCUPATIONAL ILLNESS

Stage of Assessment	Interpretation and Usefulness
Chief complaint and history of present illness	• Consider present and previous occupational exposures
Past medical history	• Consider past history of occupational diseases • Identify other potential causes for worker/patient's condition
Social history	• Understand patient's social support and potential exposures at home
Family history	• Identify other potential causes for worker/patient's condition
Occupational history	• Evaluate work-relatedness of disease
Physical examination	• Clinical diagnosis • Assess disease severity and functional impairment
Investigation (often called the "workup" of a patient)	• Clinical diagnosis • Assess disease severity and degree of exposure • Identify other potential causes for worker/patient's condition
Treatment and follow-up	• Clinical treatment of disease • Determine if response to treatment is as predicted for the diagnosis • Identify other potential causes for worker/patient's condition
Rehabilitation	• Return worker to highest possible level of function (objective is return to baseline state) • Prevention of further or future disability • Monitor fitness to work
Management of occupational aspects	
Worker management	• Notification of occupational disease • Inform worker of rights • Determine impact of illness on fitness to return to work
Workplace inspection	• Identify cause of condition • Workplace environmental assessment for exposures • Assessment of fellow workers for exposures and occupational disease • Prevention of disease or injury in others
Implementation of workplace preventive measures	• Prevention of occupational disorders at the workplace

The first part of the clinical evaluation involves making a *diagnosis*, which identifies the specific disorder that the worker has developed. At the very least, characterization of the disorder requires identifying the class of the work-relatedness of the clinical disease and the process that is occurring (toxicity, trauma, cancer, infection, and so forth). The second part of the evaluation, establishing work-relatedness of disease (often called *causation*), is critical in occupational medicine because one must know what hazardous exposure was responsible and document that it occurred as a result of work. The subsequent parts of the evaluation examine the severity of disease, the degree of impairment in relation to the nature of work, and the worker's fitness to return to work. Adequate implementation of workplace interventions and preventive measures will also prevent other workers from succumbing to similar medical problems.

Diagnosis Many disorders are obvious and can be immediately identified, such as a laceration (cut of the skin). Others, particularly occupational diseases, are harder to identify, such as a lung disease that requires an X-ray to see. Diagnosis is based on identifying a pattern that fits the known pattern of a disorder and then testing to see if the findings are consistent with that disorder.

The first step is to take the *history*, which is the story of how the disorder started and developed. This is usually taken from the worker (now a patient), if he or she can recount it. Often, this personal history is reconstructed from or supplemented by information from the medical records and sometimes by the observations of others. A systematic checklist of symptoms, called the review of systems, is filled out by the patient. The family history (what disorders close members of the family have had) and social history (what has happened in the patient's life) may be valuable.

Symptoms are the specific sensations or observations of the patient. Symptoms may include pain, shortness of breath, itching, or whatever else the patient has experienced. Symptoms cannot be objectively verified because they are the subjective experience of the patient.

Signs are the specific findings that are observed by the health professional. They may include redness, swelling, cough, skin rash, or other observations that can be objectively validated. Various clinical tests may be used to bring out important signs. For example, the health professional may move a knee in a certain way to test the strength of the ligaments or listen to the patient's chest with a stethoscope to hear breath sounds, e.g., wheezing, which occurs in asthma but also in other lung conditions. A physical examination is a systematic clinical approach to finding signs or, very importantly, verifying their absence.

Laboratory tests may be performed to identify the problem or to confirm the problem if the symptoms and signs point to a particular diagnosis. For example, a blood test may reveal anemia. A toxicological test may reveal that the patient has lead in his her blood much above what is normally observed in the population. A urinalysis may reveal that there is protein in the urine, which is often a sign of early kidney disease.

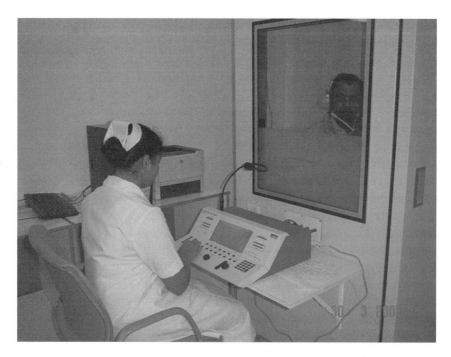

Figure 13.3 Audiometry using a soundproof booth is a more accurate form of hearing test than the portable screening audiometry shown in Figure 5.1, which is adequate for early detection of hearing loss. It is required for diagnosis and tracking the progression of hearing loss. (Photograph courtesy of Shuiaba Occupational Medical Centre, Ministry of Health, Kuwait.)

Imaging studies are tests that reveal abnormalities in structure. An X-ray is the most common imaging test. For example, a chest film may reveal the presence of pneumonia, tuberculosis, or pneumoconiosis shown by shadows on the film that are cast by abnormalities in the structure. Examples of conventional X-rays can be found in Chapter 16. Computerized tomography (often called "CT scanning"), high-resolution CT scanning, and MRI (magnetic resonance imaging) are sophisticated tests in which the body is examined using X-rays or intense electromagnetic fields (in MRIs), and the image is constructed in three dimensions using computers. Nuclear imaging is a term used for a large family of tests that rely on safe, low-level radioactive chemicals that are injected into the patient and tend to concentrate where there is inflammation or cancer. The image shows where these *lesions* (abnormalities of structure or function) are located.

Functional studies test whether parts of the body are operating as they should. Pulmonary function tests, for example, show whether the patient can move air in and out of the lungs normally and whether the capacity of the lungs to hold air is diminished. Neurobehavioral testing is a very complicated field involving the patient's ability to perform simple or complicated tasks (such as recognizing objects, remembering or tracking a moving object), the patient's ability to integrate and process information (such as tests of word recognition and association), and the patient's emotional state (depressed, easily distracted). The simplest of these tests include the ability to draw a clock, testing the patient's ability to arrange spatial relationships. Among the most complex of such tests are intelligence tests (often called "IQ tests" because the "intelligence quotient," a measure of intelligence compared to the distribution in the population, is being measured). There are many functional tests, each specific to the part of the body or the function being evaluated.

Direct visualization is possible in many organs. For example, a flexible fiber-optic tube passed into the lung can reveal the presence of lung cancer. Arthroscopy involves cutting a small hole in the side of a joint and passing a small fiber-optic tube into it to see the interior.

Infections may be evaluated by culture, in which some body fluid is put on a culture medium to see what bacteria or other pathogens grow. They may also be evaluated by serology, in which an antibody to a particular pathogen is detected as evidence that the patient has been infected in the past.

There are many other specialized tests, including skin tests of different types used to determine whether a person has been exposed in the past to the bacterium that causes tuberculosis or whether he or she is allergic or sensitized to a particular antigen, and tests for blood in the stool, used to identify cancers in the gastrointestinal tract.

Sometimes the only way to make a diagnosis is to take tissue from the patient and look at it under a microscope. This is easy in the case of blood and can be used to identify malaria or leukemia or other disorders that show up in blood. At other times, it may be necessary to take tissue during surgery or with a needle, which is called a *biopsy*. This is often required to make the diagnosis of cancer.

In complicated or unclear cases, the physician makes a list of possible disorders that are compatible with the findings. This is called the *differential diagnosis*. The physician then goes down the list, usually starting with the most potentially serious, the most treatable or the most common possibilities, and conducts tests or looks for evidence to confirm or rule out each disorder. Sometimes, there is no test, the test is unavailable, or the test does not provide a clear answer. In such cases, the physician may observe the patient to see how the disorder develops or may treat the patient for a condition thought to represent the most likely possibility and observe the response to treatment.

It is important to make a specific diagnosis because this usually determines how to treat the patient and guides the physician in knowing what the course of the disorder is likely to be in the future. Among lung diseases, pneumoconiosis looks very much like hypersensitivity pneumonitis. However, the pneumoconiosis, once it occurs, is not treatable, and the objective is to keep it from getting worse. The hypersensitivity pneumonitis, on the other hand, can be treated and may get better.

Establishing Work-Relatedness of Disease An occupational etiology should be suspected if an illness shows a temporal sequence (timing of onset and duration) that is associated with work (such as during or after work shifts), persists despite treatment and standard measures for control of personal or lifestyle risk factors, does not fit the typical demographic profile, or is of an unknown origin. Recognition is usually achieved by taking the occupational history of the patient. The ability to recognize the illness, its likely cause, and the work situation in which the exposure occurred are the prerequisites of establishing the work-relatedness of the clinical disease. Laboratory tests to document exposure are readily available for only a few occupational exposures and are not generally suitable for screening every patient who might have a work-related illness.

The Occupational History When a physician or nurse takes information from a patient, the resulting summary is called a *history*. The occupational history is a record of what jobs a worker has held, when he or she held them, what he or she did, what the worker knew he or she was exposed to, and what protective equipment was available. Typically, the occupational history is collected by a questionnaire or an interview with a nurse or physician, often in the course of a much longer interview regarding the patient's health.

A good occupational history may enable the physician to attribute a specific work-related cause to the patient's problem and expedite the best treatment. It also facilitates the implementation of appropriate workplace preventive measures, thus limiting disease occurrence in other workers.

Reasons for taking an occupational history include:

1. diagnosis of occupational disorders
2. identifying the cause of the disorder for purposes of compensation
3. identifying the cause of the disorder for purposes of prevention
4. evaluating fitness to work
5. surveillance of workers at risk
6. assessing disability and eligibility for compensation
7. health education
8. occupational health research

Structure of the Occupational History It is always important to know the occupation of a patient with an injury or illness. It is helpful in simple cases of minor injuries and diseases that may have an impact on the person's work performance. It helps the health-care professional to determine fitness to work and to provide a document (usually a "note") that the patient was known to have been ill, which is called *medical certification* of an illness. It helps to identify risks of impaired work ability (such as sleepiness) when medications are prescribed. If an injury is acute and is related to work, this will be obvious. Diseases or chronic problems are usually not so clear and require more investigation.

It is not always necessary or efficient to take a lengthy, detailed account for all patients. The occupational history may be limited simply to knowing the patient's employment status and job title, or it may be extensive, depending on the nature of the underlying medical problem.

A comprehensive and detailed occupational history is normally required in a clinical evaluation of a suspected or known occupational disorder, especially when the cause is not known. The comprehensive occupational history is best taken by using a structured questionnaire. Typically, this questionnaire consists of the following parts:

- The job history. This is a section in which the worker enters the job title, the name of the employer, the dates worked, the actual tasks performed, the exposures he or she can remember, and what protection was provided.

- Exposure inventory. This is usually a checklist in which the worker identifies exposures he or she has encountered during his or her entire working life. It is important to correlate this with the job history if the worker indicates a potentially hazardous exposure. Usually, the worker can identify more exposures on the checklist than he or she can remember job by job.
- Environmental and personal history. This section is not a complete medical history but records essential information needed to interpret the occupational history: smoking history, allergies, environmental exposures, hobbies, and military service. It typically consists of only a few questions. Some of this information, such as smoking and allergies, is usually collected as part of the overall patient history and may be recorded elsewhere in the medical record.

The health-care professional should develop a systematic approach to the occupational history and become familiar with the sources of information needed to interpret it. In a busy medical practice, it is frequently more efficient to apply a self-administered questionnaire (sample shown in Table 13.4) as a means of screening for work-relatedness. This could be administered outside the medical consultation to save time. A positive response suggests the possibility of work-relatedness and would then prompt the practitioner to take a more detailed occupational history. The completed form becomes part of the medical record. Subsequent review and periodic updating is easily done to ensure accurate records.

Interpretation

After the occupational history has been obtained, it must be interpreted. This may require further questions, such as those listed in Table 13.5. Interpretation of the

TABLE 13.4
SELF-ADMINISTERED QUESTIONNAIRE ON PATIENT'S WORK HISTORY (EXAMPLE)

Patient Name/Identity Card Number: Elliot K J Y / 9175642
Instructions: List the jobs you have had since you first started working, including any military service.

Period of work	Company details, including nature of product or services	Job title and specific duties	Major workplace hazardous exposures	Personal protective equipment
1982–1987	Fly-by-Night Paint Shop	Paint mixer	Thinners, paints, lead, solvents	None available
1987–1989	Greg & David Paint Industries: paint manufacturer	Quality Inspector	Thinners, paints, lead, solvents	Respirator, used regularly with training
1990–1995	Greg & David Paint Industries: paint manufacturer	Quality Supervisor	As above	Respirator available, rarely used
1996–2000	Greg & David Paint Industries: paint manufacturer	Quality Trainer	Computer work, work stress	None

TABLE 13.5

ASSESSING WORK-RELATEDNESS OF CLINICAL DISORDERS

- When did it start and how did it progress?
- What type of work do you do?
- Do you think your health problems might be related to your work?
- Are your symptoms different at work and at home?
- Are you currently exposed to chemicals, dusts, metals, radiation, noise, or repetitive work?
- Have you been exposed to chemicals, dusts, metals, radiation, noise, or repetitive work in the past?
- Are any of your coworkers experiencing similar symptoms?
- Do your symptoms go away when you are away from work over a weekend or on vacation? Do they return when you come back to work?
- Have you ever had this condition before?

effects of exposures requires knowledge of the disorders characteristically associated with various occupations and the effects of hazards encountered in the workplace. Table 13.6 lists examples of hazards associated with particular disorders.

Interpreting the Job History A careful description of work in present and previous employment is required to assess occupational exposures throughout a worker's lifetime. Most occupational diseases have latency periods, some as long as many years (e.g., asbestosis, silicosis, toxic neuropathies, and occupational cancers). Interaction and accumulated effects from previous workplace exposures could result in clinical disease in the present job even though exposure levels may be within acceptable limits.

Interpreting the Exposure Inventory Major exposures should be listed for each job in the job history with respect to the work processes and the work environment. These exposures may include metals, chemicals, dusts, physical factors (i.e., repetitive motion, noise, and radiation), microorganisms, and stress. Indirect exposures should also be recorded because the patient's health can be affected by exposures originating in other parts of the workplace. For example, an unprotected bystander located a few meters away from a protected welder may experience health symptoms while the protected welder does not.

Although exposure dosage is hard to assess without visiting the workplace, a preliminary assessment should be attempted based on information provided by the worker. The worker may be able to provide some details of the engineering control measures. Specific questions such as the presence of doors and windows, the use of fume cupboards, the functional status of exhaust fans, and the local exhaust ventilation systems could be asked. The worker should also be asked whether he or she uses personal protective equipment consistently, if the device is properly fitted (especially for respirators), and the frequency of equipment maintenance.

TABLE 13.6

SPECIAL CONSIDERATIONS FOR OCCUPATIONAL DISEASES

Coronary artery disease	May be aggravated with certain exposures, e.g., carbon monoxide, methylene chloride
Respiratory disease	May aggravate severity of occupational lung diseases
Renal (kidney) impairment	May be aggravated with nephrotoxic agents and increased susceptibility to toxic agents excreted via kidneys
Neurological (nervous system) diseases	May be aggravated by exposure to neurological agents; abnormal central nervous system function may reduce awareness and compromise safety
Immune deficiency states, e.g., AIDS	Increased susceptibility to infections at the workplace; may require policies to protect the health of the worker at work
Atopy (history or family history of allergies)	Higher risk of occupational asthma and irritant contact dermatitis
Skin diseases	May enhance percutaneous absorption of chemicals
Elderly	Less tolerant of extreme physical environments, physical labor, and more prone to chemical toxicity
Pregnancy	May require protection from workplace exposures to prevent exposure of fetus
Smoking	Modifies toxic exposure, aggravates effect of respiratory disease, and confers synergistic risk in certain situations
Physical fitness	Susceptibility reduced with better physical conditioning

For common industrial chemical products, the manufacturer is required in many countries to make available on request a summary of the ingredients of the product, their hazardous properties, and their possible health effects in a document called a *material safety data sheet*, often called an "MSDS." In most of these countries, it is also required that essential information be on the label of the product and that the MSDS be available at the workplace for workers to read.

Time Relationship of Symptoms to Work The timing of symptoms in relation to work is often a useful gauge for a potential occupational illness. Evidence that suggests that the disease could be work-related includes symptoms that worsen at work; symptoms that improve off-site, during vacation, or after stopping a particular job; or symptoms appearing only after starting the particular job or after a new process or material was introduced.

Such a relationship is particularly important when evaluating occupational accidents or acute poisoning where there is an obvious cause-and-effect relationship. An immediate diagnosis can often be made. One must, however, realize that the association between work and symptoms may be obscured as the disease progresses. The *temporality* (sequence of events) of the above relationship may have existed in the beginning, but when the clinical disorder becomes severe and complicated enough, symptoms often occur outside the working periods. For example, occupational asthma does not always occur on the job and sometimes disturbs a worker's sleep at night.

Symptoms Among Coworkers The probability that work is contributing to a commonly-shared illness is strengthened if the patient's coworkers are experiencing similar symptoms, as they would all have had the same occupational exposures.

Abnormal Circumstances at Work The worker is asked to consider any unusual circumstances at work that could affect the environmental exposure levels. This may include changes in personnel, machinery, or processes, breakdown or shutdown in equipment, or perhaps the need to increase work output per worker or overtime work.

Environmental and Personal Exposures To have a complete picture, enquiry should be made as to domestic exposures, hobbies, and known non-occupational causes of disease (see Table 13.7). For example, the use of headphones to listen to loud music may lead to sensorineural hearing impairment.

The smoking history is especially important. It is well recognized as a cause of ill health and may interact with occupational exposures to markedly increase the risk of disease (e.g., smoking has a synergistic effect with asbestos to increase lung cancer risk) and may also enhance absorption of chemicals (e.g., lead absorption appears to be higher among smokers).

Problems in Taking an Occupational History Occupational histories are not always easy to interpret. A particular job title may be misleading, at least to the health-care professional. Similarly, the same work process can have varying exposures, for example, if one is manually operated and the other is automated. The exposures that are characteristic of a particular job may change over time and with new technology. The interviewer should be aware of such problems. Common problems with the occupational history include the following:

- *Ambiguous job titles and processes.* An "industrial engineer," for example, will have vastly different workplace hazard exposures if he or she is a mechanical rather than a chemical engineer. A "production operator" in a car battery plant differs from a "production operator" in an electronics factory, even though they share the same job title. A "fireman" may be a fire fighter or someone who stokes a furnace with coal.
- *Multiple jobs.* The same worker may hold multiple jobs or have other part-time work.
- *Inaccurate information.* The fear of losing one's livelihood or shame sometimes makes people less than accurate in their occupational history. This is particularly common when the job is illegal (such as a sex worker) or disreputable (such as a debt collector) or is considered demeaning or held in low regard (such as a leather worker in some caste-conscious cultures). However, it also occurs when workers or, more commonly, their families try to upgrade the status of a job, such as calling a painter an interior decorator.
- *Lack of knowledge.* Sometimes workers have no idea what chemicals they are working with. This is often because the worker cannot read the label, which may be written in a foreign language or because the worker cannot read or cannot read the language in which the label is written.

TABLE 13.7

COMPONENTS OF A THOROUGH OCCUPATIONAL HISTORY

1. Present job description and nature of work

2. Hours of work and description of shifts system

3a. Types of workplace hazards

- Chemicals (e.g., formaldehyde, organic solvents, pesticides)
- Metals (e.g., lead, arsenic, cadmium)
- Dusts (e.g., asbestos, silica, coal)
- Biological (e.g., HIV, hepatitis B, tuberculosis)
- Physical (e.g., noise, repetitive motion, radiation)
- Psychological (e.g., stress)

3b. Degree of exposure (could be an estimate)

- Duration of exposure
- Exposure concentration
- Route of exposure
- Presence and efficacy of exposure controls
- Quantitative exposure data from inspections and monitoring

4. Previous occupations

- Lifetime history, with dates of employment and job duties
- Military history
- Hobbies and avocational exposures
- Sports

5. Other jobs or "moonlighting"

6. Time relationship between work and symptoms

- Symptoms occur or are exacerbated at work and improve away from work
- Symptoms coincide with the introduction of new exposure at work
- Symptoms coincide with other change in working conditions

7. Previous significant medical history

- Past injuries
- Past illnesses
- Surgery

8. Workplace protection

- Use of personal protective equipment on the job
- Methods of material handling
- Engineering protective measures

9. Presence of an occupational health program at work

- Periodic health surveillance
- Workplace environmental assessment
- Regulation of workplace exposures
- Availability of trained medical or nursing care

10. First aid and acute care provided at time of injury or illness

(Continued)

TABLE 13.7 (Contd.)

11. Similar complaints among other workers

12. Presence of any abnormal circumstances at work
- Breakdown or shutdown of machines or processes
- Increased demand for production
- Changes in personnel, materials, or processes

13. Other environmental (including domestic) exposures
- Home environment (e.g., water, air, soil contamination)
- Indoor air quality
- Dampness, mold, and allergens at home
- Social lifestyle
- Smoking habits
- Alcohol use
- Drug use
- Addictive behaviors (including gambling, compulsive spending)

- *Proprietary or protected information.* Sometimes a work process or, more often, chemical product is a protected industrial secret. The manufacturer may not be required to disclose what is in the product, and the label may be of little help.

Occupational histories, like medical histories in general, are not always completely accurate. Workers may exaggerate their functional capacity if they think that their job is in danger. They may deny prior injury or previous workplace exposures, especially during pre-employment, periodic, and fitness-to-work examinations. It may even be more so during disability assessments for compensation cases. The worker may selectively reveal his or her employment in one job but not the other, especially if the full-time employer may not approve, thus significant information on occupational exposures may be missed.

Clinical Management

Clinical management is what the physician or nurse or other health professional does in a health-care setting, as opposed to administration or hazard control. The clinical management of suspected occupational disorders begins with the assessment of present and past occupational history and exposures, which is essential to the proper management of disorders arising out of work. The time relationship of symptoms to work exposure, recent change or abnormal circumstances at work, and the presence of similar symptoms among coworkers gives valuable clues to the diagnosis. Non-occupational exposures, such as smoking, may also be relevant. An accurate diagnosis of a work-related disease allows for treatment and prevention of recurrence of the disorder in the patient. Similarly affected and exposed workers can also be treated and protected.

A disorder is any abnormal condition of the body that interferes with normal life. An injury is generally defined as a disorder resulting from physical damage to the body, usually as the result of a single event, such as a fall. A disease is generally defined as a disorder that is started by a particular cause, such as a chemical exposure, and then carries on, affecting the body for some period after the initial damage. A disease can be acute, meaning that it occurred suddenly, or chronic, meaning that it has lasted a long time. Injuries are usually acute, by definition. However, some disorders are characterized by physical damage that builds up over time with repeated injury or constant strain. These are called *cumulative injuries* and may include the musculoskeletal disorders often called repetitive strain injury or cumulative trauma disorder. A common form of cumulative injury is noise-induced hearing loss; once the damage begins, each exposure to loud noise adds to the damage, and the cumulative effect over time is loss of hearing. For convenience, in order to differentiate them from acute injuries, cumulative injuries are often classified as "diseases" for statistical purposes.

The management of an injury generally requires recognizing and diagnosing the injury, documenting how it occurred, making a judgment based on the evidence of the cause of the injury (which is usually obvious) and whether it arose out of work, following the worker/patient through recovery, providing rehabilitation or referring the worker for retraining, if necessary, and then conducting a fitness-to-work evaluation to ensure that the worker can return to the workplace and do the job safely.

The management of clinical disease generally requires making a clinical diagnosis, providing the appropriate treatment, making a judgment based on the evidence of the cause of the condition (which is often difficult) and whether it arose out of work, following the worker/patient through recovery, and then conducting a fitness-to-work evaluation to ensure that it is safe for the worker to return to the job or a disability evaluation to determine why he or she cannot. An accurate diagnosis requires taking a medical history, performing an examination, and conducting whatever tests are necessary. For example, a case of anemia in a worker who repairs automobile radiators might present with a clinical picture of weakness. A blood test may show anemia and identify it as the type typically associated with problems related to hemoglobin and not the type that is typically associated with iron deficiency. The blood lead levels may be very high, revealing the cause of the disorder. The occupational history will confirm that the worker is exposed to lead at work because lead is used in the repair of radiators. In practice, knowledge of the worker's job may have led the physician to suspect lead toxicity from the beginning.

Medical illness is characterized as *acute*, meaning that the onset is sudden, or *chronic*, meaning that it has lasted a long time. The immediate priority when treating an acutely ill or injured patient is to stabilize the medical condition, which may require a referral to a higher level of health care, most often a hospital, especially in medical emergencies. For less urgent cases, the medical examination should rule out other possible causes, including those that are not related to occupation, before concluding that it is related to a workplace exposure. A list of the clinical presentations of some common occupational diseases is included in Table 13.8.

The best medical management for the condition is then selected among the available options, including treating the immediate medical problem, preventing exacerbations, detecting complications early, and preventing disability. When the occupational health professional is unable to provide the best treatment option, the case should be referred to a clinical specialist for management of the underlying disease condition.

A psychosocial assessment may sometimes be useful. Occupational disorders are often associated with adverse psychological effects. The extent depends upon the individual response, the nature and severity of the disease, and the availability of a social support network to the worker. Conversely, the subjective expression of disease may sometimes be influenced by the individual psyche, such as degree of pain. In some situations, people who fake their symptoms (*malingerers*) must be distinguished from patients with genuine illness.

Case Study 5

Mr. Q, a young man performing general labor work at a construction site, sustained multiple abrasions (scratches) after a fall. The supervisor sent him to the company doctor, who dismissed it as an isolated incident. Mr. Q was given treatment and returned to work. The next day he fell again but hit his head on the ground. Tests showed an enlarging intracranial hematoma (blood clot pressing on the brain) and he had to undergo emergency decompression surgery.

A common mistake in evaluating suspected occupational illness or injury is to focus too narrowly. A minor accident may seem insignificant but may hide a predisposing cause. In Mr. Q's case, he was an unsuspected solvent abuser, which caused periods of drowsiness and incoordination. This is probably why he fell down in the first place.

It is important for the health professional to think broadly. A seemingly innocuous hyperpigmented skin rash may be a cutaneous sign of arsenic toxicity, or a complaint of shortness of breath may be pulmonary, cardiac, psychogenic, hematological, toxic, musculoskeletal, or neurological in origin.

Occupational Aspects of Clinical Disorders The health-care professional's job is to protect the worker from further harm and to comply with any occupational health and safety legislation or regulations that apply (summarized in Table 13.9). If the health-care professional is not adequately trained in this area, he or she should refer the case to a qualified occupational health specialist. This may be necessary if the health-care professional is unable or does not have the skills to determine whether the medical problem is work-related, is unable to manage important occupational aspects of the cases with competence (such as workplace inspections, disability evaluation, fitness-to-work examinations, and medical surveillance), or is unable to prepare the necessary reports under workers' compensation or other insurance systems. The physician or nurse or other practitioner should always be prepared to seek help when it is required.

TABLE 13.8

CLINICAL PRESENTATION OF COMMON OCCUPATIONAL HEALTH DISORDERS

Disorder	Physical Hazard	Chemical Hazard	Biological Hazard	Common Symptoms and Signs
Anemia	• Ionizing radiation	• Inorganic lead • Benzene • TNT • Arsine	• Parasites	• Weakness • Shortness of breath • Pallor (white skin color)
Jaundice		• Carbon tetrachloride • Halothane • (Other chemicals)	• Leptospirosis • HIV • Viral hepatitis	• Skin and eyes turn yellow • Urine turns dark • Stools turn light-colored
Proteinuria (protein in urine, an early sign of disease)		• Mercury • Cadmium • Aminoglycoside • Antibiotics • Gold		• Often no sign until tested • Sometimes body swelling, fatigue
Peripheral neuropathy	• Pressure on nerve • Mechanical injury to nerve	• Inorganic lead • i-Methyl-butyl ketone • n-Hexane • Carbon disulphide	• Epstein-Barr virus	• Burning pain • Loss of feeling in hands and feet • Shooting electrical sensations
Psychosis (mental disorders) Delirium (acute mental disorder due to physical causes) Dementia (loss of memory and reasoning ability)		• Inorganic mercury • Organic lead • Manganese • Arsenic • Solvents	• Cerebral (brain) malaria • Encephalitis and other severe infections (many causes)	• Behavioral abnormalities • Changes in thinking • Emotions • Personality

(Continued)

TABLE 13.8 (Contd.)

Disorder	Physical Hazard	Chemical Hazard	Biological Hazard	Common Symptoms and Signs
Respiratory disorders		• Fibrogenic dusts (cause pneumoconiosis) • Wood dusts • Animal proteins • Raw cotton • Smoke/fumes • Allergens	• Pneumonia Hypersensitivity pneumonitis • Occupational asthma	• Cough or shortness of breath (breathlessness)
Musculoskeletal disorders	• Poor workplace ergonomics • Repetitive strain • Vibration			• Pain • Soreness • Weakness
Hearing loss	• Noise • Barotrauma (increased pressure, usually in diving) • Decompression illness (decreased pressure, usually in diving)			• Loss of hearing • Loss of ability to discriminate words • Inability to hear speech over background noise
Reproductive disorders	• Microwave • Ionizing radiation	• Endocrine disruptors • Heavy metals • Solvents • Some pesticides		• Infertility
Cancers	• Ionizing radiation	• Benzene • Many other chemicals • Asbestos	• Hepatitis B • Aflatoxins	• Cancer (variable)

TABLE 13.9

STEPS IN THE MANAGEMENT OF OCCUPATIONAL DISORDERS

Protect the health of worker

Assess exposure levels at the workplace by doing a workplace inspection

Health education of worker

Evaluate urgency of the problem

- Is condition serious to patient?
- Are others in the workplace affected?
- Is there a pattern to the problem?
- Can the problem be explained by characteristics of the working population or illness in community?

Referral to qualified occupational health specialist where required

Occupational health and safety legislative procedures

Notification to appropriate labor or health agency

Proper documentation of medical report

Regular updating of medical records

Proper filing and tracking of medical records, correspondence, and documentation (for medico-legal purposes)

The occupational health professional should ensure that the workplace is safe. The incidence of occupational disease at a particular workplace suggests that exposures are in the hazardous range, thus the exposure levels should be assessed. First, any relevant material safety data sheets for workplace chemicals should be requested from the employer. A workplace inspection may follow, usually performed by a team that includes the occupational health professional accompanied by members of management. The existing control measures and their effectiveness should be documented as well as information on previous environmental monitoring results (if any). Employees working in the same vicinity should be interviewed and screened for any similar medical complaints.

In addition, the patient must be educated about his or her medical condition and treatment, workplace hazards, use of personal protective equipment, and workplace control measures as a means of increasing his or her work health awareness. It may also be necessary to advise the worker about his or her legal rights. The law usually requires the employer to take responsibility for the employees' health. The employer pays for medical costs incurred unless otherwise contractually specified. The employer does not have the right to discriminate against workers or fire them for their inability to perform when they return to work or for refusing to work in any hazardous area/situation.

Obviously, these steps are much easier if the occupational health professional works within the plant or workplace. It may be difficult or impossible for an outside health-care worker to gain access to a plant, especially if the employer is hostile. One also must be careful not to compromise the interests of the worker by approaching the employer prematurely, in a confrontational fashion, or without permission of the worker.

TABLE 13.10

AN APPROACH TO CATEGORIZING OCCUPATIONAL ILLNESS DESIGNED FOR
DEVELOPING COUNTRIES

Category	Criterion	Example
1	Work as direct and necessary cause	Mesothelioma arising from asbestos exposure; cholinergic crisis from exposure to organophosphate pesticides
2	Work as contributory factor	Shift work as risk factor for hypertension; mental illness from workplace stress
3	Existing disease aggravated by work; or latent disease precipitated by work	Varicose veins aggravated by standing work; contact allergic dermatitis from workplace exposure
4	Disease due to increased access	Alcohol dependence among bartenders; suicide using pesticides among rural farmers and farm workers

Occupational health and safety legislation often and properly requires that health-care workers report a case of suspected or confirmed occupational disease. The health-care professional may be obligated to notify the appropriate labor or health authority, which will then initiate its own investigation and enforcement action.

The evaluation of occupational health problems is not necessarily limited to identifying occupational causes of specific disorders. A non-occupational disorder may interfere with the worker's ability to do the job. An occupational exposure may aggravate the symptoms of a non-occupational disorder. Table 13.10 describes a means of categorizing diseases as they relate to occupation as a cause, as an aggravating factor, or as an obstacle to return to work.

Impairment and disability evaluation are discussed in Chapter 14.

14

OCCUPATIONAL INJURIES

Tee L. Guidotti

Traumatic musculoskeletal injuries are the most common occupational disorders. Most occupational injuries are very similar to injuries that occur in sports or in daily life. They are different in that they are connected to work, are often dealt with through special insurance systems (such as workers' compensation), and are all potentially preventable.

The term *injury* is often used differently in occupational health than it is in medicine or the other health professions. In occupational health, the definition of injury is heavily influenced by the insurance sector and the needs of statistical classification. For occupational health purposes, an injury is a disorder that happens as the result of a single event, generally as the result of trauma but sometimes as a result of other physical or chemical factors, and usually results in damage or impairment right away. A disease is a disorder that develops over time or is the result of longer-term or repeated exposure. Musculoskeletal disorders that result from chronic strain or repeated motions are therefore counted as diseases. Musculoskeletal disorders that result from trauma and that are the result of a single event are counted as injuries. Similarly, disorders resulting from chemical exposures that develop over a period of time or that are due to chronic toxicity are counted as diseases. Disorders that are the result of chemical burns or acute toxicity are counted as injuries. Poisonings may be treated as injuries or diseases, depending on whether they are acute or chronic.

This chapter deals primarily with traumatic injuries. Safety and injury prevention is discussed in Chapter 6. The effects of disability resulting from severe injuries last well beyond working life, when it can interfere with income. Box 14.1 describes how the burden carries over into retirement and causes preventable disability in life.

PATTERNS OF INJURY

Roughly-one quarter of injuries are to the back and neck. Back injuries are responsible for over 40% of claims and a large number of complaints that go unreported. Second in frequency are hand injuries, accounting for approximately one-fifth of

Box 14.1

Disability after Retirement

Occupational health and safety is an important social issue in an aging population. It is as important in preventing disability after retirement as it is in protecting the health and earning ability of current workers. In a population in which people are not only surviving to retirement in large numbers but living far beyond retirement age, controlling occupational causes of disability represents one of the few "tried and true" opportunities available for reducing the burden of physical disability in older age.

In a study in the United States in the 1980s, 6,096 women and 3,653 men completed a questionnaire on disability and occupation. The analysis took into consideration and adjusted for age, marital status, educational level, and rate of attrition. The authors concluded that occupational disorders make a much greater contribution to disability in the general population and among retirees than has previously been assumed (Leigh, Fries 1992).

Compared to men, the women had higher mean levels of disability (0.062 to 0.415 vs. 0.008 to 0.329 for men). Specific occupations associated with excess or disproportionate levels of disability, compared to the general population, were different for men and women.

For men, the occupations associated with excess disability included machinery maintenance, mining, construction and non-construction laborers, bus drivers, farmers and farm workers, shipping and receiving clerks, auto mechanics, and painters; accountants also rank surprisingly high. The least disability was observed among mechanic supervisors, educational administrators, butchers and meat cutters, civil engineers, and postal clerks.

For women, the occupations associated with excess disability included non-construction laborers, farm workers, "winding and twisting" machine operatives, private home cleaning personnel and housekeepers and servants, food preparation supervisors, laundry and dry cleaning operatives, "packaging and filling" machine operatives, nursing aides and health attendants, nurses, and dressmakers. The least disability was observed for sales personnel, child care workers in private households, designers, clerks, and data-entry personnel.

Having no usual occupation was highly associated with disability, equivalent to second rank among women and first among men. However, given the way the study was designed, it is not possible to determine whether the disability came first and interfered with employment or whether unemployment is a risk factor for chronic disability (as it appears to be for many other health problems, including risk of death).

French retirees of both sexes living at home in the metropolitan area of Paris showed increased levels of disability among those subjects who had worked outdoors and with ergonomic hazards during their working lives. In particular, exposure to awkward postures, noise, heavy loads, dust, and inclement weather were particularly associated with disability. As in the American study, the French investigators found higher levels of disability among women. White-collar (office worker) occupations showed the lowest levels of disability. Most disability was musculoskeletal, followed by cardiovascular and hearing loss.

The authors concluded that occupational hazards are associated with impairment later in life and are a substantial cause of disability among the post-retirement population (Cassou et al. 1992).

An important aspect of disability that these studies illustrate is the disproportionate burden among women. Far from being protected, women's traditional occupations, such as nursing, housekeeping, and dressmaking, are associated with higher levels of disability than many men's traditional occupations.

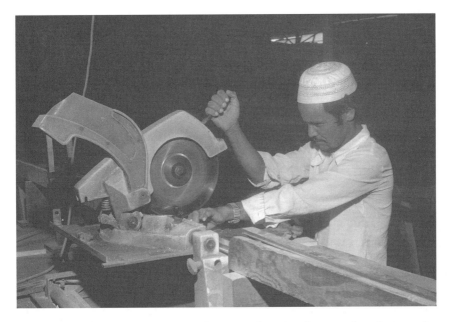

Figure 14.1 This man is cutting a metal pipe with a circular saw that does not have a guard on it. He is one loud noise or distraction away from cutting his fingers off. He also has no safety glasses to protect his eyes. (Photograph courtesy of Saudi Aramco World/ SAWDIA.)

all occupational injuries. The rest are distributed unequally among other parts of the body. Table 14.1 shows the distribution of disabling injuries by the body parts most affected in the Canadian province of Alberta.

Injuries may be categorized in various ways, but they are commonly described in these terms:

- *soft-tissue injuries* (where there is damage to a muscle, joint ligament, or tendon) are by far the most common occupational injury, about 40% of total injuries
- *fractures* (when a bone is broken) constitute only about 10% of occupational injuries
- *dislocations* (when a joint is separated)

TABLE 14.1

DISTRIBUTION OF DISABLING NONFATAL WORK INJURIES AND ILLNESS, CALIFORNIA, 1988 (n = 371,738)

Injury	% Total	Body Part Most Often Affected
Strains, sprains, hernias	42.9	Back (48%) Lower extremities (18%)
Cuts, lacerations, punctures	15.6	Upper extremities (69%)
Fractures	10.9	Upper extremities (42%) Lower extremities (38%)
Contusions, crushes, bruises	10.8	Upper extremities (28%) Lower extremities (37%)
Abrasions	4.3	Eye (81%)
Burns and scalds	2.6	Upper extremities (45%)
Concussions	0.8	Head (100% by definition)
Multiple injuries	0.6	—
Amputations	0.2	Upper extremities (97%)
Electrocution	0.1	—
Other	11.0	—

TABLE 14.2

DISTRIBUTION OF LOST-TIME CLAIMS BY PART OF BODY INJURED, WORKERS' COMPENSATION BOARD OF ALBERTA, 1982–1986

Back and Neck	27.6%
Hand (inc. fingers and wrist)	20.0%
Foot (inc. ankle)	10.2%
Trunk (excluding back)	10.0%
Leg	8.2%
Eyes	5.7%
Arm	4.1%
Multiple sites in same incident	6.6%
Other (including head)	7.6%
Total	100%

- *penetrating injuries* (e.g., when a worker steps on a nail)
- *crush injuries* (where the injury is due to pressure)
- *lacerations* (where there is a cut or open wound)
- *falls* (which may be from a height or into a hole)
- *head trauma* (which implies a risk of brain damage)

- *multiple trauma* (which occurs in severe incidents, often involving motor vehicles)
- *burns* (which may be the result of heat [*thermal injury*], electricity, or chemical injury to the skin) are uncommon (less than 5%) but often serious

The great majority of occupational disorders are soft-tissue injuries sustained in industrial or motor vehicle accidents while on the job. Crush injuries are often very painful and require long recuperation. Burns, although uncommon, often result in severe disability and therefore are discussed in some detail below.

PAIN

Many occupational injuries involve pain, and the evaluation and treatment of chronic and repetitive musculoskeletal disorders, particularly soft-tissue injuries, is dominated by issues of the management and interpretation of chronic pain.

Pain is a complex sensation, only partly the result of stimulation of particular pain receptors and transmission of nerve impulses to the brain. Pain is integrally linked with emotion. Not only is pain profoundly disturbing in itself, but it is made worse by attention and depression. It is obvious that the perception of pain may affect mood. As well, mood and cognition may affect the perception of pain. People feel less pain when their attention is distracted from it, and they feel more pain when they are anxious. Mood elevation, physiotherapy and other activities, preoccupation with other matters, and absorption with intellectually stimulating and rewarding activities all seem to reduce the perception of pain.

Unfortunately, serious occupational injuries are often associated with an intensive psychological focus on the injury. Virtually all of these complexities of pain perception come into play in occupational injuries because of the social dynamics of occupation and claiming compensation. Compensation claims are often disputed and must be appealed, physicians must be consulted, treatment must be scheduled, the worker's life is disrupted, and—at the extreme—family and friends may question whether the hapless patient is exaggerating to gain sympathy or for another reason. The result is that the injury may become the center of the injured worker's life, a source of great frustration to which is connected issues of self-esteem, community recognition, relationships with family and others, fulfillment of goals, blaming of others, and control over one's own life. In some cases chronic pain becomes the predominant symptom, often well out of proportion to the magnitude of the injury.

Chronic pain syndrome is a pattern characterized by chronic pain, continuing long after the injury should have healed, that is disproportionate to the injury and becomes the focus of the person's life. Injured workers with this problem are often depressed. The management of chronic pain in such situations should follow an integrated approach, employing both medicine and psychotherapy. Realistically, there is little hope for full resolution until the status of the claim is resolved. Dependency and depression are serious risks during this period.

The management of most occupational injuries is not different from that of injuries that occur in daily life. However, prompt treatment is usually important in recovery, and frequent evaluation can help in an early and safe return to work (see Chapter 17—"Fitness to Work"). The standard care of occupational injuries places greater emphasis on rehabilitation services to guide recovery of strength, range of motion (mobility of the joint), and coordination. The standard care of occupational injuries also emphasizes observing the progress of the injured worker as he or she recovers and determining when he or she is fit to return to work.

Effective and appropriate intervention for work-related injuries and illnesses has many benefits: earlier return to work, less disruption in the lives of workers, more individualized case management, and reduced costs to employers and the economy. Ideally, the occupational health care-system would apply the knowledge, insight, and skill of the physician toward early treatment, monitoring of functional capacity, and documentation of claims for compensation.

The primary health-care system provides most care to injured workers, especially for those in small enterprises, rural areas, and employees of industries that do not have organized occupational health services. The primary health-care system usually covers all parts of a country, controls access to hospitals and specialized services, and is the most familiar part of the health-care system for workers and their families.

In reality, however, treatment and medical care for occupational injuries often tend to be rushed, especially in community health-care facilities, because the primary health-care system is overloaded and health-care providers are always in a hurry. Injured workers often have to wait while other patients are seen first, on the assumption that their needs are not as urgent. Medical care tends to be applied in a routine manner and without consideration of rehabilitation issues and what may be required before the worker can return to his or her job. The system tends to be insensitive to the needs of individual workers and employers. For example, in a desire to give their patients the benefit of more time off or increased compensation, physicians often serve as advocates for individual claimants who also happen to be their patients for general health care, creating a conflict of interest. At the same time, primary care services often wait too long to return workers to their jobs, may not have the expertise to handle cases requiring extensive rehabilitation, and are usually unfamiliar with the hazards in local workplaces. In some countries, the system has accepted a less professional standard of medical services because this is all that is available. This is less than satisfactory because workers and their employers lose financial security, may lose income, and do not receive the best possible care, resulting in unnecessary disability.

Because of increasing costs of providing health care for injured workers and dissatisfaction over the outcome, hospitals and health services in many countries, such as Canada, have been under pressure to improve the quality of care and to do better in returning workers to their jobs. The strategies for doing this have included such innovations as:

- upgrading the quality and responsiveness of the primary care system through training and financial incentives
- encouraging the development of occupational health clinics and facilities where the local demand and market for health-care services can support them
- providing *case management*, which is a program of tracking individual injured workers through the system, monitoring their progress, solving problems involving access to care, and scheduling return-to-work evaluations as soon as the injured worker appears ready
- purchasing health services outside the government-financed primary health-care system, which has been highly controversial
- developing guidelines and protocols, or "care maps," that outline the most effective way to treat injured workers with common disorders based on the best available evidence
- sponsoring rehabilitation services through financial guarantees and contracts or direct provision of services to ensure access by injured workers when they need it

This aggressive strategy was possible because of the country's well-developed health-care system and government reforms in health care that made it easier for the workers' compensation system to make these arrangements. However, many of their methods could be used in other health-care systems.

Occupational health clinics and other facilities can improve outcomes and the quality of care by emphasizing early and effective treatment, monitoring of improvement, rehabilitation and physiotherapy if necessary, early and safe return to work, the scientific approach to fitness to work, and communicating with employers. Ideally, the objectives of the occupational health service should be:

- to return workers to work as early as it is safe to do so after appropriate care
- to provide a consistent and vigorous mechanism for performing fitness-to-work evaluations
- to provide an expeditious, effective, and efficient method of treatment of work-related injuries
- to evaluate early intervention strategies for common conditions (such as soft-tissue injuries)
- to demonstrate a process of management of work-related injuries that emphasizes a positive, goal-oriented rehabilitation model of treatment that results in an early return of the injured worker to gainful employment, whenever possible
- to provide the opportunity for outcomes research as a method of demonstrating the efficacy of this approach toward the management of work-related injuries
- to educate health-care professionals regarding the most effective care management of injured workers

Early and safe return to work benefits the worker as well as the employer. After an injury, the worker and his or her family lose income. The worker loses an important social connection, since work integrates people into their community and life. During recuperation, the injured worker may lose strength and the skills that are needed to return to the job. Rather soon, the worker becomes less able to work. Many workers become depressed, especially if the injury is severe. Prolonged time off work, beyond a month or two, is associated with a greatly reduced likelihood that the worker will ever return to work.

EVALUATION OF IMPAIRMENT AND DISABILITY

When a male worker falls off a ladder while on the job and sprains his foot, work-relatedness is obvious. There are two components to the ankle injury: healing the acute injury and recovering normal function after the initial healing process. The acute injury may be characterized by pain, swelling, and an inability to walk. The recovery phase may be characterized, in sequence, by pain when too much weight is put onto the ankle, pain when the foot is flexed or the worker stands too long, an inability to walk quickly, sufficient recovery for the worker to be able to return to normal use of the foot for daily life, fitness to return to work on limited duty because pain in the foot limits the capacity to stand or walk, and finally a return to normal capacity.

This simple example illustrates the normal course of recovery from an injury:

- the acute injury, when the damage occurs and the prevailing concern is getting away from the hazard and to safety
- initial management of the injury, including first aid (for management of bleeding, setting fractures, putting on a cast, and other immediate problems) and interventions to prevent further problems, such as immunization against tetanus or applying ice to prevent swelling and inflammation
- the healing phase, while the body handles the short-term consequences of the injury (such as swelling, pain, bruising, and sometimes infection)
- the recovery phase, while the body recovers from the longer-term consequences of the injury (such as loss of muscle strength, stiffness, pain when the body part is used, and/or joint instability)
- fitness for modified duty, when and if the worker recovers sufficiently to do some work but not enough to return to his or her usual job
- fitness for duty, when and if the worker is able to return to the regular job with all its usual duties

During the healing phase and the early recovery phase, the injured worker's functional capacity is of course reduced but is not stable. Immediately after an injury, even one that is serious, workers may be able to move around and may not realize how seriously they are injured. However, during the first few hours and even days after a serious injury, the functional capacity often gets worse, particularly as swelling and bruising become more painful. Over time, however, the functional capacity normally improves. However, it takes some time before the injured worker recovers enough to function around the house, in daily life, and to consider going back to work. In insurance terms, this shifting incapacity is called *temporary impairment*. It is usually not worthwhile to measure, or *rate*, temporary impairment because it changes too soon, and there is no point until there

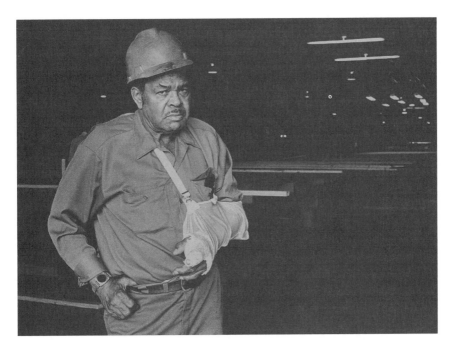

Figure 14.2 This man has experienced a serious injury to his left upper extremity, causing impairment in his ability to use his arm and hand, resulting in temporary disability while he is recovering. Because of his impairment, he is unable to do his regular job, but he is able to return to work with limited duties, so his disability is partial rather than total. If he does not fully recover and his impairment persists, he will have permanent partial disability. These definitions do not adequately describe the pain, anxiety, and financial insecurity faced by the injured worker and his family. (Photograph by © Earl Dotter, all rights reserved.)

is a clear idea of whether the worker will be able to return to work or what level of compensation will be needed for the long term. Instead, the occupational health professional waits until the worker has shown no further sign of recovery or improvement for an appropriate period. At that point, which is called *permanence*, the level of impairment is called *permanent impairment*.

PERMANENT IMPAIRMENT AND DISABILITY

Concepts of disability have evolved greatly in recent years. The current understanding of disability is as a mismatch between the capacity (what the person can do, the opposite of impairment) of the person and the requirements of the activity in which he or she wishes to participate. There are three obvious approaches to limit disability:

- Preserve capacity to the maximum extent possible (reduce the level of incapacity) through effective medical treatment, rehabilitation, and retraining.
- Modify the environment to reduce barriers that limit participation, such as ensuring access for persons in wheelchairs with or other mobility issues or

making accommodations in the workplace that make it easier for a person with disabilities to work.

- Change the requirements for participation, by allowing work from home or facilitating communication by the means most suited to someone with a communicative disorder, for example, by using dictation software and voice recognition for persons who can contribute in roles that normally "require" writing.

All people pass through certain phases of life in which they do not have the capacity to take care of themselves or to play a role as a worker or independently functioning member of society, if only in infancy. For most, aging brings increasing limitations in capacity. For a few, congenital conditions may result in lifelong dependency and disability. For many, injury or illness may bring disability earlier in life than it should occur.

Disability results from impairment, which is a deficit, or loss, of normal function. What the worker could do before the injury (such as walk and flex the foot all the way up or down) is that worker's normal *functional capacity*. The difference between the worker's previous functional capacity and functional capacity after the injury is the degree of impairment that can be apportioned to the injury. Impairment can be measured in many ways, such as how much less the ankle can flex at all, how much less it can flex without pain, how much strength it has lost, and how well a person can walk on it. The measurement of impairment is usually done for purposes of compensation by an occupational health professional who evaluates the functional capacity of the worker against a guide, which usually features a series of standardized tables. In North America, the standard guide is the *American Medical Association Guide to the Evaluation of Permanent Impairment.*

Because the level of permanent impairment is important for insurance purposes in determining the level of compensation needed and when the worker is fit to return to work (see Chapter 17), there are many terms regarding aspects of impairment that are borrowed from the insurance industry. *Partial impairment* is, as the wording implies, a functional loss that is limited to a body part (or a *regional impairment*) or that involves partial loss of function of the whole body (or *total person*). Partial impairment usually, but not necessarily, implies that the person can at least look after him- or herself at home and may be able to work at some jobs. An example of partial impairment would be loss of the ability to use the thumb on a hand, which makes it impossible to pick up small objects and to use the hand normally. *Total impairment* means that the person is unable to work and, in many cases, cannot look after himself or herself at home. An example of total impairment is quadriplegia, a spinal cord injury at the level of the neck in which patients lose the use of their arms and legs.

However, impairment by itself is not very informative in determining what an individual can do and whether he or she can return to meaningful work. Impairment has to be matched with what the job requires and the prospects for employment. *Disability* in the insurance (workers' compensation) sense occurs when the effects of an injury or illness reduce the ability of the worker to compete on the open labor market in the occupation for which the worker is trained and is well suited otherwise. The impairment rating or measurement is only one of several factors that go into rating disability.

There are many ways to calculate disability, and different countries, insurance organizations, and social security systems use different methods. Most, however, take into account the degree of functional impairment, the worker's training and skill, the condition of the labor market in his or her occupation, and the availability of alternative employment for someone with the same level of impairment. For example, consider an injury to the fifth finger on the left hand in a right-handed person that results in an inability to flex this finger normally. This is a small degree of impairment. For most people, this degree of impairment would not translate into significant disability. However, for a concert pianist, this permanent impairment may ruin a career by making it impossible to perform and therefore result in total disability for that occupation.

Disability is also described as temporary or permanent, partial, or total. Temporary disability is when the injured worker is recovering but cannot yet return to work. Disability is permanent when no further change is expected in the patient's capacity for work. Total disability does not mean total incapacity to do any meaningful work but an inability to compete in the labor market in one's own occupation or closely related work.

The physician does not decide the degree of disability under workers' compensation or other disability programs. The role of the clinician is to supply accurate information on three of the several determinants of disability: work-relatedness, impairment, and prognosis.

It is not unusual for a worker to experience more than one injury to the same body part, especially in a high-risk industry. In such cases, it is useful for insurance or compensation purposes to establish the impairment caused by the latest injury by determining how much additional loss of function has occurred.

PSYCHOLOGICAL ASPECTS

Most occupational injuries are accompanied by a psychological reaction that can range from denial through minor annoyance to shock and depression. The degree of the emotional response does not seem to correlate closely with the degree of the injury, although serious injuries are more likely to result in depression and blaming. The psychological response that an injured worker will experience is conditioned by personality factors, individual and collective beliefs, the exposure situation, who is perceived to be responsible for the injury, and the perceived responsiveness of the employer. The presence of a strong psychological component in a case of suspected occupational disorder is normal. If there is no visible reaction, then the worker is probably in denial and either involuntarily masking the behavioral response or voluntarily choosing not to show a reaction.

Blaming is one of the most important psychological issues when a worker is injured because it is natural for people to want to assign responsibility for the injury. This may lead to rage against a supervisor, employer, or coworker. Sometimes, the worker blames him- or herself, but this can become self-destructive. Self-blame often results in a loss of self-esteem and depression.

The presence of the short-term disability resulting from the injury immediately sets the worker apart from his or her working peers and establishes new dynamics within the family. Routines are upset, and the recovering injured worker may be underfoot at home. The injury may threaten the well-being and even survival of the family. The family is often not capable of providing the unconditional support the injured worker expects to receive.

The injured worker, of course, wants to talk about the injury and may want to talk about who is to blame. Very quickly, family, friends, and community tire of the story and the blaming. They may turn away and stop listening. They may even accuse the injured worker of laziness or faking the impairment.

Most injured workers accept their condition for a while, recover, and return to independence, within the limits of whatever permanent disability they may suffer. Some do not and either overreact to their new dependent state with anger or become passive and chronically dependent. Some develop exaggerated reactions, including depression, post-traumatic stress disorder, somatization, symptom exaggeration, and chronic pain syndromes.

Post-traumatic stress disorder (PTSD) is a psychological reaction that occurs when a person has experienced an emotionally overwhelming, profoundly threatening, or frightening experience outside the experiences of daily life. He or she cannot stop thinking about it, has recurring dreams about it, panics when he or she returns to similar situations, and is nervous and on edge. The frequency of PTSD in the general population is now known to be much higher than previously recognized.

Somatization is a state in which a person projects anxiety onto his or her body and experiences what to that person are physical symptoms. Somatization is common in medicine generally. Somatization needs to be distinguished from symptom exaggeration, which is the normal tendency to overstate pain and other symptoms related to an injury when an injured worker is depressed or wants to communicate to another person how bad it is. Symptoms actually feel worse when the injured worker is sad or anxious and is focused on the injury or the resulting impairment. He or she feels better when distracted and in good spirits. Many injured workers feel worse at night because when they go to bed at night they feel the pain more severely and lay awake thinking about their injury. Symptom exaggeration is not the same as *malingering*, which is intentional misrepresentation.

The psychological path of an injured worker need not be a downward spiral. Prompt care, a positive attitude oriented toward recovery, a commitment on the part of the employer to take the worker back, and effective rehabilitation can change the lives of injured workers for the better.

15

MUSCULOSKELETAL DISORDERS

Thomas Läubli and Craig Karpilow

Musculoskeletal disorders, as a class, are distinct from injuries in the standard classification of occupational disorders, even though injuries usually affect the musculoskeletal system. Injuries are generally defined as one-time events associated with trauma, but the category of so-named *musculoskeletal disorders* involves conditions that are chronic in nature and usually develop over time due to ergonomic factors, although their symptoms may come on suddenly. Musculoskeletal disorders affect muscles, nerves, and connective tissues, but not usually bone. There are many challenges that face the occupational health professional in managing this important aspect of occupational health.

Musculoskeletal disorders are very common. For low back pain the point prevalence (percentage of those who have pain on the day of the interview) seems to be 15%–30%, the one-month prevalence (percentage of those who had pain within the last month before the interview) 19%–43%, and the lifetime prevalence about 60%–70%. A slightly lower prevalence is reported for neck pain.

It is difficult to obtain accurate information on the amount of work lost due to work-related musculoskeletal disorders. The European Agency for Safety and Health at Work published data that are based on the Fourth (2005) European Survey on Working Conditions (see Table 15.1). There are huge differences among the member states: the prevalence of work-related low back pain is low in United Kingdom and the Netherlands but somewhat high in Portugal, Slovenia, and Estonia; absence from work is rather low in Sweden and is highest in Finland. This is a clue that there are also social and cultural factors at work, as described below.

Musculoskeletal disorders account for approximately one-third of all occupational disorders, according to compensation records in many countries. A much larger number probably go unrecorded because many workers tolerate minor injuries and the pain and discomfort associated with musculoskeletal disorders, if not disabling, without seeking medical care. Often, there is also a significant incentive from supervisors for employees not to report injuries or minor discomforts.

TABLE 15.1

PREVALENCE OF MUSCULOSKELETAL DISORDERS IN EUROPE

	European Union	Range Among Member States
Prevalence of backache	25%	11%–47%
Prevalence of muscular pain in arms or legs	17%	6%–29%
Prevalence of health-related absence from work over the past 12 months	23%	14%–45%

The employer obviously wants to maximize its profits and production quotas, which is felt at all levels of production and service industry sectors. The worker wants to be able to bring home a paycheck for an extended period of time and support his or her family in a reasonable manner.

In the workplace, there are many factors that contribute to an increased risk of musculoskeletal problems. These include highly repetitive work, rapid change of direction, forceful gripping, forceful or awkward movements, prolonged static or awkward postures, insufficient rest or recovery time, heavy or frequent lifting, use of vibration tools, and poor job satisfaction. Some musculoskeletal problems even are associated with cigarette smoking and depression. As a consequence of this multifactoral picture (see Chapter 3 for a discussion of multifactoral disorders), many of these factors are addressed in a fragmentary way by various specialties within the field of occupational health, including occupational medicine, ergonomics, physiotherapy, hand therapy, occupational therapy, exercise physiology, and others. However, they are more effectively managed by an integrated approach.

Occupations with a high risk of musculoskeletal injury include carpentry, food processing (such as meatpacking), construction work, mechanics, harvesting (such as asparagus cutters, strawberry pickers), sheet metal work, welding, nursing and nursing assistants, long-distance driving, delivery of packages, janitorial services, assembly line production, lift operators, various office workers, data input workers, and supermarket checkout clerks. This is not an exhaustive list by any means. One can find ergonomically inappropriate (see Chapter 7) working positions in all occupations and professions.

There are many types of musculoskeletal disorders. The disorders involve muscles, tendons, joints, discs, nerves, and blood vessels. They do not usually involve bones.

Chronic musculoskeletal disorders are commonly associated with ergonomic hazards, including the following:

• compressive and shear forces at the low back
• whole body vibration
• heavy and exhausting work
• repetitive movements

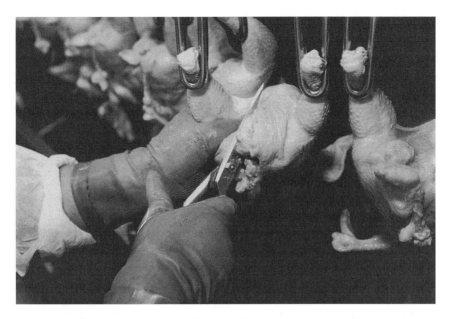

Figure 15.1 Poultry workers and other workers in the meat-packing industry have high rates of musculoskeletal disorders as well as injuries. This worker is cutting chicken on an assembly line, which involves repeated gripping of the scissors, repeated flexion of the wrists, holding slippery objects, rapid pacing of work, and working in cold temperatures, all of which contribute to the risk of musculoskeletal disorders. The glove is reinforced with steel mesh to prevent serious hand injury, but injury protection is inadequate in many other workplaces in the industry. (Photograph by © Earl Dotter, all rights reserved.)

- hand-arm vibration
- abnormal positions of the neck
- compression of nerves (especially in carpal tunnel syndrome)

EVALUATING A MUSCULOSKELETAL DISORDER

Evaluation of musculoskeletal disorders is done by qualified health professionals with appropriate training, such as physicians and nurses, and so the details of clinical examination will not be described in detail here. The occupational health professional's first task is to determine what happened (or did not happen) in the workplace. In the health professions, this is called *taking the history*. Some very astute health-care professionals can be nearly 99% sure of the diagnosis after taking a very careful history. How well the worker can relate what happened is, of course, a major issue in how accurate the history is. Various prompts are used to try to delve into the environment in which the worker carries out his or her job and the way it is carried out. Oftentimes it is also helpful to question supervisors, coworkers, and family members, who can all contribute pieces to the puzzle as to what happened to the worker. Once all of this information is gathered, the occupational health professional proceeds with an examination of the worker and, often, the workplace.

The occupational health physician or nurse will use the clinical and laboratory tools that are available to determine what has happened to the worker. Although there are many high-tech devices available, expensive testing is not always needed and is seldom allowed by those paying the bill.

In musculoskeletal disorders, only a small percentage of cases have obvious physical findings. Although trauma to an extremity, such as a wrist, hand, arm, or leg, will often produce obvious fractures that can be seen on an X-ray, chronic repetitive motion or vibration on the same extremity often will not produce a visible sign. They may produce symptoms of pain, relatively mild degrees of swelling and inflammation, and slowed electrical changes in nerve conduction (NCV), and they may occasionally change in an ultrasound evaluation, but these are not obvious on examination. More often than not, there will be no obvious physical findings. Instead, the worker will present with complaints (*subjective findings*) of discomfort, which are usually not able to be substantiated by clinical or laboratory findings. Because of this, the greatest challenge is to distinguish real from imagined and determine if there are other factors that are contributing to the presenting complaint. Job satisfaction, financial gain, retaliation against an employer, inability to do the requested or required work, or just not wanting to work can all be factors.

The most common complaint is pain. Pain and muscle spasm often go together, especially in the back.

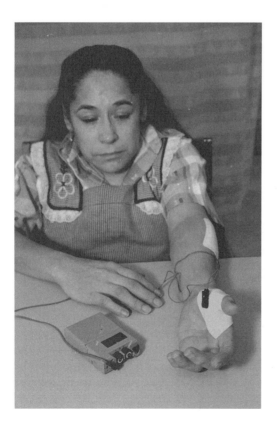

Figure 15.2 A garment worker in San Antonio, Texas (USA), is evaluated for repetitive strain injury by nerve conduction velocity. The device measures the speed of electrical impulses from the hand to the arm below the elbow. Injury to the nerve shows as slowing of the conduction velocity. This type of work involves sewing, cutting fabric, and repeatedly lifting piles of clothes. She did in fact have a repetitive strain injury. (Photograph by © Earl Dotter, all rights reserved.)

The occupational physician has to consider all the other possible disorders that could be causing the condition. There are several factors that determine how injured the worker is and how long it will take him or her to recuperate and be able to return to work.

- How long has he or she been having the problem?
- How serious was the injury initially?
- What underlying factors does the worker have (diabetes, arthritis, etc.)?
- How motivated is the worker to get better?

Diagnosis is made with a thorough physical examination to locate muscle spasms and determine the limits of ability to move an extremity (due to stiffness, weakness, or pain), neurological examination (examining how nerves work), radiographic examinations (X-rays), laboratory tests, electromyography (evaluation of the electrical impulses in muscle tissue), ultrasound, etc. A precise diagnosis is needed for correct treatment, together with assessment of the workplace and of fitness to return to work.

Patterns of Pain and Discomfort

Usually, the area of pain is directly related to the positions that the worker must maintain throughout the day:

- Prolonged standing (for 8 to 12 hours), especially on uneven surfaces, often results in back or hip pain.
- Repetitive bending or lifting often results in low back pain.
- Reaching or lifting above the shoulder often results in pain in the neck with tightness and pain in the shoulders and interscapular (between the shoulder blades) region.
- Repetitive, forceful work with the upper extremities, particularly the hands and wrists, often results in pain and numbness in the extremities.

The common musculoskeletal disorders tend to follow characteristic patterns.

Muscle Tension and Spasm

These conditions occur when a muscle becomes stiff and painful and often result from prolonged contraction or a sudden spasm of the muscle. They are common conditions and usually minor but can be painful at the time.

- *Writer's cramp* is a spasm in the hand familiar to anyone who has ever written a long document by hand.
- *Neck tension syndrome* or *postural neck pain* is pain related to a spasm or tonic contraction of muscles in the neck and upper back. It is often associated with anxiety or stooped posture and often is accompanied by a tension headache. The pain can radiate down one of the arms to the fingers and produce numbness due to nerve root compression.

Tendonitis and Tenosynovitis

Tendinitis, or inflammation of the tendons, is commonly seen in the shoulder, elbow, and wrist (e.g., inflammation of the tendons of the shoulder joint in welders, sheet metal workers, and mechanics). Inflamed tendons in the forearm, hands, or wrists give rise to pain and tenderness when the tendons are moved. Tendons are wrapped within a sheath called the synovium that also covers the joint. Inflammation of tendons within the tendon sheath, or *tenosynovitis*, may result in nerve compression at the wrist, which gives rise to the carpal tunnel syndrome. This results in tingling, numbness, pain, and weakness of the hand, making it difficult to handle small objects. Common forms of tendonitis and tenosynovitis include:

- epicondylitis, which involves the elbow
- trigger finger, which is a tendonitis involving the finger that is characterized by a popping sensation
- De Quervain's syndrome, often called "trigger thumb," which is a minor condition involving the thumb characterized by a popping sensation
- hand-arm syndrome, which is a common but poorly defined problem involving multiple sites of tendonitis and soft-tissue inflammation in the upper extremity; a characteristic repetitive strain injury of people who use their arms for prolonged periods without support or rest periods
- supraspinatus tendonitis, which causes pain only when the arm is raised beyond a certain point and the affected tendon (of the supraspinatus muscle) is compressed against a bone; the characteristic tendonitis of welders and riveters
- rotator cuff tendonitis, which is an inflammatory condition of the soft tissues surrounding the shoulder, which often includes supraspinatus tendonitis
- frozen shoulder, which is a condition in which the soft tissues surrounding the shoulder become stiff and painful to move, resulting in loss of motion and strength; tends to occur when the shoulder is kept immobile, not moved normally for a long period of time, and also occurs spontaneously (and reversibly) in many women in middle age for reasons that are not yet understood; rarely an occupational disorder in the direct sense but sometimes occurs because a worker has kept the arm immobilized after an occupational injury
- bicipital tendonitis, which causes tenderness over the shoulder due to inflammation of the tendon of the biceps muscle; very common

Nerve Damage

Nerves are closely associated with soft tissue of the musculoskeletal system. They are often damaged, sometimes permanently, by soft-tissue injuries and inflammation that primarily involves surrounding musculoskeletal structures. As a result, symptoms and signs of peripheral nerve damage, such as numbness and abnormal sensation, slow conduction of nerve impulses, and shooting pains, often accompany musculoskeletal disorders.

Nerve root irritation, or *radiculopathy*, occurs when there is irritation of the peripheral nerve as it passes out of the spinal column. This irritation may be mechanical, the result of *nerve root compression*, but is more often the result of inflammation and the effects of the chemical signals, called *cytokines*, that go along with inflammation. Radiculopathy is usually associated with soft-tissue damage around a vertebral joint and especially with damage to one of the pads, called an *intervertebral disc*, between the bones of the spine, or *vertebrae*. There are many different bioactive substances in herniated disc tissue that could have a damaging effect on the nerve root. This would also explain why radiculopathy and pain can develop without signs of nerve root compression.

Nerve entrapment syndromes are a set of conditions that are characterized by pressure on the nerve. The pressure occurs as a result of inflammation and swelling at a place where the nerve is easily compressed or pinched, usually where it passes through a narrow opening or under a tendon. This pressure damages the nerve and causes slowing of nerve impulses. They are characterized by numbness and *paresthesia*, an abnormal tingling sensation that is often painful. They may occur in acute injury, especially in crush injuries, but are more characteristic of the long-term swelling and inflammation in chronic musculoskeletal injury. The most common nerve entrapment syndrome is carpal tunnel syndrome, described below, which involves the median nerve as it passes under a tendon in the wrist. The ulnar nerve, which supplies the side of the hand opposite the thumb, mostly over the palm, is also susceptible to entrapment at both the elbow and wrist.

Vascular Compromise

Like nerves, blood vessels are also closely associated with the musculoskeletal system and can be affected by entrapment and compression, causing reduced blood flow to the tissue supplied by the blood vessel. In a muscle, this reduction of blood flow results in weakness, difficulty sustaining contraction, and pain. Vascular compromise can also occur in acute injuries as a result of entrapment syndromes, but is more characteristic of compression by adjacent muscle, long-term swelling, and inflammation in chronic musculoskeletal injury.

The most common form of vascular compromise due to compression is *thoracic outlet syndrome*, an uncommon disorder in which the blood vessels that supply the upper extremities are pinched in the shoulder area by the action of muscles when a worker pushes against heavy resistance or lifts his or her arms over the head.

Another common form of vascular compromise is *vibration vasculitis*, a disorder in which vibration induces spasm in the blood vessel and cuts off circulation. This results in characteristic signs of reduced blood flow and sensitivity to cold.

Repetitive Strain Injury

Repetitive strain injury (RSI) is a class of musculoskeletal disorders in which chronic discomfort, pain, and functional impairment may result from numerous repeated movements of an upper extremity. Swelling is often present as well. There are many synonyms for repetitive strain injury, including "overuse syndrome" and "cumulative trauma disorder," although *cumulative trauma* is more properly used to describe a theory of causation that includes noise-induced hearing loss and other conditions in which repeated but very small degrees of physical trauma are thought to play a role. Most of the musculoskeletal conditions described in this chapter are associated with repetitive movement rather than a single initiating event.

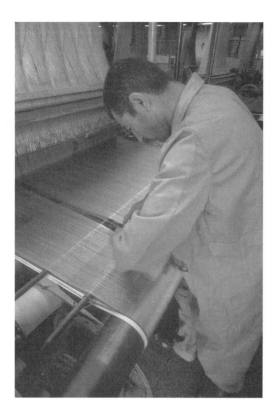

Figure 15.3 Rapid and repeated motion of relatively weak body parts, such as the fingers or wrist, causes a type of musculoskeletal disorder called "repetitive strain injury." This weaver in Syria is at risk for this condition. (Photograph by Robert Azzi, Saudi Aramco World/SAWDIA.)

Women are most commonly affected, in large part because of the nature of the jobs that present a high risk.

Occupational factors associated with RSI include a sustained and awkward posture, excessive manual force, use of intrinsically weak body parts in unusual or forceful movements, inadequate time for recovery or breaks in the work, and high rates of repetition of the movement. Other occupational conditions, such as cold working conditions and vibration, may make the condition worse.

The frequency of reported repetitive strain injuries has increased dramatically in recent years. This is partly due to increased recognition and attention to the disorders, but the increase in incidence is also real and due to the increasing number of jobs that require execution of a limited number of fine motor movements of the hands and arms, such as keystrokes, assembling small parts, cutting fabric, and packaging small items. Occupations with particularly high rates of RSI include airline reservation agents, telephone operators, insurance claim and other data input workers, stockbrokers, secretaries, and newspaper reporters, although some less automated industrial jobs such as meat packaging and textile manufacturers have also experienced elevated rates of RSIs.

COMMON SYNDROMES

A syndrome (as discussed in Chapter 16) is a collection of specific symptoms and signs that suggest a particular disorder when they occur together in a pattern.

Neck, Shoulder, Arms

Cervical (neck) *nerve root irritation* occurs when damage to the nerves that run down the arm is located in the neck or due to nerve irritation in the shoulder area. The pain can radiate down one of the arms to the fingers and produce numbness due to nerve root compression. This can result from chronic irritation of supporting tissues, arthritic changes, or acute trauma. The same pattern of pain can be produced from problems arising at the wrist, including work requiring high-strength grips, repetitive movements of short cycles with the wrist in awkward postures, and use of vibrating tools or vibratory equipment.

Fibromyalgia is a poorly understood condition in which the worker experiences chronic widespread pain and exquisite tenderness in several specific "trigger points," mostly in the back and shoulders. Fibromyalgia is also associated with debilitating fatigue, sleep disturbance, and joint stiffness. Fibromyalgia is considered a controversial diagnosis, with some physicians contending that the disorder is a "non-disease," due in part to a lack of objective laboratory tests or medical imaging studies to confirm the diagnosis.

Carpal Tunnel Syndrome

Carpal tunnel syndrome is a specific disorder in which the median nerve that supplies the thumb-side of the hand, mostly over the palm, is compressed under the tendon that holds it down as it passes through the wrist in a space called the carpal tunnel. Because there is little extra room between the bones of the wrist and the tendon, swelling in this area compresses the nerve and first causes reversible injury and later, if uncorrected, may cause permanent damage. The effects are first perceived as numbness and tingling in the hand where the median nerve provides sensory innervation, clumsiness in writing and handling small objects, and often pain at night while trying to sleep. It frequently affects both hands.

In its occupational form, the symptoms of carpal tunnel syndrome first come and go, depending on how much the worker has used his or her hands, but later symptoms become permanent if ergonomic corrections are not made (see Chapter 7). Occupational carpal tunnel syndrome is associated with repetitive movements such as typing, using scissors, using a computer mouse, and repeatedly using tools with a twisting motion.

Carpal tunnel syndrome is not caused only by work-related repetitive strain. There are many non-occupational causes. Anything that can cause swelling in that anatomic space in the wrist, or that causes the nerve to become unusually susceptible to injury, can cause carpal tunnel syndrome, including pregnancy, diabetes, endocrine abnormalities, osteoarthritis, rheumatoid arthritis, and vascular diseases.

Carpal tunnel is usually treated with anti-inflammatory medications, rest periods in between periods of work, splints if necessary, and, in cases that cannot be managed otherwise, surgery.

Low Back Pain

Low back pain is one of the most common medical conditions, afflicting approximately 85% of all persons at some time during their lives. It is one of the most

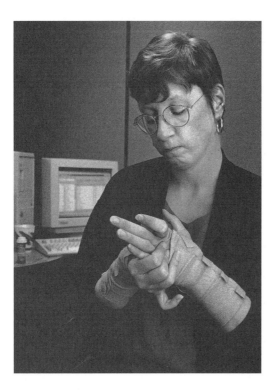

Figure 15.4 This worker has developed carpal tunnel syndrome and is using a splint to reduce her pain. This nerve entrapment condition results when the median nerve is compressed due to swelling in the narrow space in the wrist through which it passes. It may be caused by many medical conditions but is also a repetitive strain injury and is much more common among workers who use a keyboard and a mouse for long work sessions without rest periods and with poorly designed work stations. (Photograph by © Earl Dotter, all rights reserved.)

common problems in occupational health. Work-related low back pain occurs more often in jobs with high physical demand, prolonged static work postures, bent-over postures, and sudden unexpected high physical loads, such as in truck driving, nursing, and material-handling jobs.

The most common physical finding that goes with low back pain is muscle tightness and pain. The onset may be acute or gradual. This can occur suddenly, even without strain such as heavy lifting or obvious injury. Low back pain can also occur suddenly after a minor injury. The common physical injuries that cause low back pain are strains or tears in the back muscles, tendons, ligaments, or the discs that separate the bones (vertebrae) that make up the spinal column. Pain in the back may be associated with radiation down one or both legs (the pain feels like it is shooting down the leg) due to irritation of one of the nerves (the sciatic nerve); this condition is called *sciatica*.

Many people have *degenerative spine disease* by the time they are a few decades old. This very common condition involves wear and tear on the vertebrae and may make it more likely that the worker will develop low back pain. However, the presence or absence of degenerative spine disease does not appear to predict who will get low back pain. Inflammation and the accompanying chemical signals, called *cytokines*, may play an important role in degenerative spine disease. There are many different bioactive substances in herniated disc tissue that could have a damaging effect on the nerve root and would also explain why radiculopathy and pain can develop without signs of nerve root compression. On the other hand, small, unmyelinated nerve fibers are abundant in most structures surrounding the disc and the end plates as well as in muscles, tendons, ligaments, and joint capsules. Thus, all structures of the lumbar spine can be sources of pain.

There are a few serious conditions that produce low back pain. These include:

- central disc herniation or prolapse, which involve massive displacement in the structures around the spinal column that can pinch adjacent nerves and cause severe pain and even paralysis
- spinal stenosis, an unusual narrowing of the space within the spinal column
- infection in the spinal column
- osteomyelitis of a vertebra, an infection of the vertebra
- metastatic or primary cancer that affects the spinal column
- fracture of the vertebrae in the spinal column, which is uncommon and usually occurs in major trauma

These conditions are uncommon, however, and generally easy to identify. The physician looks for signs or indicators of these serious conditions, such as fever, paralysis, and interference with nerve function. If they are not present, management should be kept as simple and as uncomplicated as possible.

The vast majority of low back injuries are self-limited and do not result in permanent disability. Most employees can return to work quickly or within a few days. Nonsteroidal anti-inflammatory drugs and muscle relaxants are usually all that is required. Rest for a day or so may be useful, but prolonged bed rest makes low back pain much worse and interferes with return to work. Almost all cases of uncomplicated low back pain respond well to this conservative treatment. Contemporary treatment of low back pain emphasizes avoiding both bed rest and surgery because they can do more harm than good.

Returning to work after an episode of back pain or after surgery can be facilitated by a period of accommodation: lighter duties, with restrictions on repeated bending, stooping, and twisting. The importance of early return to work cannot be overemphasized. Workers with back complaints who are away from work for over six months have only a 50% chance of ever returning to work. If they are off work for over one year, this possibility drops to 25%, and if more than two years, it is almost zero. Psychological and social issues may be more important than physical issues for pain, and even more important for preventing long-term disability.

Arthritis

Many workers complain about stiffness after working for a period of time. This can be a minor adjustment to a new job or new aspect to an old job. It can also be an indication of more chronic problems. Arthritis is a disease that affects the musculoskeletal system. There are basically two common types of arthritis: osteoarthritis and rheumatoid arthritis. These two kinds of arthritis are very different, and a physician is needed to differentiate between them.

Osteoarthritis is a very common condition that comes with advancing age and overuse, especially of joints. There are many theories as to why it occurs, but essentially the joints wear out and cause stiffness and pain. It can be caused by using a particular part of the body too much or in an inappropriate way in the workplace. Typically, a person develops osteoarthritis in the large joints (such as the knees and hips); pain and stiffness improve after rest and get worse with activity. The condition may be disabling and ultimately require the worker to move to a different type of work. Osteoarthritis may have an occupational cause in workers who have carried heavy loads or who have otherwise placed strain on their joints for a prolonged period of time.

Rheumatoid arthritis is not an occupational disease, with rare exceptions related to its association with certain lung diseases. It is an inflammatory disease with autoimmune aspects. It can start at a young age or occur later in working life. The patient's work history has no bearing on how the disease develops or how severe it can become. Typically, rheumatoid arthritis starts in the smaller joints of the hand and fingers. The joint tends to become stiff with rest and moves more freely when used. It is treated with completely different drugs than osteoarthritis. However, the disease can be very incapacitating to the worker and may even force the worker to retire.

TREATMENT OF COMMON MUSCULOSKELETAL DISORDERS

Effective diagnosis, evaluation, and treatment of an injured worker with a musculoskeletal disorder are true challenges in occupational health. However, it is possible to achieve good results when the whole health team contributes to the process.

Treating musculoskeletal disorders often requires taking the worker out of the ergonomically incorrect position that caused the problem in the first place, with a period of rest or assignment to alternative work (see Chapter 7).

Physiotherapy, occupational therapy, and hand therapy are all techniques of rehabilitation that have been developed over the years to restore function in injured muscles, joints, and other soft tissues of the musculoskeletal system. The therapist, under supervision of a physician, employs special techniques to stretch, strengthen, decrease contractures (areas of tightness where the worker cannot fully use the extremity in its normal range of motion), and stimulate muscles and nerves to function more normally.

If the worker cannot tolerate the pain associated with the injury or condition, pain-relieving drugs (called *analgesics*), anti-inflammatory drugs, and/or muscle relaxants will usually be prescribed by the physician. Taken too early, before a diagnosis is made, these drugs can confuse the picture and make it harder for the physician to come to a correct diagnosis. These drugs have various side effects that the physician must manage and balance against the benefit to the worker:

- *Analgesics* are given for pain. Mild pain-relieving drugs such as acetaminophen (paracetemol) and the nonsteroidal anti-inflammatory drugs (see below) are preferred in managing chronic musculoskeletal disorders.
- *Muscle relaxant*, or relaxing, drugs are often employed in musculoskeletal disorders (methocarbamol, diazepam, baclofen, etc.) to allow the tight or strained muscles to relax. These drugs make some people sleepy, while others tolerate them with no problems. The worker's response to the drug will determine if the worker will be able to continue at his or her work.

- *Nonsteroidal anti-inflammatory drugs* (ibuprofen, aspirin, naproxen, etc.) are the most common class of drugs used to treat musculoskeletal disorders. (Steroids have too many side effects when taken orally, so only nonsteroidal drugs are used for this purpose.)

The nonsteroidal anti-inflammatory drugs have an advantage because they are both effective analgesics and act to reduce inflammation. These are often taken at home by workers before they come to the health center in an attempt to self-medicate. They are not addictive and do not cause any sleepiness that can affect the worker on the job. These drugs are often all that is necessary for simple stiffness and other minor joint conditions. This class of medications ranges from inexpensive to very costly. Some have side effects that can prevent continued use (such as bleeding of the stomach, if used to excess and taken without food). There are many competing brands, and the occupational health-care worker must balance the use of the simpler drugs or the expensive ones with the real efficacy and the cost to the worker or employer.

Other effective techniques include:

- heat for relaxing muscles where there is spasm
- ice for acute pain and inflammation and to prevent inflammation from developing after a strain
- strengthening exercises
- ultrasound treatment, to slow or treat minor aspects of the problem
- job modification to reduce the factors causing the problem

In some cases of severe or intractable issues, such as work-related carpal tunnel syndrome or trigger finger, when conservative treatments (splints, therapy, medicines, and rest) have not alleviated the problem, surgery may be necessary. There are various surgical techniques that are used by orthopedic and hand surgeons to assist the physician in treating the intractable cases and get the worker back to work. After surgery, there will be a mandatory period of rest, then therapy and retraining before the worker can return to his or her usual job. Depending on the circumstances, the occupational physician may recommend that the worker be placed in a different type of job after recovery from the surgery to prevent the same problem from arising again.

PROGNOSIS, IMPAIRMENT, AND DISABILITY

Impairment and disability are measured and defined for chronic musculoskeletal disorders as described in Chapter 14 for acute injuries. The difference is that in chronic musculoskeletal disorders, recovery and rehabilitation is often a slower process, and the worker may experience frequent setbacks, such as:

- a variable time course, during which the condition often gets better, then worse, and the worker may have "good days" and "bad days" for no obvious reason

> **Box 15.1**
>
> ## Rheumatoid Arthritis: A Non-Occupational Disorder That Interferes with Work
>
> As an example, consider a 67-year-old jeweler in Italy who makes high-quality jewelry for sale in his own store to local residents and tourists. Over a period of several years, he developed pain and stiffness in his fingers and knuckles. At first, he ignored the problem and thought he was just getting old. However, one day he found that he could not solder a clasp on a necklace without dropping it and almost burned himself. He was very worried because the economy was poor, his business could not be easily sold, and he did not feel that he had the resources to retire comfortably. He saw an occupational physician, thinking that his problem was work-related from years of working with his hands. However, the physician diagnosed rheumatoid arthritis, a disease that was not work-related but could interfere with work. Because of her experience with the treatment of work-related musculoskeletal disorders, the occupational physician recommended a physiotherapist and referred the worker to a primary care physician who could manage the underlying disease. The jeweler was able to continue working without pain for another four years, by which time the economy was better and he was able to sell his jewelry shop and retire.
>
> The occupational health team can implement protective devices such as cockup splints (adjustable to different anatomical positions) and elastic bandages to limit the progression of pain from a sore wrist. If the pain is severe or causes enough impairment that the worker cannot use the hand for a period of time, muscles will weaken and the hand will lose its grip strength. Tendons may shorten and ligaments may stiffen, and the hand will lose its range of motion and dexterity (ability to make coordinated fine movements). Physiotherapy, hand therapy, and occupational therapy, depending on need, may be required after the acute injury heals and the worker enters the rehabilitation phase. These treatment modalities will restore strength, dexterity, and coordination to the hand. If the arthritis is effectively treated and is not too severe, the worker will be able to return to work.

- exacerbations and secondary injury, which are common and often lead to a reluctance to use the body part out of fear of re-injury
- varying perception of pain, as described below

Prognosis is a prediction of the probable outcome, especially whether the worker will be able to go back to work. In general, minor conditions of the muscles and joints should have a good prognosis: the worker should be able to return to his or her usual job without problems after sufficient time has passed for recovery. Just like serious injuries (e.g., falling off a building and breaking many bones), severe musculoskeletal disorders may have a poor prognosis: the worker may not be able to return to the usual work due to the long-term problems from the injury.

In some cases, where a worker has significant musculoskeletal problems, a program designed to increase strength and capacity to do the specific work required by the job, known as a *work-hardening program,* may be useful to prepare the worker for returning to work. This is an intensive therapy program based on a simulation of the workplace as part of the therapy.

It is important to learn what the worker's job requires to be able to determine if he or she is fit to return to work (see Chapter 17). Some companies delineate this process, but most do not. The functional abilities of a particular job can be evaluated and documented by a physiatrist (a specialist in rehabilitation), a kinesiologist (a professional specialized in exercise and body movement), or other qualified individuals. Given the lack of objective criteria for determining fitness to return to work in many situations, it is important to ensure that the worker is returning to a job situation that will not provoke a recurrence of musculoskeletal symptoms. This is where the whole therapeutic team needs to participate in the evaluation of the workplace.

Social factors may influence the return to work. This is discussed at length below and in Box 15.2.

One of the most important factors in prognosis is early return to work. This cannot be overemphasized. The longer the worker stays away from work, the less likely he or she is to return to the workforce. The reasons for this are complicated but include a loss of physical conditioning (loss of strength and stamina) while the worker is resting at home and not working, loss of social integration in the workplace, loss of motivation (and often developing depression), and loss of skills due to lack of practice. Some companies have devised elaborate programs to get the worker back to the workplace to do anything—even the simplest and least demanding tasks—just in order to keep them in the habit of going to work.

Box 15.2

Understanding Social Influences on Outcomes

Psychological and social factors clearly have a strong influence on both individual cases of chronic musculoskeletal disorders and the overall pattern of outcomes seen in occupational disease statistics. Understanding these social influences may provide a key to lowering the high rate of disability due to musculoskeletal disorders.

In one excellent prospective study, the investigators studied the prevalence and coincidence of symptoms or signs of degenerative changes in the back, shoulders, hips, and knees in 575 fifty-five-year-old residents of Malmö, Sweden. They analyzed the relationship of these symptoms to a set of predisposing factors, mostly measured much earlier in life. Back pain was the most common complaint—nearly 1/3—in men and women. Locomotor discomfort coincided more often and was more frequent in women. Overweight was related to knee and back complaints in men. Men with shoulder complaints were more often smokers. Men with knee complaints had higher levels of serum glutamyl-transferase, indicating a higher alcohol intake. Sleeping disturbances were more common in subjects with shoulder, back, and knee complaints. Subjects with moderate or heavy workloads had more locomotor complaints, particularly in the back, hips, and knees. Of all the factors studied, job dissatisfaction was the variable with the strongest independent association with locomotor discomfort in both genders (Bergenudd and Nilsson 1988, 1994). These findings suggest that better outcomes, including return to work and the ability to walk without pain, can be achieved with a better working environment and that workers can reduce their risk of musculoskeletal disorders by good general health habits.

It is difficult to formulate preventive strategies without good research, and the quality of many scientific studies is limited. More research is needed before proposing evidence-based changes in social policies. To achieve clear understanding of individual predictive factors, long-term prospective studies are necessary (see Chapter 3), but there are few long-term cohort studies, such as that cited above. Even fewer of these studies have lasted longer than five years or confined the analysis to a specific diagnosis (e.g., sciatica due to proven disc herniation). Neck pain, in particular, has not been much studied. From the various reports in the literature, it has been impossible to differentiate between individual risk factors for first-time occurrence of low back pain and risk factors for recurrence and chronicity, thus many questions remain open for further investigation.

PAIN AND CHRONIC MUSCULOSKELETAL DISORDERS

Pain is a critically important dimension in chronic musculoskeletal disorders. In addition to being a symptom, it is deeply connected to the psychological issues that are inherent in these disorders. The management of pain is not simple and requires a deep understanding of the physiology and pathology of pain by the treating health professional.

Treatment of pain in these conditions should be as conservative as possible. It is dangerous to over-treat the pain of chronic musculoskeletal disorders. Pure pain-relieving drugs such as the opiates (codeine, morphine, oxycodone, etc.) should not be used. These *strong analgesics* are appropriate for severe pain in acute trauma but are addictive, have significant side effects, and are stronger than required for chronic musculoskeletal disorders. They also present a risk for re-injury because their use may alter the worker's sensory perception of pain, which may allow the worker to be injured again or "overdo" an activity that perpetuates the damage.

Pain is a multidimensional, subjective sensation. Pain may be a useful warning signal or an indicator of a health problem, or it may become a problem in its own right. In chronic musculoskeletal disorders, the pain serves no useful purpose in alerting the person to injury. Instead, its constancy tends to wear people down and contribute to depression and anxiety. Conversely, depression and anxiety can also amplify the perception of pain.

Experimental studies and clinical experience show that pain is perceived through a simple system and well-defined chains of neurons. In most pain states, both neurophysiologic and emotional factors influence the perception of pain. The initial pain stimulus, such as a pinprick or touching a hot surface, can be described in terms of stimulation intensity. Depending on the intensity of the stimulus, more or fewer nerve impulses are generated to be carried by nerves to the brain. These impulses are a coded pain message to the brain that describe the nature and intensity of the pain. However, how the brain perceives the pain message depends on the state of the brain at the time, and this is, at least in part, determined by the individual's emotional state. The emotional component makes pain a subjective, individual experience. How the person handles the pain, emotionally as well as physically, generally plays a greater role in chronic or recurrent pain than the immediate emotional reaction to acute pain (see Chapter 14). With recurrent pain, individual coping strategies become critically important and may determine the level of the resulting disability.

It is common to distinguish among different types of pain that are common in musculoskeletal disease:

- *Nociceptive pain* is caused by activation of pain receptors that are present in most tissues. This is the most common type of pain in musculoskeletal disorders.
- *Neurogenic pain* originates in the peripheral and central nervous system. The different pain mechanisms may simultaneously be present. It occurs in injuries in which nociceptors are activated, but nerves are also injured.
- *Psychogenic pain* is an uncommon type of pain. It appears in cases of deep depression and schizophrenia and appears to arise solely from psychological factors.

Research on pain sensation in work-related musculoskeletal disorders is advancing very quickly. There are several mechanisms that can explain the development of pain in work-related musculoskeletal disorders. The existence of these mechanisms has been proven, but it is still an open question as to whether they constitute the main reason for musculoskeletal pain. Diagnostic tools are not yet available that would identify the most relevant pain mechanism in individual patients. Pressure on a nerve or a nerve root, e.g., from disc hernias or increased pressure in the carpal tunnel, does not directly cause pain. Continuous pressure causes only a brief discharge of impulses. If there is demyelinization or inflammation, pressure causes prolonged discharges.

Pain receptors are free nerve endings called nociceptors. By a mechanism not fully understood, they are capable of distinguishing between innocuous (harmless) and noxious events and of encoding in their rate of discharge the intensity of a noxious stimulus. The *sensibility* (threshold of sensitivity to stimulation) of a nociceptor is not constant and may be lowered (the phenomenon is called sensitization) by previous noxious stimulation, making the nociceptor unusually sensitive if it has been stimulated recently. This is in contrast to the usual neurological response, *tolerance* or *adaptation*, which occurs when the nociceptor gets used to a familiar non-noxious stimulus, such as touch or mild levels of heat or cold, and increases its threshold of sensitivity so that the feeling diminishes.

Inflammation also reduces the threshold, making the nociceptor more sensitive. Endogenous substances that normally are present during inflammatory processes (described briefly in Chapter 16) may also increase the sensitivity of nociceptors. In inflamed tissue, nociceptors have an increased background activity as well as a lowered threshold for mechanical stimulation. This may explain why inflammation causes spontaneous pain, even without stimulation. The lowering of the mechanical threshold also means that more nociceptors can be activated by weak mechanical stimulation when inflammation is present. Therefore, the pain stimulus may be perceived as much greater than it really is. In animal models it has been shown that there are large genetic differences in pain perception, and many positive or negative influences on pain transmission are known.

The nociceptors, such as nerve endings in the skin, are in the same cell as long fibers (called *axons*) that conduct nerve impulses. When a stimulus is detected by the nociceptor and it is encoded into nerve impulses, these impulses are transmitted up the peripheral nervous system by so-called *afferent* fibers, which carry information about sensation to the central nervous system. (*Efferent* fibers, on the other hand, travel from the central nervous system and mostly control movements.) Nociceptive afferent fibers terminate in a relay connection in the spinal cord (the dorsal horn, anatomically), where they activate second-order neurons that relay the nerve impulses carrying the pain message to the brain.

The afferent fibers also connect with motor nerve cells, which control reflexes and *muscle tone* (degree of contraction at rest, or how "tight" the muscle is), and with the sympathetic nervous system. There is intensive debate over how these connections may be related to changes in muscle tone and the delivery of blood to the tissues. There may be a positive feedback loop, or vicious circle, that increases muscle tonicity, which in turn would activate its own nociceptors. This could perpetuate muscle guarding and tension and interfere with adequate delivery of blood to the overly tight muscles. Research continues on this subject.

In acute pain, the central nervous system can override the pain message. Descending (efferent) pathways projecting from several areas of the brainstem can modify the ascending transmission of signals. A well-known example of these pain-modifying mechanisms is illustrated by the injured car driver who, after a car accident, runs along the street to get away from the fire and who does not feel pain in that moment. Chapter 14 discusses other aspects of acute pain.

Chronic pain involves neuroendocrine abnormalities that are correlated with lowered pain thresholds. Patients with fibromyalgia and sometimes those with chronic low back pain show elevated cerebrospinal fluid levels of neuropeptides SP and NGF. *Neuropeptides* are small, protein-like molecules that have specialized roles in the nervous system. SP is a neuropeptide that is released when axons stimulate sensory nerves in transmitting the nerve impulses. SP causes the release of signals that promote inflammation and may have a role in some forms of depression. The neurotropin NGF is released during growth or damage to sympathetic nerves and is essential to recovery and healing. However, NGF also lowers the pain threshold (which makes the nociceptor more sensitive) and seems to reduce activity and cause fatigue when it is given to humans or animals.

These findings provide an explanation of why it is common for workers with chronic musculoskeletal disorders to experience fatigue, depression, and changes in their perception of pain that are often out of proportion to the inflammation and impairment that can be observed objectively. Beyond a certain point, which varies with the worker's personality and often the degree of depression, the pain itself may take over as the major problem and the primary cause of disability. The so-called *chronic pain syndrome* is a condition in which the pain perpetuates itself out of proportion to the actual injury. This is discussed in Chapter 14 as it applies to acute injuries, but it is also a factor in chronic musculoskeletal disorders.

Box 15.3

A Case of Work-Related Musculoskeletal Disorder

The worker was a 41-year-old former employee of a garment manufacturing company from 1977 to 1988 in Edmonton, Alberta, Canada. She immigrated to Canada as a young adult and had less than a high school-equivalent education prior to leaving her native country.

On September 15, 1986, she experienced the onset of left shoulder and neck pain and subsequently noticed numbness in an ulnar (little finger side) distribution of her left hand, primarily involving the fifth digit. This was worse when she used her hands repeatedly. She was initially given wrist supports, but these made her condition worse. She also noticed the onset of right-sided discomfort and numbness affecting digits four and five of her right hand. She was evaluated with nerve conduction studies, which showed slowing of nerve conduction. The diagnosis was entrapment of the ulnar nerve on both hands and a carpal tunnel syndrome of her left wrist. She is right-handed.

She underwent surgery twice—in June 1988 for release of a nerve entrapment at her left elbow and wrist and in February 1989 for release of nerve entrapment at her right elbow only. Since then, she has been much improved with respect to the pain in her upper extremities, but she still has pain in her left shoulder and neck, particularly with exertion.

Her duties at the company involved working on a sewing machine stitching jeans. She worked hunched over the machine, using her left arm and hand repetitively and vigorously to handle the heavy fabric while it was being sewn. In order to hold on, she had to grip very tightly and continuously through the operation. She noticed little vibration, however, as she did not touch the machine but held on to the garment by the fabric.

A claim to the Workers' Compensation Board was initially denied on the grounds that her conditions were related to other medical problems, specifically her thyroid condition. She had undergone radiation destruction, or "ablation," of her thyroid with radioactive iodine, presumably for early thyroid cancer, and has done well on thyroid replacement since. Hypothyroidism, a condition in which the gland is underactive, is known to be associated with carpal tunnel syndrome. However, there is no evidence that thyroid ablation with replacement of the hormone is associated with the condition.

On physical examination, the scars from her surgery are visible. Two clinical tests, one for compression of blood vessels in the shoulder area (Adson's maneuver) and one for entrapment of the median nerve (Phalen's test), were negative at the time of the examination, but Phalen's test was positive in the past. She appeared to be depressed and tearful, and her English skills were poor.

Nerve entrapment syndromes from repetitive strain and overuse are common, and the garment industry is notorious as a source of these problems. The constant gripping and repetitive movement in an awkward position are very compatible with the subsequent development of this patient's nerve entrapment problems and certainly the musculoskeletal complaints affecting her neck and shoulders. It is noteworthy that her problems are particularly severe on her left side, although she is right-handed. This is easily explained by the requirements of her job, and there is no other plausible medical reason for this localization.

It makes little sense that her musculoskeletal and nerve entrapment problems would be associated in any way with her thyroid condition. In the first place, the presentation of any thyroid disease, including extreme hypothyroidism, in this form in isolation would be such a remote possibility as to be inconceivable. Radionuclide ablation of the thyroid with appropriate hormone replacement is an extremely benign treatment with few side effects. It is not credible to think that her neck pain is associated with a thyroid disorder. Nothing else in the patient's medical history suggests an alternative cause for her musculoskeletal pain.

There is no reasonable doubt that her nerve entrapment and musculoskeletal pain is a direct consequence of her work. She experienced considerable relief following surgery, precisely as would be expected from nerve entrapment associated with overuse and repetitive motion. She has had residual pain in her neck and shoulder localized to the site primarily involved in her work. This has not been affected by surgery, and indeed one would not expect it to be relieved in this manner.

Musculoskeletal disorders of this type, affecting soft-tissue structures primarily, persist quite long after the offending motion and load at work have ceased. She is permanently/partially impaired by her residual chronic pain and neck and shoulder discomfort. It was strongly advised that she not return to work requiring heavy and repetitive use of the upper extremities. Her lack of command of English and her limited educational level made it difficult for her to find another job. Eventually, she was awarded permanent disability following an appeal to the Workers' Compensation Tribunal.

PSYCHOLOGICAL FACTORS

The psychological and social issues that arise from chronic musculoskeletal disorders have features in common with that of severe acute injuries (Chapter 14) but also important differences. Some of these psychological and social factors may be of importance only in certain cases. Others are more generally applicable.

There is extensive evidence that social factors (culture, family and social support, social class, education, involvement in the workers' compensation system, need for social security benefits, conflict over medicolegal proceedings) may influence the reporting of back pain, pain behavior, disability, and sickness absence. These social influences are complex and interact and are very powerful overall. For example, unemployed persons or workers who have taken early retirement have a prevalence of back pain that is comparable to the working population in general, but medical care or sickness certification for low back pain is increased.

Social factors that may influence return to work include:

- culture and perception
- family and social support
- social class, education
- workers' compensation or social security benefits
- medicolegal issues

These social influences are complex and interacting. Some are powerful as determinants and predictors of outcome on a population level; others may be of importance only in certain workers. The strongest relationships seem to be with the prevalence of disability. This is discussed at length below and in Box 15.2.

Individual psychological characteristics generally are of limited value in predicting the response to chronic musculoskeletal disorders. Increased pain and disability from musculoskeletal disorders and poor return-to-work rates have been related to high job demands, low job control, monotonous work, high perceived workload, work under time pressure, and poor social support by colleagues or superiors.

The strongest associations between psychological and social factors and outcome seem to be with the prevalence of disability. Individual psychological characteristics generally do not predict chronic musculoskeletal disorders very accurately. However, some evidence exists that type A behavior, a personality type that is characterized by impatience and a feeling of urgency, seems to be correlated with an increased risk. Consistent relationships have been shown between many psychosocial factors at work and increased musculoskeletal disorders: high job demands, low job control, monotonous work, high perceived workload, work under time pressure, and poor social support by colleagues or superiors. Musculoskeletal disorders are also correlated with the stress symptom, tension/anxiety (Bongers et al. 1993). This means that these conditions are also one of many manifestations of stress (see Chapter 11).

When pain progresses from an acute phase into a chronic or recurrent state, difficulties may arise in getting support at the workplace or at home, and problems may develop such as job loss and financial distress. This is similar to the psychosocial adjustment issues observed in acute injury, as discussed in Chapter 14. In chronic musculoskeletal disorders, however, there is an additional complication because there is usually no obvious injury that can be seen by other people. Claims for compensation in these cases are often rejected by insurance systems, such as workers' compensation, because they are hard to prove objectively. This often results in suspicion on the part of family members, friends, and neighbors that the worker with a chronic musculoskeletal disorder is exaggerating or faking the pain.

If the worker's responses are maladaptive, he or she may experience increased stress, "learned helplessness," depression, anxiety, and somatization, which can all worsen the perception of pain. One way of looking at this is as an equation: mechanical factors plus global pain sensitivity plus psychosocial factors equal the degree of functional impairment and pain that a patient experiences.

PREVENTION

Prevention is the ideal approach to reduce the prevalence of work-related musculoskeletal disorders. Although prevention appears to be a straightforward in concept, it is important to define and understand preventive strategies.

- Primary prevention aims at the whole population. At the workplace, the objective is to reduce exposures (e.g., heavy loads, one-sided or repetitive tasks) and/or to improve individual capacities to deal with exposures.
- Secondary prevention is directed toward detection of disease in persons who are not suffering from symptoms and giving them the benefit of early treatment at a time when the disease is easier to cure or control. (Some authorities use the term to mean detecting potentially harmful health-related behaviors or exposures and intervening to stop or reduce them, but most prevention scientists do not use the term this way.)
- Tertiary prevention is prevention of disability and re-injury. Rehabilitation that is directed toward reintegration at the workplace may be considered tertiary prevention.

It is important to be clear on what is being prevented. A given program may, for instance, have an effect on pain perception, but not on sick leave; it may primarily aim at return to work, but not on pain reduction.

The scientific evaluation of prevention programs is a very demanding task. The recurrent nature of musculoskeletal disorders creates difficulty in measuring and defining effects. Moreover, because the factors controlling back and neck pain are not entirely clear, it is difficult to know exactly what to do. Prevention studies also need long follow-up periods to observe adequately the possible benefits of the program. Many factors, such as economic developments, cannot be adequately controlled by the investigator, so randomized controlled studies are difficult (see Chapter 3).

Back schools are common preventive measures. They are based on the assumption that musculoskeletal overload can be reduced and controlled by improved knowledge on the part of workers about body mechanics, stress, lifting techniques, optimal postures, and other issues. Back schools usually involve several sessions to discuss anatomy, biomechanics, lifting, and postural changes related to work as well as a program of exercises. They are attractive because they use educational principles and are inexpensive. The method makes sense to participants, seems logical, and participants report great acceptance and satisfaction. However, most randomized studies have not shown any beneficial effect of back schools (Linton and van Tulder 2000).

Lumbar supports, which are wide belts or girdles around the waist, are supposed to prevent low back pain by three mechanisms:

- by supporting the trunk and preventing excessive flexion
- by reminding the wearers to lift properly by enhancing the normal sensation of joint position (a sense called proprioception)
- by increasing intra-abdominal pressure, which may decrease intradiscal pressure

However, there is no consistent evidence that lumbar supports prevent low back pain. In fact, a large study conducted by the National Institute of Occupational Safety and Health in the US showed no benefit.

Exercises have been used successfully in rehabilitation and in secondary prevention. There is clear evidence that physical therapy is a successful method to improve function and return the worker with chronic low back pain to the job. It may also work as a method of primary prevention. Medical/physical therapy training differs from self-guided sports activities. Muscle imbalances and muscle shortening are identified, and the goal is to achieve an optimal body posture. Self-guided training can easily increase these dysfunctions and is of limited value to prevent musculoskeletal disorders.

Ergonomic interventions are described in Chapter 7. The potential value of interventions designed to improve the psychological and cultural aspects of the workplace are described in Chapter 8.

16

OCCUPATIONAL DISEASES

Gregory Chan Chung Tsing and David Koh

Occupational diseases are illnesses that are associated with a particular occupation or industry. They result from chemical, physical, biological, or psychological hazards or factors in the work environment and although they may occur due to other causes, are not a special risk in the workplace if there is no such exposure. These diseases are preventable if the hazardous exposure is eliminated or reduced to a level that protects workers.

Occupational diseases exist on a continuum, starting with purely occupational diseases at one end of the spectrum where the relationship to specific workplace causative factors is well established; through occupational contributions to multi-factorial diseases, in which work-related factors contribute to the risk; through work-related diseases, where there is a possible causal role for workplace factors that aggravate disorders that a worker may have from other causes; to general diseases, for which there is little association with workplace factors other than the question of fitness to work (see Chapter 17). Table 16.1 outlines the differences.

The pattern of occupational disorders is constantly changing due to changes in the economy, in industrial processes, and in the workforce. However, these changing patterns are often overlooked because work-related diseases are rarely monitored. Occupational diseases often go unrecognized, known occupational diseases are consistently underreported in every country, and new occupational diseases are introduced from time to time by changing technology. The list of notifiable occupational conditions recognized at any one time by governments, insurance companies, or compensation agencies is never complete.

In general, occupational diseases cost more than injuries to workers and to the economy because they tend to be chronic and often lead to permanent disability. Severe or fatal occupational injuries are also costly, but the average cost of an injury on the job is much less than the average cost of an occupational disease. Occupational diseases, therefore, produce a significant cost burden for workers in medical expenses, loss of earnings, reduced life expectancy, physical or psychological suffering, loss of future earnings, and financial and social difficulties. Employers also face costs in compensation for lost earnings, disability and death, medical costs, time lost, decreased productivity, decreased employee morale, and unfavorable public relations. The prevention and control of occupational hazards

TABLE 16.1

CHARACTERISTICS OF OCCUPATIONAL, WORK-RELATED, AND GENERAL DISEASES

Occupational Diseases	Work-related Diseases	General Diseases
Occurs in working population, specific to occupations	Occurs in working and non-working people	Anyone can be affected
May be common or rare in the occupation	Usually common	May be common or rare in general population
Cause-specific	Multifactoral	May be multifactoral or cause-specific, but cause is not occupational
Example: asbestosis	Example: low back pain	Example: diabetes
Work exposure is essential	Work exposure may be a factor	Work is incidental; principal occupational concern is fitness to work
Notifiable, compensable	May be notifiable and compensable	Not compensable
Affects fitness to work	Affects fitness to work	May affect fitness to work
Preventable by controlling hazards in the workplace	May reduce risk by controlling hazards in the workplace	No relationship to hazards in the workplace

decreases the risk of developing both occupational and work-related diseases, and the benefits of such a program generally far exceed the costs.

For workers, occupational diseases may be catastrophic, resulting in loss of income for the family, expenses for medical care, and severe disability that may make it impossible to hold a well-paying job in the future. Some occupational diseases lead to early death, and most lead to significant impairments in daily life.

This chapter introduces some of the occupational and work-related diseases and their management and prevention, particularly skin diseases, lung diseases, hearing loss, nervous system disorders, cancers, musculoskeletal disorders, and reproductive system disorders.

OCCUPATIONAL SKIN DISEASES

Occupational skin diseases are defined as skin diseases induced or aggravated by exposures to agents in the work environment. They comprise a third to half of all occupational illnesses in some countries. While most skin conditions do not cause obvious disability, and only rarely cause death, they do contribute to productivity losses, loss of wages, and sickness absence. Studies have shown that they may severely interfere with the quality of life and may even affect mental health.

Occupational skin diseases are often seen in construction, metal, engineering, electronic industries, and service industries such as hairdressing, health care, and restaurants. They can be broadly divided into three groups

- Dermatitis (skin inflammation)—The most common is contact dermatitis (irritant and allergic contact dermatitis), which accounts for 90% of all occupational skin diseases.
- Skin damage—This includes a collection of "benign" (not malignant) conditions, such as skin infections and damage from various physical agents.
- Skin cancer (malignancy)—The most common is squamous cell carcinoma and basal cell carcinoma, and the most serious is melanoma, which is often fatal.

All occupational skin diseases are preventable. Principles of prevention apply beginning with substitution or removal of causative agents, engineering control measures, and isolation of the worker. Good hygiene and personal protection should be applied, including the use of impermeable but cool and comfortable gloves (kept clean on the inside) and work clothing, including aprons.

Dermatitis

Contact dermatitis is a skin inflammation caused by direct contact with an environmental irritant or allergen. It is distinguished from endogenous dermatitis, which is a hereditary class of skin disease that, while not recognized as occupational, is usually aggravated by working in wet, hot environments. Dermatitis is clinically characterized in the acute state by redness, swelling, small fluid-filled blisters, and oozing. In the chronic stages, the skin can be scaly, thickened, or fissured with pigmentary or color changes. Subacute dermatitis occurs when there are mixed features of acute and chronic dermatitis. Contact dermatitis may be irritant or allergic. It is very important to distinguish which is which in the individual case.

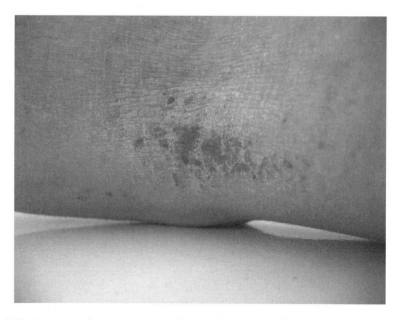

Figure 16.1 Eczema is the most common form of occupational skin rash and can be caused by allergy or irritation. (Photograph courtesy of iStockphoto.)

Heat, humidity, and physical abrasion aggravate both allergic contact dermatitis and irritant contact dermatitis.

Irritant contact dermatitis is caused by substances that directly damage skin at the site of contact following single or repeated exposures. It is not caused by an immunological reaction. Irritants that cause irritant contact dermatitis fall into two categories: strong and weak. Strong irritants include strongly reactive chemicals (such as ethylene oxide), acids, and bases that will induce skin irritation in almost everyone. The skin reaction to strong irritants is usually immediate and obvious. Weak irritants include weak acids, solvents, soaps, and detergents. Most people can work with weak irritants without difficulty, but some workers have susceptible skin and will experience irritation. The skin reaction to weak irritants may build up over time but usually occurs soon after the worker starts using the chemical. Irritant contact dermatitis is controlled by preventing exposure to the irritating exposure. This is usually possible by changing the chemicals used on the job or by introducing a barrier, such as gloves, between the skin of the worker and the chemical. When the irritation is prevented, the worker can usually continue working in the same job.

Allergic contact dermatitis is caused by an immunological reaction and is always acquired after first exposure to the chemical. Sensitization to an agent often does not occur for months to years, particularly from workplace agents. Common sensitizers include nickel, fragrances, hexavalent chromium (Cr^{+6}), rubber chemicals, and epoxy resins. After sensitization occurs, only minimal contact is needed to produce a skin reaction, which usually appears in 36 to 48 hours. The reaction may also spread to previously normal skin, distant from the initial eruption. Allergic contact dermatitis can be confirmed with a skin test known as a patch test. Once the chemical that causes the reaction is identified, the worker can be advised to avoid the exposures (both work and domestic). However, because only a very small exposure will produce an allergic contact dermatitis, it is much more difficult to control than irritant contact dermatitis. Reducing exposure may not be enough, and it may be necessary to prevent the worker from even coming into contact with the chemical; thus a job change may be required.

Contact urticaria (*urticaria* means "hives") is an immediate wheal and flare reaction of the skin that is itchy and usually subsides after a few hours. It occurs rapidly on contact with certain agents, such as rubber latex (gloves, boots, aprons), raw food (meat, seafood, eggs, vegetables, fruits), antibiotics, amines, animal proteins or secretions (e.g., from caterpillars, arthropods), and industrial chemicals (e.g., formaldehyde, benzoic acid). Contact urticaria may be immunologically mediated and may progress to a systemic *anaphylactic reaction*, a severe allergic reaction that can be very dangerous and even life-threatening. However, chronic cases are mostly self-limited and only make the worker/patient uncomfortable. Workers should be tested with a skin prick test if they are working with a substance that is known to cause this condition, and if positive, removed from exposure to the offending agent. Non-immunologically mediated contact urticaria is usually localized and not life-threatening. Unlike contact dermatitis, it is often not possible to identify the antigen responsible for urticaria.

Phototoxic contact dermatitis is a condition in which the skin rash is caused by sensitivity to ultraviolet radiation in sunlight. It is not immunologically mediated and occurs as a result of exposure to a phototoxic substance, such as industrial chemicals (e.g., tars), certain chemicals produced by plants (especially limes and celery), and medicines (e.g., tetracyclines, phenothiazines).

Photoallergic contact dermatitis is immunologically mediated, and the allergen is activated only in the presence of ultraviolet light. Photoallergens include medicaments, fragrances, sunscreens, and antiseptics. A photopatch test may be done to diagnose photoallergy.

Acute dermatitis should be treated with potassium permanganate wash to dry up the dermatitis. Sometimes there is an infection on top of the dermatitis that may require antibiotics, but the antibiotics do not treat the underlying problem. Pruritus, or itch, may be symptomatically treated with antihistamines. Chronic dermatitis is managed with topical steroids, creams, or ointments, but the use of combination creams such as steroid/antibiotic/antifungal preparations is best avoided. Any exposure to the agent would need to be minimized.

Skin Cancer

The risk of skin cancer is increased in outdoor jobs and jobs that require exposure to ultraviolet light, polycyclic aromatic hydrocarbons (as in roofing or laying asphalt), or chemicals that photosensitize the skin. Most skin cancers are either of the squamous or basal cell type. They tend to be very slow growing and can be treated by surgical removal. However, some people with skin that is easily damaged at the cellular level, or who have genetic defects that result in an inability to repair the damage, may develop many cancers wherever they are exposed to sunlight. A few people develop melanoma, a much more aggressive form of skin cancer that is often fatal. People with light skin and who sunburn easily are more susceptible to melanoma.

Skin Damage

This category of occupational skin diseases includes everything other than dermatitis and cancer and comprises less than 10% of all occupational dermatoses. It can be divided into three groups. One group is caused by physical environmental factors that directly damage the skin, such as ultraviolet light, ionizing radiation, heat, cold, and mechanical factors. These injuries to the skin result in a variety of disorders, such as ulcers, calluses, blisters, abrasions, and scars. Chrome ulcer is one example. Another group is caused by infections and infestations. A third group results in disorders of the *sebaceous gland*, the organ in the skin that produces oils, and examples include acne and chloracne, caused by organochlorine exposure.

Treatment of all occupational skin diseases begins by removing exposure to the causative agent. A job change may be necessary for severe cases. Other occupational skin diseases are managed according to the nature of the diagnosis. Infections require antimicrobial therapy; physical agents such as ultraviolet radiation and heat need barriers to reduce exposure, etc.

The lungs are an entry point for environmental agents and also a target organ for their toxic effects. Inhaled hazards produce a wide range of respiratory and systemic disorders. Traditional lung diseases such as silicosis and asbestosis are gradually on the decline as exposure to silica and asbestos declines. However, occupational lung diseases remain almost as common as they used to be in the past because occupational asthma is on the rise. The increased appearance of occupational asthma primarily relates to the increased use of sensitizing chemicals. Some gaseous chemicals inhaled into the lungs pass into the bloodstream without affecting the lungs and cause *systemic toxicity* (poisoning in other parts of the body).

Occupational lung diseases may affect the *airways* (the bronchial tubes that conduct air into the lungs, leading to the *alveoli*, or air sacs), the *interstitium* (the tissue that supports the walls of the air sacs), or both. Depending on the response to an inhaled toxic agent, the resulting disease may be a *restrictive* or an *obstructive* lung disorder or a *malignant* (cancerous) or a *benign* (non-cancerous) process. A restrictive disease is one that interferes with the ability of the lungs to inflate fully and is usually caused when the lung tissue is affected by scar tissue or *fibrosis*. An obstructive disease is one in which there is increased resistance to the flow of air, which makes it difficult to empty the lungs of air. *Reversible airway obstruction* occurs when the obstruction is caused by a temporary narrowing of the airways through constriction or inflammation, as in asthma. Fixed airway obstruction occurs when the obstruction is permanent, as in emphysema. A classification of occupational and work-related lung disease is shown in Table 16.2.

TABLE 16.2

TYPES OF OCCUPATIONAL LUNG DISORDERS

Disorder	Agent	Examples
Asthma Allergic response (high molecular-weight antigens)	High molecular-weight antigens	• Wood dust: Western red cedar • Foodstuff: grain dust, flour, coffee beans, shellfish • Animal products: dander, secretions • Pharmaceuticals: antibiotics, other drugs • Detergent enzymes: *B. subtilis* proteases
Allergic response (low molecular-weight chemicals)	Low molecular-weight antigens, which chemically combine with serum proteins to form complete antigen	• Adhesives: isocyanates, formaldehyde, epoxy resins • Acid anhydrides, aliphatic amines • Soldering fluxes: colophony • Welding fumes • Metals and their salts: platinum, nickel, chromium

(Continued)

TABLE 16.2 (Contd.)

Disorder	Agent	Examples

Irritant response
  Cough
  Irritant asthma
  Reactive airways dysfunction
  syndrome
	Chemicals that are
	  irritating but not highly
	  toxic
		• Solvents
		• Fumes
		• Isocyanates (chemical reaction)
		• Trimellitic anhydride

Toxic inhalation
Respiratory irritation
  Acute pulmonary edema
	Toxic gases	• Sulfur dioxide, chlorine, ammonia
		  (tends to affect upper respiratory
		  tract and airways)
		• Phosgene, ozone, nitrogen dioxide,
		  hot mercury, cadmium fumes (tend
		  to affect lower lung and cause
		  pulmonary edema)

Infections Pneumonia Other infections	Microbes	Viruses, bacteria, fungi

Hypersensitivity pneumonitis
(many specific disorders, may
  become chronic)
	Biological dusts	Spores, mold, bird droppings,
		  organic dusts

Fume fevers
(self-limited, characterized by
  systemic toxicity but not life-
  threatening)
	Chemicals that provoke a
	  short-lived but intense
	  inflammatory reaction
		Metals: zinc, copper, cadmium
		Products of certain plastic polymers
		Welding, cutting, and brazing fumes
		  (depends on metals being worked)

Chronic Respiratory Disorders		

Pneumoconiosis
  Coal workers'
  pneumoconiosis
  Asbestosis
  Silicosis
  Beryllium disease
  Many others
	Mineral dusts
	Metal dusts
	Organic dusts
		• Coal, asbestos, silica
		• Iron, tin, barium,
		• Cobalt (also associated with a form
		  of asthma)
		• Beryllium (also associated with an
		  immune disorder resembling the
		  disease sarcoidosis)

Lung cancer	Carcinogens	Asbestos, arsenic, chromium, coke
		  oven fumes, nickel, subsulfide
		  radionuclides

Mesothelioma (a cancer of the lining of the thorax and lungs)	Asbestos	Asbestos

Occupational Asthma

Occupational asthma is a disease that is characterized by variable airflow limitation and airway hyper-responsiveness. During episodes of asthma, the airways constrict due to inflammation or contraction of smooth muscle in the wall of the airway in response to chemical mediators released by a trigger. Triggers are usually antigens, and the response is usually allergic. In allergic occupational asthma, the worker must work around the antigen for a while before becoming sensitized to it. Sensitization is very specific: although a worker may be allergic to more than one antigen, he or she will be allergic to just those antigens and may be allergic to only one. It is not possible to predict who will become sensitive to a chemical in the workplace on the basis of a past history of allergies or asthma.

Irritant occupational asthma includes asthmatic responses caused by inflammation resulting from irritation from chemicals that do not provoke an allergic response. In general, the allergic form of occupational asthma requires removal of the worker from the workplace if the responsible chemical cannot be removed, because he or she will respond to very low levels of exposure to the antigen. Irritant occupational asthma may respond better to control of whatever in the workplace is causing the problem.

Asthma appears as a cough (especially at night), tightness of the chest, wheezing, and shortness of breath. Asthma is a very common disease and is not necessarily work-related. It can be triggered by allergens in the home and in the environment outside the workplace or by a chest infection. Severe cases can result in death, although this is rare. The disease can usually be managed by medications that reduce the inflammation in the airways and that block the constriction of the airway in response to the allergic response or irritation.

In *aggravational* or *work-related asthma*, workers who already have asthma or conditions that cause reactive airways have more frequent or more severe asthmatic attacks because of irritant exposures in the workplace. However, the workplace exposures do not cause the asthma in the first place. It is common for people with very mild asthma, or with allergies that give them a tendency toward reactive airways without actual asthma, to start wheezing, coughing, or becoming short of breath in a workplace with irritant chemicals or a high level of dust.

Occupational asthma can be identified in many ways and distinguished from asthma that has no relationship to work. The symptoms generally improve on days off work or longer holidays, although not always. Frequently the attacks occur right after the worker has been exposed to one specific chemical or has been engaged in one specific work process. Sometimes, the attacks occur at night or hours afterward, but on days that the exposure has taken place.

The diagnosis depends on demonstrating that workplace factors are causing variable and reversible airway obstruction. This normally requires an occupational history and serial lung function assessments. The evaluation should seek to establish the following:

- exposure to substances that may be acting as allergens or irritants
- presence of a temporal relationship
- natural progression of the disease, e.g., rhinitis, cough, wheeze
- aggravating and relieving factors
- use of medication, which may mask effects of the workplace

Early detection and removal of the worker from exposure is important, as prolonged exposure may lead to permanent disability.

Toxic Inhalation

Toxic inhalation is a specific term used to describe a potentially very serious, even lethal, lung toxicity caused by a variety of gases and metal fumes. A gas that is chemically reactive causes an acute inflammatory reaction in the respiratory tract. Gases also often irritate the eyes, airways, and respiratory units of the lungs. If the gas is relatively soluble in water, it does not penetrate very far into the lung and tends to cause its effects in the upper airway (nose and throat) and not further down. However, if the gas is not soluble in water or if the exposure is intense, it penetrates into the lung and can produce severe lung damage. The clinical manifestations may be that of an acute upper respiratory tract irritation, chemical pneumonitis (lung inflammation), and *pulmonary edema* (filling of the lung tissue with fluid that occurs over a period of hours). Pulmonary edema is often fatal. Later, if the worker/patient recovers, there is often lung scarring and there may be fixed obstruction of injured airways.

Toxic inhalation is sometimes seen together with smoke inhalation, especially in fires that involve burning chemicals or plastics. It often occurs in situations where a worker has been working in a *confined space*, such as inside a tank or in the hull of a ship with inadequate ventilation. Certain hot metal fumes, such as hot mercury (but not iron), can cause severe toxic inhalation. One cause of toxic inhalation is hot cadmium fumes, but this causes a severe lung disease and should not be confused with metal fume fever (described below).

Lung Infections

Infections are discussed in greater detail in Chapter 10. Pneumonia is an infection that involves the air sacs of the lung. There are many causes of pneumonia, most of which are not work-related. A *lung abscess*, like abscesses elsewhere in the body, is a localized infection that is sealed or walled off in its own space. They are also rare as occupational infections. *Bronchitis* is an inflammation of the airways that is very common with colds or influenza and not usually occupational, but it can also be caused by irritation from chemicals and dust and so is usually not the result of an infection when it is work-related. *Tuberculosis* is a serious and transmissible disease that has its own pattern of X-ray appearance resulting from the lungs' attempts to wall off the infection. Tuberculosis can be transmitted wherever infected people come into contact with others, including the workplace.

Hypersensitivity Pneumonitis

Hypersensitivity pneumonitis, often called *extrinsic allergic alveolitis*, is an immunological disease of the gas-exchanging parts of the lung due to an immune response to inhaled large organic particles, such as mold spores or grain dust. The lung reacts to these antigens with intense inflammation and in the process may damage the lung itself. This disease results from diffuse inflammation of the interstitium, the lung tissue forming the structure of the wall of the air sac, and may be complicated by *granulomas*, which are small, localized scarring reactions and generalized scarring (fibrosis). It typically begins with a flu-like illness 4 to 10 hours after exposure and may last for several hours or days. At this early stage, it may resemble asthma and there can be wheezing, an obstructive defect in lung function, and coughing.

If exposure continues, fibrosis may set in, causing irreversible lung damage and scarring in the interstitium. The chest X-ray may show a pattern that initially looks like pneumonia and later looks like pneumoconiosis. The process results in a restrictive lung function pattern, and reduced diffusing lung capacity can be detected. Repeated attacks can lead to chronic pulmonary fibrosis. Diagnosis is made from a combination of the occupational history and clinical features and is often supported by the presence of antibodies revealed by specific blood tests. Treatment is primarily by medications that reduce inflammation during acute attacks. Identification and removal of the agent or isolation of the worker is essential to prevent hypersensitivity pneumonitis from becoming a chronic, disabling illness.

Fume Fevers

Metal and polymer fumes produce an acute, febrile, self-limiting illness with muscle aches and influenza-like symptoms. In most cases, the symptoms occur within eight hours following exposure and normally last up to two days. Diagnosis is based primarily on the clinical history and the time relationship between exposure and onset of symptoms. There is no confirmatory test, and treatment is largely symptomatic. Repeated exposures may lead to tolerance. The main means of prevention is through the control of exposure to the implicated dust products and metal or polymer fumes. Metal fume fever, not to be confused with toxic inhalation, results from exposure to high concentrations of zinc. It most often occurs when inexperienced welders try to weld or cut metal that is galvanized or of mixed composition. It may also occur in response to copper and, confusingly, to cadmium fumes. Cadmium can produce several lung disorders, including this mild one. Fortunately, it is an uncommon exposure in the workplace.

Pneumoconiosis

Pneumoconiosis (pneumoconioses is the plural) is a general name for a collection of similar diseases of the lungs caused by inhaled mineral or organic dust and the reaction of lung tissue to the presence of the dust. The normal reaction of the lung to dusts is to remove it by means of coughing, carrying it up and out with sputum in the airways, and by engulfing it and carrying it out in specialized cells called macrophages. When there is too much dust, when the dust is hard to remove, or when the dust has toxic properties that interfere with the macrophage, it accumulates in the deep lung and provokes an inflammatory reaction. For complicated reasons that relate to the immunological response to the inflammation caused by the dust, many pneumoconioses are associated with disorders elsewhere in the body and certain types of arthritis. All pneumoconioses can be prevented by dust control and worker protection.

For most dusts, this inflammatory reaction is mild. For some dusts, however, it can be severe and may lead to scarring of the lung (*fibrosis*) where the dust is concentrated. On a chest X-ray, these areas of fibrosis appear as little dots that may grow together as the disease progresses. Initially, the dust irritates the airways and may cause an obstructive defect. Later, however, the fibrosis may produce a restrictive defect. Unfortunately, the dusts that cause extensive fibrosis are common.

Most pneumoconioses are detected on an X-ray of the chest before they produce symptoms in the workers. The sign of a pneumoconiosis is an early pathological change (in medicine, any pathological change is called a *lesion*) in the lung tissue that eventually is seen on the X-ray as a visible shadow, called an *opacity*.

A clinical and occupational history is required for diagnosis, backed by evaluation of the exposure risk and pulmonary investigations including a chest X-ray, lung function tests, and spirometry. Treatment is symptomatic and supportive (as for coal workers' pneumoconiosis). Prevention requires control of airborne exposure, respiratory protection, and medical surveillance.

Silicosis Silicosis is the pneumoconiosis caused by inhalation and deposition of dust containing silica, typically in its most common form, which is called α-quartz. It is the most common occupational lung disease worldwide, especially in developing countries, and one of the most serious. Severe cases can be disabling and even fatal. Occupations at risk include mining, quarrying, tunneling sandblasting, foundry work, handling crushed silica flour (which is used in many manufacturing processes), brickwork, and pottery making. There are several variants of the disease.

Typical, chronic silicosis occurs after several years of exposure, takes several years to develop, and is associated with a restrictive lung function that becomes

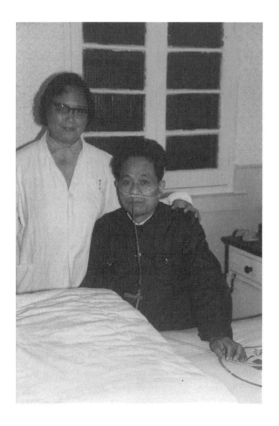

Figure 16.2 Patient with severe asbestosis, Harbin, Heilongjiang (China), in 1987. Notable signs include facial expression (reflecting stress of being unable to breathe comfortably), expanded chest, "clubbing" shape of his fingernails, and bluish tinge to his lips and fingernails (*cyanosis*, a sign of insufficient oxygen), despite supplemental oxygen. (Photograph by Tee L. Guidotti, University of Alberta.)

increasingly severe and may progress even without continued silica exposure. Diagnosis is based on a history of silica exposure and the classic X-ray findings that include widespread rounded dot-like nodular opacities in both lung fields, especially in the mid and upper zones, sometimes with visible deposits of calcium, called *calcification*, in the lymph nodes. Under a microscope, the lung tissue shows that each focus of fibrosis begins as a concentric, fingerprint-like lesion consisting of collagen fibers with crystals of silica trapped inside. Later, these *silicotic nodules* come together into larger masses of scar tissue that, if the disease progresses, cause an increasingly severe restrictive defect and shortness of breath. Management is supportive because there is no definitive treatment. The disease cannot be stopped, reversed, or cured. In order to prevent more rapid and severe progression, the worker should be removed from further exposure to silica, but the silicosis will continue to progress.

There is a form of *accelerated silicosis* in which this all happens within a few years instead of slowly and which is often fatal. Accelerated silicosis occurs when exposure to silica has been very high. *Acute silicosis* may occur within weeks of intense exposure and consists of an acute, severe inflammatory reaction that is usually fatal. *Silicotuberculosis* is a disease that occurs when a worker with silicosis is infected with tuberculosis, which accelerates the process of fibrosis. It tends to progress more rapidly than chronic silicosis and is difficult to treat. Silicotuberculosis is a particular problem where the rate of tuberculosis infection is high in the general population or among coworkers. Silica exposure is also associated with lung cancer, a type of arthritis called systemic sclerosis (or scleroderma), and a form of kidney disease, which is usually mild.

Asbestosis Asbestosis is a particular pneumoconiosis that is defined as a chronic diffuse fibrosis of the lung tissue caused by inhaled asbestos fibers. Occupations at risk include shipbuilding and repair, production of asbestos cement products, mining and processing of asbestos fibers, insulation workers, and demolition workers. Perhaps the greatest source of exposure today is work that requires removal of asbestos insulation. However, people who live around asbestos mines are sometimes exposed. Historically, the families of asbestos workers have developed asbestosis from exposure to dust brought home on the clothes of workers. Asbestos is a group of *silicate* (meaning composed of an oxygenated form of silica) minerals with magnesium and often other chemicals in a particular structure that forms fibers. Asbestos fibers are very long and narrow, easily breathed in, and persist for a long time in the lung (see chapter 9). Generally, a large cumulative exposure, over many years, precedes the development of asbestosis, which takes several years itself to manifest. (See Chapter 9.)

There are two main types of asbestos. First, there is a family of minerals called the *amphiboles*, which form solid, shorter and straight fibers, and which includes crocidolite (blue asbestos), amosite (brown or gray asbestos), anthophyllite (also called brown asbestos) and tremolite (not commercially used but present as a contaminant in chrysotile), and. Amphibole asbestos is difficult for the lung to remove. Second, there is serpentine asbestos, which exists in sheets that roll up to form very long, hollow, curly fibers and includes *chrysotile* (white asbestos).

Chrysotile is also difficult for the lung to remove but tends to dissolve slowly over time. Not all types of asbestos are equally harmful, and the risk is probably greater in crocidolite and amosite than chrysotile asbestos. However, exposure to any form of asbestos can cause asbestosis and cancer.

Asbestos is carried by macrophages through the lungs and into the *pleura*, the membrane that covers the lungs in the thoracic cavity. Thus, its effects are not limited to the lung itself. It causes severe inflammation that, if there has been enough exposure, leads to widespread fibrosis. Symptoms of asbestosis include shortness of breath during exertion and cough. Unlike silicosis, where the silicotic nodule is distinct, asbestos causes a more diffuse fibrosis that starts as microscopic scars around collections of fibers and progresses to long and dense scar tissue in the lung. Asbestos fibers, often coated with iron in the form of asbestos bodies, can be seen in the lung under a microscope.

The chest X-ray initially shows many ragged, thread-like irregular opacities, mostly in the lower lungs; this damage progresses to diffuse fibrosis.

Asbestosis often causes a number of secondary changes that lead to physical signs that a physician can recognize, such as clubbing (a condition in which the tips of the fingers look swollen under the nail) and inspiratory rales or crackles (sounds that can be heard in the lung using a stethoscope). There are usually visible scars on the pleura called *pleural plaques*, which may calcify. Pleural plaques may occur without asbestosis and are a reliable marker that the worker has been exposed to asbestos. Exposure to asbestos also causes cancer of the lung and cancer of the pleura,

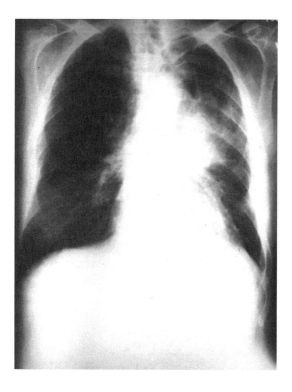

Figure 16.3 Chest X-ray of a patient with asbestosis (note linear lung markings, more easily seen in the right lower lung field, which, because of how the image is taken, is on the left in X-rays) and a large lung cancer in the left lung at the hilum (middle right side in the photograph; the "hilum" is the knobby structure seen on an X-ray where the airways and blood vessels branch into the lung).

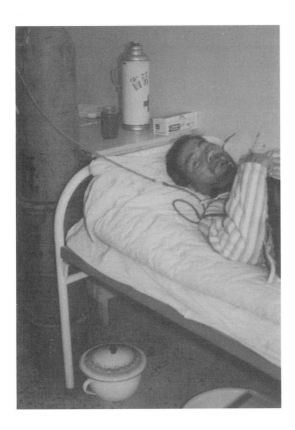

Figure 16.4 A patient with severe silicosis, Harbin, Heilongjiang (China), in 1987. Because silicosis cannot be reversed, medical management relies on managing complications and supplying oxygen when the disease is advanced; there have been no significant advances in treatment. Silicosis is entirely preventable but remains the most common serious occupational lung disease worldwide. (Photograph by Tee L. Guidotti, University of Alberta.)

called mesothelioma, which can also occur without asbestosis. Workers with asbestosis are at risk of developing lung cancer and pneumonias and have diminished reserve to fight off other lung diseases. It is, of course, always important to discourage smoking and even more important in people with lung disease. However, workers with asbestosis are at a heightened risk. There is a strong synergistic interaction between cigarette smoking and asbestos exposure that greatly magnifies the risk of lung cancer, much more than the usual risk of smoking alone.

Coal Workers' Pneumoconiosis Coal workers' pneumoconiosis is another chronic fibrotic lung disease. It is almost always seen in underground coal miners and is caused by inhalation and deposition of coal dust. The coal dust is carried around the lungs by macrophages, and where it collects there is a fibrotic reaction that produces a lesion called a coal dust macule. This lesion is not as dense as a silicotic nodule and grows more slowly. Although no symptoms may be present during the early stages, workers exposed to coal dust at high concentrations and for prolonged periods may develop progressive disease. Shortness of breath on exertion and bronchitis occur in the advanced stages due to chronic fibrosis. Chest X-ray findings are characteristic, starting with small rounded opacities called *simple coal workers' pneumoconiosis*. The disease usually does not progress rapidly, but if the opacities become large, the disease is called *complicated coal workers' pneumoconiosis* and carries a worse prognosis or expectation for future progression. In some workers, for reasons that are not well understood, the fibrosis progresses rapidly and produces a syndrome called *progressive massive fibrosis*, which can be severely disabling and even fatal.

Coal workers' pneumoconiosis is often found together with silicosis in the same worker, especially in miners who have drilled tunnels and shafts as well as mined coal. Rheumatoid arthritis is sometimes seen together with coal workers' pneumoconiosis.

There is no treatment for coal workers' pneumoconiosis. Workers with coal workers' pneumoconiosis should be removed from further excessive exposure to reduce the risk of progression.

Other significant pneumoconioses *Beryllium disease* is a special type of pneumoconiosis caused by exposure to dusts of beryllium metal. It results from an immune reaction that strongly resembles a particular type of lung disease called sarcoidosis.

Hard metal disease is a special type of pneumoconiosis resulting from exposure to metal alloy containing cobalt. This unusual pneumoconiosis may also feature asthma-like reactions.

Inert dust pneumoconiosis results from the inhalation of inert dusts such as titanium or plastic polymers or other materials that are not chemically reactive and do not induce fibrosis. The chest X-ray may show opacities, but these pneumoconioses are rarely associated with symptoms, chest physical findings, or pulmonary function abnormalities.

NOISE-INDUCED HEARING LOSS

Noise-induced hearing loss is a form of progressive deafness caused by exposure to noise. Although there are many sources of noise in daily life, severe noise-induced hearing loss is almost always the result of exposure in the workplace. It results from the cumulative effects of injury to the small hair-like structures in the inner ears that receive sound energy and convert it into a nerve impulse. This injury occurs with greater frequency and in more people when the noise is above 85 *dBA* (which refers to *decibels*, a measure of sound intensity, adjusted by the sensitivity of the human ear). As a general rule of thumb, when two people with normal hearing are standing a meter away from each other but cannot understand each other's speech easily because of the background noise, the noise level (about 85 dBA) is loud enough to cause hearing loss over time. (See Chapter 8.)

Noise-induced hearing loss is usually the result of years of exposure to continuous loud noise. The hearing loss begins in the high frequencies and soon begins to impair hearing in the medium-high frequencies, which happen to be those of greatest importance in human speech. Thus, noise-induced hearing loss tends to impair the worker's ability to understand speech relatively early. This can cause serious communication, social, and psychological problems, particularly as the worker gets older.

Hearing loss is measured with an instrument called an audiometer, which works by testing how loud a tone has to be before the worker can hear it. The instrument produces a graph, called an *audiogram*, of how well the person hears at various frequencies. Noise-induced hearing loss characteristically first affects hearing at a frequency of 4,000 Hz. (Hz, or Hertz, is a measure of frequency and equals cycles per second.) As hearing loss progresses, the loss of hearing at that frequency becomes more and more pronounced, and hearing is lost at frequencies above and below 4,000 Hz. The audiogram of a person with noise-induced hearing loss classically shows bilateral, symmetrical reduction in hearing with a maximal dip at 4,000 to 6,000 Hz. This change is permanent and is called neural hearing loss because it affects the sensory structure and nerve.

An especially loud continuous noise can also cause transient hearing loss, which is called a *temporary threshold shift*. Workers who have been in noisy areas, usually for several hours, will find they do not hear as well as usual after the noise stops or upon going into a quieter area. Hearing returns within a few hours. In extreme cases, it may take more than a day for speech comprehension to return. A temporary threshold shift is the body's reflex response to protect the ear from further damage. It is a sign that the worker has been exposed to dangerously loud noise. It should be considered a warning that the worker is at risk of rapidly losing hearing with continued noise exposure. Very loud, sudden noise, called *impulse noise*, or a low-intensity explosion can also cause serious hearing loss due to direct acute damage to the ear. The sudden loud noise can rupture the eardrum or cause dislocation of the ossicles, bones in the ear that conduct sound, resulting in conductive deafness across all frequencies.

Noise-induced hearing loss almost always occurs in both ears, usually roughly equally, with one exception. Unilateral hearing loss is common when firearms are frequently used on the job, for example, among police officers who do not use hearing protection during target practice.

Other effects of noise include tinnitus and vertigo. *Tinnitus* is a ringing noise in the ears and is frequently high-pitched. It can occur for many reasons but in a normal, healthy worker is usually a sign of excessive noise exposure. Vertigo, or a sensation that the surrounding environment is spinning around the patient, is uncommon and occurs usually after extreme noise exposure, such as unprotected hearing in the presence of firearms or jet engines. Noise can also aggravate preexisting medical conditions such as high blood pressure.

The diagnosis of occupational hearing loss is based on a history of work-related noise exposure, exclusion of other causes of hearing impairment (including through ear examination), and an audiometric examination. Prevention can be very effective. A hearing conservation program consists of noise exposure mapping, engineering controls to reduce exposure, administrative measures to reduce noise exposure, periodic surveillance of exposed workers with audiograms, provision of personal protection such as ear plugs and ear muffs (choosing those that are rated to block noise effectively), and training in how to use them properly.

DISORDERS OF THE NERVOUS SYSTEM

Nervous system disorders can be broadly classified as central or peripheral nervous system disorders or dysautonomias. Because the nervous system is extremely complicated, explaining how these disorders occur can be difficult. However, in practice, most of the common occupational disorders of the nervous system are relatively simple, at least as far as the symptoms and signs they present. Acute neurological conditions are often treatable, and the patient may recover fully or partially when removed from the exposure, depending on the cause. Unfortunately, chronic nervous system disorders often do not respond well to treatment and are usually permanent by the time the physician makes the diagnosis.

Central nervous system disorders affect the brain and sometimes the spinal cord. They often present themselves as behavioral disorders (as in toxic organic psychosis, toxic encephalopathy). Others affect certain parts of the brain more than others and cause very specific neurological signs (such as the abnormalities of gait and movement seen in workers exposed to manganese who develop a condition similar to Parkinson's disease but are otherwise normal).

Peripheral nervous system disorders affect the nerves outside the brain and spinal cord. One set of nerves, called *afferents*, carries sensation (such as pain, touch, temperature, pressure, and vibration or position) from the body to the brain via the spinal cord. Another set of nerves, called *efferents*, carries signals for muscles to move from the brain to the body.

Dysautonomias involve a third set of nerves existing within the central nervous system and also outside it, alongside the peripheral nervous system. This is called the *autonomic nervous system* because it carries the signals that regulate bodily functions automatically, such as breathing, the dilation (opening) or constriction (partial closing) of blood vessels, sweating, dilation or constriction of the pupil (by muscles in the iris of the eye), secretion of some glands (such as salivary glands), and the movements of hollow organs with smooth muscle, such as the intestines. Dysautonomias, while they do occur in occupational medicine, are much rarer than disorders of the central or peripheral nervous systems.

Central Neurological Disorders

Central nervous system disorders from workplace exposures are often acute and often due to brief exposures to high concentrations of a toxic agent, such as organic solvents (e.g., toluene or xylene), toxic gases (e.g., carbon monoxide or hydrogen sulfide), and some pesticides (e.g., organophosphates). Symptoms may include confusion, dizziness, headache, poor concentration, tremor, convulsions, vomiting, excessive bronchial secretion, and muscular tremor and cramps, depending on the agent. Treatment is primarily supportive with removal of the exposure. Prognosis depends on the severity and nature of acute exposure. A number of neurotoxic agents have been implicated in both acute and chronic central neuropathies including solvents, lead, pesticides, carbon disulfide, white spirit, and styrene.

Chronic central nervous system disorders occur as a result of repeated or prolonged exposure. These conditions are usually permanent. They often appear first as memory loss, but because memory loss is very nonspecific and can occur when the individual is simply distracted or depressed, they are often hard to spot.

Toxic organic psychosis describes a group of severe organic mental disorders characterized by personality and behavioral changes. The onset is gradual and occurs over months to years. The disorder may progress to overt psychosis in the form of hallucinations, depression, and suicidal tendencies. Exposure to carbon disulfide can do this, as can very high exposures to mercury.

Among the more potent neurotoxins are the metals mercury and manganese. Occupations at risk for mercury inhalation include dental assistants, research laboratory personnel, and instrument and measurement equipment workers. Manganese exposure, for example, in welding ferromanganese alloys (most common on railroads), is frequently associated with symptoms similar to Parkinson's disease—a movement disorder characterized by difficulty in walking.

Peripheral Neuropathies

Damage to the peripheral nerves, or neuropathy, can cause sensory or motor impairment or a combination of both.

Motor neuropathies present as muscle weakness, wasting, and diminished tendon reflexes. Lead poisoning has been a common toxic cause of motor neuropathy. Injury to the nerve can also do this, especially where the nerve is close to the surface and vulnerable to trauma, as at the elbow (which can cause hand problems) and the side of the leg (which can cause foot problems).

Sensory neuropathies are more common. They usually present as abnormal sensations, often burning and numbness to pain and vibration. This occurs earliest in the hands and the feet and is called a "stocking-glove" distribution. The extremities are affected first because the nerves to them are the longest in the body. Therefore, if there is injury that interferes with nerve impulse transmission, the nerves of the hands and feet are more likely to show symptoms early, as the distance the nerve impulse must travel is lengthy.

Peripheral neuropathy is usually a result of chronic exposure to a neurotoxic agent over months or years. The causal agents include heavy metals (e.g., lead, mercury, arsenic), solvents (e.g., n-hexane, methyl-butyl ketone, carbon disulfide), and pesticides (e.g., organophosphates), each of which may produce quite different clinical pictures. Historically, the heavy metals are the most common cause of toxic peripheral neuropathy.

Nerve conduction studies are useful confirmatory tests for neuropathies affecting accessible nerves. They show slowing of the nerve impulses, which is evidence of a damaged nerve. Electromyography (EMG) is less often helpful but shows evidence of damaged muscle.

OCCUPATIONAL CANCER

In industrialized countries, about one out of every three people will develop cancer during their lifetime. The causes of cancer are multifactoral and involve genetic, environmental, and lifestyle factors. About 5% to 10% of cancers are attributable to occupational exposures but some authorities believe that this is an underestimate. All occupational cancers, like all other occupational diseases, are preventable. Only a few chemicals—out of the many that are used in industry and the over 860 chemicals (including chemical classes and mixtures) that have been extensively tested—are known to cause cancer.

Taking age into consideration, the risk of cancer overall has remained fairly constant for a decade or more in most countries. Modest increases in sites such as the pancreas have been balanced by declines at sites such as the stomach. However, the public perception is that cancer is dramatically increasing. This is largely because the population in most of the world is aging, and age is the single most important determinant of the risk of cancer.

Cancers associated with personal choices of lifestyle, such as cigarette smoking, contribute the greatest fraction of preventable malignancies in industrialized countries, such as North America. Cancers associated with occupational exposures (e.g., chemicals known to be carcinogenic) are a much smaller fraction of preventable cancers, but are of particular concern to society because they are all theoretically preventable. Occupational causes of cancer are preventable and affect certain identifiable groups disproportionately. Some carcinogens associated primarily with occupational exposures, particularly asbestos and radon, may contribute significantly to national or regional cancer rates because of the widespread distribution of the hazard, the large number of workers exposed, the potential for wider exposure among the general population, and the synergistic effect with cigarette smoking.

Cancers that are caused by occupational exposures may, rarely, be a characteristic *histological* (tissue) type that is rarely seen associated with occupational exposure, as is the case with hepatic angiosarcoma and vinyl chloride or pleural mesothelioma and asbestos. When the cancer is unusual, making the association with occupational exposure is much easier and more certain. More often, occupational cancers are more common histological types. Occupational causes of more common cancers are much more difficult to identify. For example, a common type of lung cancer, squamous cell carcinoma, may be caused by asbestos, arsenic, chromates, nickel, coal tar, acrylonitrile, and vinyl chloride, among other exposures. Occupational cancers may affect multiple sites, such as the lung, the pleura, and the gastrointestinal tract in the case of asbestos. Occupational cancers are treated the same way as similar cancers that are not related to work.

After exposure to a carcinogen, a period of time (called the *latency period*) must elapse before a cancer develops, if it does. Occupational causes of cancer typically are associated with a latency period of over 20 years from exposure until clinical appearance of the malignancy, but there are many exceptions. The latency period may vary between 5 to more than 50 years, depending on the intrinsic carcinogenicity of the substance, the degree of exposure, the age of the individual, exposure to promoting agents during the latency period, the type of cancer, and the time required for clone of *neoplastic* (in this meaning, cancerous) cells to grow into a clinically detectable cancer. The latency period is not fixed rigidly but depends on the agent, the individual, the circumstances, and the intensity of exposure, especially exposure early in one's working career. Many occupational cancers do not appear until the exposed worker is much older and may have already retired.

The characteristics of chemical carcinogenesis, the long latency period, and the lack of specificity make identification of human carcinogens very difficult and lead to considerable confusion over which exposures cause cancer and which do not. By the time an individual develops a cancer, an on-the-job exposure may be long past and poorly remembered, or the picture may be clouded by many different exposures, including cigarette smoking. A worker may be exposed to several of these substances in the course of employment or military service and may also smoke and have a hobby involving exposure to hazardous substances. Thus it is difficult to sort out the exposures responsible in a given case, and one must rely on epidemiological approaches to get a population-based perspective on risk.

Table 16.3 lists occupational exposures known or strongly suspected to cause cancer in humans. Many other chemicals, such as 4-aminodiphenyl and β-naphthylamine, are known to be potentially carcinogenic and have been withdrawn from commercial use. Some chemicals, such as dioxins, are known carcinogens in animal studies but have not yet been demonstrated to be carcinogenic to humans. Arsenic, for example, is known to be a human carcinogen, but animal studies have not reproduced the carcinogenic effect. The reason is that human beings metabolize (chemically modify) arsenic differently than animals. Other chemicals, such as lead, beryllium, the phenoxy herbicides, and ethylene dichloride, are suspected of being carcinogenic, but the evidence is not clear. The International Agency for Research on Cancer (IARC) is a scientific body that reviews the evidence for carcinogenicity of compounds. Their reviews or monographs are used extensively by cancer investigators and regulatory agencies worldwide. For example, asbestos has been recognized as a human carcinogen by IARC for many years.

TABLE 16.3

KNOWN OR HIGHLY SUSPECT CARCINOGENS IN THE WORKPLACE

Substance	Where Encountered
Asbestos	Very widespread until the late 1970s, especially in • Construction • Auto repair • Shipbuilding • Present in many products • Cement pipe (mostly used for water distribution)
Coke oven emissions	• Steel mills • Coke ovens
3,3'-Dichlorobenzidine	• Pigment manufacturing • Polyurethane production
Radium	Limited use
Uranium and radon	Underground mining
β-Naphthylamine	• Chemical industry • Dyestuffs industry • Rubber industry
Ultraviolet light	Ubiquitous
Auramine and magenta	Dye manufacturing
Carbon tetrachloride	Very widespread

(Continued)

TABLE 16.3 (Contd.)

Substance	Where Encountered
Benzidine	• Clinical pathology laboratories • Chemical dyestuffs • Plastics • Rubber • Wood products
β-Propriolactone	• Plastics • Chemical industry • Pharmaceutical industry
Vinyl chloride	• Petrochemical industry • Plastics industry • Rubber industry
Chloromethyl methyl ether (CMME)	Chemical industry
Bis(chloromethyl) ether (BCME)	• Chemical industry • Nuclear reactor fuel processing
Ethyleneimine	• Chemical industry • Paper industry • Textile industry
N-nitrosodimethylamine	• Chemical industry • Rubber industry • Solvent industry • Pesticide industry
Chloroprene	Synthetic rubber industry
Trichlorethylene	Previously very widespread use as solvent and degreasing agent, now withdrawn from use
Benzene	Very widespread in industry as solvent and chemical constituent
Polychlorinated biphenyls (PCB)	Very widespread, particularly in • Utilities and electric power • Chemical industry • Wood products industries (Suspect, not confirmed in human studies)
Chloroform	• Chemical industry • Pharmaceutical industry • Textile industry • Solvent industry
Acrylonitrile	• Plastic industry • Textile industry
Leather dust	Leather goods industry
Wood dust	Hardwood furniture industries
Chromate (hexavalent)	• Electroplating • Metal products • Photography industry • Textile industry
Nickel salts	Widespread, especially in • Metal products • Chemical industry • Battery industry
Ionizing radiation	Very widespread, especially medical and industrial X-ray

(Continued)

TABLE 16.3 (Contd.)

Substance	Where Encountered
Arsenic	Very widespread
Cutting oils	• Machining • Metal working trades
Hydrazine	• Mechanical applications • Pharmaceutical industry
Ethylene dibromide	• Foodstuffs (fumigation) • Gasoline; additive industries
Pesticides	Agriculture and pesticide manufacturing • Aldrin • Dieldrin • DBCP • others

Occupational carcinogens vary greatly in their potency. Bis(chloromethyl) ether (BCME) (used in the nuclear industry in preparing ion-exchange columns to refine fuel-grade uranium) is a highly potent carcinogen producing small cell carcinoma of the lung in a high percentage of workers exposed to the chemical. The dust of hard woods, on the other hand, is a low-level carcinogen. Exposure may result in carcinomas of the nasal cavity and sinuses in a small number of cases, but the risk is low compared to other occupational carcinogens.

Identification of Occupational Carcinogens

Detection of occupational causes of cancer is based on three scientific approaches: epidemiological studies of workers exposed to a particular agent or working in a particular industry, animal studies to determine the carcinogenicity of a substance in a controlled experiment, and laboratory studies of the biological properties of the substance. Each approach has certain strengths and weaknesses.

Epidemiological studies are difficult to perform due to latency periods and obstacles to getting access to suitable groups of exposed workers. In addition, they are difficult to interpret because additional exposures may occur on the job, smoking and other lifestyle habits may confound the data, and because of the statistical uncertainty in estimating the number of cancers that would be expected without the exposure having occurred. On the other hand, epidemiological studies give direct information about human health risks. In epidemiological studies, several criteria are applied before concluding that an exposure may be carcinogenic for humans. The most generally accepted criteria are those of Sir Austin Bradford Hill (see Chapter 3). IARC and regulatory agencies such as OSHA take such criteria into account when weighing the evidence in considering whether to treat a substance as a carcinogen.

Animal studies are expensive and depend on very high exposure, which shortens the latency period and increases the cancer rate so that a cancer risk can be detected with a relatively small number of animals (dozens rather than tens of thousands). The risk of cancer from a chemical exposure at a given level varies considerably among different animal species and among strains of a given species, making extrapolation to humans difficult. Much of this variation is due to differences in the metabolism of the biological properties of suspected carcinogens. Animal carcinogenicity studies are very helpful in identifying substances likely to cause cancer but do not prove that carcinogenicity will occur in humans.

It is not possible to determine any one individual's personal risk of developing cancer. Too many variables are involved that modify the probability of developing cancer in a single individual. For example, family history is a very important factor in the overall risk of developing cancer, but its influence varies by the site and type of cancer, the degree of relationship, and the pattern of inheritance. Family history itself is only a crude indicator of genetic predisposition because a tendency to develop cancer may result from various genetic traits, at least in theory, and not all of these are likely to be expressed in an individual's accessible family tree. Furthermore, many genetic traits do not reveal themselves until the individual is challenged by an environmental exposure, because the genetic trait is only a susceptibility—or potential "weakness"—that does not become apparent unless a person is exposed to a carcinogen. For example, there is a strong genetic pattern of susceptibility to lung cancer, but it is usually not seen except among smokers. If everybody smoked, lung cancer would be considered to be primarily a genetic disease. If nobody smoked, the pattern of susceptibility would be invisible. Because some people smoke and some do not, there is a confusing picture that, once sorted out, reveals an interaction between heredity and the smoking habit that accounts for many and perhaps most cases of lung cancer.

Similarly, individual variations in diet, lifestyle, hygiene, and medical care affect cancer risk, often in ways that are difficult to quantify. In particular, the effect of many of these factors is to modify the risk associated with other factors. For example, certain foods high in vitamins A and C appear to reduce the risk of cancer by chemically modifying the response to carcinogens in the body. Other foods have traces of naturally occurring carcinogens or promoters in them and may or may not elevate the risk or interact with stronger carcinogens. These numerous individual influences cannot be measured accurately nor interpreted for specific individuals. It is possible only to estimate individual risks based on population measurements.

Although the risk for a specific individual cannot be determined, it is relatively easy to determine cancer rates for a population, a group of individuals living in a community, or a group sharing some common feature. The risk of developing cancer, the probability that one of a certain group of people might develop cancer at a certain age, is reflected by the rate of cancer incidence in the population, or how many people (per 100,000) get cancer in a year in that designated group.

Cancer *incidence* is the frequency of appearance of new cancers. Cancer *prevalence* is the frequency of individuals in a population who have cancer at a given time. A population may have a constant incidence rate, but the prevalence rate might change considerably as a result of earlier detection, longer survival, or higher cure rates. When cancer incidence changes, it may be the result of changing exposures or lifestyle patterns, but it may also be the result of changes in the population's composition (aging, immigration, out-migration), changes in the reliability of diagnosis or reporting, or changes in the death rate from other causes. Obviously, the earlier a person dies, the less likely he or she is to develop a type of cancer usually appearing at an advanced age. Conversely, the longer a person lives, the more likely he or she is to develop such a cancer, whether or not it is ultimately the cause of death. Cancer rates for two comparison populations are statistically "adjusted" to take into account differences in the age structure.

These complications should serve to illustrate why cancer rates must be considered very carefully. They cannot be applied as risk estimates for individuals without taking into account the individual's personal health characteristics. Cancer rates should also be compared between populations with great care. Cancer rates for a population are only an aggregated estimate of the risk of developing cancer for an individual member of that population. There are too many uncertainties to forecast risk for a single individual with any degree of accuracy.

Cancer risks, and indeed the risk of developing any disease, should be considered a matter of probability, not a matter of certainty. Exposure to a carcinogen such as cigarette smoke or asbestos may raise the chances of getting cancer minimally or significantly, depending on the exposure, but the modified risk for each individual would vary.

Asbestos-Associated Cancer

Asbestos is quantitatively the single most important occupational carcinogen. The two characteristic cancers associated with asbestos are bronchogenic carcinoma of the lung and pleural or peritoneal mesothelioma. In addition, other cancers are thought to be associated with asbestos exposure, including cancer of the larynx and, less strongly, colon cancer, some lymphomas, and ovarian carcinoma.

Asbestos-related lung cancer is highly synergistic with cigarette smoking and has a latency period between exposure and detection of the malignancy of two or three decades. In evaluating a possible occupational association with a patient's malignancy, a complete and accurate history of the patient's employment and the specific jobs performed is critical. Relatively brief employment decades ago may be responsible for causing cancer. Asbestos and smoking together raise an individual's risk of cancer much more than the sum of either alone, to as much as l00 times that for nonsmokers. Lung cancer associated with asbestos cannot be distinguished from lung cancer from smoking cigarettes.

Pleural mesothelioma is a particularly aggressive and incurable malignancy that is closely associated with asbestos exposure. This tumor often results from modest exposure and may have a latency period of several decades. It is not associated with smoking. Mesotheliomas occur rarely in the general population without asbestos exposure because they are almost always associated with asbestos exposure. They may occur in families living near sites where asbestos was used or in which a member was employed in an occupation involving exposure to asbestos and brought asbestos fibers into the home on his or her contaminated work clothes.

Table 16.4 lists occupations that are identified by the International Agency for Research on Cancer (a constituent organization of the World Health Organization) as associated with an elevated cancer risk among workers. This is only a partial list, as other industries probably also have elevated risks but have not been studied by IARC. Several of these occupations have changed their processes and may no longer confer an elevated risk, as in the case of isopropyl alcohol manufacturing.

REPRODUCTIVE DISORDERS

Chemical, physical, or biological agents can cause reproductive impairment or adverse developmental effects. Most of the concern for reproductive effects in occupational health is centered on chemical exposures. The major physical hazard for adverse reproduction outcomes is heat, which is associated with low fertility among men and a risk of fetal malformations in pregnant women. The major biological agents associated with reproductive impairment are those causing sexually transmitted diseases, but those are not within the scope of this chapter. See below for others of significance in occupational exposures.

Reproductive toxicity is the occurrence of adverse effects on the reproductive system resulting from exposure to chemical agents. Adverse birth outcomes are the occurrence of adverse effects in the fetus and include fetal death, structural abnormalities or birth defects, functional deficiencies, and altered growth. Developmental toxicity may occur during prenatal development in the womb or may occur after birth and up to the time of sexual maturation. The adverse effect(s) may result from the mother's exposure before conception but usually results from exposures during the pregnancy.

There are many mechanisms by which reproductive toxicants act, including disruption of the neuroendocrine pathway, disruption of genetic material with resulting mutation or cancer, and disturbance of the fetal developmental process

TABLE 16.4

OCCUPATIONS ASSOCIATED WITH CANCER RISK (INTERNATIONAL AGENCY FOR RESEARCH ON CANCER)

Aluminum production

Boot and shoe manufacture and repair

Coal gasification

Furniture manufacture

Hematite underground mining

Iron and steel foundries

Isopropyl alcohol manufacturing (strong-acid process)

Manufacture of auramine

Manufacture of magenta

Nickel refining

Painting

Rubber industry

resulting in congenital malformations or fetal death. Most chemical reproductive hazards cause infertility (particularly in males), spontaneous abortion or miscarriage, and early fetal death because the chemical is directly toxic to sperm-forming cells, the embryo, or the fetus, respectively. Most spontaneous abortions are not detected by the women who have them and instead are experienced as abnormal or skipped menstrual periods. Chemicals that are less toxic may result in survival of the embryo or fetus but may have a toxic effect at a critical period in organ formation, usually in the first trimester (the first three months of a normal nine-month pregnancy). These chemicals are called *teratogens* and can cause birth defects. A few chemicals resemble hormones and appear to interfere with normal action, either by acting like hormones themselves or blocking the activity of the natural hormones. They can produce either fertility problems or birth defects and are called *endocrine mimics*.

It is very difficult to know for sure when a chemical has had an effect on reproduction. Human reproduction is a very uncertain process for a number of reasons. Fertility is highly variable from one population to another and varies with age. Spontaneous abortions are very common naturally; in fact, it is estimated that almost one half of all conceptions are lost, although a woman who was pregnant may not be aware of the loss unless it occurs after two or more months. Birth defects affect almost 2% of all live births. Most defects are minor, but some, such as Down syndrome and incomplete spina bifida (defects in the spinal column), are both common and major. The majority of birth defects appear not to be related to chemical exposures, but some are associated with alcohol consumption during pregnancy, some with drugs, and others with malnutrition. Against this background of commonly occurring reproductive problems, it is difficult to study reproductive hazards. Epidemiological studies must be very carefully designed to detect and distinguish these adverse outcomes from the normal background incidence.

The agents known to cause birth defects are wide ranging. Those causing fetal congenital malformations, for example, are physical (e.g., radiation and heat), microbial (e.g., rubella, cytomegalovirus, toxoplasmosis), and chemical (e.g., penicillamine, tetracyclines, thalidomide, polychlorobiphenyls, cocaine).

In general, the male reproductive system is more vulnerable to chemical and physical hazards. Disruption of the male reproductive system almost always expresses itself as infertility. Male fertility disorders can be caused by physical agents (e.g., chronic low-level radiation and heat), chemical agents (e.g., dibromochloropropane, kepone, lead, carbon disulfide, estrogens, vinyl chloride, tetraethyl lead), or factors such as overwork and stress. Some neurotoxins can produce impotence in the male.

Female disorders and their possible causal agents are summarized in Table 16.5.

Transmission of reproductive toxicity by males to females occurs through transmission in the semen. In females, reproductive toxins can directly impact the reproductive system or the ova or be transmitted to infants via the mother's breast milk.

Occupational cancers in infants or an increase in cancer risk in childhood can occur due to parental germ cell damage or transplacental exposure or exposure through lactation (mother's milk). Children may also be exposed to carcinogens brought home on contaminated clothing.

Diagnosis of exposure to a reproductive hazard requires a comprehensive reproductive and occupational history and an exposure assessment. Each case and exposure situation must be assessed individually in an attempt to quantify exposures to potential reproductive hazards.

Prevention of reproductive disorders necessitates overcoming many obstacles. Safe levels that protect the mother and fetus are likely to be different and lower than customary occupational exposure levels for various workplace toxicants. Furthermore, safe levels for reproductive concerns have not been reliably established for most chemical exposures. Moreover, it is not possible to exclude all

TABLE 16.5

HEALTH EFFECTS ON FEMALE REPRODUCTIVE SYSTEM

Disorder	*Examples of Causal Agents*
Menstrual Disorders	Metals: *lead, mercury* Solvents: *styrene, mixed organic solvents, benzene, carbon disulfide, toluene* Physical agents: *ionizing radiation, noise*
Infertility	Metals: *lead, mercury, multiple metals* Steroids: *androgens, progestins, estrogens* Anti-cancer agents: *methotrexate, cyclosphosphamide* Other therapeutic agents: *halothane, L-dopa, opioids, psychiatric drugs, tranquillizers* Industrial chemicals: *formaldehyde, aniline, plastic monomers, polyaromatic hydrocarbons* Personal habits: *solvents, alcohol* Physical hazards: *ionizing radiation, noise*
Spontaneous Abortions	Metals: *arsenic, lead, mercury, multiple metals, antimony* Solvents: *styrene (laboratory workers), carbon disulfide, benzene* Physical agents: *ionizing radiation*
Female Malignancies	Cervical cancer: *solvents (trichloroethylene, carbon tetrachloride)* Breast cancer: *ionizing radiation (radiographers), radium*
Preterm and Low-Birth-Weight Babies	*Heavy physical work, whole-body vibration, noise, lower socioeconomic status*
Congenital Malformations	Metals: *lead, mercury, multiple metals* Solvents: *mixed organic solvents (laboratory workers, printing industry)* Physical agent: *ionizing radiation, heat, noise*
Childhood Cancers	Leukemia/lymphomas: *petrol-related paternal occupation* Central nervous system: *mother in chemical industry; father exposed to solvents in aircraft industry*
Breast Milk Contamination	*Solvents, heavy metals, organochlorines, viruses*

persons of reproductive age from jobs with risk, particularly if such a policy discriminates against a particular age group or gender (usually women). This means that control measures should minimize the levels of toxic risks to protect all workers, irrespective of gender. An effective program to prevent reproductive disorders includes the following:

- removal of hazards and exposures, particularly through engineering and administrative controls
- preventing domestic exposures
- protection through the duration of breastfeeding
- temporary job reassignment in pregnancy, preconception, and for cases of subfertility or failure to conceive
- medical surveillance and early notification of pregnancy
- health education and risk communication
- legislation for safe use and monitoring of reproductive hazards

For pregnant employees, special consideration must be given to physical hazards in jobs that require lifting, standing, walking or climbing, including adjustment of physical demands, working at heights (ladders, platforms, poles), and the operation of certain types of heavy machinery. Pregnant workers should have adequate space to work, proper-fitting uniforms, regular shifts, ready access to toilet facilities, adequate rest, and should not stand for prolonged hours. Breastfeeding can be facilitated by giving new mothers flexible work hours, provision of an area to express milk, and a refrigerator to store breast milk. Medical surveillance may assist in early pregnancy notification and alternative placement during pregnancy as well as for a reassessment of reproductive risk at the workplace.

OTHER OCCUPATIONAL DISORDERS

There are many other classes of occupational disorders, including:

- Blood disorders, such as anemia and hematological malignancies, caused by chemicals normally present in rubber, dyestuff, and explosive industries, and inorganic lead
- Cardiovascular disorders caused by occupational exposure to carbon disulfide, nitrates, methylene chloride, and carbon monoxide
- Liver disorders due to chemicals or infectious agents. Liver toxicity from chemical exposures is called *hepatotoxicity* and usually presents as a form of hepatitis. It is a particular problem with some solvents and chlorinated chemicals.
- Renal dysfunction, due to exposure to occupational and environmental toxins such as heavy metals (arsine, cadmium, lead, mercury, beryllium, vanadium), petroleum hydrocarbons and organic solvents (carbon tetrachloride, ethylene dichloride, chloroform, trichloroethylene, dioxane, toluene, phenol, alcohol), pesticides, and silica. Kidney toxicity due to chemical exposures is called *nephrotoxicity*.

- Occupational infections due to work-related exposures to microbial agents (discussed in Chapter 10)
- Endocrine disorders, while unusual, can occur as a result of exposure to certain chemicals.
- Eye disorders due to trauma, foreign bodies, chemicals and radiation; occupational eye diseases, including allergic conjunctivitis and acquired work-related infections like toxoplasmosis and Newcastle virus disease; "arc eye" or "welder's eye," due to ultraviolet radiation exposure without adequate eye protection or, less commonly, due to an arc flash; and "glassworker's cataract" due to infrared radiation

While this chapter has reviewed the more common disorders, almost all other organ systems can be adversely affected. In all cases, the accurate diagnosis of occupational and work-related disorders and their causal agents is critical, and management of these disorders should include preventive measures as well as treatment. This is because prevention not only avoids, in many cases, the re-emergence of the disease, but also ensures that other exposed workers at risk of similar disorders are protected.

17

FITNESS TO WORK

John W. F. Cowell

Fitness to work (FTW) describes the match between the capabilities of the worker and the work that the worker is being asked to do. In order to determine the precision of the match, the occupational health professional needs to know the worker's physical state, mental capacity, skill level, and conditions that could place him or her at unusual risk in the work environment. The occupational health professional also needs to know the demands of the job, which may include requirements for physical strength, alertness, coordination, good eyesight or hearing, the ability to see colors, stamina, or any number of other capabilities. Ordinarily, the occupational health professional is not called upon to assess the educational level, skill level, or language ability of the worker, but these too are important in fitness to work and to protect the worker's health. A worker with limited education, or who cannot understand the training that he or she is given, may not be able to work safely. FTW is often called "fitness for duty." Some authorities prefer this term because it avoids confusion over whether a worker is fit to work at a particular job, which is the true meaning, or for work in general.

Some disorders, whether acquired from occupational exposures or injury or from other causes, interfere with the ability to work. These are discussed in Chapter 16. The occupational health professional may be called upon to assess the ability of workers with these disorders to do their jobs safely, without presenting an unacceptable risk to themselves or others. Such evaluations are often required when workers are recovering and are due to return to work if able.

The assessment of fitness to work (FTW) is called a *fitness-to-work evaluation*. The purpose of an FTW evaluation is to both determine whether workers can do the job and to protect workers' health, in relation to the requirements of the work. It is intended to ensure that workers are not placed at unnecessary risk or through their inability to do the job become a hazard to themselves or others.

An FTW evaluation may be performed at various times and for various reasons prior to and during employment. They are most common in the form of *pre-placement* or *pre-employment* evaluations (pre-placement is preferred and is legally required in many countries) and *return-to-work* evaluations.

A properly performed FTW evaluation strikes a fair balance between the rights of the worker and those of the employer. On the one hand, it provides the worker with an assessment of his or her medical capacity to perform the assigned work in a healthy manner. In addition, the evaluation documents the worker's health status at particular points in time, so that future claims of injury or illnesses in relation to the work can be dealt with on the basis of the factual medical record. From the employer's perspective, it provides assurance that the worker will not pose a threat to himself or herself or others and that the worker will be able to perform the work safely and as required.

In FTW evaluations, the examiner is asked to render an informed opinion about the worker's health and functional capabilities in the context of the working conditions. The examiner is not expected, nor is it appropriate, to render an opinion about the worker's health status outside of the context of the work. Specifically, an FTW evaluation is not intended to be a comprehensive evaluation designed to explore all aspects of a worker's health; rather, it is focused specifically on the question of matching the worker's health to the working conditions.

An FTW evaluation should be performed only by an occupational health professional who is familiar with the working conditions and job demands. To be useful, the evaluation must be directly related to the precise job requirements and working conditions and must consider the limitations of currently available evaluation procedures and diagnostic techniques.

Most FTW evaluations are performed by either a physician or a nurse and involve testing for medical conditions that might interfere with work. Clinicians performing the evaluations must strictly adhere to their professional codes of ethics; in particular, the medical findings must remain confidential between the examiner and the worker.

A *functional capacity evaluation* is performed by a physical therapist or a specialist in work capacity known as a *kinesiologist*. The most sophisticated of these evaluations use standardized protocols, such as the Isernhagen protocol, which apply specialized and calibrated equipment to determine strength, flexibility, gait, and endurance. They reliably identify physical limitations on the ability of a worker to do the work, whether the worker is healthy or recovering from injury or illness.

The examiner's judgment will affect the rights and obligations of the employer, the worker, and the insurer, if the worker is covered by insurance. There may be legal requirements for FTW evaluations, particularly in jobs that involve the safety of others. Therefore, the evaluation carries a high ethical responsibility for the practitioner and must be performed (and be seen to be performed) with great competence and objectivity.

A major limitation on FTW evaluations is the sensitivity and specificity of available screening tests. *Sensitivity* refers to the ability of the test to identify individuals who have a disease or impairment. *Specificity* refers to the ability of a test to rule out the disease or impairment in a person who is well. Most tests that are generally available for FTW evaluations are adapted from clinical tests used by physicians to assess people with illnesses. They were originally designed to assist in making a diagnosis in a clearly ill person presenting to the physician. They are seldom very sensitive and are often not even very specific. When one applies these tests to a group of patients who are being investigated precisely because they are likely to have the disease in question, the lack of specificity presents relatively little difficulty. Knowing that an individual has a high likelihood of having the disease or impairment in the first place, the physician uses the test for guidance in selecting among alternative diagnoses that are highly probable.

When a nonspecific or an insensitive test is applied to the general population, however, there is a potential for difficulty. Most groups of workers are relatively healthy and have a low prevalence of the conditions for which they are being tested. FTW evaluations have an inherent problem with the screening tests' low predictive values. The predictive value of the test is a function of the sensitivity (how readily the test detects a problem), specificity (how likely it is that the test is detecting the disease or problem for which it was designed), and the prevalence of a condition in the population being screened (how common it is). For most clinical tests, sensitivity is relatively high but specificity is much lower. In this case, the test will be much better at picking up individuals who have the disorder than in ruling out people who do not. In a population of generally healthy workers, all or most of the truly diseased individuals may be detected (true positives), but a very large number of non-diseased persons will be incorrectly identified as having the disease or impairment (false positives). Usually, the false positives will greatly outnumber the true positives in a healthy population. This may lead to great confusion and often to legal problems. If an individual is excluded from a well-paying job solely on the basis of an imperfect screening test, there may be grounds for legal action. Choosing the best clinical screening tests for an FTW evaluation must be done with care, and the opinion must not be based solely on the results of the clinical test results. (See Chapter 5.)

The point of an FTW evaluation is to match the job description and its health requirements with the worker's capabilities and health. This is achieved by comparing the health findings obtained during the evaluation to the working conditions that are represented in a set of health standards supplied to the clinical examiner. The examiner is expected to provide a clinical opinion of fitness in relation to the specific working conditions. The opinion will be expressed as "fit," "unfit," or "fit subject to work modifications" and will be further qualified as temporary or permanent. Clearly FTW evaluations must be work-specific and should be done only with an accurate description of the work and preferably with a set of validated health and performance criteria derived from an analysis of the tasks required by the work.

FTW EVALUATION

There are several types of evaluations undertaken in assessing fitness to work.

- pre-placement (preferred) when a worker has been offered a full- or part-time job, subject to passing a relevant medical evaluation
- pre-employment (not allowed in many countries)— when a worker must pass a medical evaluation in order to be considered for a job or to be hired at all
- return to work—when a worker is returning to work after recovery from an illness or injury or when the worker has returned to a modified job and is being re-evaluated for return to unmodified duties

- continuing clinical impairment—when a worker remains absent from work and must be assessed for continuing disability coverage for short-term, long-term, or workers' compensation insurance coverage
- job transfer—when a worker transfers to a job where the working conditions are significantly different from the existing job
- change in working conditions of existing job—when the existing working conditions have been significantly altered
- change in health status in existing job—when new health problems develop that may be aggravated by existing working conditions
- performance-initiated review—when health reasons are identified as the cause of failing job performance, and a medical review has been suggested (job security not yet at risk) or is required (job security is at risk) by the employer

Pre-employment Health Examination

For many years, employers required prospective employees to pass a medical examination before they could be hired. This *pre-employment health examination* is a medical evaluation to decide whether a person is healthy enough to work and, therefore, employable. Pre-employment examinations began as a way to protect the worker from harm, to protect other employees, and to protect the interests of the employer. The objective was to identify and exclude from work those who were sick or too weak to work. They were called examinations, rather than evaluations, because they were primarily based on a physical examination to identify obvious clinical illness and disability. These examinations were not very sophisticated and were based on standard medical examinations rather than screening tests. They were most effective in identifying workers who had chronic diseases or obvious disability and, generally, ineffective in matching work capacity to the job requirements. As health improved in the general population and the prevalence

---

BOX 17.1

Modified Work Following Occupational Injury

Data provided by the Workers' Compensation Board of Alberta, Canada, for the period of July 1 to September 30, 1998, showed that 47% of their injured-worker clients returned to work, but only 19% of them returned to their former, pre-injury level of work. The other 28% of workers returned to a modified level of work.

This reflects the results of an extensive program introduced by the Board to persuade employers to accept injured workers back into the workplace as soon as they are ready to return.

Contributed by Harold Hoffman

---

of diseases like tuberculosis declined, such "medical clearance" examinations became less important, and the pre-employment examination was replaced by the pre-placement evaluation. In recent years, new thinking about disability (conceived as a problem with the environment rather than with the worker) and of fairness to workers with limited impairment has led to recognition that a worker does not have to be healthy or fit all around to do a job; he or she only has to meet the requirements of the job itself. Under the Americans with Disabilities Act, pre-employment examinations are not allowed in the United States because they may lead to discrimination against disabled workers. Other countries have similar legislation, making pre-employment evaluations against the law in those countries.

Pre-placement Evaluation

In many countries, such as United States, UK, and Canada, the pre-employment examination has been replaced by the *pre-placement evaluation*. The purpose of the pre-placement evaluation is to determine if the worker being considered for a particular job is physically and psychologically fit to carry out that job and to ensure that this job will not be of any danger to the worker's health. Pre-placement evaluations are often called "post-offer" or "post-hire, pre-assignment" evaluations, in order to emphasize their timing: after a decision has been made to hire the candidate but before they are actually assigned to do the work. Under the law in many countries, this is an important distinction that separates pre-placement evaluations from pre-employment examinations.

The pre-placement evaluation is carried out after it has been determined that the candidate for a job is qualified and is conducted in order to ensure that the new hire has the capacity to do what is required and, if not, what accommodation or modification in the work environment may be needed. The offer of a job is made contingent on the candidate being able to carry out its duties. The pre-employment examination is carried out before a decision is made to hire the person and may result in bias against an otherwise qualified candidate. The same tests should always be given, consistently, to all job applicants in order to avoid discrimination. The criteria used should apply to all workers in that job category, without selectivity or discrimination.

Pre-placement evaluations may also be given when an existing employee is reassigned or when the job tasks change notably. This is not necessary when the new job has the same or less stringent requirements.

Health problems may make some jobs hazardous for the worker or cause a risk for other workers or the public. Thus, for example, it is often necessary to exclude a worker with epilepsy and unpredictable seizures from working at heights or with unstable diabetes from jobs that require driving. However, such conditions must be well documented and must directly and obviously present a risk to others. Workers should never be excluded from the workplace as a way to avoid controlling work hazards.

Both the worker and the employer should get copies of the written report of the evaluation. The information given to the employer should not include any data of a medical nature, including the diagnosis. The employer only needs to know whether the person is fit for the specified work tasks of the job and to be apprised of any limitations (conditions and job tasks that are medically unsuitable, either permanently or temporarily).

Periodic Health Evaluation

Period health evaluations are examinations performed at intervals, usually every year, to identify work-related illness. They are required by law in many countries as part of a comprehensive occupational health program. The purpose is to monitor workers' health, to detect as early as possible any sign of ill health related to the job, and to verify workers' fitness for the job. Periodic health evaluations are necessary when a job includes exposure to potential hazards that cannot be eliminated by preventive measures. They are also useful to ensure that occupational health protection is working.

The frequency, content, and methods of periodic health evaluations depend on the quality and quantity of the exposure(s). The examinations are conducted every month or every few years, depending on the nature of the exposure and the biological response expected. They may be limited to only one test (e.g., blood lead in lead exposure, audiometry in noise exposure), or they may be comprehensive (e.g., clinical examination, spirometry, chest X-ray, and audiometry are all part of a standard evaluation for miners). Guidelines for these examinations are available from many sources, including the International Labour Organization.

Return-to-Work Health Evaluation

A *return-to-work evaluation* is primarily intended to "clear" a worker to go back to his or her usual job after an inquiry or illness. It establishes that there is no longer any medical objection to prevent the worker from working at a certain job and it also represents a formal notice to the employer that the injured worker is ready to go back, having completed treatment and rehabilitation. It marks the beginning of reintegration of the worker into the workplace, which is often an important step toward full recovery.

A return-to-work health evaluation is required after a disabling injury or a long absence for health reasons. The idea is to determine the worker's capacity to perform his or her work tasks and to identify possible needs for accommodation, reassignment, or rehabilitation. The decision to allow the worker to return to the job is not made by the physician or nurse; it is a decision made by the employer. The health provider clears the employee on medical grounds by establishing that the injured worker is fit to return to the work, can physically do the job, and will not, through weakness or incapacity, become a threat to him- or herself or to other workers. For example, a worker who loses his or her coordination or sense of balance (which sometimes happens from illness and occasionally injury) should not climb a ladder, work on a scaffold, or drive a motor vehicle unless the sense of balance is restored. Not only might the worker hurt him- or herself by falling, but other workers could be injured.

There are two common problems with return-to-work evaluations. The first is that many medical practitioners and many employers use the term "light duty" to refer to a temporarily diminished workload without describing exactly what they mean. If the worker is not ready to return to full duties, the physician should specify exactly what restrictions apply, such as limits on heavy lifting, on the number of hours that can be worked, or an accommodation that is needed. The other problem is that many employers claim not to have "light duty" or restricted work available, either because of the nature of their work (for example, it is difficult to place restrictions on a construction worker working on site) or because the manager or (usually) supervisor does not want to take responsibility for any worker who cannot do the full job without restrictions. This may reflect an attitude that workers who are on "light duty" will be resented by other workers who have to carry a greater load, fear that workers will abuse the restrictions, or concern that the worker may injure him or herself again. Actually, employers who have a policy of facilitating return to work and who cooperate with health providers to achieve early and safe return to work usually have good results in getting their employees back to work with few problems.

Job Description

An adequate job description is essential to an FTW evaluation and should be provided by the employer prior to the evaluation. A job description should include the following:

- a description of the job function and precise job performance requirements
- location of the work
- hours of the work
- occupational safety and ergonomic hazards
- occupational health hazards
- psychosocial demands of the job
- special or unusual requirements of the job

Job descriptions may include the following information, depending on the job:

- *Physical features*
  - working near moving equipment
  - bending, lifting, pulling required
  - working in awkward or cramped quarters
  - working with hand tools
- *Critical exposures and work characteristics*
  - ergonomics
  - vibration
  - solvents
  - noise
- *Health standards*
  - good hearing (tested by an *audiogram*)
  - no medical condition precluding working alone
  - no medical condition interfering with detailed, close-up work
  - musculoskeletal strength, flexibility, and dexterity

Once the process of comparing the findings of a clinical evaluation with the health standards appropriate to the particular working conditions is completed, the clinical examiner is required to render an opinion of fitness to work. There are three possibilities—fit, unfit, or fit subject to work modification or accommodation.

Fit This judgment means that the worker is able to work in the assigned job without restriction, is not likely to pose a threat to self or others in performing the work tasks, and is not likely to suffer adverse health consequences in the performance of normal duties. The worker can perform all the tasks in the job description, without reservation.

Unfit This judgment means that the worker is not able to work in the assigned job, despite reasonable work modifications. The worker cannot do everything in the job description and is incapable of performing the essential functions of the job, so an accommodation would not help. This judgment may be temporary or permanent, depending on the severity of the medical condition.

Fit Subject to Work Modification or Accommodation The worker is not able to work in the assigned job without changes in either the working environment or the way the work is performed. Once these changes are made, the worker can perform the essential functions of the job. If the medical condition would have put him or her or others at risk, the accommodation is sufficiently reliable to ensure the safety of the worker and others. The worker may not be able to perform all of the tasks in the job description, even with accommodation, but can manage the essential functions and requires relatively minor degrees of assistance to do what is required. This characterization may be classified as either temporary or permanent, depending on the severity of the medical condition and the nature of the working conditions.

Clinical evaluations for FTW should be performed in an appropriate clinical setting, giving the worker privacy and dignity. The actual medical findings must be shared with the worker/patient being examined, but not with the employer unless the worker has given his or her express consent. Only the worker has the right to authorize release of the medical findings. The employer needs to know the FTW determination (fit, unfit, or fit subject to work modification, with a statement of what that modification should be) so that the worker can be placed appropriately in the workplace. The disability insurer or workers' compensation insurer may, with the worker's written permission, receive the full medical record.

Performing objective and useful FTW evaluations is not an easy task. However, done well and with the highest level of clinical competency and ethics, they provide an invaluable tool for worker, employer, and insurer alike.

Accommodation A modified level of work involves an *accommodation* proportionate to the impairment. Accommodation is an intervention that restores the capacity of a worker, who is otherwise qualified and able to do the work, to overcome the specific limitations that stand in the way. Accommodation may be permanent, in the case of a worker with permanent impairment, or it may be temporary, e.g., an injured worker who has recovered from the injury but is not fully rehabilitated (see Chapter 14).

The three general conclusions regarding fitness to work—fit to work, unfit for work, and fit to work with accommodation—are usually applied to new hires or to injured workers at the point where they are being considered for return to work; however, they may be applied in any FTW evaluation as summarized above. Fitness-to-work recommendations are made by occupational health professionals, such as physicians and nurses, but the actual decision on placing a worker is made by the employer's representative, such as the human resources officer or supervisor.

What accommodation may be necessary depends on what the worker may require:

- improving access to facilities by means that reduce physical barriers, such as ramps to go around stairs for workers who use wheelchairs
- devices or equipment that compensates for the impairment, such as amplifiers for the telephones of workers who are hearing-impaired
- provision of staff who can help in the work, such as people hired to read material to a worker who is blind
- job restructuring and reorganization, such as reassigning some tasks to other workers but giving the impaired worker tasks they are capable of doing
- "light duty," in which an injured worker may do only some of the normal duties, or may do other tasks that are less demanding, during the recovery period
- modification of work hours, such as converting to part-time or a modified work schedule
- transitional work, in which an injured worker who has recovered but is not ready to return to full duty may do something else for a period of time
- training materials or policies, such as ergonomic training for workers who have a musculoskeletal impairment

In every case, the best approach to accommodation is a flexible one, on a case-by-case basis, because the needs of each worker with impairments are very different.

Accommodation needs to be considered in the context of impairment, disability, and handicap, which are also discussed in Chapter 14.

- *Impairment* is a loss of the capacity to function. It is objectively measured against what is normal for an uninjured, normal individual.
- *Disability* is a loss of the capacity to perform a person's social role, which may be personal, family, cultural, or occupational demands (see Chapter 14). It is specific to the job or to the activity (e.g., what is required on the job or for activities of daily living). Occupational disability reflects the implications of the impairment for the worker's ability to earn a living. As such, it is heavily influenced by what jobs are available on the job market and what jobs the worker can be expected to do.

- *Handicap* is the difference between the individual's capacity and what is required to function to an acceptable degree of performance. The handicap is therefore an estimate of the degree of accommodation required to make up for the loss of capacity.

An accommodation is, therefore, a means of making up the difference between disability and expected performance, which is measured by the handicap.

Some employers are committed to a proactive approach in managing the injured worker's return to work. However, many supervisors and junior-level managers do not want workers to return until they are fully capable of performing all the tasks required of them. They are concerned about:

- lost productivity, because workers who come back from an injury may not be able to work as hard as another worker
- employee morale, because other workers may resent the special treatment that the injured worker receives
- reinjury, if the injured worker is likely to hurt himself or herself again on the job

Because the decision to return an injured worker to his or her job is a business management decision made by managers rather than a medical decision made by occupational health professionals, otherwise capable workers may be denied the opportunity to go back to work as soon as they are able. However, some managers realize that returning injured workers to their jobs is actually good business because:

- Rapid reintegration into the workforce improves outcomes; the longer a worker stays off work, the less fit he or she will be to return after the rehabilitation phase.
- Rapid reintegration into the workforce reduces costs of medical care and lost wages; in countries that have compensation systems that provide pensions or wage replacement, costs tend to be driven by time off work, and the longer injured workers stay off the job, the less likely they are to return at all.
- Early and safe return to work ensures that the worker will be able to continue as an employee and the investment in training and experience will not be lost.
- The cost of training a substitute worker can be very high.
- In some countries, the employer may face legal action if the worker is not allowed to return.
- Product spoilage may occur when an inexperienced new worker has to take the place of the injured worker.
- Accommodation and early return to work tell the other employees that the employer cares about their future.
- Return to work enhances what some have called "occupational bonding," which is the degree to which a worker feels integrated into and part of the working group as a social community; it is a powerful force for productivity and job satisfaction.

In the case of injured workers who are under consideration for return to work, accommodation will be temporary and should be reviewed periodically to determine when it is no longer needed.

The concept of accommodation also applies to decisions based on pre-placement evaluations, when an applicant for a job is otherwise qualified and can do the job with reasonable accommodation. In this case, the accommodation should be assumed to be permanent and has to be sustainable and reasonable in cost. In the United States, the Americans with Disabilities Act, for example, states that the employer has a duty to provide reasonable accommodation for qualified applicants for a position unless this would impose "undue hardship" upon the employer, taking into account the cost of the accommodation, the financial resources of the employer, and the type of operation or operations involved.

18

HEALTH PROTECTION, HEALTH PROMOTION, AND DISEASE PREVENTION AT THE WORKPLACE

René Mendes and Elizabeth Costa Dias

The field of health promotion seeks to improve the level of health in a population by preventing diseases, controlling hazards, improving fitness and well-being, and enhancing the capacity of workers, and indeed all members of society, to function without impairment due to health problems.

Thus, health promotion is not limited to disease and injury prevention. It is also a strategy to improve the ability of workers to live their lives and to function in their family and community roles. The key insight of health promotion in the context of occupational health is to perceive the workplace as a community. On the one hand, when work is associated with health hazards, it can cause or contribute to occupational diseases or aggravate existing ill health of a non-occupational origin. On the other hand, when work is meaningful and valued by society and meets the social, financial, and personal needs of workers, it can be a positive force for growth and social security and can even help alleviate the consequences of ill health.

The workplace is not exclusively a setting of hazardous exposures. It is also a rich social environment in which people produce goods and services of value to others in a relationship defined by employment that creates a form of community through a shared work experience and, often, social class. The workplace may also be seen as an excellent opportunity to promote health, and this idea is implicit in the concept of healthy work. The organization of the workplace, and the possibility it provides for educating and reaching large groups of people, provides a means for health protection and disease prevention.

At the international level, the International Labour Organization (ILO), since its inception in 1919, and the World Health Organization (WHO), established in

1948, have been refining approaches to improving health and the quality of working life. In 1988, the WHO Expert Committee on Health Promotion in the Work Setting (hereafter called the WHO Expert Committee) declared that "the work environment constitutes an important part of man's total environment, so health is to a large extent affected by work conditions. . . . [W]ork is a powerful force in shaping a person's sense of identity. It can lend vitality to existence, and establishes the cyclical patterns of day, week, month and year."

There is a continuous two-way interaction between a person and his or her physical and psychological working environment: the working environment may influence the person's health either positively or negatively, and productivity is influenced by the worker's state of physical and mental well-being. Work, when it is well-balanced and productive, can be an important factor in promoting health and well-being as well as preventing disease. For example, partially disabled workers may be rehabilitated by undertaking tasks suited to their limited physical and mental capacities, which may increase their working capacity and allow them to support themselves and their families with dignity. However, the positive influence of work on health has not yet been fully exploited. Knowledge of work physiology and ergonomics has contributed greatly already to the prevention of disease. These fields need to be further developed and applied for the benefit and enhancement of workers' health.

The WHO Expert Committee refers to the positive influence of work on health, which is included within the concept of health promotion, and contrasts it to three broad categories of adverse effects associated with work—occupational diseases and injuries, contributions to the multiple causes of other diseases, and the potential to aggravate existing ill health of "non-occupational origin" (see Chapter 16). "WHO has repeatedly emphasized that occupational health programs should not be limited to the prevention and control of work-related hazards, but should deal with the full relationship between work and health and include general health promotion." This interesting concept will be used in this chapter as the basis for a discussion on concepts and practices of health protection and disease prevention in the workplace.

Some employers have established programs for health promotion in their workplaces, and some unions have developed such programs for their members. These programs use the workplace and the access to workers that it provides as a way of enhancing the health of workers through fitness activities, disease prevention, and education.

Many factors may lead to the establishment of health promotion activities in the workplace. In some countries, the primary driving force for the introduction of workplace health promotion programs is economic; a successful program provides quantifiable savings to the enterprise. In other countries, programs are introduced predominantly for social reasons as part of national policies for health. In yet others, there are statutory requirements for regular medical examinations of all workers, or of specific occupational groups, at which informal discussions about lifestyle may take place. However, outside of certain industries in developed countries, planned health promotion programs are rare.

The rationale for employer sponsorship of health promotion programs includes:

- preventing loss of worker productivity due to avoidable illnesses and disability and their associated absenteeism
- improving employee well-being and morale
- improving the quality of life for workers and their families
- controlling the costs of employer-paid health insurance
- reducing the level of health care services required
- reducing impairment and disability due to injuries and illness

Similar considerations have stimulated union interest in sponsoring programs, particularly when union members are scattered among many organizations too small to mount effective programs on their own. Employers, for their part, have become increasingly interested in the relationship between the health of their workers and productivity. Box 18.1 sets forth the economic context within which workplace health promotion programs were introduced in North America, comparing how the forces leading to workplace health promotion programs in two otherwise similar countries were very different.

However, according to the WHO Expert Committee, "this does not imply that economic justification is paramount." Examples of effective programs evaluated on non-economic grounds are also necessary to encourage the global development of workplace health promotion. Many more studies need to be undertaken to assess the positive value of workplace health promotion in terms of improved health and healthy behavior, reduced health-care costs, less frequent disability, increased productivity, reduced absenteeism, and reduced employee turnover. Concrete evidence is, however, difficult to obtain because such studies are methodologically complex, organizationally difficult, and, in some ways, ethically controversial because of confidentiality issues and the boundaries that define the legitimate interest of the employer in the personal life of workers.

Box 18.1

The Economic Context of Workplace Health Promotion

Health promotion programs are most likely to be introduced when economic forces demand it. In the United States in the 1980s, for example, the following economic trends pushed health promotion programs forward:

- high and rising cost of insurance provided to employees by their employers
- increasing losses due to absence, low productivity
- competition for talented workers in high value-added industries
- the expense of providing other benefits to employees, which made health promotion programs attractive

- the availability of a trained workforce of managers of health promotion programs who were graduating from exercise science and kinesiology graduate programs
- increasing interest in fitness on the part of employees

It became very popular for business groups to form to study these issues, such as the Washington Business Group on Health. These groups formed in most major cities and advocated more direct involvement by employers in the health of their employees. They promoted many innovations, such as case management (see Chapter 14), and led in the complicated negotiations for health-care insurance that resulted in large health provider organizations replacing individual physicians as the dominant way that health care was provided in the country. Individual employers often offered health education programs and new fitness centers for their employees at the same time that they were reducing the amount they spent on health insurance. However, by the early 1990s, employers were dissatisfied with the results because fitness centers seemed to benefit primarily those who were already fit and active, and they were beginning to question the wisdom of providing health promotion to employees who later left the company. Health promotion is an investment for the long term, and because of the high turnover in many sectors of the U.S. economy, the fear was that those workers would leave after a few years and the investment would be lost.

In Canada, by comparison, employers did not spend nearly as much on the health care of their employees because health care was managed in each province with a public, single-payer insurance system that covered all residents. Costs were much lower and removed from the direct control of employers. As a result, health promotion programs were more often community-based in the 1980s, and did not become as popular among employers until the early 1990s. At that time, there was great interest in reducing the costs being incurred from injury, both work-related and not. There was also great interest, due to reforms in the health-care system, in reducing the demand for health services in the community. At that time, many employers engaged in programs to improve the health of workers, and some did so in coordination with programs in the community.

One such program was a cooperative program between an oil company, Syncrude, and the community of Fort McMurray, Alberta. Syncrude noticed that many of their employees had injured themselves playing sports. Together with the community, they started a model injury prevention program that later resulted in Fort McMurray becoming the first community in North America to join the WHO Safe Community Network. (Guidotti 2000)

DEFINITIONS AND CONCEPTS

For the purposes of this chapter, the concept of health will be defined as the extent to which an individual or group is able, on the one hand, to realize aspirations and satisfy needs and, on the other hand, to change or cope with the environment. Health is a resource for everyday life, not the objective of living; it is a positive concept emphasizing social and personal resources as well as physical capacities.

In the context of health promotion, positive health is a state of health beyond an asymptomatic state. Concepts of positive health usually concern quality of life and the potential of the human condition. Notions of positive health may include self-fulfillment, vitality for living, and creativity. Moreover, positive health is concerned with thriving rather than mere coping.

"Health protection comprises legal or fiscal controls, other regulations and policies, and voluntary codes of practice, aimed at the enhancement of positive health and the prevention of ill-health" (Downie et al. 1996). Health protection, applied to occupational health, is an approach to maintaining the health of a population of workers and their families by introducing public health measures or prevention-oriented health care that controls or eliminates hazards and creates a safe and healthy working environment. Disease prevention is a closely related approach that seeks to target specific diseases and prevent them through specific interventions that remove their causes. Health protection and disease prevention are fundamentally strategies to prevent something bad from happening, whereas health promotion is basically a positive strategy to improve or enhance health in a community or population.

Health promotion is the process of enabling people to increase control over, and to improve, their health. To reach a state of complete physical, mental, and social well-being, an individual or group must be able to identify and realize aspirations, satisfy needs, and change or cope with the environment. Therefore, health promotion is not just the responsibility of the health sector, but goes beyond healthy lifestyles to well-being (see the WHO's Ottawa Charter for Health Promotion).

In the context of occupational health, the WHO Expert Committee on Health Promotion in the Work Setting has defined health promotion as a continuum ranging from the treatment of disease to the prevention of disease (including protection against specific risks) to the promotion of optimal health. Achieving optimal health includes improving physical abilities in relation to sex and age, improving mental ability, developing reserve capacities and adaptability to changing circumstances of work and life, and reaching new levels of individual achievement in creative and other work. In a work setting, these health indicators may be evaluated quantitatively by indices of *absence* (the word is preferred to *absenteeism*), job satisfaction, and work stability.

Even within WHO, different concepts are used in official documents; e.g., the concept of health promotion may include components such as treatment of disease and prevention of disease (see above), and the definitions may be used differently in various textbooks. Thus, it is often helpful to think of these terms as reflecting different schools of thought or points of view that can overlap. Health promotion has been the preferred approach by WHO and many governments since the 1980s. Health protection is an older approach that was adopted by governments in setting up pre-1080s regulatory systems and safety standards. Disease prevention is the traditional approach taken by public health agencies and preventive and primary care medicine.

Disease prevention relies heavily on the principles of applied *prevention*, which is the concept of reducing the risk of occurrence of a disease process, illness, injury, disability, handicap, or some other unwanted phenomenon or state. Prevention strategies are classified as "primary," "secondary," and "tertiary." Primary prevention is the strategy of preventing the disease in the first place, through measures that remove the hazard (such as malaria control), reduce exposure (such as clean water, pasteurization of milk or quarantine from highly infectious diseases), or prevent an individual from contracting the disease even if he or she is exposed (such as immunization). Secondary prevention is the strategy of screening people for early signs of risk (such as high blood pressure) or the early stages of the disease itself (e.g., treatable forms of cancer such as skin cancer or colon cancer) and then treating them before the disease manifests or grows worse. Tertiary prevention is the prevention of disability resulting from a disorder, such as rehabilitation to prevent permanent impairment after an injury.

Downie et al. (1996) conclude that "health promotion comprises three overlapping spheres of activity: health education (or more precisely, that part which contributes to the overall goal of health promotion), prevention, and health protection."

The classic Leavell and Clark (1965) model, established in the 1960s, describes primary prevention as composed of health promotion and specific protection. However, by common definitions such as those that have evolved in the *Dictionary of Public Health* and *the Dictionary of Epidemiology*, primary prevention is the protection of health by either personal or community-wide interventions such as preserving good nutritional status, physical fitness, and emotional well-being, immunizing individuals and entire communities against infectious diseases, and making the environment safe, for example by treating drinking water. Within the Leavell and Clark classification, immunization constitutes a good example of specific protection against infectious diseases (the second level of primary prevention). For them, health promotion constitutes the first level of primary prevention. It is not targeted against disease, but in favor of health.

Primary prevention includes those activities that are intended to prevent the onset of disease in the first place. The classic example of primary prevention is immunization against infectious diseases, but the use of seat belts, the installation of air bags in automobiles, the avoidance of tobacco use, the minimal intake of alcoholic beverages, and the inspection and licensure of restaurants are all examples of common public health activities that exemplify primary prevention.

Secondary prevention can be defined as "the measures available to individuals and populations for the early detection and prompt and effective intervention to correct departures from good health" (Last, in the 1995 edition of the *Dictionary of Epidemiology*) and refers to techniques that find health problems early in their course so that action can be taken to minimize the risk of progression of the disease in individuals or the risk that communicable illnesses will be transmitted to others. Examples of this principle include the early diagnosis of hypertension with follow-up treatment to minimize the risk of future vascular disease and the early diagnosis and treatment of sexually transmitted diseases to minimize the transmission potential of those conditions to others.

Tertiary prevention consists of the measures available to reduce or eliminate long-term impairments and disabilities, minimize suffering caused by existing departures from good health, and promote the patient's adjustment to irremediable conditions. This extends the concept of prevention into the field of rehabilitation. Tertiary prevention ". . . is focused on rehabilitation, in an effort to prevent the worsening of an individual's health in the face of a chronic disease or injury. Learning to walk again after an orthopedic injury or cerebrovascular accident is [such] an example" (Scutchfield and Keck 1997).

The "Health Field Concept"

Most of today's policy discussions about health promotion were shaped by the 1975 publication of the report *A New Perspective on the Health of Canadians*, often called the "Lalonde Report" after the minister responsible for developing it, Marc Lalonde. The report describes the major determinants of health in a population as being the outcome of factors operating in four broad fields: human biology, health services, environmental influences on health, and health-related behaviors. The Lalonde Report established priorities for improving the health status of the Canadian people, building on the health field concept. It described the relationships among access to health-care services, human biology, environment, and individual behaviors, and estimated the relative contribution to outcomes that progress in each of these fields might make. The report concluded that advances in modifying personal risk, improving the environment, and adding to our knowledge of human biology were more likely to improve health status than further work on the quality and efficiency of the medical care system. The report is now credited with establishing health promotion as a major component of strategies to improve health and for stimulating research on the determinants of health-related behaviors for risk reduction.

Heightened interest in risk reduction paved the way for the creation of the Canadian Task Force on the Periodic Health Examination, whose 1979 report represented another major contribution to health promotion and disease prevention by introducing a method of applying "evidence-based" decision rules to setting priorities for clinical preventive services. The task force used data on the burden of suffering to determine those conditions or risk factors most needing preventive interventions.

In line with the Lalonde report, the WHO Expert Committee of 1988 (see above) stated that disability, disease, and death can be viewed within the framework of the four main "health fields," which are human biology, environment, lifestyle, and health-care organization; each health problem is affected by factors from one or more of these elements. This division into four elements, when applied to occupational health, can be very useful in identifying preventable problems and their contributing factors. With regard to workplace health problems, it is important to identify both those whose causes include work activities or exposures, and those that have other causes but may be effectively screened, treated, or reduced in severity through interventions in the workplace.

This statement offers an initial criterion for the definition of the scope and comprehensiveness of health promotion in workplaces, using a flexible definition of the meaning of health promotion. According to this Expert Committee statement, at least two dimensions deserve attention at the workplace:

- "health problems. . . whose causes include work activities or exposures" (see Table 18.1)
- those problems "that have other causes but may be effectively screened, treated, or reduced in severity through interventions in the workplace" (see Tables 18.2 and 18.3)

Accordingly, the Expert Committee points out that "WHO has repeatedly emphasized that occupational health programs should not be limited to the prevention and control of work-related hazards, but should deal with the full relationship between work and health and include general health promotion." For the Expert Committee, as the concept of occupational health care has been expanded, a commitment to the overall health of the worker has been introduced (World Health Organization 1988).

This concept of occupational health care as embodying both health protection and health promotion has been accepted by many governments and employers. For example, the UK Employment Medical Advisory Service stated in a triennial report that "the workplace has come increasingly to be seen as a base for general health promotion. . . . The distinction between disease and ill-health arising from the workplace and that arising from other causes is increasingly difficult" (World Health Organization 1988).

Professor Richard Schilling, a famous teacher of occupational medicine in the United Kingdom, pointed out that ". . . while the worksite is the obvious place for controlling work-related disease and injury, for which managers have a legal and moral responsibility, it is also an appropriate setting for a much broader approach

TABLE 18.1

CATEGORIES OF WORK-RELATED DISEASE

Category	Examples
I. Work is the necessary cause.	<ul><li>Silicosis, asbestosis</li><li>Lead poisoning</li><li>Irritant dermatitis</li><li>Occupational asthma</li><li>Other</li></ul>
II. Work is a contributory causal factor, not a necessary one.	<ul><li>Coronary heart disease</li><li>Musculoskeletal disorders; low back pain, carpal tunnel syndrome, etc.</li><li>Malignant tumors; lung cancer, leukemia, etc.</li><li>Other</li></ul>
III. Work provokes a latent disorder or aggravates established disease.	<ul><li>Peptic ulcer</li><li>Chronic bronchitis</li><li>Contact dermatitis</li><li>Asthma (previous)</li><li>Some mental disorders</li><li>Other</li></ul>

Adapted from Schilling, 1984

TABLE 18.2

OPPORTUNITIES FOR HEALTH PROTECTION, HEALTH PROMOTION, AND DISEASE PREVENTION

Category of Work-related Disease	Opportunities for Health Protection, Health Promotion, and Disease Prevention at Workplaces
I. Work is the necessary cause.	• Reduction or elimination of occupational hazards that act as determinants of disease or work injuries (emphasis on physical and chemical hazards)
II. Work is a contributory risk factor or determinant in multifactoral pathological processes or entities.	• Reduction or elimination of the fraction of risk attributable to work environment and/or working conditions (emphasis on organizational and ergonomic conditions) • Reduction of risk factors related to individual biology (genetic, familial, age-related, sex-related, race-related, degenerative processes, etc.) • Reduction of risk factors related to lifestyles (taken in the sense of general way of living based on the interplay between living conditions as a whole, and individual patterns of behavior as determined by sociocultural factors and personal characteristics • Reduction of risk factors related to the access to and quality of health services
III. Work provokes a latent disorder or aggravates established disease.	• Reduction or elimination of occupational hazards that act as triggers or aggravators of pre-existing diseases • Reduction or elimination of the fraction of risk attributable to working environment and/or working conditions • Reduction of risk factors related to individual biology (genetic, familial, age-related, sex-related, race-related, degenerative processes, etc.) • Reduction of risk factors related to lifestyles (based on the interplay between living conditions as a whole, and individual patterns of behavior as determined by sociocultural factors and personal characteristics) • Reduction of risk factors related to the access to and quality of health services

Adapted from Schilling, 1984

to preventing unnecessary disease and disability" (Schilling 1984). This comprehensive concept gives occupational health an excellent framework within which to act to promote health.

THE OTTAWA CHARTER

The *Ottawa Charter for Health Promotion* was a key document in the development of WHO's approach to health promotion. Since 1986, the *Ottawa Charter for Health Promotion* has been an essential reference for the conceptual development of

TABLE 18.3

EMPLOYERS' RESPONSIBILITIES FOR HEALTH PROTECTION, HEALTH PROMOTION, AND DISEASE PREVENTION

Actions or Activities	Employers' Responsibility
Reduction or elimination of occupational hazards that act as determinants of disease or work injuries (emphasis on physical and chemical hazards	• Ethical • Legal
Reduction or elimination of occupational hazards that act as triggers or aggravators of pre-existing diseases	• Ethical • Social (shared) • Legal (in specific conditions)
Reduction or elimination of the fraction of risk attributable to work environment and/or working conditions (emphasis on organizational and ergonomic conditions)	• Ethical • Social (shared)
Reduction of risk factors related to individual biology (genetic, familial, age-related, sex-related, hereditary, degenerative processes, etc.)	• Social (shared)
Reduction of risk factors related to lifestyles (based on the interplay between living conditions as a whole, and individual patterns of behavior as determined by sociocultural factors and personal characteristics)	• Social (shared)
Reduction of risk factors related to the access to and quality of health services	• Social (shared) • Legal (in specific conditions)

health promotion, particularly by the World Health Organization and countries that follow the WHO model.

Box 18.2 presents a passage from the charter that describes actions required to achieve health promotion. This health promotion dimension may include, for example, worksite wellness programs such as cessation of tobacco use, physical exercise, nutrition, weight management, injury prevention, family planning, sexually transmitted diseases, substance use and abuse (alcohol and other drugs), oral health, immunizations, chemoprophylaxis, and self-examination of the breasts, skin, and testes, among others.

Health promotion, health protection, and disease prevention at worksites should be dealt with not only with the comprehensive view of occupational health as total health of workers (either work-related or not work-related), but also with the understanding that workplaces are social and political spaces where workers may exercise active roles, putting into practice the full idea of *empowerment*, which is the core of the modern understanding of health promotion.

The workplace has several advantages as a location for health promotion activities and the delivery of preventive health services. For example, workers are easily accessible and environmental monitoring is facilitated, which makes it possible to control at the source various industrial environmental pollutants.

Occupational settings are appropriate sites where health-related activities can take place. These may include health assessment, education, counseling, and health promotion in general. From a public policy perspective, worksites provide an efficient locus for such activities involving as they often do a far-ranging aggregation of individuals. Moreover, most workers are in a predictable work location for a significant portion of time almost every week. Also, the workplace is uniquely advantageous as an arena for health protection and promotion. It is the place where workers congregate and spend a major portion of their waking hours. In addition to this propinquity, their camaraderie and sharing similar interests and concerns facilitate the development of peer pressures that can be a powerful motivator for participation and persistence in a health promotion activity. The relative stability of the workforce—most workers remain in the same organization for long periods—makes for the continuing participation in healthful behaviors necessary to achieve any benefit. (This assumption may need to be revisited given recent economic upheavals and unemployment.) The workplace affords unique opportunities to promote the improved health and well-being of the workers.

However, the concept of health promotion as applied to workplaces goes beyond these features, putting the worker, either alone or organized, in the middle of the process as an active subject and not a passive target. This belief fits within the concept of self-empowerment, i.e., the achievement of personal autonomy through the development of and use of life skills for health. Self-empowerment is a process designed to restore decision-making capabilities and to equip individuals with a belief in their autonomy, together with the skills necessary to enable them to decide what to do about their own health, their family's health, the health of the community, and their health at work. It means to enable workers to take control and responsibility for their health as an important component of everyday life. Self-empowerment is a crucial resource for such control, responsibility, and action.

Richard Schilling proposed a classification of work-related diseases that is summarized in Table 18.1. Work-related disease could be grouped into three categories, in which work is (1) the necessary cause, (2) a contributory cause, and (3) an aggravating factor.

Table 18.2 presents practical ways of achieving these objectives. Table 18.3 shows some employers, responsibilities (ethical, legal, and/or social) for health protection, health promotion, and disease prevention at the workplace according to the nature of actions or activities.

Warshaw and Messite (1998) described the outcomes that should be seen as the result of effective health promotion in the workplace:

- cognitive/emotional: knowledge, motivation, well-being, self-efficacy, self-esteem
- behavioral: immediate (0–3 months), short term (3–6 months), intermediate term (6–8 months)
- physiological: blood chemistries, anthropometrics, heart function, physical disease

- financial: medical utilization (inpatient, outpatient, diagnosis specific, etc.); medical costs (total, outpatient, diagnosis specific, etc.); absenteeism; disability (claims, costs)
- health status: quality of life, morbidity, mortality

Box 18.2

What Health Promotion Means in Practice (according to the Ottawa Charter)

Health promotion means. . .

Build healthy public policy. Health promotion goes beyond health care. It puts health on the agenda of policy makers in all sectors and all levels, directing them to be aware of the health consequences of their decisions and to accept responsibilities for health. Health promotion policy combines diverse but complementary approaches including legislation, fiscal measures, taxation, and organizational change. It is coordinated action that leads to health, income, and social policies that foster greater equity. Joint action contributes to ensuring safer and healthier goods and services, healthier public services, and cleaner, more enjoyable environments.

Create supportive environments. Changing patterns of life, work, and leisure have a significant impact on health. Work and leisure should be a source of health for people. The way society organizes work should help create a healthy society. Health promotion generates living and working conditions that are safe, stimulating, satisfying, and enjoyable.

Strengthen community action. Health promotion works through concrete and effective community action in setting priorities, making decisions, planning strategies, and implementing them to achieve better health. At the heart of this process is the empowerment of communities and their ownership and control of their own endeavors and destinies. This requires full and continuous access to information and learning opportunities for health as well as funding support.

Develop personal skills. Health promotion supports personal and social development through providing information, education for health, and enhancing life skills. By so doing, it increases the options available to people to exercise more control over their own health and over their environments, and to make choices conductive to health. Enabling people to learn throughout life, to prepare themselves for all of its stages, and to develop coping strategies to deal with chronic illness and injuries is essential. This has to be facilitated in school, home, *work*, and community settings. Action is required through educational, professional, commercial, and voluntary bodies and within the institutions themselves.

Reorient health services. The responsibility for health promotion in health services is shared among individuals, community groups, health professionals, health service institutions, and governments. They must work together toward a healthcare system that contributes to the pursuit of health. The role of the health sector must move increasingly in a health promotion direction, beyond its responsibility for providing clinical and curative services. Health services need to embrace an expanded mandate that is sensitive and respects cultural needs. . . (Extracted from the Ottawa Charter for Health Promotion, 1986. Source: Pan American Health Organization, 1996; emphasis added)

During the late 1970s and early 1980s, costs for health care in the United States began to rise. In the United States, insurance is paid for workers and their families primarily by employers. Access to health care is therefore tied to employment, and the employer has a strong interest in the health care that workers receive because they are paying for it.

The response to this increase in costs consisted mostly of three changes: employers began to form organizations that would seek ways to contain health costs, they began to offer new forms of insurance in which access to care was managed, and they began to introduce "worksite health promotion" programs on a large scale.

The first generation of programs consisted mostly of screening programs to detect health problems. The worker would undergo a set of tests, and the results would be sent to his or her personal physician. However, the worker's physician usually did not pay much attention to the results. Health education classes were introduced; weight loss and smoking cessation were usually the most popular. Exercise programs were introduced, and some employers even built gymnasia and exercise rooms in their buildings, usually at the corporate headquarters.

The results were disappointing. In the beginning these programs were very popular, but soon employers noticed that the workers who used them most were the workers who were younger and in good physical shape—those who needed them the least. Even so, they had become very popular, and employers often found that they could not eliminate them if they wished to compete with other firms for the best employees. Health-care costs continued to rise.

In the 1990s, companies began to concentrate more on "wellness" and case management for workers with health problems. This strategy involves programs that encourage workers to stay healthy by their own efforts and to manage their diseases carefully.

Health Programs

The most popular types of health programs that have been offered by employers to their workers in North America are health education, fitness, disease screening, smoking cessation, and obesity and dietary management. These individual programs can be packaged into programs such as those listed below.

Fitness centers are employer-sponsored facilities that have exercise equipment and space to hold educational sessions. They are usually located at corporate headquarters and in larger facilities operated by the employer. They tend to attract participation from workers who are health conscious and want to maintain their fitness level.

Health fairs are events held at the worksite or in the community under the sponsorship, usually, of a major employer or health-care institution. The health fair is an opportunity for participants to obtain a set of screening tests, basic health education, and general advice in a convenient, often public setting. Sometimes influenza immunizations or other preventive services are offered as well. The health fair is usually staffed by a nurse with a physician on call or on site but not

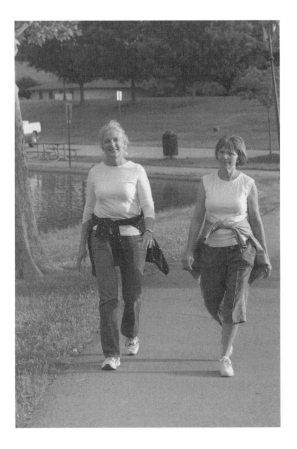

Figure 18.1 Employer-sponsored wellness and health promotion activities should emphasize inclusiveness and accessibility to workers at all fitness levels rather than athletic training, in order to encourage participation by those who need them most. They do not need expensive equipment. Organized lunchtime walking groups have been very popular where they have been organized, and the activity can be done indoors in building corridors in inclement weather.

necessarily involved in every encounter. Some health-care facilities offer basic health fairs once a year as a free service to employers, in part as a marketing promotion and in part to encourage workers to obtain their own and their family's care at the same facility. Health fairs offer very useful opportunities for health education and probably raise initial awareness of health issues among workers.

Periodic health evaluations are of value, but the "annual physical examination" is now considered obsolete as a strategy for periodic health evaluation. Most screening tests are not required as often as once a year, especially for younger workers. The physical examination in itself, even when combined with standard clinical laboratory tests, is now recognized as an inefficient means of detecting health risks or the earliest stages of most treatable disorders. However, the cachet enjoyed by the physical examination after years of promotion and its status as an employment benefit have made it difficult to deny to managers and service employees.

The "executive physical" is a periodic, comprehensive medical evaluation for executive and other key personnel whose health is thought essential to the employer's future. It is also a popular job benefit.

The pattern of health promotion programs in North America deviates from the provisions of the Ottawa Charter and represents a more prescriptive, directive attitude toward the health of workers. This difference is partly the result of the employer's payment for the cost of health care and partly due to differences in attitudes toward health promotion, which in the United States tend to emphasize guidelines, restrictions, and prescriptions rather than change in the environment to support healthy behaviors. However, this difference in perception of what health promotion means in practice has led to a wider range of health promotion programs that have been developed for delivery to the worksite in the United States.

19

INDUSTRIES AND WORKPLACES

Hugo Rüdiger, Michael Nasterlack, Andreas Zober,
and Tee L. Guidotti

This chapter describes the common hazards and health problems for particular industries. Although the descriptions are not comprehensive, nor is the list of industries discussed exhaustive, the major issues in each sector are highlighted. For a more complete overview of a particular industrial sector, the standard reference work in English is *Patty's Industrial Hygiene and Toxicology*; concise descriptions of many industries are also provided in the *International Labour Organization Encyclopaedia of Occupational Health and Safety*.

Some occupational hazards and health problems are to be found almost universally in business and industry, e.g., noise, stress, ergonomic problems, low back pain, and substance abuse issues. Others are sufficiently typical in manufacturing, construction, and service sectors to be considered common, e.g., safety problems and disorders such as hand injuries, dermatitis, and repetitive motion injuries. Issues related to indoor air quality or "sick buildings" and repetitive strain injuries are common in office work. Others are characteristic of the industrial sector.

However, workers who hold jobs within a given industry are not necessarily exposed to the characteristic hazards of that industry. It depends on the specific job. Certain jobs within each industry (e.g., welding) present hazards unique to the occupation and are generally the same regardless of the industrial setting. Other jobs may be generally unremarkable except for exposures characteristic of the particular industry, such as janitorial services, in which the only unusual hazardous exposures are those present in the specific workplace being cleaned. In still others, jobs that appear to be unrelated to production may still involve exposure to hazards in the industry. Maintenance crews or millwrights, who take care of factories, may encounter almost every chemical used in the plant and especially may be exposed to asbestos when it is present. Workers in a mine are mostly miners, but some of them are electricians and welders.

The recognition of a hazard in a new industry, such as biotechnology or microelectronics, is frequently a surprise to those working in the industry. For experienced occupational health and safety personnel, however, the emergence of these problems is predictable. In the development of a new industry, the emphasis is always on new technology and markets; rarely are the principals in a new industry interested in looking backward to historical hazards, nor do they have the time (or interest) to investigate hazards in unrelated industries. To entrepreneurs and pioneers in industry, health and safety hazards are seen as obstacles to the main goal of production and to be dealt with only as they arise. Moreover, professionals in one industry do not usually talk to their counterparts in other industries about occupational hazards. Occupational health and safety personnel over time often become highly specialized in their particular industry. The result is that hazards are rarely anticipated early enough.

For example, hydrofluoric acid (HF) is a very hazardous substance used to etch glass, silicon chips for computers, and the walls of glass tanks in chemical plants. HF causes deep burns and tissue damage and may cause permanent scarring or even loss of a hand or other body part. These burns require immediate and highly specific treatment. When the semiconductor (silicon chip) sector of the microelectronics industry was just starting to expand on an industrial scale, there were many injuries involving HF that resulted in severe injury and disability. The hazards associated with HF came as an unpleasant surprise in the new microelectronics business because few in the industry were aware that hydrofluoric acid presented serious hazards, although this had been known in the glassmaking industry for many years. Similarly, when biotechnology took off as an industry, there were again avoidable hydrofluoric acid burns because the hazard was not appreciated, although it had become well known a few years earlier in the microelectronics industry.

These experiences lead to a virtually ironclad rule of occupational medicine: Old hazards never disappear for long; they reappear in new industries.

BIOMEDICAL RESEARCH, BIOTECHNOLOGY, PHARMACEUTICALS

Biomedical research, biotechnology, and pharmaceuticals now appear to be merging into one large industry or enterprise to a degree that would have been inconceivable just 20 years ago. In addition to the obvious connection between biomedical research and the development of new products, production on an industrial scale may present the potential for significant exposures to chemical hazards previously limited to much smaller-scale laboratory operations. Occupational health and safety management in this sector is complicated by its newness, which has resulted in the entry of many junior workers and development-oriented scientists inexperienced with health and safety hazards and unfamiliar with safety procedures in the respective industries.

Biomedical Research

The occupational hazards involved with laboratory research and development of new techniques are specific to the organisms or methods being used and depend on whether or not human tissue or blood products are used. However, there are hazards common to many biomedical research activities.

Physical hazards are very common in research laboratories and include electrical hazards, ignition sources, mechanical equipment with exposed blades or grinding surfaces, heat sources, liquid nitrogen and other cryogenic sources, ultraviolet and infrared radiation, and radiation. Most laboratory settings have had stringent guidelines for controlling radionuclides and radiation sources, but, until recently, general occupational safety measures were often relatively weak.

Chemical hazards in biochemistry research laboratories have not generally been as severe as in chemistry laboratories but are significant. Many organic solvents are used heavily, including methanol, and there is a potential for high exposures, particularly in operations such as thin-layer chromatography. Other specific chemical hazards depend on the research being carried out, but many include a number of corrosive agents (such as potassium dichromate, frequently used for cleaning pipettes), strong acids and bases, oxidizing agents (such as hydrazine), carcinogens (such as dioxane), and other toxic substances.

Research laboratories in universities and similar academic settings have particular occupational health and safety problems. They are often shared by many investigators with little overall supervision. Graduate students, postdoctoral fellows, and undergraduate students come and go, often with minimal orientation and rarely with intensive training in laboratory safety. Laboratory technicians tend to be more permanent and over time usually become the mainstay of enforcing health and safety measures; there may be considerable turnover, however, if faculty leave or if grants terminate. The intense pressure for academic productivity and achievement sometimes leads to shortcuts and unnecessary risks being taken, especially by junior investigators in unsupervised situations. These same pressures, combined with the distractions of more lofty intellectual pursuits, sometimes lead to an attitude of neglect by senior investigators. In recent years, academic laboratories have often strengthened enforcement of safety guidelines and have expanded their health and safety offices in response to perceived problems in laboratories, sometimes over the objection of senior scientists who are accustomed to high degrees of freedom in their academic pursuits.

Occupational health and safety measures for laboratories cannot rest on strict guidelines and regular inspection alone because of the constantly fluid and adaptive nature of research. Rather, emphasis is increasingly placed on training all users of laboratory facilities, especially students. Reagents must always be completely labeled, with standardized symbols for their hazard potential. Hazardous chemicals and pressurized tanks of gas should be stored in appropriate cabinets. Personal protection is essential for any process in which splashes or spills may occur. Equipment should be certified and regularly inspected for electrical safety and performance; fume hoods should be tested regularly to ensure that airflow is adequate. Decontamination procedures following spills should be spelled out and readily available; chemical decontamination procedures have been developed for the safe disposal of small quantities of hazardous materials. Emergency procedures, such as evacuation plans, should be clearly posted. The management of laboratory safety is a highly specialized area and should, whenever possible, be under the supervision of a safety officer with specific experience in laboratories and in dealing with research scientists.

Biotechnology

The technologies most closely associated with the revolution in biotechnology presently underway are genomics, informatics, cloning, recombinant DNA, monoclonal antibody production, and fermentation. In a typical application, bacteria or yeast species are transfected with DNA coding for a desirable peptide gene product and are then cultured in fermentation tanks to produce large quantities of relatively pure product with agricultural or biomedical uses. However, the most significant hazards are often encountered in research on a laboratory scale and in operations involving testing and quality assurance. Many other biological mechanisms are being exploited to produce new products.

Although biotechnology is a new industry sector, it has already received close examination for its hazard potential because of concern that infective-engineered microorganisms might be released into the environment. This resulted in a voluntary moratorium against research involving genetic manipulation of microbes in the early 1980s supported by prominent investigators associated with the Asilomar series of research conferences. This moratorium was called off when no evidence of a risk was forthcoming. The organisms now transfected with altered genetic material are of very low infectivity and are carefully controlled.

Physical hazards associated with biomedical technology can be substantial. These include exposure to very low temperatures in cryogenic operations, with the potential for tissue damage much like thermal burns. Radionuclides and radiation sources are common in laboratory and testing operations, as are ultraviolet radiation sources to reduce airborne contaminants.

Chemical hazards in biotechnology that are uncommon in smaller-scale laboratory practices include exposure to acetonitrile, sodium azide, and hydrazine. Acetonitrile (CH_3CN) is used as a solvent and reagent in high-pressure liquid chromatography; it is reported to be the most frequent toxic exposure in biotechnology. Apparently, acetonitrile is metabolized to cyanide and produces an asphyxiant effect at the cellular level (cytochrome inhibition), much like that of cyanide. The mechanism of action of acetonitrile has not been extensively investigated, however, and little is known of the effects of chronic, long-term exposure. Azide is a commonly used preservative in cultures. Azide acts as both an arterial vasodilator, much like nitroglycerin, and is a cytochrome inhibitor, although less potent than cyanide; patients recovering from azide intoxication have been reported to experience behavioral changes. Hydrazine, used in cleavage reactions, is explosive, very irritating, and highly neurotoxic. Other common chemical exposures include ethylene oxide formaldehyde, acrylamide (a potent neurotoxin), hydrofluoric acid (which produces deep and severe burns), tetramethylene diamine (a severe mucosal irritant and sensitizing agent), and ethidium bromide (a probable mutagen and possible carcinogen).

Biological hazards have thus far not been a problem because of the selection of microorganisms with intrinsically low infectivity. At present, concern is focused primarily on the theoretical possibility that altered genes introduced into one microorganism may, through conjugation, enter another in which the effects would be unpredictable. The release of genetically altered organisms into the environment has already occurred, the prototype experiment having been the release of so-named Frostban® "ice-minus" plant frost damage-inhibiting bacteria on test plots. Regulation of the release of genetically altered microorganisms into the environment in the United States rests with the Environmental Protection Agency under the Federal Insecticide, Fungicide, and Rodenticide Act (FIFRA) and the Department of Agriculture. Other aspects of biotechnology in the United States are regulated by the National Institutes of Health, the Food and Drug Administration, and the Occupational Health and Safety Administration. Europe is expected to take a more consolidated approach.

Despite the high level of technology in the industry and the training workers in biotechnology receive, there is surprisingly little knowledge about many of these hazards. Ethidium bromide and acetonitrile, for example, are heavily used, although the toxicological literature is scanty on both. Biotechnology workers may be unfamiliar with common hazards in the industry, having often been recruited from more traditional research laboratory settings or directly out of a university. Personal protective measures, including gloves, aprons, and eye protection, and worksite hazard control, including adequate ventilation, proper spill control procedures, and engineering controls, are essential in biotechnology operations as in all industry and laboratory research.

Pharmaceuticals

In general, drug manufacturing is heavily contained and controlled so that the product is not handled by workers. This is primarily for reasons of maintaining pure drug standards. Drug manufacturing plants are typically very clean, and workers usually wear gloves and protective clothing in operations where they may come into contact with product. However, these protective measures are primarily aimed at protecting the product from contamination and not protecting the worker from hazards. The potential exists for workers to have toxic and particularly immunologic responses to the drug being produced and/or to the chemicals used in its manufacture.

Drugs are chemical hazards in themselves and are made from chemicals that may present their own hazards. Large pharmaceutical plants are much like chemical plants in their risk profiles. Materials handling and packaging the finished product may result in problems common to other industries, such as back strain and minor injuries.

It is difficult to generalize about health problems in the pharmaceutical industry because much depends on the feedstocks used and the product. For example, male workers in one plant manufacturing oral contraceptives developed gynecomastia, the abnormal development of breast tissue. In general, allergic sensitization to the product is a bigger risk than toxic effects because of the magnitude of exposure, and seems anecdotally to be more common with antibiotics. Severe reactions, such as hypersensitivity pneumonitis, have been reported but are rare.

CHEMICAL INDUSTRY

Chemical hazards in the workplace are generally on the decline, at least in developed countries, and this is true as well in the chemical industry. As a consequence, health hazards for employees in this industry today may not be much different from those in other industries. This means that—as almost everywhere—musculoskeletal disorders and skin diseases of different origins as well as impaired hearing are the leading work-related disorders and, together with an increasing importance of stress-related health problems, are concerns for chemical industry employees. Besides these unspecific occupational health hazards, however, a few are typically related to the industrial production of chemicals. Some of these are not only important in occupational medicine but more so in the field of environmental medicine.

Chapter 9 discusses potentially harmful substances in detail. The section below describes established principles of health protection and surveillance of workers in the chemical industry.

Production-Related Hazards

Problems associated with the chemical industry can be divided into those associated with handling and transportation of feedstocks, the manufacture of chemical products, and distribution of chemical products.

Basic Chemicals on Large Scale The whole range of chemical products, including pharmaceuticals, is mostly derived from relatively few raw materials: air, water, crude oil, and salt. They are used to synthesize about 300 parent compounds that serve to build a multitude of different consumer products. Many of these parent substances bear inherent hazards such as flammability, explosiveness, toxicity, or carcinogenicity. Therefore, for industrial settings where such chemicals are produced and stored, precautionary measures must be established that include developing simulation models to estimate the probability, size, public health, and environmental impact of an accidental release and developing emergency response programs. Emergency preparedness would, for example, include storage of antidotes or medication, organizing their distribution in an emergency situation, and setting up communication channels with the neighbors of the facility.

The following two examples are given to illustrate the problems that can arise from the handling of potentially dangerous substances. These substances can be handled safely, provided that appropriate technology is applied together with adequate emergency preparedness.

Monomers

The organic chemistry that is the basis of all sorts of plastics is based almost entirely on products from crude oil, mostly short-chained aliphatic compounds. All synthetic plastic materials are polymers (i.e., multiples of smaller monomeric compounds that form huge molecules that give the products their unique and desired properties). Many of these monomers are by nature highly reactive and, once incorporated, may bind to biological structures such as DNA, causing irreversible damage. Some monomers, such as vinyl chloride or ethylene oxide, are proven or probable human carcinogens. On the other hand, the polymeric products no longer contain significant monomeric residues. They are largely inert and nontoxic and can be used in a wide range of applications, including medical equipment and food packaging. Because polymeric plastic materials are indispensable and abandoning their manufacture is not realistic, their production must not pose a significant health risk to employees, neighbors, or the environment. That requires control of the monomeric feedstocks. The measures to achieve this goal are discussed below.

Chlorine

Chlorine, which is produced from salt, is the most important inorganic compound in chemical production. It is used in at least one step of the synthesis of approximately three-quarters of all chemicals produced, although only 40% of the finalized products still contain chlorine. Because elementary chlorine is highly reactive and toxic to living organisms, it cannot be handled openly in workplaces. Chlorine intoxication generally occurs as a result of accidental releases. The most relevant and common route of exposure is inhalation. Chlorine is corrosive when it contacts moist tissue such as the eyes, skin, and upper respiratory tract, causing eye irritation, coughing, chest pain, and dyspnea. Bronchospasm, laryngospasm, and pulmonary edema may occur even after a symptomless interval of several hours and may cause death. Thus, chlorine is an example of a highly dangerous substance that is nevertheless irreplaceable in modern chemical technology.

Special Groups of Hazardous Substances

Some potentially hazardous substances in the chemical industry deserve special attention because estimating safe exposure limits has not been possible. These substances can largely be grouped into the following categories:

Carcinogens The German Commission for the Investigation of Health Hazards of Chemical Compounds in the Workplace has defined 268 substances proven or suspected to be carcinogenic. For more than half of these, the scientific designation of a maximum workplace concentration (MAK) or a threshold limit value (TLV) was not possible. Among these are important chemicals such as benzene; vinyl chloride; hydrazine; 1,3-butadiene; some synthetic fibers; and technically important metals such as nickel, chromium, or cobalt. When it is necessary to use such substances, special measures are required for protection and monitoring. These include routine analyses of workplace air and biological material (e.g., blood, urine) by analytical methods and special medical supervision of exposed individuals. Special techniques for genotoxic monitoring (such as chromosome analysis, sister chromatid exchange, micronucleus assay, comet assay, or the determination of DNA- or protein adducts) are valuable for surveillance of carcinogen-exposed workers.

Allergenic Substances Although many substances may be capable of causing allergy, a substance is called an occupational allergen only if it causes an allergy in more than 1% of the exposed workers. Allergy in the workplace mostly affects the skin or the respiratory tract. In most cases, a strictly maintained MAK or threshold limit value (TLV) protects employees from becoming sensitized, with the exception of genetically predisposed individuals. However, sensitized individuals will often develop symptoms even if the MAK/TLV is maintained.

Neurotoxic Substances There is an increasing number of investigations that have described acquired cognitive deficits in long-time exposed workers using sensitive neuropsychological testing instruments. High exposures to organic solvents have been identified as the cause. These cognitive deficits are mainly subclinical but may cause impairment or disability in severe cases. Probably, most cases that are diagnosed today are due to high past exposures, where the respective TLVs were exceeded, sometimes to a considerable extent. It has been hypothesized that combination effects of solvent mixture exposures may occur. This means that detectable nervous disturbances may occur, even if the MAK/TLVs of the individual substances are in compliance with regulations. However, this has been demonstrated only for peripheral neurotoxic effects (polyneuropathies) caused by mixtures of n-hexane and methyl ethyl ketone.

Reproductive Toxicants MAK/TLVs are defined for the healthy adult worker and do not preclude toxic effects to the unborn fetus. About 20 substances with proven or suspected fetotoxicity below valid MAK/TLVs have been designated by the German Commission for the Investigation of Health Hazards of Chemical Compounds in the Work Area. Examples are lead, methyl mercury, and diethylene glycol dimethyl ether. As yet, scientific attempts to define special MAK/TLVs for pregnant women have not been successful for any of the fetotoxic substances.

Some chemicals may irreversibly influence male fertility, the most prominent substance being dibromochloropropane (DBCP). DBCP was used in agriculture to kill roundworms and was found to cause infertility in male workers who applied it. Others are DDT and ethylene glycol monomethyl ether. Various substances, either from natural sources or industrial chemicals, exhibit hormonal activities, so-called xenoestrogens, e.g., polychlorinated biphenyls or bisphenol-A (also known as biphenyl-A, a monomer used in the manufacture of epoxy resins and polycarbonate) and some persistent organochlorine pesticides.

Occupational Toxicology in the Chemical Industry

The chemical industry offers a good example of the application of the principles of hazard control and management outlined in Chapters 2, and 12.

Exposure Reduction The protection of workers' health from adverse effects of raw materials, intermediates, or products is based on three principles that must be applied hierarchically according to feasibility: (1) substitution of toxic substances with less hazardous ones, as available; (2) introduction of technical measures to prevent contact with hazardous substances; and (3) use of personal protective equipment.

Replacement of hazardous substance. The first and most effective way to prevent adverse effects due to a chemical is by substituting it with a different, less hazardous material. This has occurred in the past with many substances, especially carcinogens. Examples for such replacements are asbestos (by glass wool, rock wool, etc.), benzene (by other organic solvents), and n-hexane (by iso-hexane).

The limitations of this strategy include a lack of available alternatives, technical requirements, and sometimes economic considerations. The decision to abandon the use of a given chemical should always be based on a prior risk-benefit analysis. This includes an assessment of the potential risks associated with the availability of a substance or product and the hazards inherent to the intended substitute, which may be less well understood due to a lack of research and experience.

Safe production measures. The second priority is to control and minimize exposure. Reduction of workplace exposures is a crucial step in the planning of modern production and processing units. In past decades, considerable progress has been made in the reconstruction of production units with the aim of achieving closed systems where the operating staff has virtually no contact with hazardous products or intermediates. Thus, even highly toxic substances, which are nevertheless technically irreplaceable (e.g., chlorine, cyanide, many monomers), can be used safely in the production of many products of everyday life (e.g., plastics, medications). In general, engineering control strategies have led to a marked reduction in exposures that can be measured not only at workplaces but also in surveys of background exposures for the general population.

Personal protective equipment. If sufficient exposure control is not technically achievable, the use of personal protective equipment is necessary. It must be selected after assessing workplace health risks. Additional workplace characteristics such as heat, light, confined space, and the individual worker's state of health have to be taken into consideration when deciding the appropriateness and feasibility of certain protective measures. Furthermore, it must be ensured that the use of the equipment not only protects against the identified risk, but also does not impose an additional risk of its own. The employees have to be aware of the risks to be prevented and trained in the use of the protective device. In several countries, protective devices are legally categorized with respect to the risks they protect against (e.g., minor hazards such as dirt; medium hazards such as irritation, noise, bruises; major hazards with irreversible or deadly effects), and different quality standards are set for the approval of these devices. Providing employees unapproved protective devices would be considered unlawful and eventually lead to liability claims.

Surveillance

Where relevant health risks cannot be confidently reduced or eliminated, surveillance measures that can be targeted to exposures as well as to health effects are mandatory.

Air monitoring. Exposure to chemicals is usually assessed by air monitoring. Stationary devices can continuously monitor workplaces or be placed in the vicinity of potential sources of contaminants, such as chemical reactors, hazardous material stores, etc. Personal air sampling in the worker's breathing zone is more appropriate for individual exposure assessment, as those results reflect individual characteristics such as height, working position, varying distance from the source of exposure due to the physical movement of employees in carrying out required daily tasks.

Air monitoring has some limitations. First, the sample collection enables only an estimation of the mean exposure during the time of observation (e.g., a work shift). This may lead to an underestimation of potentially harmful peak exposures that could be particularly important in the development of sensitization or neurotoxicity outcomes for some chemicals. However, with adequate technical equipment, air monitoring may reveal peak exposures occurring during particular jobs or tasks. Second, the method neglects routes of exposure other than inhalation, such as dermal absorption and ingestion of particles. Third, factors such as physical workload and body fat content may alter the uptake and retention of inhaled chemicals.

Biological monitoring. Biomonitoring can determine the body burden of a chemical. Either the unchanged chemical or its metabolites are measured in body fluids (blood or urine), fat, or exhaled air. Given sufficient knowledge about the distribution, metabolism, and routes of excretion of the chemical in question, the results of biomonitoring yield additional information beyond ambient air monitoring. For example, determining alkoxy-acetic acids in urine reflects not only inhalational exposure to glycolethers but dermal exposure as well.

Recent advances in biomonitoring are aimed at measuring not merely the body burden of a substance, but its effects as well. Such biomarkers could be early indicators of biologically relevant effects before signs of overt toxicity appear. The measurement of adducts formed at hemoglobin, DNA, or other relevant biological structures has been introduced as a step toward effect monitoring. However, because the sites of these adducts may not match the target organs of toxicity, adduct monitoring must still be considered a type of exposure, rather than effect, monitoring.

Standards and Guidelines for Exposure Control

TLVs are maximal airborne concentrations of substances in the workplace to which workers may be repeatedly exposed for a definite time period without adverse health effects. Well-known examples are the German MAK-values (maximum concentration values in the workplace) and the respective TLV-TWAs created in the United States as time-weighted average concentrations for a conventional 8-hour workday and a 40-hour workweek. Short-time exposure limits (STELs) are used to control the frequency and extent of peak exposures. They are usually limited to the two- to four-fold TLV and may not last longer than 15 minutes.

For substances with the potential for skin absorption, TLVs usually provide no protection. Here, the significance of exposure is assessed by comparing biomonitoring data with a biological exposure index (BEI) (*biologischer Arbeitsstoff-Toleranzwert* [BAT]) as described above.

The most valuable data for setting such occupational exposure limits would be obtained from epidemiological or industrial toxicology studies carried out under conditions comparable to those for which the recommendation is intended. However, even TLVs or BEIs based on such nearly optimal conditions cannot be considered predictive for the whole working population because there may always be some workers hyper-susceptible to specific substances who might show health effects at or below the generally well-tolerated TLVs.

If the above-mentioned data are not available, human exposure data obtained with the desired substance might be extrapolated to define a threshold value.

Another possibility would be to rely on data of a substance with similar chemical, physical, and toxicological properties selected on the basis of structure-activity relationships. However, in many cases, human toxicology data for determining threshold values are nonexistent. Thus, in practice, relevant parts of the TLV-setting process often rely on data from animal studies.

ENVIRONMENTAL PROTECTION

Sustainable Development

The use of renewable natural resources must account for the system's capacity to regenerate in order to avoid depletion. Some nonrenewable resources have to be left for future generations. This vision of sustainable development is not being achieved in our modern society. However, during recent decades, the idea of environmental protection has gained a broad acceptance in our societies, including industry. In its study entitled *Limits to Growth* (1972, updated 2004), the Club of Rome (an influential global think tank) pointed out that human activity must make due allowance for the limited availability of natural resources. The guiding theme of sustainable development is a logical extension of this principle.

At the United Nations Conference on the Environment and Development in Rio de Janeiro in 1992, this principle was adopted as binding among the community of nations. The aim is to satisfy the economic, ecological, and social needs of our society without jeopardizing the development prospects of future generations. Today, in most countries, industrial impacts on the environment through emissions into the air, water, and soil are regulated by national laws and international treaties. Furthermore, industries make voluntary commitments beyond legal requirements. This has led to remarkable and demonstrable reductions in environmental pollution in many heavily industrialized regions during the last few years. Nevertheless, it is undisputable that in many parts of the world there is still an urgent need for protective action. Here globalization may provide a chance to prevent developing countries from repeating the mistakes that the "first world" committed during the period of industrialization.

Responsible Care Product Stewardship

Responsible Care® is a worldwide initiative of the chemical industry. It consists of the participating companies' voluntary public commitment to safety, health, and environmental protection. Depending on the support of the management boards, concrete achievements under the framework of Responsible Care® require the participation of all employees within all their activities, from research and manufacturing to sales and distribution. Responsible Care® involves a wide array of different tasks that include environmental conservation; industrial health and safety; prevention of accidental releases; emergency response programs; dialogue with the public, authorities, neighbors, and scientists; and product stewardship. Product stewardship is defined as the responsible and ethical management of the health, safety, and environmental aspects of a product throughout its life cycle. Thus, it comprises the initial concept and design of a product as well as research and development, manufacturing, storage, distribution, applications, foreseeable use, recycling, and disposal. Beyond the producers' employees themselves, suppliers of raw materials, contractors, carriers, and customers have to be involved in order to minimize the potential adverse impact of products.

Special Concepts of Health Surveillance in the Chemical Industry

General Health Surveillance Regular medical surveillance in modern working environments can be instrumental in recognizing occupational health effects. To provide a high standard of occupational health and safety, health evaluations for employees in factories have been a longstanding practice. This tradition started as early as 1866 in BASF Aktiengesellschaft, Germany, with the hiring of a plant physician for the 130 workers employed at that time.

Occupational medical surveillance is regularly provided in many countries, at least in the larger companies, although not necessarily for the multitude of workers in small firms. In 1985, the International Labour Organization issued recommendations on occupational health services that as of 2001 had been ratified by only 20 of its 150 member states. In several countries, occupational health services are legally required, with a trend to include all workers, irrespective of the size of the employing company or the type of industry. In an effort to standardize different national legislation on this topic, the European Commission passed the framework Directive 89/391 in 1989. This directive clearly stated the employer's responsibility, both for health and safety at work and for the provision of an occupational health service.

Special Concepts and Best Practice Guidelines A body of regulations exists in several countries regarding the type and extent of occupational medical surveillance of workers, which is mandatory for all employed persons exposed to certain hazardous materials. In Germany, these are the *Berufsgenossenschaftliche Grundsätze* issued by the Employment Accident Insurance Fund (*Berufsgenossenschaft*). These regulations cover 45 physical or chemical exposures, workplace conditions, and specific endpoints that are particularly relevant for the occurrence of work-related diseases. Some of these exposures, such as β-naphthylamine, vinyl chloride, or asbestos, are no longer used in developed countries. However, they are still associated with the majority of occupationally induced cancers in the chemical industry due to the long latency periods in carcinogenesis. Thus, occupational medical surveillance serves not only to prevent new disease, but also to identify and reduce adverse effects of past exposures.

ELECTRONICS

The modern electronics industry is the result of advances in physics and inorganic chemistry since 1948. In the last four decades, the industry has transformed itself several times over with advances in basic science, technology, product design, and especially information technology. Because the occupational hazards of software development and product design are not noteworthy for occupational hazards, this section will emphasize production in the microelectronics industry.

The industry includes many sub-industries manufacturing peripherals and accessory equipment, producing software, and operating telecommunications. The more characteristic toxic hazards are found in the microelectronics segment of the industry, particularly silicon chip manufacturing.

When it was first introduced, the microelectronics industry was hailed as a highly desirable clean and safe industry to be located near residential communities. Within 10 to 15 years, however, cases emerged of serious environmental pollution and occupational health problems. Such an experience is not unusual for industries just starting up, and the microelectronics industry has, to its credit, responded through organizations such as the Semiconductor Safety Association. Today, the industry remains highly sought after by local communities, but it is much more highly regulated and monitored.

The clean image of microelectronics results from the meticulous preparation required in the production of chips and microscopic integrated circuits, which can be completely spoiled by tiny specks of dust. As a result, chips and semiconductors are manufactured in "clean rooms" and employees wear clean overalls (often called "bunny suits") to protect the product. These measures provide no personal protection against toxic gases or spills, however.

The principles and function of microelectronic components are far beyond the scope of this discussion, but a brief description is required to understand the occupational health implications. Chips are miniaturized circuit systems that replace entire boards of electrical wiring; they look like small rectangles only millimeters in size. They exist in the form of solid blocks but consist of a complexly organized

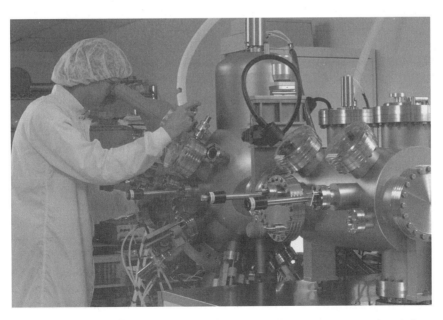

Figure 19.1 Electronics and semiconductor manufacturing has a variety of toxic hazards. This device coats silicone chips with gallium arsenide, an arsenic compound. (Photograph by Chris Rogers, iStockphoto.)

array of electrically conductive pathways controlled by semiconductor regions constructed into the structure of the chip. They are constructed layer by layer, with photographic duplication of the circuit diagram on a microscopic level creating an image or mask, called the "photoresist," that is etched to outline the circuit. Semiconductor regions are created within the structure of the chip by treating it with "dopants," controlled levels of impurities; these regions are the size of micrometers and are layered on top of one another, separated by the insulating base material of the chip. Silicon is by far the most heavily used substrate for chip production; it must be immaculately pure. The chip is produced from silicon metal by layering it over the substrate with other substances that are then sandwiched between layers of silicon, deposited from silane (SiH_4) or silicon halides. The production of other devices involves gallium arsenide (for light-emitting diodes) and germanium.

Physical hazards in the microelectronics industry include ionizing radiation and electromagnetic fields. However, the most common physical problems are probably ergonomic in origin—arising from the assembly, packaging, and shipping of product. Repetitive strain injuries are also reported to be a problem in the industry.

Chemical hazards in the microelectronics industry are varied and often exotic. Potentially significant exposures that are commonly encountered include arsine, boron trifluoride, boron trichloride, chlorine, dichlorosilane, germane, hydrogen chloride, hydrogen fluoride, oxides of nitrogen, nitrogen trifluoride, phosphine, phosphorus, silane, silicon tetrachloride, and silicon tetrafluoride. The list of metals that can be used as dopants reads like the periodic table of the elements, but prominent among them are arsenic, antimony, gallium, and germanium, usually in the form of their oxides; the list of non-metal dopants is more restricted but includes phosphorus and boron compounds. With the exception of silicon hexafluoride, which is also encountered in the power industry for high-tension switching mechanisms, these chemicals are virtually unique to this industry. All are potentially toxic; several (including arsenic pentafluoride, arsine, diborane, diethyltelluride, germane, and phosphine) are among the most toxic compounds in common use in industry. Many are very poorly characterized toxicologically, and several have no established occupational exposure levels in the United States or Canada. The industry also uses a number of inert gases and chloro- and fluorohydrocarbons of less toxicological concern, although their decomposition products may be toxic. A great deal of hydrogen is used in the production of extremely pure silicon from silicon halides and silane; hydrogen and silane both present a substantial hazard of fire and explosion. Organic solvents are heavily used at various stages in the process. Unusual photosensitive organic compounds are used in the preparation of photoresist; several are suspect carcinogens or reproductive hazards.

Metals used in the doping process range from the common to the highly exotic. Even the common metals are used in the form of unusual and often highly toxic compounds. The hazards of arsenic and its oxides are well known: it is a highly toxic metal that causes systemic toxicity, peripheral neuropathy, anemia, skin changes, and cancer. Arsine (AsH_3) is one of the most toxic gases known and produces an acute and usually lethal hemolytic anemia on inhalation. Antimony is similar to arsenic in its toxicity and is a suspected carcinogen; the toxicity of stibine (SbH_3) is similar to that of arsine. Gallium and germanium are not well characterized toxicologically, but their compounds are associated with irritant effects such as dermatitis, renal failure (gallium), and hematological effects. Germane gas (GeH_4) is hemolytic, similar to arsine and stibine; neurotoxic effects have been suggested.

Phosphorus compounds are highly toxic in a variety of ways. Phosphine, an unwanted by-product of the process, may induce acute pulmonary edema or more subacute central nervous system, cardiac, and hepatic toxicity. The toxicology of phosphine is not well understood despite its extensive use as a fumigant. Boron itself is relatively nontoxic (although there is a suspicion of association with infertility), but its compounds—boric acid (H_3BO_3), the boranes, and boron halides—are highly toxic with neurotoxicity and irritant effects.

Hydrofluoric acid is a common and serious chemical hazard shared with certain other industries, including biotechnology, geological and mineralogical research, oil well drilling, and glass etching. In the microelectronics industry, it is used to etch the surface of the chip. It is a highly corrosive, deeply penetrating acid that causes severe tissue necrosis by binding intracellular calcium due to its acidic character (which, paradoxically, is relatively weak in the dilute forms in which it is normally used, although these dilute forms can still cause extensive injury). On skin, it penetrates rapidly and deeply but preserves the appearance of normal skin so that the extent of tissue damage is often not visible for hours or days. The onset of pain is typically delayed by some hours. There are several highly specific measures that should be taken with hydrofluoric acid burns, and physicians who may encounter them should be prepared in advance, as timely treatment is essential to minimize tissue loss and scarring. This means that the specific treatment (calcium gluconate gels and injectable solution) must be on hand in advance and readily available. Once acute measures are begun, physicians unfamiliar with these injuries should immediately seek knowledgeable consultation. Severe exposures are serious medical emergencies and may require extreme interventions, including in-hospital monitoring for systemic toxicity due to fluorosis and pulmonary edema following inhalation. Experienced medical consultation should be sought for all hydrogen fluoride exposures.

Given the nature and level of potential exposure to toxic substances in the industry, it is not surprising that the risk of cancer, reproductive effects, and other occupational disorders would be of concern. To date, however, there have been few studies of the health experience of workers in the microelectronics industry. The risk of systemic toxicity and dermatitis appear to be better documented.

ENERGY TECHNOLOGIES

Energy is a product, a commodity, and a necessary resource. Reliable supplies of energy are needed to power industrial activity, transportation, home cooking and heating, and communications. The cost of energy is a major factor in economic growth and development and influences technology. Energy sources on a large scale can be broadly classified among the following:

- combustible nonrenewable fuels (oil, natural gas, coal, peat, and oil sands) that were created millions of years ago ("fossil fuels")
- combustible renewable sources or biomass fuels (wood, charcoal, animal dung) that were created recently ("biomass fuels")
- hydroelectric (using dams and waterfalls to generate electricity)
- alternative (wind power, solar energy, geothermal, photovoltaic)

Of these principal types of fuels, oil is the most heavily consumed, traded, and extracted, representing 34% of the world's energy supply in 2009 (all figures reported by the International Energy Agency 2009). Coal is next, at 42%, followed by natural gas at 20.7%, renewables and combustible waste at 2.5%, nuclear at 6.8%, hydroelectric generation of electricity at 16%. There is great variation around the world. For example, Russia has huge coal, oil, and gas reserves. Japan has little of each. France has many nuclear reactors generating electricity, while the United States and Canada have many hydroelectric dams.

Energy use correlates with economic development. In 1999, countries of the Organization for Economic Cooperation and Development (OECD), with a combined population of 1.1 billion, consumed slightly under a third of the world's energy, three times as much as China, with a population of 1.3 billion. China is today the world's largest consumer of total energy, and of energy from coal, renewable sources, and biomass.

Energy is converted from one form to another. Falling water pushes a turbine that generates electricity. Heat from a furnace may be used for heating a building, a process known as *cogeneration*. Synthetic fuels may be made from other fuels, such as liquefied coal, which closely resembles crude oil and is easier to transport than coal itself.

Historically, the major energy industries have each had very different occupational health problems. Technologies that are relatively small in scale at present, such as solar energy, photovoltaic, or wind power generation, are beyond the scope of this chapter. Energy industries also present environmental challenges. Global ecological changes, such as the accumulation of carbon dioxide resulting in the "greenhouse effect" with heat retention and climatic changes, are not considered here, only because the focus in on occupational health.

Coal

Coal is by far the most widespread fuel worldwide. Most coal is consumed locally. It was once on the decline worldwide because cleaner fuels are more readily available but is now rapidly increasing its share of world energy consumption.

Coal is mostly broken-down vegetable matter that has been turned from peat (a loose form of compacted organic matter) into a rock-like mineral. Millions of years ago, forests on the surface of the earth grew and died and left behind their organic remains. When the organic material was compacted underground, it transformed into coal. There are three types or "ranks" of coal, which in decreasing order of density and economic value are anthracite, bituminous, and lignite, which is barely denser than dried peat. Anthracite is used mostly for steelmaking and heavy industry; bituminous is used for heating and power generation; and lignite is mostly used for power generation. (Peat, where it exists, is usually burned as biomass in homes.)

Coal is composed mostly of elemental carbon with small quantities of minerals, sulfur, water, and metals. Coal also has some quartz in it, but how much depends on where the coal is mined. To dig coal underground, miners must go through rock layers, and this also exposes workers to quartz dust or silica.

Underground coal mining has been, with logging, among the most hazardous of industries. There are many safety hazards in the normal operation of a mine, ranging from drilling and reinforcing the mine shaft, cutting the coal from out between rock layers, explosions to loosen up coal seams, flooding (when the mine is below water level, water seeps in and has to be pumped out), high temperatures (in deep mines), and often electrical and diesel vehicles underground. There are many things that can go wrong and limited ways to escape. The fatality rate among coal miners varies from country to country and with the characteristics of the mine. Common problems include roof-falls (when the rock above a mine shaft starts to give way and rocks begin to fall), cave-ins (when the rock above a mine shaft drops down into the mine), explosions (when methane is released), fires and accumulation of toxic gases, and sometimes low oxygen levels.

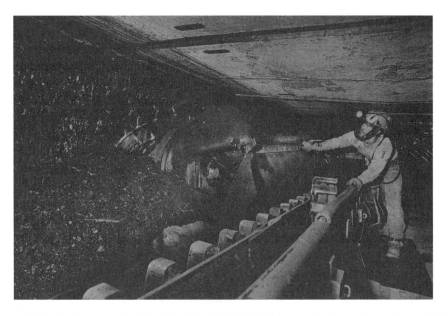

Figure 19.2 Coal mining in West Virginia (USA) is highly mechanized. A machine called a *continuous miner* digs out the coal from between layers of rock, and the coal is then brought out of the mine by a conveyor belt. Historically, coal mines have had many serious hazards, both for injury and for occupational disease, mostly coal workers' pneumoconiosis resulting from inhalation of dust. Note that this miner is wearing face protection and a light on his hard hat (helmet) and that the ceiling (called the "roof") is reinforced to prevent rock from caving in. (Photograph by © Earl Dotter, all rights reserved.)

The major health hazard of underground coal miners has been the inhalation of coal dust. Coal miners historically have been at risk for at least three serious lung diseases: complicated coal workers' pneumoconiosis resulting from exposure to coal dust; silicosis resulting from exposure to quartz dust by rock drilling and tunneling; and tuberculosis, common in disadvantaged coal mining regions and made worse by silicosis. Coal workers' pneumoconiosis, widely known as "black lung," is the characteristic occupational disease of coal miners.

Surface mining is safer for the miner than underground mining but often does more environmental damage. Surface miners are not at great risk for coal workers' pneumoconiosis.

Petroleum

Petroleum, or crude oil, is the most heavily consumed form of energy. The cost and occupational risks of oil production are rising sharply as easy reserves are depleted. It provides gasoline for transportation and heating oil and a variety of non-energy products such as lubricating oil and chemicals from which plastics are made. The petroleum (and gas) industry is divided into two major segments, the "upstream" (drilling, well servicing, pumping, maintaining collecting systems) and the "downstream" (refining, product manufacturing, marketing).

The upstream segment is relatively small in terms of number of people employed, and the hazards are mostly physical. Oil wells are like hazardous construction sites, and the oil that comes up is often under great pressure. Well blowouts can be dramatic and dangerous. Fire is an ever-present threat. A toxic gas, hydrogen sulfide, is a serious problem in some fields. Oil and gas wells are often located in remote areas, including offshore platforms; therefore, access to medical care may be difficult in an emergency. The single greatest hazard in the upstream industry, however, is injury due to motor vehicle incidents, because servicing wells and conducting exploration activities to find oil and gas often involve long distances in rough terrain.

The downstream segment of the industry is larger and more likely to present opportunities for chemical exposure. Small pinhole pipeline leaks are common, but large leaks that allow significant amounts of oil or gas to escape are rare. Shut-off devices, responding to reductions in pressure inside the pipeline, generally limit the damage.

Refineries are usually very large chemical plants that distill petroleum products in tall, pressurized towers. These include lighter products such as gasoline and diesel fuel, heavier products such as kerosene and jet fuel, heavy products such as fuel oil for heating, and asphalt, which is the tarry substance left behind. Refineries present a number of physical hazards involving fire and explosion, chemical hazards (mostly benzene and hydrogen sulfide), and hazards associated with maintenance and modifying equipment (particularly involving confined spaces, or chemical hazards such as hydrofluoric acid). Because of these risks and the potential for catastrophic incidents, occupational hygiene and safety procedures at refineries are usually well developed.

Although a variety of hydrocarbon products produced from petroleum have specific toxic effects, the toxicity of crude petroleum is relatively low. A large

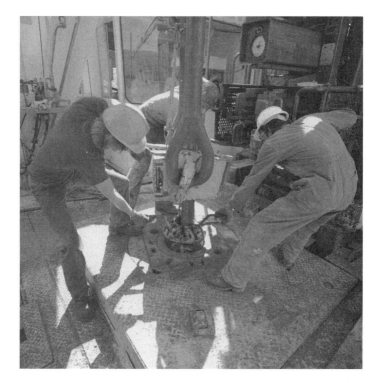

Figure 19.3 Roustabouts are laborers who handle drilling operations and pipe on an oil well. They are often at risk of serious injury and frequently work under hazardous conditions in extreme climates or offshore. (Photograph by Westphalia, iStockphoto.)

variety of chemicals are used in the production of petroleum, however. Changes in procedures and exposures over time make it difficult to link exposure to specific procedures or chemicals with health outcomes data.

Natural Gas

Natural gas is becoming more important because of concerns over climate change. It is primarily used for heating, generating electricity, and industry. Due to its chemical structure, it produces less carbon dioxide for the energy it produces than any other fossil fuel. Natural gas is found at various locations around the world, including North America, Russia, the North Sea, and the Middle East. A major problem with natural gas throughout history has been getting it to market. Natural gas is more difficult to handle than petroleum. It has to be compressed and then pumped through pipelines or refrigerated and moved as a liquid. Recently the discovery and aggressive exploitation of "shale gas" (natural gas found in deep shale beds) has opened new sources of gas in North America, Europe, and Asia closer to major markets.

Gas operations present many of the same problems as oil wells and pumping stations. Natural gas presents a constant fire hazard. Most of the hydrocarbon content in natural gas consists of short-chain alkanes, which are generally not toxic.

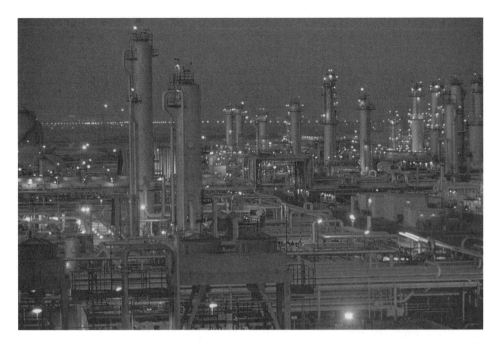

Figure 19.4 The oil refinery in Ras Tanura, Saudi Arabia, is one of the largest in the world. Refineries are basically elaborate plants for distillation of petroleum into lighter fractions, such as gasoline, and heavier fractions, such as kerosene, which are then sold or shipped as different products. Occupational health management has to be strict in a refinery because of hazards involving safety, fire, and toxic chemicals. (Photograph courtesy of Saudi Aramco World, SAWDIA.)

Sulfur-containing or "sour" gas deposits may release the highly toxic gas hydrogen sulfide when tapped. This has resulted in fatalities among gas workers in the upstream industry and occasional risks to nearby communities. Periodically, highly visible accidents have turned public attention toward the sour gas industry in particular, and this has sustained public pressure to assure safety and the protection of the environment.

Oil Shale and Oil Sands

Oil and gas in shales and sands were formed from organic matter in ancient oceans. These fossil fuels have a smaller share of world energy consumption and supply. Oil shale and oil sands contain large quantities of complex hydrocarbons embedded in a mineral deposit. Oil shale is a slate-like rock abundant in parts of Colorado, Utah, and Wyoming in the United States; Scotland; and Estonia. Although the potential for energy development is great, economic considerations have sidelined oil shale development because it costs too much to produce. Studies done in the past suggest that there may be a higher cancer risk from shale oil than other petroleum products. Oil sands are different geological formations in which the bitumen is locked in a sandy matrix which is easier to handle. Oil sands are soft deposits found in the United States, Siberia, and elsewhere, but exist in vast deposits near the surface in western Canada. The technology of extracting hydrocarbon from oil sands is in operation today. New methods of extracting the oil *in situ*, by liquefying it underground are being tested. The mineral is strip-mined and easily crushed. The sites where oil sands are mined and extracted do not appear to show unusually high rates of injury or disease, but a comprehensive study has not been performed. Shale gas, as noted, is natural gas trapped in the spaces within shale rock.

Nuclear Energy

Nuclear energy is an important source of electricity in some countries. Almost all large nuclear-generating capacity is located in OECD countries, but there are smaller-scale reactors in many developing countries.

All nuclear reactors work by generating heat from fission ("splitting") of unstable radioactive isotopes that are contained in fuel rods organized in structured "piles," in which intense fission activity occurs in a "core" by creating a chain reaction. Chain reactions occur when neutrons from the fission of one atom bombard other atoms, and their fissions in turn release many more. The generation of heat is controlled by managing the chain reaction, usually by physically moving pellets of uranium or inserting into the pile materials that absorb neutrons. Electricity is produced by heating water or other substances to create steam, or its equivalent, which runs a turbine.

Older nuclear reactors were not well contained and did not have adequate backup mechanisms to prevent a chain reaction from going out of control, a situation often called "meltdown." Modern nuclear reactors are typically built with many backup systems and safety devices and are enclosed in a very strong structure designed to withstand an explosion from within and to contain any radioactivity that might leak out in an incident. The most modern reactors are designed to shut down and cool the core automatically, without operator effort, if anything goes seriously wrong. All of these designs share certain problems, however, including that of disposing of the used or "spent" fuel after it is mostly used up and is no longer efficient. The fuel is still highly radioactive and must be reprocessed to produce richer fuel from what remains in the old fuel, or stored until the radiation decays over tens or hundreds of years.

Health concerns associated with nuclear fission include short- and long-term environmental contamination associated with uncontrolled emissions during accidental release and the possibility of rare but catastrophic accidents. Such an accident occurred in 1986 when a Soviet reactor at Chernobyl, in Ukraine, experienced a meltdown and released radiation over Eastern Europe.

Nuclear workers in conventional power-generating reactors do not appear to be at high risk for occupational injuries or disease, including radiation-associated risks. Isolated incidents do occur, such as an uncontrolled chain reaction on a small scale that occurred at a reactor in Japan in 1997 that exposed several workers to high radiation. Workers in the nuclear industry may be at risk for chemical exposures that involve a toxicity hazard rather than radiation. For example, some workers in the nuclear industry in the United States were found to have had exposure to asbestos and to beryllium, a metal used in nuclear reactors that causes a lung disease and may cause cancer.

In response to considerable public skepticism over the safety of nuclear energy, the nuclear power industry has developed a new generation of prototype technology for improved and safer reactors, featuring passive systems that are designed to shut down and cool off in the event of a mishap. However, a major drawback to expanded use of nuclear energy is the problem of transporting and storing used fuel and radioactive waste. While many innovative technologies have been developed to store the highly radioactive waste of the industry safely and securely, each has problems, and none are universally accepted.

Proponents assert that safer reactor technology will permit expansion of nuclear power capacity at a level of risk acceptable to the public and to the degree required to offset global ecological disturbances resulting from fossil fuel combustion. Skeptics doubt that substitution of nuclear power for traditional sources could alleviate more than a nominal fraction of the greenhouse effect and point out that the problem of safe disposal of high-level nuclear waste and the decommissioning of obsolescent nuclear facilities has not been solved.

Nuclear fusion, a completely different nuclear technology from fission, remains a distant but intriguing possibility. Fusion energy involves the forced union of hydrogen atoms to create inert helium, a process that releases large amounts of energy but little radiation. Active research is underway in the United States and Russia to develop fusion as a viable energy source. Occupational health problems associated with fusion are expected to be similar to other large industrial processes. Environmental health effects and catastrophic effects are thought to be highly unlikely with this technology.

Electricity Generation

Large-scale generation of electricity worldwide is primarily produced by hydroelectric and thermal power. Increasingly, electricity is also being produced by "alternative" technologies such as wind power and geothermal wells, but the bulk of electricity worldwide is produced by conventional (thermal) power plants, hydroelectric dams, and nuclear reactors in some countries, such as France.

Thermal power depends on the production of heat through the combustion of fossil fuels or through nuclear fission. Traditionally, the thermal power industry has not been considered high risk for occupational health problems compared to other industries. It is not clear that this situation will continue, however. Industries in most sectors of the economy have substantially improved their occupational health and safety performance in recent years. By comparison, the thermal power industry no longer appears to be so favorably positioned. Today, industries and individual companies are expected to demonstrate their safety explicitly rather than relying on the absence of complaints and thus, the assumption of low risk.

The occupational hazards associated with hydroelectric power are the same as those of any large construction or industrial operation. Massive ecological changes resulting from dam building and flooding have made hydroelectric power increasingly controversial.

In the past, studies suggested a risk of cancer that appeared to be associated with the electromagnetic fields and residential household wiring. This finding stimulated much research, with the eventual conclusion that there is probably little or no actual risk.

Biomass Fuels

Biomass fuels are not practical for most industrial applications but are common household fuels in most of the developing world. Indoor air pollution associated with biomass fuels can lead to respiratory disease and even lung cancer, and in some countries it is a serious hazard for those working in the home.

METAL FABRICATION AND MANUFACTURING

Various manufacturing plants have different safety hazards and health risks; this depends more on the nature of the initial materials and on the manufacturing processes than on the final product. Common hazards encountered in metal fabrication involve falling objects, confined spaces, high temperatures, solvents, electrical current, and compressed gases; asbestos exposure may still be encountered in older plants. Shift work is common, and the industry often experiences cycles of high activity followed by layoffs. In this industry, more than in most others, it is necessary to examine the particular processes used and the experience of the particular subsector before drawing general conclusions.

Heavy Manufacturing

The operation of heavy equipment typically involves predictable safety hazards and noise exposure. The risk of injuries in the manufacturing sector is usually high, and the severity of the injuries is greater than in most other industries. There is obviously a great deal of difference between manufacturing an automobile engine and building a ship, but the hazards of metalworking tend to be similar.

Foundry casting is associated with an elevated risk of lung cancer, thought due to polycyclic hydrocarbons released from the mold (and binding compounds used to hold the sand together in the mold) during the pouring process and possibly to silica dust exposure. Casting into sand and subsequent removal of the casting from the fractured sand creates an opportunity for exposure to silica dust and for silicosis. The potential for burns from the molten metal is high because casting is not so easily automated as steelmaking; in the past, gloves were made of asbestos and presented a hazard of exposure to this dust. When the casting is removed from the mold, it is in rough form. Extra bits of metal from the pouring channel and air vents may be chipped away with an air hammer (a process known in England as "fettling") and this presents a hazard of vibration white finger disease. The casting may also be ground, presenting a hazard of flying metal sparks and shards, or sandblasted, presenting a risk of silicosis or abrasive pneumoconiosis. Occasionally, a grinding wheel may shatter, presenting a risk of severe injury from flying fragments.

Metal parts may require turning on a lathe or other forms of machining. Machining is associated historically with a risk of skin and lung cancer thought to be due to the spray of droplets of machine oil used for lubrication and cooling. Occupational dermatitis is also a common problem in machining operations for the same reason.

Pickling is a process of treating steel by immersion in acid baths; these can be highly irritating and present a hazard of chemical burns. Metal parts may also require degreasing in solvents (presenting a hazard of solvent exposure), galvanizing (presenting a risk of metal fume fever), metal plating or coating (sometimes presenting a risk of toxicity from nickel or chromates), and hardening (in some processes presenting a hazard of cyanide exposure).

Electroplating is a common industrial process requiring the preparation of the metal surface with solvents and degreasing agents, pickling, and immersion in an acidic plating solution. These solutions are very irritating and corrosive. Today, plating baths are usually enclosed and are ventilated, but in the past exposure levels were often very high in metal plating shops. Chromic acid solutions contain hexavalent chromate and are associated with an increased risk of lung cancer, as well as mucosal irritation and dermatitis (chromate burns are ulcers that are very slow to heal).

Assembly work is highly variable, depending on the product, but may pose a risk of repetitive strain injury, if the movements required are repetitive and fine, or of back injury or sprain, if the movements are awkward and weight bearing. These are fundamentally ergonomic problems (see Chapter 7). Some tools, such as air hammers and socket wrenches, may expose workers to vibration and the risk of vibration effects. Welding, and its attendant hazards, is a common process in assembly operations in heavy industry.

Shipyards

Shipbuilding is a special case of metal fabrication involving building a structure out of metal on site. In this respect, the relationship between shipbuilding and heavy metal fabrication is much like that between building construction and the manufacture of wood products.

Shipyards engage primarily in ship repair and alteration. Major repairs to the hull require a dry dock. The larger shipyards may engage in shipbuilding; this industry is increasingly dominated by South Korea because larger-capacity cargo and tanker ships cannot be accommodated by many North American shipyards. Ship breaking is the dismantling of a ship for scrap and is done by smaller operators, often in developing countries, sometimes under poor and even dangerous conditions. Shipyards are very hazardous workplaces, and occupational health and safety management has been a difficult challenge.

Ships present particular design problems that are reflected in their construction. They are subject to serious corrosion. Therefore, all metal surfaces must be stainless steel, brass, or painted steel. Ships have intrinsic problems maintaining temperature because they are floating metal objects sitting on an infinite heat sink in the form of deep water. They must therefore be extensively insulated. Ships must be wired for power and electrical control systems. In constructing a ship, there are many more activities occurring simultaneously than just metal fabrication, and shipyard workers are often exposed to hazards other than those primarily characteristic of their own work. The principal activities that go into constructing a ship include welding, painting, electrical wiring, insulation, and mechanical installation. Welders on a ship, for example, are exposed to their own welding emissions as well as particles from insulation materials, noise, solvents, and paint fumes generated by other workers in close proximity.

Physical hazards characteristic of shipyards include scaffolding and high-voltage electrical hazards as well as significant hazards of fire and explosion. Noise levels are often exceedingly high, making hearing protection essential. Because intensive industrial activity is carried out below deck and between bulkheads (interior walls on a ship), the potential for confined space incidents is very great. High levels of fumes and toxic gases may accumulate in spaces without adequate ventilation. Chemical hazards may include a variety of solvents, glycols, welding and burning fumes, and insulation materials. Historically, heavy exposure to asbestos has occurred among many shipyard workers.

The average life of a large ship is only a few decades. The ship usually passes through several owners as it gets older and less reliable. When it is no longer seaworthy, it is broken apart for salvage and scrap metal. Ship breaking is a particularly hazardous operation. In this part of the industry, intact ships are stripped of their fixtures and then cut apart for scrap or reassembly; this work has a high potential for serious occupational health and safety problems. Metal fume fever, lead toxicity, combusted paint fume accumulations in confined spaces, and other disorders are occasionally seen in ship breaking operations.

Light Manufacturing and Metal Forming

Light manufacturing may be associated with a number of hazards, depending on the materials that are used the process used to make the product. The hazards common to most light manufacturing industries are ergonomic in nature and are described in Chapter 7. Metal forming is a particularly common type of light manufacturing and so will be described in more detail.

The production of products from rolled sheet metal and wire involves some risk of injury, but usually the injuries sustained by workers who fabricate the metal parts are less severe than in heavy industry and tend to involve the hands, with a higher frequency of lacerations. Gloves are obviously required in such situations.

Certain processes of metal forming have particular hazards. Metal stamping is sometimes performed with a drop hammer or with hydraulic pistons using lead molds, because lead tends to "give" and thereby avoids the tearing that occurs in brittle metals (such as titanium) from being stamped. Lead dust is a hazard in such operations, particularly with drop hammers, which also produce impact noise.

The assembly of small metal parts may be associated with repetitive strain injury. Solvents and degreasing agents are often used in these industries, and if the parts are small, the concentrations in the breathing zone may be high when the worker leans over the work. Similarly, these parts must often be painted and coated, and this is often done by spray painting, introducing a hazard of solvent exposure.

Increasingly, metal and plastic composite materials are used in applications requiring low weight and high strength, as in the manufacture of airframes (aircraft bodies). These composites have been associated with dermatitis, and there

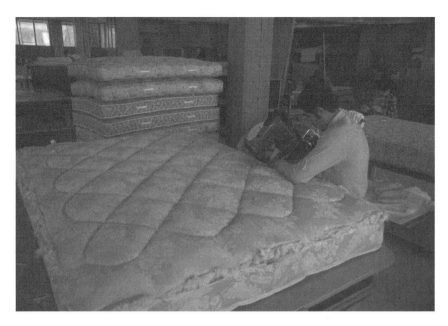

Figure 19.5 These workers are manufacturing mattresses in Lebanon. (Photograph by Khalil Abou El-Nasr, Saudi Aramco World/SAWDIA.)

has been some concern over the toxicity of their constituents, but to date these have not been extensively studied.

MINING AND SMELTING

Mining and smelting are often done in close proximity but usually involve different groups of workers. These industries have historically been associated with very high frequencies of occupational injuries and illnesses. While both industries have improved their performance in recent years, they should still be considered high risk.

Mining

Mining as an industry has probably been more influential than any other in shaping attitudes regarding occupational health. Historically, mining has been one of the most dangerous common occupations (the others being logging and commercial fishing). This largely reflects past conditions in underground mines, but the hazards of mining today remain substantial.

Mining operations can be divided for occupational health purposes into aboveground (or "surface") and underground. Aboveground operations are generally much safer and involve the same types of hazards as large construction projects and heavy industrial sites. Open-pit mines (mining by digging from the surface), auger mines (drilling into the side of a hill), and quarrying are examples of mining operations that are entirely above ground. Asbestos mines present the most serious hazards in aboveground mining. These mines are usually open-pit but involve exposure to asbestos fibers.

The most serious hazards involved in the mining industry are generally underground. Underground mining typically involves sinking a vertical shaft from which a horizontal corridor follows the underground stratum in which the mineral deposit of interest is located. The plane at which active mining is taking place is called the "face" of the mine. In coal mining, this follows a seam of coal pressed between rocks; in metals mining, this follows an ore deposit within the rock itself. The mineral deposit is removed by digging, drilling, and blasting with explosives. The ore is removed from the mine in small electric trains, wagonloads, or by conveyor belts. (Many years ago, miners often used small wagons pulled by donkeys or children.) In modern coal mines, a machine called a "continuous miner" chews away at the face of the coal seam, and the broken coal and rock is taken away by conveyor belt.

Tunneling and shoring are among the most hazardous processes in an underground mine. Whenever the mining passes through rock, particularly in drilling the shaft, creating tunnels, and through ore deposits, there is a potential risk of silica dust exposure. The hole that is dug out has to be reinforced to ensure that it does not collapse. The ceiling of the tunnel has to be reinforced with timbers, steel beams, or "roof bolts" (long retaining bolts screwed into the rock) to keep fractured rock from falling on the miners and to keep the tunnel from caving in. Many serious and often lethal mine accidents are the result of cave-ins, roof falls, or collapsing tunnels. Sometimes these incidents occur spontaneously, but they can also occur following mine explosions. They are particularly a problem when the rock is fractured.

The hazard of explosives is well recognized in mines. For safety, explosives that do not detonate easily are used in modern mines. These are typically packed in concentric circles and other patterns in holes drilled into the face and timed to explode so that the adjacent rock will be minimally disturbed, yet the interior of the pattern is reduced to rubble. The area of the mine in which the explosion is to occur is evacuated, and the miners do not return until the fumes have been blown out by the ventilation system. Early return to the face after explosion risks exposure to high levels of explosive combustion products (in the past, nitrogen dioxide was a common hazard) or depleted oxygen levels. The rock may be damaged following the explosion, making the roof potentially unstable.

Intentional mine explosions may misfire or cause unexpected safety problems. There is also a risk of unintentional explosions underground. These occur when there is methane gas ("firedamp") underground, usually released from the coal seam. Some mines and coal formations are said to be more "gassy" than others, reflecting the release of methane. High levels of coal dust are also explosive underground.

As the mineral is dug out, the corridor increases in length (and sometimes size) and must be structurally reinforced to prevent its collapse. The ceiling or roof of a mine corridor carries the weight of many tons of earth above it and may collapse easily, depending on the composition and fracturing of the rock stratum. Roof falls are among the most common and feared safety hazards. Thus, roofs are reinforced by the insertion of long steel bolts with plates at the near end called roof bolts. In coal mines, the fossilized remains of tree trunks are common just above the coal seam (a fossilized swamp); when undercut, these trunks tend to fragment and fall abruptly, sometimes causing fatal injuries.

Underground corridors or chambers may be very small, sometimes only high enough to crawl through, or huge, with interior space equal in size to a large house, especially in the case of salt mines (which are easily dug). Reduced lighting, the traffic of mine vehicles, and the many electrical cables and water drainage lines in a typical mine combine to present many of the same hazards as a busy manufacturing plant. Ventilation is supplied by large ducts, usually consisting of plastic and fabric on a wire frame. These ducts can contribute to high noise levels.

Mines of many types are at risk for flooding and may have high levels of radon daughters. Radon daughters are gaseous radionuclides (occurring from the disintegration of radium) that may be present from rock or carried in by underground streams. Radon daughters are a particular problem in uranium mines and are associated with an increased risk of lung cancer. Underground hazards that are particular problems for coal mines are (1) the accumulation of methane to levels that are explosive or that may cause asphyxiation; (2) coal seams that can, though rarely do, catch fire underground and may smolder for months or years, producing carbon monoxide in the oxygen-deprived atmosphere; and (3) coal dust associated with coal workers' pneumoconiosis ("black lung"), a problem brought largely under control by the suppression of dust in mines.

In hard-rock mines, the principal exposure risks tend to be associated with physical hazards, silica dust, and radon. The toxicity of the mineral being mined is not a major hazard until the ore is refined and smelted.

Primary Smelting

Nonferrous metals tend to occur together in ores, and the objective of the smelting process is to separate them from each other and from the rock in which they are contained. Ferrous (iron-bearing) ores are smelted more easily than nonferrous ores and typically do not have the other, more toxic heavy metals as major constituents. Most ferrous ores are smelted in a blast furnace to make steel (see Steel below).

Smelting is a complex industrial process with many opportunities for toxic exposure. Recent studies have reported an elevated risk for lung cancer and obstructive airways disease among smelter workers. There is also the possibility that smelting activity can affect non-worker residents of smelting communities from emissions and "tailings" (spent ore from which the mineral has been extracted).

Smelters may emit a large amount and wide variety of pollutants, among them cadmium, lead, arsenic, and sulfur oxides (with sulfide ores) unless tight controls are in operation. Sulfate and sulfide are associated with particulates of respirable particle size, and free sulfur dioxide (SO_2) is released, particularly from copper smelting, in which the ore itself is a sulfide. Reduced pulmonary function and symptoms of bronchial irritation have been reported in workers in copper smelting operations and have been related to SO_2 exposure.

Secondary Smelting

The recovery and recycling of lead from old automobile batteries and of copper from wiring and plumbing fixtures is a common small business frequently associated with junkyards and auto wrecking operations. Because these businesses tend to be small operations that operate sporadically as they receive shipments of raw material, they sometimes present occupational and environmental hazards. Lead emissions have been a serious problem with some secondary lead smelters. Recovery of copper from insulated wiring and other materials that include plastic can be complicated. Despite these problems, secondary smelters perform highly valuable functions by recycling resources. Their operation can be made safe with proper engineering controls, but they must be carefully managed.

Aluminum Reduction

Aluminum reduction is a particular smelting technology that differs greatly from other types of smelting. The essential features of aluminum reduction plants are massive electrolysis batteries that require enormous amounts of electricity; for this reason, aluminum reduction plants are almost always located near cheap sources of electricity, usually hydroelectric power plants.

The potential toxicity of aluminum itself does not appear to be a problem in aluminum reduction plants. The most characteristic exposure is to heat and volatile organic hydrocarbons in the vessels in which aluminum is produced, called "pots."

The electrolytic cells have electrodes coated with organic material. The cathode is lined with a thick layer of carbon, and the anode is coated with tar. Under conditions of operation, these become quite hot and release volatile hydrocarbons, including benz(a)pyrene. Fumes from these electrodes are irritating and can cause airway sensitivity called "potroom asthma." These fumes are thought to be responsible for the excess of lung cancer and bladder cancer reported among aluminum reduction workers. A less serious but cosmetically undesirable and sometimes anxiety-provoking finding among these workers is multiple telangiectases (often called "broken blood vessels"), possibly associated with the combined exposure to hydrocarbon (perhaps with photosensitivity playing a role) and to heat. Heat stress is also a common problem in workers in the potroom.

There is evidence for a possible excess risk of mortality from lymphoma among aluminum reduction workers.

PAPER AND PULP

The process of making paper on an industrial scale is one of separating individual vegetable fibers from wood, rags, or recycled paper, which makes the pulp, and reforming them into paper.

Wood consists of cellulose fiber and lignin, a form of biological glue. Lignin is brownish in color and darkens with age and exposure to light. Pulp and paper is therefore bleached chemically to make it whiter and more stable in light. Hardwoods make finer papers; certain types of softwood, such as aspen, are lighter than others and require less bleaching.

Although an increasing amount of paper is made by recycling existing paper stocks, especially newsprint, most new paper manufacturing requires large quantities of wood pulp. It is therefore common for the pulp and paper industry to be integrated with other forest products in the same firm or through local trade. For example, a sawmill may sell its chips to a pulp mill and its sawdust to a pressboard mill. However, most pulp mills still make pulp from new wood and must receive timber at the plant site. The hazards of this activity are similar to those mentioned below in the subsection on forest products.

Pulp and papermaking is a very old industry. Many plants are nearing obsolescence and consist of old-fashioned working environments that are difficult to bring to contemporary standards of safety. The more modern plants, however, are heavily automated and keep processes almost entirely enclosed; these plants often have very small workforces.

All pulp-making processes require the separation of individual cellular fibers by breaking down the chemical and mechanical bonds between the fibers and liquefying the lignin. The lignin becomes a mixture of complex organic compounds; residual lignin is also present in the pulp produced and in the water squeezed out of the pulp during papermaking. Because wood naturally has a high water content, the process of making paper actually results in a net gain in water, which must be cleaned up safely.

There are three major processes used in making pulp: sulfite, Kraft, and thermomechanical (TMP). The sulfite process, now largely obsolete, requires steeping the wood chips in a hot acidic solution of sodium bisulfite made from caustic soda and sulfur dioxide gas; this process has been associated historically with water and air pollution and foul odors. Hydrogen sulfide may be produced at hazardous levels.

The Kraft process, today by far the most common and still the standard for high-quality papers, involves digestion in a hot alkaline sulfate solution made by mixing sodium hydroxide and sodium sulfide. The digestion "liquor" is regenerated by burning the organic content derived from lignin and treating the recovered chemicals with calcium hydroxide. Therefore, the Kraft process tends to be more energy-efficient because it utilizes the considerable organic content of the lignin for heat, and this provides Kraft plants with a considerable economic advantage. A modification of this process used mainly for hardwoods uses soda ash (sodium carbonate) instead of sodium sulfide; the digestion occurs solely because of the alkaline reactions. Kraft plants virtually always bleach the pulp with chlorine or hypochlorite. The presence of chlorine results in the production of organochlorines (including dioxins) from the complex cyclic organic products in the residual lignin. These organochlorines are washed out in the water removed from the pulp and have been a source of effluent water pollution in rivers and lakes. Because of the bad reputation of the Kraft process for polluting, the industry has been making a concerted effort to control effluent and identify sources of chlorinated organic compounds (including dioxin) production. Uncontrolled release of chlorine and hydrogen sulfide (from digestion) may present a serious inhalation hazard. Mercaptans produced in the process may cause an odor problem.

The most recent pulp-making process is the thermomechanical process (TMP). A small amount of sulfite may be added to facilitate mechanical separation rather than to digest the wood (in which case the technology is called the "chemothermomechanical process," or CTMP). The wood chips (usually of smaller dimensions than in a Kraft mill) are fed with water through a mechanical device consisting of two grooved discs that tear the fibers apart from one another but do not shred them. During this process, they are also heated above boiling so that as steam is released the chip explosively expands, further separating the fibers. The TMP process leaves more lignin in the pulp, which must therefore be bleached more heavily to obtain a grade of paper comparable to the Kraft process. Bleaching with hydrogen peroxide or sodium hyposulfite avoids the production of organochlorines. TMP is very well-suited to the production of newsprint, and technical improvements have made it possible to produce increasingly finer grades of paper by this process. But at the present state of development, TMP-produced paper cannot match the highest-quality grades produced by the Kraft process. The technology has considerable environmental advantages in producing a more benign effluent but is not as energy-efficient as the Kraft process.

Pulp may be pressed to 10% water content and shipped to papermakers, or it may be used to make paper on site in a continuous process. The process of papermaking can be customized for the grade and type of paper desired. Fundamentally, however, this involves mixing the pulp with a quantity of water, settling it onto a screen, and removing water by suction, pressure, and heat. The paper is finished by pressing the surface between rollers for smoothness and applying a coating if needed for printing or display purposes. It is typically cut and packaged on site, in the case of writing papers, or shipped in huge rolls for printing. The occupational hazards associated with pulp and paper manufacturing are predominantly physical. These are typically very noisy plants, requiring strict compliance with hearing conservation and noise control programs. High temperatures and steam releases are serious hazards in the boiler and digester areas. Safety hazards are particularly significant when plants receive timber and chip their own wood; on the papermaking side, the complex and continuously operating papermaking machines have numerous rollers, pinch points, and exposed blades. Water puddles are common. Working conditions are often hot and humid. The plants generally hum with a constant vibration. When oxygen and hydrogen peroxide are used as bleaching agents, there is a potential for explosion and fire.

Chemical exposures include the hazard of uncontrolled chlorine leaks and toxic inhalation. Exposure to wood dust, lime, and other irritants in the front end of the process is associated with chronic sinusitis, a common complaint of workers exposed to wood dust. The same exposures to irritants and wood dust are also thought to be associated with an increased risk of nasopharyngeal cancer (see Wood below). An association with lung cancer has not been demonstrated, and its absence may be due to the relatively large particle size of the wood dust. The presence of sulfur compounds, especially in the sulfite and Kraft processes, provides the opportunity for exposure to hydrogen sulfide and sulfur dioxide. Chlorine gas leaks may result in potentially fatal toxic inhalation, but usually result in a severe acute bronchitis and eye irritation.

The characteristic occupational disorder in the pulp and paper industry is sinusitis; this may be closely related to the increased risk for nasopharyngeal cancer, although the latter is still a rare disease among these workers. There is also evidence for progressive impairment in respiratory function that may continue after cessation of exposure. This has been variously attributed to exposure to sulfur compounds and to chlorine. Recent evidence suggests an increased mortality from cardiovascular causes among pulp mill workers; the likely cause is not clear.

In the past, mercury compounds were used to control algae growth in effluent ponds from pulp mills. These are no longer used today. Some mills use bromine-containing compounds that may sensitize skin, causing allergies. Mercaptans (sulfur compounds that give off a foul odor) are also produced as by-products of the Kraft process and may sensitize skin. Generally, the most modern plants deal with their effluent by using current primary and secondary treatment methods before discharge.

PLASTICS AND RUBBER FABRICATION

Natural rubber is a natural polymer, consisting of linked, interconnected molecules of latex derived from rubber trees. Synthetic rubber duplicates this structure using synthetic materials, principally 1,3-butadiene. Plastics are polymers of smaller, synthetic chemicals, derived from petroleum. Plastics have become indispensable in modern life, and many varieties have been developed to exploit various desirable properties.

Plastics

Plastics are polymers, connected sequences of much smaller molecules called monomers, and come in two varieties, thermoplastics and thermosets. Thermoplastics are linear or branched polymers that can be repeatedly softened by heating and reworked; they include polyethylene, polyvinyl chloride, polystyrene, and polypropylene. Thermoplastics are typically produced by polymerizing the monomeric feedstock and supplying the manufacturer with bulk plastic material that is then heated and formed. Thermosets are cross-linked, creating much greater structural rigidity, resistance to heat, and bonding strength; they include epoxy resins, polyamides, polycarbonates, and polyurethanes. Thermosets must be created in place by combining the raw materials. The formation of polyurethane requires urea formaldehyde or isocyanates. Many chemicals are added to the plastic, depending on the purpose. These include colorants, antioxidants (to prevent cracking), isocyanates, metals, and hardeners. Glues and solvents may be used to fuse plastic parts.

The manufacture of thermoplastic products involves heating the plastic, which is usually provided in the form of small pellets or powder, and reforming it by extrusion (as in tubing), calendaring (rolling to form sheets), laminating, film casting (creating a thin layer of hot plastic on a drum than can be applied to paper), or molding (as in solid parts). A common physical hazard in these situations is heat from the plastics molding apparatus. Spills of hot plastic may cause burns and may adhere to burned skin.

As in all manufacturing industries, a common problem is back injuries from handling product and materials. Ergonomic problems are common because trimming and finishing operations are performed by hand.

The characteristic chemical hazards of the plastics industry are those of the monomeric (single unit) feedstock. Monomers are single, potentially toxic molecules. Polyvinyl chloride is made from vinyl chloride, which is associated at extremely high exposure levels with a bone disorder in the fingers (acroosteolysis) and a disorder of blood vessels in the hands (Raynaud's phenomenon), at high exposure levels with hepatitis and a rare form of liver cancer (angiosarcoma), and may be associated with cancers at different sites and possibly a form of arthritis-like autoimmune disease (mixed-connective tissue disease). Polystyrene is made from styrene, which is associated at high exposures with solvent toxicity effects, liver function abnormalities, and chronic central nervous system effects. Acrylonitrile is associated with adrenal toxicity (an uncommon outcome) and is a suspected liver and lung carcinogen. Because of these hazards, the manufacture of plastics is usually tightly controlled.

The polymer formed from the monomer is usually chemically unreactive and therefore nontoxic. In general, there is little monomer left in the plastic polymer (multiply-bonded molecules form the solid plastic) when it arrives for use at the plant. Monomer may be released when the polymer is heated or burned at high temperatures, but almost none persists into the final plastic product.

Solvents, epoxy resins, isocyanates, and dust are common problems in the plastics industry and are often associated with dermatitis. Epoxy resins and isocyanates can sensitize workers and cause allergies, which may be severe. Inhalation of dust from ground plastic such as polyvinyl chloride has been described as causing pneumoconiosis, but this is rare, apparently not progressive or severely restrictive, and probably occurs only with high exposures to dust.

Synthetic Rubber

Most synthetic rubbers are made from 1,3-butadiene monomer: polybutadiene alone, mixed polymers of styrene and butadiene, polyisoprene (methylbutadiene), or polychlorobutadiene (neoprene). Another important class of synthetic rubber is the polysulfides, made from ethylene dichloride (1,2-dichloroethane). Each polymer has particular desirable characteristics. Styrene-butadiene "rubber" is the most heavily produced and is primarily used in making tires.

The monomeric feedstock for polybutadiene, 1,3-butadiene, is a nonspecific irritant and a suspected human carcinogen on the basis of positive animal studies. Chloroprene is associated with central nervous system depression and hepatotoxicity and is suspected to be a human carcinogen on the basis of case reports. Ethylene dichloride is a strong irritant and hepatotoxin and known animal carcinogen; it is presumed to be a human carcinogen. These carcinogenic effects were only recently identified, and the industry is still responding with appropriate control measures.

Rubber Products

The rubber products industry has been dominated historically by the tire industry. Today, synthetic rubber is more commonly used than natural rubber.

Natural rubber, in the form of latex, or increasingly synthetic rubber, is compounded with carbon black, antioxidant compounds, coloring agents, and other ingredients intended to prolong useful life, increase strength, and prevent cracking. The rubber is then molded to make tires and cured or vulcanized, a heat treatment with sulfur that cross-links the rubber polymers and results in a stronger and more elastic material. Layers of rubber are laminated and finished by trimming and grinding. These processes typically take place in close proximity, and individual steps in the process are not easily isolated. Because of the vulcanization treatment, the rubber tire does not have the same tendency to induce allergy as latex itself, although allergic reactions may still result and are often associated with the sulfur compounds in tire rubber.

Ergonomic problems are common in the industry because of the hand trimming required. Chemical hazards are numerous and, despite extensive research, poorly characterized because of the many possible reactions and as yet uncharacterized products of heat treatment. The chemical exposure of greatest concern in the industry has been nitrosamines, which are known to be produced at certain steps in the tire-building process. Nitrosamines, as a class, are potent carcinogens. Workers in the rubber industry have been shown to have an excess of certain types of cancer, particularly lung and prostate, and this has been attributed to exposure to nitrosamines. The role of the nitrosamines as the agent responsible for the observed cancer excesses has never been confirmed.

STEEL

Steel is an alloy of iron and carbon made at very high temperatures in forced air, open hearth, or blast furnaces.

Gaseous emissions from the blast furnace can be lethal if not adequately controlled. Carbon monoxide is produced in the blast furnace, and potentially serious toxicity occurs if ventilation is inadequate. Particulate matter is associated with chronic "industrial" bronchitis among workers. The ash of coke ovens is of greater concern due to its content of potential carcinogens; there may be 1% benz(a) pyrene in such particles.

There is a substantial physical hazard from fires, explosions, and heat in steel mills. Flue dust fires may occur after cyclone separation or carbonaceous dust particles ignite. Metal fires from furnace processes may also oxidize or ignite explosively. The intense heat generated by the blast furnace produces intense infrared exposure that can burn. Hot steel is extremely dangerous, and direct contact with molten steel is, of course, usually fatal.

Coke oven fumes constitute a major occupational hazard and are associated with an excess risk of lung cancer among workers assigned to these batteries. Refractory brick (high-temperature-resistant "firebrick") has a high silica content. Particles from crumbling firebrick may aerosolize in the respiratory range and are a cause of silicosis in workers who rebuild blast furnaces. Asbestos has been used in heat shields and in various uses around the plant. The role of asbestos could be important in accounting for a reported cancer excess in a particular plant. Most of these hazards are now historical in developed countries. Steelmaking has adopted new "continuous" technologies that are cleaner.

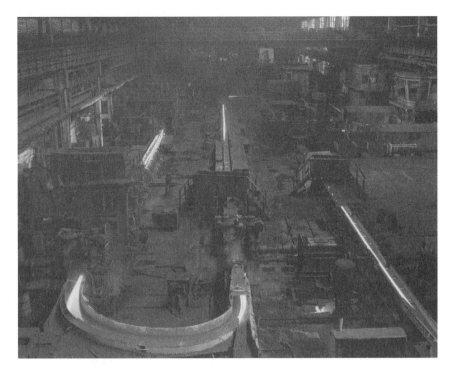

Figure 19.6 A continuous rolling steel mill in Ukraine, making pipe. (Photograph by Oleg Fedorenko, iStockphoto.)

Steelworkers, despite these considerable hazards, tend to be healthy and have overall cause-specific mortality rates substantially lower than the general population. Their causes of death are parallel to those of the general population, except that they have a disproportionate rate of accidents.

A large body of work has been accumulated on cancer mortality among steelworkers. It is now well established that workers in the coke ovens, who constitute a small fraction of steelworkers as a whole, are at high risk for lung cancer. This association is exposure and cumulative-dose related. There is a lesser excess of cancer of the rectum. There are highly suggestive, but not definitive, associations for cancer of the kidney (hypernephroma—an uncommon tumor) and bladder, and a possible association with cancer of the pancreas in workers associated with other, mostly finishing, processes. However, steelworkers in general historically have a lower mortality from cancer at all sites than the general population.

TRANSPORTATION

Transportation is a broad industry that includes commercial trucking, commercial passenger car services, automobile rentals, bus and van service, air transport, trains, metropolitan subway or light-rail train service, passenger and cargo ships, ferries, pipelines, and much more. Within this very diverse sector of industry, however, there are some common features. Almost all transportation modalities depend on an operator (who may be called a driver, captain, pilot, or other name depending on the mode of transportation) who must remain alert and in control at all times in order to ensure the safety of passengers and crew. All transportation equipment requires regular maintenance for safety and long use.

Many modes of transportation involve long distances and remote locations, such as cargo ships. This creates a requirement for emergency medical services for the crew and passengers and possibly a means of evacuation for life-threatening medical cases, as in the case of ships. Shipboard occupational health is a well-developed specialty within the field. Box 19.1 describes the risk of occupational injury in dockyard workers who handle cargo.

In the transportation industry generally, the major hazards to workers are associated with maintenance of the equipment (including solvents, exhaust from diesel engines, and physical hazards associated with injury), noise (a problem in almost all transportation subsectors), heat, and the ergonomic challenges of driving or operating equipment. The occupational health issues of individual drivers are discussed in Chapter 24.

However, the most critical occupational health concerns in transportation involve making certain that passengers and the general public are safe. Because of the obvious implications for public safety, governments generally require regular medical evaluations for drivers of vehicles used in commerce (long-haul trucks and buses and boats) and pilots. The U.S. Department of Transportation also requires urine drug testing for commercial drivers. Local governments sometimes add additional restrictions for drivers of ambulances, taxicabs, and transit buses. The intent of these evaluations is to detect early conditions that may interfere with safe performance, but they also serve as an opportunity for a relatively mobile group of workers to attend to medical problems before they get out of control.

A problem that frequently arises is the appropriateness of restrictions on drivers who have common illnesses, particularly epilepsy and diabetes. Studies of unselected civilian drivers have shown that the frequency of citations for speeding or unsafe driving is approximately the same among drivers with diabetes and epilepsy as for the general driving population, after adjusting for age. However, both groups were cited more often for violations involving alcohol or drugs (or similar impaired behavior which may have been mistaken for abuse) and for apparently careless (or otherwise affected) driving, particularly drivers with epilepsy. Both disease-affected groups showed higher rates of incidents involving personal injury and, to a lesser degree, property damage. As a consequence, uncontrolled diabetes and epilepsy are usually considered grounds for prohibiting commercial drivers from operating their vehicles. However, drivers with the conditions can safely drive when they are treated effectively and have a history of good control.

A central issue in the restriction of driving privileges is the degree of control the affected individual has over the condition. There is little disagreement that persons with frequent seizures or hypoglycemic events should not be driving or flying. Ordinarily, persons with epilepsy who have been free of seizures for long periods and those with diabetes who do not use insulin are not restricted from personal driving. Many employers do not allow either to drive on the job, however. In long-haul transport, the situation for the worker with epilepsy or diabetes is further complicated by disruptions in the cycle of meals and sleep, distance from sources of help in the event of an emergency, stress, and the effects of medications.

In common practice and on the weight of the evidence, it appears justified to suspend all driving privileges of individuals with uncontrolled diabetes or epilepsy or other conditions leading to unpredictable temporary incapacity; many jurisdictions have laws requiring that patients with such conditions be reported to the motor vehicles bureau. Brittle (insulin-dependent) diabetes and epilepsy with recent seizure activity should be considered a contraindication to driving on the job. Personal driving is a matter for state and provincial authorities, but the physician may be required by law to report such patients. Individuals with adult-onset diabetes under reasonable control and other chronic disorders should be evaluated with respect to fitness to work as outlined in Chapter 17.

BOX 19.1

Shipping and the Safety of Dock Workers in India: Improvements in the Past Decade

India has a long coastline that includes 163 ports. These ports not only provide employment for local residents but are a critical part of the economic infrastructure supplying goods to all Indians. The majority of workers are employed by the governing bodies of the ports (the "port trusts"), by dock labor boards, and by private businesses.

Cargo traffic in and out of these ports has increased over the years, leading to problems of safety, increasing injuries, and hence a revision of working procedures. The initial 1948 Indian Dock Labourers Regulation was limited in scope in that it provided safety only for workers employed on board or alongside ships, omitting workers in other areas of the port, such as warehouse workers. The 1961 Dock Workers Scheme addressed safety measures regarding all workers, including those not covered under the 1948 regulations.

The Directorate General Factory Advice Service and Labour Institutes (DGFASLI), a technical section of the Government of India's Ministry of Labour, enforces matters related to the health, safety, and welfare of workers employed in docks, ports, and factories. In addition, they are responsible for enforcing the Marking of Heavy Packages Act and the Manufacturing, Storage and Import of Hazardous Chemicals Rules. The role of the DGFASLI has been significant over the past decade in inspecting docks and ports, ensuring compliance with statutory requirements, investigating work-related accidents, recommending preventive measures, and assisting with advice on safety and health concerning port users and authorities.

Training and promoting activities in safety and conducting studies in the field of safety and health in the ports have become new objectives of inspectors, who are responsible for enforcing the acts.

Achievements of the DGFASLI have included:

- decreasing rate of accidents
- increasing safety awareness among workers through education and training
- mandatory use of personal protective equipment (PPE)
- appointing safety officers to carry out inspection of workplaces, cargo handling equipment, and facilities
- panels of doctors to conduct medical examinations of workers in all major ports
- testing and certification of ships' cargo by competent persons
- safety performance report of stevedores
- publication of safety manuals to convey technical information required by inspectors in performing their jobs

Despite these achievements, the incidence of fatal injuries is on the rise. Maintenance of a high safety and health level for dockworkers can be satisfactory only if the safety management system is restructured to meet the emerging challenges.

Adapted from: Nagarajan, P. 2001. "Occupational Health and Safety of Dock Workers: Strides Made by India in the Past Decade." *Asian-Pacific Newsletter on Occupational Health and Safety* 8(2):38–43.

WOOD PRODUCTS

Wood is a compacted mass of connected cellulose fibers glued together by lignin (see pulp and paper above). In the modern forest products industry, trees are cut, branches lopped off, and the trunks debarked before the trunk is fed into saws for production of lumber. Because trees vary considerably in dimensions, sawmills are often highly automated, and cuts are made that maximize the yield from each trunk. The green lumber is graded and dried in kilns. Some may be treated with preservatives for exposed, outdoor use. The chips and sawdust are usually collected and sold to pulp mills; sometimes chips are used to make fiberboard. The fabrication of wood products takes many forms, from manufacturing to carpentry to fine cabinetmaking. The common exposures are to wood dust, glues, and solvents associated with painting, paint stripping, and finishing.

Woodland Harvesting

Forestry practices have become very controversial because of public concern over the impact of logging on the environment (including erosion and disturbances of animal habitats), industry concern over the sustainability of yield from the remaining forests, disagreements over the practice of "clear-cutting" (logging entire swaths of forest non-selectively), and the wisdom of cutting virgin stands and old-growth forest. As a consequence, the logging and forest products industry has had to overcome considerable negative publicity and has attempted to do so by ambitious programs of reseeding and reforestation.

The cutting of trees, which is called *logging*, has always ranked among the most hazardous occupations. Logging as a subindustry tends to be dominated by small enterprises with all of the usual problems of limited resources they experience. In Canada, for example, it is usually performed by small teams employed by independent contractors who supply larger companies with wood on contract.

The most obvious and lethal hazard of logging is to be hit by a falling tree. When the final cut is made, local mechanical stress factors may make it difficult to predict where a tree will drop, although notches are cut to control the fall. Sometimes the trunk will split and twist. In dense growth, trees may deflect off or hang up in the branches of other trees, one reason why selective cutting is more difficult than clear-cutting.

To fell a large tree usually involves manual cutting with a chainsaw. The trunks and branches of trees in the forest may have grown to incorporate rocks, and human activity sometimes leaves fragments of metal embedded in the trunk. When chainsaws encounter these they may kick back or send the object flying. Chainsaws are also prone to kick or buck abruptly and can cause serious, sometimes fatal injuries. They are extremely noisy and produce flying chips, splinters, and dust. The vibration produced by chainsaws may cause vibration vasculitis (a potentially serious disorder of blood vessels in the hand and arm), especially with prolonged cutting and in circumstances of extreme cold. In recent years, new designs for chainsaws (particularly Canadian and Swedish models) have resulted in much-dampened vibration, diminished risk for vasculitis, and reduced noise levels.

Smaller trees can be cut by "mechanical tree-felling machines", which grasp the tree with a metal clamp and then cut the stem with a mechanized saw. These devices are very efficient and fast. The principal hazards involving their use involve the vehicle tipping over or flying chips or debris that are propelled around the machine. There is also concern that this practice could accelerate undesirable cutting and depletion of forest resources.

Logging crews should wear hearing protection, eye protection, gloves, and hardhats; the industry is formulating guidelines, but it has been difficult to enforce personal protection standards consistently because of the dispersed and remote nature of logging operations.

Removal of the cut trees from the site involves loading logging trucks, which frequently must negotiate narrow unpaved roads through forest with poor visibility. Complaints about the traffic hazard caused by logging trucks on highways and especially on logging roads are common in areas where this is a significant industry, but to date no economically viable alternative means of getting the wood out has been devised. In some areas logs are still floated down waterways. When they jam, the logs must be separated by hand by workers who walk out on the logs and pry them apart using long poles. In large log jams, this can be very dangerous.

Sawmills

Sawmills receive the tree trunks, remove the bark (debark) from them by machine, and feed them into saws that cut them to preset length and width dimensions designed to obtain the highest yield of desirable lumber. Older sawmills are crowded and busy workplaces, with workers constantly unjamming the machinery and correcting the placement of trunks that have failed to fall properly. Newer, more modern sawmills are heavily automated, with laser-controlled cutting and machine-readable marking of lumber grades. The most characteristic physical hazards of sawmills are the mechanical hazards and noise. There are innumerable pinch points, exposed blades, and drops or step-downs in a sawmill that require guards on the equipment and constant vigilance by workers. Sawmill injuries tend to be severe by comparison to other industries. Noise levels in sawmills can be extreme, well over 110 dBA; effective personal hearing protection is essential. Total body vibration is also constant but not often complained about.

The most characteristic exposure is to wood dust, a by-product of the sawing operations. This is discussed in detail below.

Wood Preservation

Wood for exposed outdoor or underground use must first be treated to prevent it from rotting, drying, cracking, and from attack by mold, insects, and other pests. In the past, this was done by soaking the lumber in creosote, a tar-like complex mixture of hydrocarbons, in large tanks. This material, similar to roofing tar, may

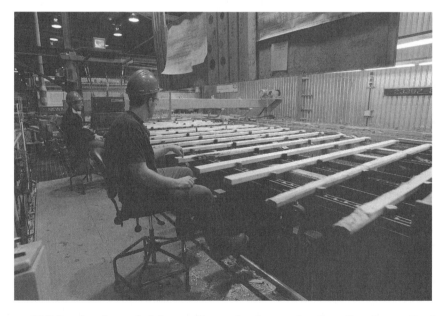

Figure 19.7 Lumber is graded for quality and price at the Canadian Forest Products (CANFOR) sawmill in Grande Prairie, Alberta (Canada). (Photograph by Greg Southam, *Edmonton Journal*.)

cause dermatitis and photosensitization on skin contact. Inappropriate disposal or spillage of creosote has caused serious environmental problems, and some old wood-preserving sites have contaminated groundwater that then migrates underground to rivers or is pumped up in wells.

Pentachlorophenol ("penta") and the other chlorophenates have largely replaced creosote as the preservative of choice, although chromate and copper compounds are used in some applications. Penta may undergo a chemical reaction under conditions of low-temperature combustion to produce large quantities of dioxins. These compounds have toxicological effects much like those of other chlorinated cyclic hydrocarbons and may induce chloracne; there is a suspicion of an association between occupational exposure to these agents and risk for soft-tissue sarcomas.

Personal protection to avoid skin contact and inhalation of wood preservative compounds is essential, as these are irritating and potentially toxic agents. Adequate ventilation is also essential, thus wood-preserving operations are always performed outdoors. Control of spills and collection and safe disposal of used or spent preservative is critical. Preserved wood should never be burned and should never be made available indiscriminately to the public without strong warnings that it should not be used in fireplaces. This has been a particular problem with old railroad ties. Old railroad ties are very popular for building gardens, but they should never be used inside homes or burned in fireplaces because they may release toxic chemicals.

Wood Products

Wood is a relatively soft material, and products made of whole wood are usually sawn, drilled, routed, planed, sanded, and otherwise finished. This produces wood dust with a size distribution determined by the hardness of the wood and the process being carried out (sawing, drilling, or sanding), respectively, producing increasingly fine dust. In general, the dust produced in these operations tends to be larger than dust in other industrial operations, so the particles tend to deposit in the upper rather than the lower respiratory tract, including the sinuses. There are pneumoconioses resulting from the inhalation of wood (and other organic) dusts and certain woods are important causes of occupational asthma. Some evidence suggests the possibility that airways reactivity and progressive airflow obstruction is associated with general wood dust exposure. An excess risk of lung cancer has been suggested. There is likely to be an association with the type of wood. Airways reactivity to a constituent of Western red cedar, a popular wood for interior paneling and trim in North America, is a well known condition with unusual features and can be severe in affected workers.

Several common woods are highly sensitizing and therefore are likely to cause allergies, particularly cedar, Western red cedar, mansonia (a substitute for walnut), redwood, rosewood, and teak. (Fortunately, pine is not highly sensitizing.) The antigens are mostly quinones and other complex aromatic chemicals impregnated in the wood. Sensitivity may be expressed as contact dermatitis, asthma (from inhaled wood dust), and even hypersensitivity alveolitis. Some woods may also contain irritants causing contact dermatitis, but this appears to be less common.

More characteristic of workers exposed to wood dust, however, are sinus problems. Chronic sinusitis is a common and persistent complaint of workers in many industries where exposure to wood dust occurs. A rare but characteristic association in occupations with exposure to wood dust is cancer of the nasal sinuses. It was previously believed that only adenocarcinoma was associated with wood dust exposure, but recent studies have also demonstrated an association for squamous cell carcinoma.

Many occupations involved in the fabrication of wood products also involve gluing, painting, and cleaning, with the potential for exposure to solvents. Construction may also involve exposure to other building materials and chemical hazards in the building trades.

In addition, wood product fabrication operations present fire risks. Wood dust suspended in air is extremely flammable and may explode with considerable force in a confined space. Maintenance to keep dust levels down, ventilation, storage of solvents in safe places, isolation of sources of ignition, a non-smoking policy, and adequate cooling on lathes and other rapidly turning machining devices can keep the risk of fire to a minimum.

Fiberboard and Plywood

Plywood is a layered sandwich of wood veneers bonded by glues. Fiberboard and chipboard are composite materials made of wood substance bonded in resin. They are used as replacements for wooden boards or (with outside ornamental veneer) as paneling, mostly in furniture. To make fiberboard, wood chips are digested into fiber, poured and rolled into thick sheets, cut, dried, compacted, and finished to a smooth surface.

Physical hazards of these processes include high noise levels and heat; fiberboard operations may be very humid, like pulp mills. Dust levels are often high, and the dust may be of smaller particle size than is usually the case in wood product fabrication and sawmills. Chemical hazards may include the bonding agents; allergic sensitization to the resins may result in occupational asthma or dermatitis. Plywood manufacture may result in exposure to formaldehyde or a similar compound, glutaraldehyde, and at low levels to some pesticides, which are used to protect the product. Wood dusts, in addition to their own hazards, may act as carriers for these other chemicals and for solvents adsorbed to the surface and, potentially, absorbed into the wood. In plywood and chipboard plants, the most common problems are dermatitis and irritation of the eyes and upper respiratory tract. Many wood dusts are sensitizing, and the fine dirt from manufacture of these products gets into clothes easily.

20

HEALTH-CARE WORKERS

Tee L. Guidotti

Health-care workers are exposed to many hazards on the job. This should be no surprise, as they take care of sick people, handle bodily fluids, and use potent chemicals and devices that were designed for treatment of patients, not for safety. However, many health-care facilities, clinics, and hospitals do not provide the same level of protection for their workers as a factory of similar size in the same community. Occupational health management in the health-care sector is an important problem worldwide and health-care facilities often set the pattern and tone for providing occupational health services in their communities.

Occupational health services for health-care workers generally face more complicated challenges than those serving other employers of comparable size. Chapter 24 discusses general aspects of healthcare work as a service occupation. The characteristic exposures encountered in hospitals are infectious agents and allergens (see Chapter 10). However, there are many others, including chemical, radiological, ergonomic, mechanical, and stress hazards.

Hospitals, in particular, consist of distinct zones of hazard:

- high-risk areas, such as the renal dialysis ward, where there is a high level of exposure to hazards such as hepatitis B virus and a high risk of occupational disorders
- special hazard areas, where there is a predominant hazard that requires special control measures, such as hoods to protect pharmacy and laboratory workers or lead aprons to shield workers from ionizing radiation in the X-ray department
- patient support areas, where there is contact with sick patients but not a high level of exposure to chemicals other than latex; predominant hazards tend to be ergonomic; hospital laundries have a particular risk of injury and transmission of disease from needles left in bedding and laundry
- administration and support services, which resemble other institutional settings in their risk profile

These zones are not absolute. For example, radiology has become a major risk zone for exposure to blood-borne pathogens as more invasive procedures are conducted that require X-ray imaging.

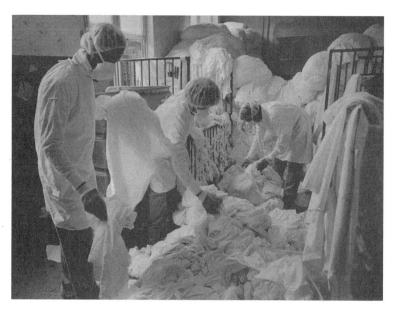

Figure 20.1 Workers in a hospital laundry in New York sort through used and potentially contaminated bedding, towels, drapes, and garments. (Photograph by © Earl Dotter, all rights reserved.)

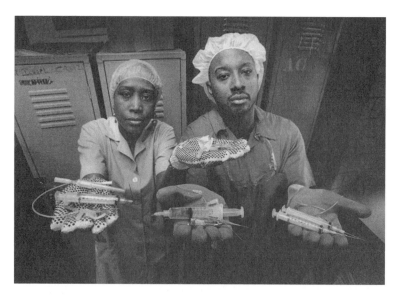

Figure 20.2 Workers in the same hospital display some of the needles and sharp objects they have encountered in the laundry. (Photograph by © Earl Dotter, all rights reserved.)

Critical Pathogens

The most characteristic hospital occupational health problems, although not the most common, are those involving exposure to agents of infectious disease, called pathogens. Table 20.1 lists common pathogens that are known to be a potential hazard in hospitals and health-care facilities and their mode of transmission.

TABLE 20.1

PATHOGENS THAT MAY BE TRANSMITTED IN A HOSPITAL OR HEATH-CARE SETTING

Organism	Disease It Causes	Health-Care Workers (or Patients) at Greatest Risk
Blood-borne Pathogens		
Hepatitis B virus	Hepatitis B	All, especially dialysis unit and surgery; dentists
Hepatitis C virus	Hepatitis C	All, especially dialysis unit and surgery; dentists
Human immunodeficiency virus (HIV)	Acquired Immune Deficiency Syndrome (AIDS)	All exposed to body fluids
Viruses causing viral hemorrhagic fever (many)	Viral hemorrhagic fevers	All, primarily a risk during local epidemics
Airborne Pathogens		
Adenovirus (many)	Adenovirus infections	All, especially pediatric units
Cytomegalovirus	CMV infection, can cause birth defects	All, especially pediatric units
Herpes virus Type 3	Varicella: chicken pox or herpes zoster ("shingles," a form of nerve infection)	All
Influenza virus (many)	Influenza	All
Measles virus	Rubeola (measles)	All, especially pediatric units
Meningococcus (a bacterium, *Neisseria meningitides*)	Meningococcal meningitis and meningococcal septicemia (tends to be an epidemic disease of young people)	Mostly emergency medical staff
Mumps virus	Mumps	All, especially pediatric units
Pertussis bacterium (*Bordatella pertussis*)	Pertussis, also called "whooping cough"	All, especially pediatric units
Parvovirus B19	Parvovirus infection, a disorder characterized by rash and aching pains and risk of bone marrow failure	All with patient contact

(Continued)

TABLE 20.1 (Contd.)

Organism	Disease It Causes	Health-Care Workers (or Patients) at Greatest Risk
Respiratory syncytial virus	RSV infection, a form of respiratory tract infection	All
Rubella virus	Rubella, may cause birth defects	Patients; risk of transmission to pregnant women (with risk to fetus) by health-care workers who are not immunized or lack immunity
Tubercle bacillus (*Mycobacterium tuberculosis*)	Tuberculosis	All
Fecal-Oral Pathogens		
Helicobacter pylori (a bacteria in the stomach and GI tract)	Ulcers, gastritis (very common)	Endoscopy technicians
Hepatitis A	Hepatitis A	All
Norwalk virus	Diarrhea (one of many causes of diarrhea but particularly infectious and common in institutions)	All
Poliovirus	Polio	All, but risk of polio is currently confined to very few locations in the world because of WHO eradication program
Salmonella species (bacteria)	Salmonellosis (diarrhea, can be a severe infection), typhoid (if *S. typhi*)	All, including laundry workers
Shigella species (bacteria)	Shigellosis (diarrhea, sometimes bloody)	All, especially pediatric units
Skin-Contact Pathogens		
Herpes simplex	Whitlow (a painful skin disease)	All, including dentists
Several "dermatophytic" fungal species	Tinea corporis (ringworm)	All
Staphylococcus aureus	Staph infections	Patients; risk tends to be from health-care workers who have the organism in their nose but may be asymptomatic

Blood-borne pathogens are transmitted by blood and body fluids and are controlled by a series of measures called *universal precautions* that are intended to prevent inadvertent exposure to body fluids, to isolate patients who are infected with highly communicable pathogens, and to prevent infection from needlestick injury and contact with other sharp objects. *Airborne pathogens*, such as tuberculosis, are transmitted primarily as aerosols and are controlled by ventilation, personal protection, and ultraviolet sources (see Chapter 8) that kill the microbes in air. Airborne pathogens are generally controlled by the use of respiratory personal protection, such as disposal air filtration respirators (most commonly the N95 type, which filters out particles in the inhalable range).

HIV/AIDS, hepatitis B, and hepatitis C are potentially serious threats to health-care workers, especially in countries where there is a high prevalence of infection in the general population.

HIV/AIDS especially has been the cause of considerable anxiety on the part of health-care workers. The virus can be spread among patients when medical objects such as syringes are not properly sterilized and are used on more than one patient. Among health-care workers, the primary mode of infection is a blood-contaminated sharp object. The greatest risk occurs when a relatively large quantity of infected blood or other contaminated body fluid is injected or contaminates an open wound. This situation tends to occur most often in surgery or procedures that involve large-bore needles or instruments. Minor injuries involving no transfer of blood or that do not break the skin present little or no risk. Needlestick injuries from syringes and mucosal contact with blood (such as splashes into the eye from an open tube in the laboratory or by mouth pipetting) must be prevented, but the risk of infection depends on the amount of blood that is actually transferred. Significant exposure includes the inadvertent injection of blood or body fluids, prolonged contact with mucosa or abraded skin, and deep wounding with blood-contaminated instruments.

Health-care workers who are significantly exposed to the HIV/AIDS virus are treated prophylactically (before they develop signs of illness) with antiviral drugs, but these drugs have potentially serious side effects. Primary prevention by control of exposure remains the best approach. HIV is less easily transmitted than hepatitis B and C, and measures adequate to protect against hepatitis B will also protect against transmission of HIV and hepatitis C. Health-care workers who are infected with HIV/AIDS are not thought to pose a risk to others, as long as their duties do not involve invasive procedures, and no basis exists for mandatory screening or excluding them from work because of the risk of infecting patients.

Hepatitis B, a highly infectious and serious form of hepatitis, is a major practical problem in hospital occupational health practice. It has been unfortunately common for nurses, surgeons, and other health-care professionals to become infected in certain areas of the hospital, particularly the renal dialysis and kidney transplantation units. Immunization of the workers with vaccine against hepatitis B virus is effective and safe in preventing the infection. The best control over hepatitis B, however, is control of potential exposure by enforcing precautions in the handling of blood specimens and in disposing of contaminated objects. Within nursing units, for example, the single most effective measure seems to be control of the disposal of "sharps" (needles, blades, and other sharp objects), the safe disposal of plastic syringes (not reusing them), and effective sterilization techniques. Hospital control of hepatitis B rests on immunization, education, and selective serologic testing. Hepatitis C, which is less communicable than hepatitis B, is controlled in the same way.

Tuberculosis has declined in prevalence in most parts of the world but remains a hazard in hospitals. Multiple-drug-resistant tuberculosis has been rising in frequency in many parts of the world due to incomplete treatment or lack of compliance by patients. Routine screening of hospital workers who have contact with patients, using a skin tuberculin test (Mantoux) or one of the newer tests, protects both patients and staff but is generally unnecessary for office workers and others at low risk.

Methicillin-resistant *Staphylococcus aureus* (MRSA) is a variant of a familiar bacterium (staph) that is resistant to antibiotics, including methicillin, which was previously used as a backup for staph resistant to other antibiotics. Treatment of deep MRSA infections is difficult, prolonged, and may involve using antibiotics with potentially serious side effects. MRSA is a common problem in hospitals because staph, which colonizes and then stays in the nose of carriers, is easily transmitted. Staph that is picked up in hospital settings tends to be selected for drug resistance because of the number of patients on antibiotics. MRSA can be transmitted on contaminated surfaces or on the hands of carriers and infects people in places where skin is broken, for example, where there is a cut, scrape, scratch, or burn. Transmission can be prevented by very rigorous cleaning (including equipment and hospital room furnishings), not sharing personal items such as towels or razors, identification and treatment of carriers with topical antibiotics in the nose (because staph carriers are so common, this is not practical as a routine and is done only when there is an outbreak), and universal precautions. (Vancomycin-resistant staph is also an emerging infection in hospitals but so far does not present a serious hazard to health-care workers.)

Rubella is a viral disease that is a danger to all women of child-bearing age because of the grave risk of birth defects following exposure during pregnancy. Hospital workers of both sexes should be screened by serology before assignment, and those not demonstrating antibody should be immunized. The point of this is not only to protect the individual worker but to create what epidemiologists call "herd immunity" (when an unimmunized individual is protected because those around him or her are immunized) so that a susceptible woman will not be inadvertently exposed to rubella during the infectious stage by a hospital worker carrying the virus from another patient or from outside the hospital.

Emerging infections, as a class, are those that were previously unknown, rare, confined, or declining infections that emerge as outbreaks and potential threats to the community and, invariably, to health-care workers, such as MRSA. Some emerging infections, such as HIV/AIDS, emerge and then become endemic and pose a persistent risk to health-care workers. Others, such as West Nile virus, do the same but do not pose a risk to health-care workers because they are not readily transmissible in the health-care setting. In recent years, hospitals and health-care institutions have faced these emerging infectious threats:

- SARS (severe acute respiratory syndrome) was a serious pneumonia-like respiratory disease caused by a coronavirus (a class of virus that previously rarely caused serious human disease) that emerged in 2002 in Guandong Province, China, and within months infected thousands and caused almost 800 deaths, most in China, Singapore, Hong Kong, and Canada. Many health-care workers were infected during the course of the outbreak. Management of the outbreak was helped by isolating suspected cases, recognition that the virus was spread by airborne droplets, monitoring health-care staff for febrile illness, and worldwide disease tracking. The experience with SARS has provided a template for managing emerging infections on a global scale.

- Pandemic influenza occurred in 2009, with a worldwide epidemic of an influenza strain (H1N1) that was unfortunately called "swine flu" at the onset, because it originated from a virus in that animal. Although less troublesome than initially feared, H1N1 did cause many deaths. In the event, the management of H1N1 was a success because a vaccine became available and was widely disseminated relatively quickly, global monitoring tracked the spread of the virus with unprecedented accuracy, and contingency plans for maintaining business continuity in a serious outbreak were tried out and found to be effective.

- Avian influenza is a much-feared risk associated with the possibility that a certain type of influenza that affects birds (H5N1) may jump the species barrier, as it already has several times since 1997, to infect human beings with a highly transmissible form of the disease in a worldwide outbreak (pandemic) similar to the pandemic of 1918, which caused many deaths among otherwise healthy and young people and which left some survivors with a chronic neurological disorder resembling Parkinson's disease. Hospitals, clinics, and public health agencies have made contingency plans to deal with a pandemic, emphasizing triage (sorting cases by severity) and keeping less severe cases out of hospitals, social isolation (discouraging people from congregating in large groups and encouraging distance work and similar measures), immunization (predicated on anticipating the right strain and producing large quantities of that vaccine), and highly selected use of antiviral medication.

CHEMICAL HAZARDS IN THE HOSPITAL

The hospital setting poses many chemical hazards, but four present the most significant problems to large groups of workers. Table 20.2 lists some of the more common. Each involves exposure to chemicals, drugs or otherwise, that are essential to patient care and therefore not easily replaced. Emphasis must be on safe handling of the chemicals to ensure the safety of hospital workers while preserving the continued use of these valuable agents. This requires both physical protection to prevent exposure and education to ensure safe work practices; neither is sufficient alone.

Ethylene oxide (EtO) may be the greatest chemical hazard, historically. Used for cold gas sterilization, EtO is usually centralized to a few locations in the hospital, particularly the central sterile supply unit. EtO is acutely toxic as a skin and respiratory irritant and is strongly suspected of causing leukemia in humans. Recently, there has been some concern regarding the possibility of neurotoxicity induced by EtO. Unfortunately, it is often handled rather carelessly in hospitals, typically being vented from gas sterilizers directly into the room, where it can be

TABLE 20.2

CHEMICAL HAZARDS COMMONLY FOUND IN HOSPITALS AND CLINICS

Chemical Hazard	Special Risk	Most Common Locations	Special Measures
Anesthetic gases	Liver toxicity, neurotoxicity, reproductive hazard	Operating rooms, recovery rooms	Venting and ventilation systems
Antineoplastic (anticancer) drugs	Birth defects, possible cancer risk	Oncology wards, pharmacy	Hoods, special preparation areas
Disinfectants	Skin irritation	All	Wear gloves while using disinfectants; hand washing is required and so cannot be avoided
Ethylene oxide	Severe skin blisters, possible cancer risk	Central sterile supply (where instruments are sterilized), cold sterilization units	Venting and ventilation systems
Formaldehyde and glutaraldehyde	Skin rash	Endoscopy units, pathology and autopsy units	Rinse thoroughly, avoid hand contact
Latex	Latex allergy	All (see Box 20.2)	Use alternatives to latex gloves and devices where latex is not needed
Mercury	Mercury toxicity	Dental offices	Special measures for handling dental amalgam; ventilation
Methacrylate cement	Allergies, liver toxicity	Operating room (used in orthopedic procedures)	Venting and ventilation systems
Nitrous oxide (anesthetic gas)	Possible cancer risk	Operating room, dental office , emergency room, burn unit	Venting and ventilation systems
Pharmaceutical agents	Wide variety of effects depending on drug: toxicity, allergy	All	Safe handling of pharmaceuticals

breathed at high peak levels by hospital employees. EtO should be vented to the outside, and levels should be monitored by periodic measurement under the most hazardous conditions, such as changing tanks and opening the sterilizer.

Antineoplastic agents have saved or improved the quality of life of millions of cancer patients but may many are carcinogenic or reproductive hazards themselves and pose a significant risk to hospital workers. Oncology nurses, pharmacists, and hospital workers handling body wastes from such patients are exposed to significant quantities of various chemotherapeutic agents, by skin contact or inhalation. This exposure has been associated with an elevated rate of miscarriages and the detection of potential carcinogens in urine. Faced with these findings, hospitals are installing vertical laminar-flow hoods in pharmacies and oncology wards and are initiating protective procedures to reduce employees' exposure to the drugs and to patient wastes contaminated with significant quantities of the drugs or their metabolites. Mixing chemotherapeutic drugs on the ward without special cabinets and training is no longer acceptable, as it was in the past, because of the hazard to the individual health-care worker drawing up the drug and to everyone else in the area. An unexpected benefit from control of exposure and centralizing their mixing has been the considerable savings from reduced waste of these expensive drugs.

Anesthetic gases have been historically associated with spontaneous abortions and liver disorders among operating theater personnel. This is now a well-recognized hazard that is easily controlled by scavenging systems that trap waste and expired gas and vent them outside the building. Nitrous oxide is a particular problem due to its reproductive toxicity and its frequent use in conditions difficult to control closely, as in emergency rooms and burn units. Many such units now routinely exclude pregnant women from assisting in procedures requiring its use.

Latex allergy has become a serious problem in hospitals, although its frequency is declining with the use of better quality latex gloves. (See Box 20.2) When "universal precautions" were first introduced to prevent viral transmission and to control the risk of HIV/AIDS and hepatitis to health-care workers, the demand for latex gloves and barriers greatly increased. Quality assurance was relaxed, and many products exposed health-care workers to excessive amounts of free latex dust and particles. This, together with much more frequent and prevalent use of latex gloves, created an epidemic of latex allergy in the 1980s and 1990s among health-care workers. Manufacturing standards improved later but not before many health-care workers were forced out of their jobs. Latex allergy can express itself as hives, skin rashes (sometimes severe), rhinitis (runny nose) and sneezing, acute asthma, and life-threatening anaphylaxis. Sensitivity to latex may also involve cross-reacting responses to other organic allergens, including antigens in bananas, kiwi, and avocados, which is called *latex-fruit syndrome*. In order to prevent serious latex allergy, hospitals and clinics now usually use non-latex gloves (usually PVC) wherever it is feasible to do so and reserve latex gloves for situations in which they are indispensable.

Finally, a variety of common agents cause contact dermatitis among hospital personnel, such as pharmaceuticals and medications (especially antibiotics) among nurses, cleaning solutions among domestic workers, and solvents among laboratory and maintenance workers. When these dermatitides (plural of dermatitis) are the result of an irritant effect, they can be controlled easily by personal protection such as wearing gloves; when they result from sensitization, they are usually much harder to manage because exposure to only a small amount of the substance is sufficient to induce the allergic reaction. Thus, it is preferable to avoid sensitization in the first instance, by maintaining good technique (antisepsis and personal protection), by never squirting excess medication out of a syringe except into a folded gauze square, and by frequent but not excessive hand washing. This is a problem in the health-care environment because frequent hand washing is necessary to prevent transmission of infection but may also perpetuate an irritant rash in the health-care worker. Alcohol-based hand-washing products appear to be less irritating than soaps.

Box 20.1

Providing Health Care at Home

As the cost of institutional medical care rises, alternative arrangements for providing care outside of the hospital are becoming more popular. A new category of domestic worker, called "homemakers" was tried out in the 1980s in San Diego, California (USA), to provide homemaking services to the disabled and elderly poor. Their services remove the need for hospitalization for clients who cannot maintain their homes independently but can otherwise take care of themselves.

Nearly all were women. Table 20.4 presents the characteristics of the clients served. The four most common characteristics of the clients were that they were elderly, disabled, ill, and blind. The homemakers provided a wide range of household services for clients, as presented in Table 20.5. Half, however, encountered safety hazards in the homes of clients, including pests, flammable trash piles, non-electrical safety hazards, garbage, and frayed electrical cords. A fairly high percentage, 8.5%, reported having experienced at least one work-related injury. Verbal or physical abuse from clients was reported by 15%.

TABLE 20.4

CHARACTERISTICS OF CLIENTS REQUIRING SERVICES OF DOMESTIC WORKER FOR HOME HEALTH CARE, REPORTED BY HOMEMAKERS

	Percent
Disabling conditions of clients	
Elderly	83.5
Physically disabled	65.9
Illness	46.3
Blind	25.9
Mental illness	13.6
Alcohol abuse	10.3
Drug abuse	2.6
Other	5.5
No response (homemaker did not know)	2.4
Illnesses reported among clients	
Hepatitis	2.2
Pneumonia	8.4
Tuberculosis	2.6
Bedsores	7.9
Cancer	17.3
Other	0.5
No response (homemaker did not know)	74.3
Use of medical equipment	
Oxygen extractor or tank	24.0
Leg brace	12.5
Ventilator/inhalation therapy	9.6

TABLE 20.4 (Contd.)

	Percent
Other	8.2
Humidifier	7.4
Sitz bath	7.2
Ileostomy/colostomy	6.5
Aids to mobility	4.3
Hemodialysis	1.9
Feeding tubes	0.7
No response (homemaker did not know)	57.3

TABLE 20.5

SERVICES PERFORMED AND WORKING CONDITIONS OF DOMESTIC WORKERS PROVIDING HOME CARE

Service Provided	Percent
General cleaning	95.4
Laundry	94.7
Food shopping	87.3
Meal preparation	77.9
Bathe/dress	50.4
Transportation	37.6
Feeding	24.7
Move in/out of bed	21.6
Give medication	8.6

TABLE 20.6

PERSONAL HEALTH PROBLEMS REPORTED BY DOMESTIC WORKERS AND A NEIGHBORHOOD COMPARISON GROUP IN DIFFERENT SURVEYS

	Domestic Workers	Neighborhood Comparison**	
Problem	Percent	Percent	P
All musculoskeletal complaints	26.1	7.77	0.006*
Back problems	15.1	3.8	0.047*
Body aches, pains	14.1	1.9	0.02*
Headaches, nausea, dizziness	11.5	23.1	0.03*
Muscle strains	9.4	0.0	0.04*
Skin irritation	6.0	3.8	0.77
Breathing problems	3.1	5.8	0.55
Other	0.7	21.1	<0.0001*
No response (none)	64.5	65.4	0.95
Total population responding	100.0	100.0	

*Significant at $p < 0.05$ by χ^2_1. Differences in survey technique should be considered in interpreting the results. Overall significance for χ^2_8: $p \ll 0.00001$.

**Females 25 to 70 in a socioeconomically appropriate neighborhood in southeast San Diego, 52 total. Age distribution of comparison population is 25–44, 26.9%; 45–64, 63.5%; 65–70, 9.6%. Five women reported their occupation as "homemaker."

A large majority of homemakers considered themselves to be in good health (Table 20.6). Subjectively reported health problems may be a conservative estimate of health risk in a population such as this one. Homemakers considered themselves in good overall health (80%), but a quarter reported musculoskeletal disorders, principally back problems, significantly more often than expected compared to a comparison group of age-matched women from a socioeconomically and culturally appropriate neighborhood. In spite of the hazards, most homemakers declared themselves satisfied with their jobs. (Note that the survey instrument had a design problem: it could not distinguish between absent responses and negative responses.)

Adapted from Zechter, J.F. and T. L. Guidotti. 1987. "Occupational Hazards of Domestic Workers Providing Home Care." *Public Health* 101: 283–291.

Physical Exposures

Radiation hazards of the ionizing variety (see Chapter 8) are largely confined to radiology suites, nuclear medicine laboratories, and radiation oncology treatment areas.

The increasing use of lasers in ophthalmology, dermatology, surgery, and otolaryngology has greatly increased the hazard from this form of high-energy light. This risk is primarily to the eyes, because the focused light can damage the retina of persons exposed in the face to the beam or its reflection, causing permanent loss of vision. Older laser devices frequently lacked adequate containment and safety features.

Microwave radiation produces heat, particularly in water-containing substances, and this is the basis for its use in ovens. Increasingly used for applications where rapid warming is required, as in kitchens or the blood bank, commercial microwave devices are generally safe except to persons with cardiac pacemakers, which can be thrown off by the magnetic forces generated.

Safety and Injury Prevention

Hospitals in general have a poor record of safety. Although needlestick injuries are the most characteristic hospital injuries and carry a particular risk of infection, the most common serious injury in hospitals is back strain. Chronic back pain accounts for the largest proportion of workers' compensation claims among hospital workers, particularly nurses. Such back problems are largely preventable through education and the use of proper techniques for lifting and rolling patients. Many hospitals conduct "back schools" through their physical therapy departments to instruct employees in lifting techniques, an intervention that has not been shown to work, and many hospitals are purchasing hydraulic lifting devices for moving heavy or unconscious patients.

Recent surveys of safety problems in hospitals suggest that hazards are by no means confined to older facilities—newer hospitals are not particularly safe either. Burns, slips and falls, electrical shocks, and cuts are particular problems associated

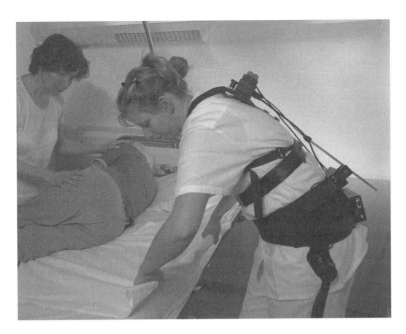

Figure 20.1 Nurses moving a patient. The most common occupational injury in hospitals is low back pain among nurses; the nurse on the right is wearing a device to monitor trunk movements for a research project. (Photograph by Dr. Sonja Freitag, reproduced by permission, *Annals of Occupational Hygiene*, Oxford University Press.)

with laboratories and food-preparation areas, wet floors, poorly repaired or poorly grounded electrical equipment, and glass ampoules and careless handling of surgical instruments, respectively. These are all problems that can be reduced by simple measures. Fortunately, fatal or major accidents in hospitals are rare, but the toll of the less severe accidents is seen in days lost to work, workers' compensation claims, increased expenses, and reduced productivity. Table 20.3 presents the distribution of injuries reported to the occupational health service of one hospital over one year. Although reporting was incomplete, the distribution accurately reflects the high frequency of back injuries and needlestick injuries in the hospital setting. Eye splashes are also common problems, seldom appreciated by the public or management.

Violence is a common problem in hospital settings. Violence is generally a greater problem in psychiatric wards, admissions offices, and in emergency departments. Many medical conditions are associated with confusion, irritability, and mental symptoms. In addition, hospitals tend to be places where emotions run high and people are angry and frustrated over what has happened to them and impatient after waiting. Lines are often long and facilities are often overcrowded. Many people are brought to the hospital under circumstances of conflict or stress and end up fighting with staff, family members, visitors, or other patients. The risk of violence is highest when the hospital or a health-care worker declines to provide a service the patient wants, denies access to drugs, or inadvertently causes pain to a patient. The risk is also increased when the patient or visitor has abused alcohol or drugs and is either intoxicated or withdrawing from substance abuse. Violence is most likely to occur when patients are admitted, transferred to another facility, waiting in line, or being served meals. Sadly, some hospitals and clinics that have poor security have had problems with assaults on patients and staff by outsiders, some of whom are motivated by the opportunity to steal money or drugs.

Stress

Stress in the health-care setting, especially in hospitals, can be intense. Shift work, emotional intensity, rapid pacing, rigid reporting and supervisory structures, frequent emergencies, and boring routines combine to create a highly stressful work environment. This high stress level is often made worse by the culture of health professionals who, being dedicated to the health of their patients, often consider it unprofessional or a sign of weakness to complain. These findings have implications for the management of hospitals, where regimentation and the need for flexibility of scheduling make it difficult to accommodate personal needs of the health-care worker. The factors discussed in Chapter 11 all apply to the hospital and health-care workplace.

Occupational Health Services for Hospitals and Clinics

Hospital and clinic employee health services require the same skills and leadership as occupational health facilities for other major employers. However, they are often underdeveloped compared to other sectors. This is often due to funding constraints but also because of the false idea that hospitals are clean, safe workplaces (they are not). The mission of a hospital or clinic is to take care of sick people, and all attention is usually devoted to that goal. The protection of the

TABLE 20.3

INJURIES REPORTED TO THE EMPLOYEE HEALTH SERVICE OF ONE HOSPITAL IN CANADA OVER A PERIOD OF ONE YEAR

Back injuries and muscle strains	147[a]	41%
Needlesticks	106	29%
Lacerations	42	12%
Assaults	36	10%
Eye splashes	20[b]	6%
Burns	6	2%
Eye injuries	3	1%
Total[c]	360	100%

Notes:
[a]76 back injuries not related to patient care
[b]17 eye splashes involved contact with body fluids
[c]May not sum to 100% because of rounding

people who work there is often overlooked. Health professionals often foster this attitude because as a group they tend to be very dedicated to their work and to accept that certain risks come with the work.

Health-care workers vary in their degree of risk and are exposed to different hazards:

- Nurses are exposed to biological, chemical, and physical hazards and, most frequently, ergonomic hazards and a risk of injuries. The single largest group of health-care workers in any hospital or large clinic is nurses.
- Physicians are exposed to similar hazards, and surgeons, especially, are exposed to the hazard of blood-borne pathogens.
- Laboratory staff are characteristically exposed to chemical hazards as well as biological hazards.
- Pharmacy workers, who are unlikely to be exposed to biological hazards, are at risk of exposure to chemicals, particularly pharmaceutical agents.
- Patient-care personnel, orderlies and nursing assistants, respiratory therapists, occupational and rehabilitation therapists, custodial staff and maintenance workers, and many other occupational groups that are required to deliver health care each share ergonomic risks, but their exposure to other hazards varies.
- X-ray technicians and radiologists are, of course, exposed to ionizing radiation as well as biological hazards. Because radiology increasingly requires invasive procedures, the hazard of exposure to blood-borne pathogens is generally increasing.
- Central sterile supply workers use ethylene oxide to sterilize heat-sensitive devices and equipment. In the past, they have been exposed to high levels of the gas during exhaust of the sterilization chambers. Local exhaust ventilation has improved the situation in modern hospitals.

Some hospitals, clinics, and other health-care organizations have effective occupational health services, but most do not give occupational health a priority except for mandatory standards. In the absence of effective occupational health services (usually still called "employee health services" in hospitals) and of genuine commitment from the administration, health-care workers within health-care institutions usually rely on informal advice and treatment from their colleagues. This system is actually counterproductive. Treatment may be given without reporting the hazard, so it remains uncorrected. Managers have no way of knowing when a problem exists if it is not reported. Few health-care workers have special training in occupational health and so this aspect of the problem is usually overlooked. Occupational injuries and health issues tend to be underreported.

Hospitals and clinics require certain basic systems for managing occupational health among their employees. These include, but are not limited to, the following:

- in-service education, emphasizing how to use personal protection and universal precautions and how to work safely
- infection control tracking and procedures, to monitor and prevent *nosocomial infections*, which are infections that result from exposure to pathogens in the hospital

- incident reporting systems, which collect information on injuries to workers, patients, and visitors, especially but not limited to needlestick injuries
- fitness for duty (see Chapter 17) to conduct pre-placement evaluations and to ensure that workers stay off the job, for example, if they are ill during the period that they are infectious and return when it is safe for them and they no longer pose a risk to others
- immunization and tuberculosis testing, periodic review, tracking, and follow-up
- safety audits, to identify and correct hazards in the workplace
- employee assistance (see Chapter 18), with support available for problems involving substance abuse and stress; health-care workers often work under great stress and have access to drugs, so it is not surprising that drug abuse tends to be a problem in this population

---

Box 20.2

Latex Sensitivity among Health-Care Workers

Health-care professionals have been developing allergies to latex in much greater numbers in recent years because of requirements to follow universal precautions to prevent the spread of blood-borne diseases such as HIV/AIDS and hepatitis. In order to protect themselves and other patients, health-care workers must wash their hands frequently and use personal protection such as gowns, masks, and latex gloves. Latex gloves are the greatest source of allergy, but other constituents of rubber also cause allergy.

Studies in Finland have estimated the prevalence of latex allergy among the general population to be <1%. The prevalence among health professionals was much higher: 2% of medical students, 3% of doctors and nurses, up to 12.5% of nurses in operating rooms (a finding replicated in France at 10%), and 7% of surgeons. Many of these professionals have had to leave their jobs because they could not function in a health-care workplace. Claims for compensation have averaged about US$83,000 each in the state of Oregon in the United States, reflecting medical care costs and loss of wages; this figure does not include direct costs to the worker, discomfort, and the disruption of having to change jobs or even careers. There have been at least 15 fatalities reported from latex-induced allergic reactions. Thus, the cost and personal impact of latex allergy is very great.

Natural rubber is produced from the sap of the tree *Hevea brasiliensis*. Natural rubber is a polymer consisting primarily (30%–40%) of cis-polyisoprene, plus various natural substances, mostly proteins. The various hydrocarbon chains in these rubbers impart physical properties to the rubber. Mixed polymers of latex and synthetic rubbers are also common. Natural rubber melts and tears easily and over time becomes brittle because of chemical reaction with oxygen. In order to ensure that it retains its strength, rubber is vulcanized. Vulcanization is the reaction of natural rubber with sulfur accelerators so that the polymer chains are cross-linked for strength and flexibility.

The problem with allergy is related to the presence of free molecules (monomer) of unpolymerized latex protein. Powdered, unwashed (but sterile) gloves are particularly a problem because free latex is present in particles that are easily inhaled. People who have latex allergy are often also allergic to bananas, chestnuts, and avocado because the proteins in these natural products resemble the latex protein and the body cannot tell the difference.

When the body becomes sensitized to latex, two types of allergy are most common:

- Allergic contact dermatitis, of the delayed type. After sensitization, a reaction typically occurs 48 to 96 hours after re-exposure. It is characterized by skin redness and inflammation and often progresses to blisters and eczema. The hand is the most common site. This reaction may be due to the sulphur compounds in the vulcanized rubber.
- Contact urticaria, an immediate hypersensitivity reaction that occurs within a few minutes in the form of hives and severe itching. The hand is the most common site, but the reaction can spread to other areas of skin and can also affect the eyes. This reaction is due to sensitivity to the latex protein itself.
- Occupational asthma, an immediate hypersensitivity reaction in the lungs.
- Occupational allergic rhinitis, which is also an immediate hypersensitivity reaction but one that affects the nose. It resembles hay fever or a cold.
- Anaphylaxis, which is a severe form of the same type of immediate hypersensitivity as the contact urticaria reaction and is due to hypersensitivity to the latex protein. Within minutes of exposure, the worker may have itching all over their body, have a runny and congested nose, feel short of breath and lightheaded, and may develop swelling around the lips and throat. This is a very dangerous reaction, sometimes fatal, because swelling in the throat may prevent him or her from breathing. This is a medical emergency and requires immediate treatment.

Workers who are sensitized to rubber and particularly to latex itself should use other types of gloves, such as those made of polyvinyl chloride (PVC), polyethylene, or elastryren (a form of synthetic latex). Unfortunately, these substitutes cost almost twice as much as conventional latex gloves, and some hospitals and clinics will not purchase them for this reason. Others do not want to stock nonlatex gloves alongside latex gloves because doing so would double their inventory costs.

Prevention of latex allergy is simple: avoid using latex gloves, and particularly powdered latex gloves, whenever it is possible to do so and still provide acceptable medical care. Latex gloves are preferred for many uses in hospitals because they are thin and flexible and it is easy to feel through them. It is much harder to feel and to perform complicated tasks such as surgery with gloves made of stiffer materials such as PVC. However, latex is not required for many routine health-care purposes that do not require manual dexterity or a fine sense of touch. Unfortunately, few hospitals provide alternatives to latex gloves in all areas of the hospital where it is practical to do so. Hospitals and health-care institutions should not be using powdered gloves because this increases the risk for their workers.

Written hospital policies on occupational health and safety are usually weak and unavailable when they are needed. Often a copy is not conveniently at hand. The hospital policy on occupational health and safety usually needs to be reviewed, rewritten, and approved at the highest level of the hospital administration. The revised policy should emphasize a commitment on the part of the medical center to the health and well-being of all employees and should explicitly make the connection between this commitment and the delivery of the highest quality of medical care to patients. The policy should be broad, a part of the basic policy document governing the hospital, and not overly burdened with details of medical screening or specific measures, as these are subject to change. It should contain the following points:

- Health-care personnel should not be expected to sacrifice or risk their own health and safety when this is avoidable in the care of others.
- Employees should be able to perform their duties without hesitation free of concerns that could cause them to hold back or to modify their duties out of fear for their own personal safety or the risk to their own families.
- Hospital employees also represent a community served by the hospital and should be afforded the same respect for quality of care as provided to other patients and clients.
- The new policy should be widely publicized and made available to each employee and member of the staff as they join the organization.

A critical component of the employee health service is a secure, confidential record-keeping system segregated from the medical records of patients and inaccessible to unauthorized parties, particularly the hospital's personnel department and unit supervisors. If confidentiality is not both assured and obvious, employees and the hospital will be poorly served because the potential for violation of personal privacy will lead to withholding of important information. A chart-based record-keeping system is usually adequate for clinical purposes, but key data need to be computerized to help in prevention-oriented services and more intensive case management. Records of employees exposed to potentially toxic substances should be kept at least 30 years, since adverse health effects may be long delayed.

These administrative and reporting arrangements are much more critical to the success of a hospital employee health service than are its physical equipment or staffing. However, to function well, the service should be centrally located, close to the center of the hospital traffic, and convenient to personnel as they come on or off shift.

21

AGRICULTURE AND RURAL DEVELOPMENT

Jyrki Liesivuori and Tee L. Guidotti

Agriculture has provided the necessities of life for farmers and their families for thousands of years. During the last 100 years, the nature of agriculture has changed in most of the world from small-scale, family farms that produced a small excess that could be sold to a model of high-volume production creating large surpluses. This has been made possible by the invention of new machines, tools, and chemicals that increase productivity. Agriculture is a heterogeneous and complex occupational sector applying multiple technologies in very different environments and in extreme weather conditions. The methods are totally dissimilar in industrialized vs. developing countries, ranging from highly mechanized agriculture in commercial plantations to traditional intensive methods in small-scale family farms. Despite the progress from new techniques, agricultural work depends on weather conditions and is necessarily undertaken in rural environments.

The huge variety of production methods and crops illustrates the complex nature of agriculture, which involves many specialized subsectors.

Agriculture produces the raw materials for food, feed, and fiber production. Crop processing and packaging, grain storage, irrigation, pest management, meat production (poultry, swine), fishery, manure, and associated domestic tasks (carrying water or fuel-wood) are all dependent on agricultural production.

AGRICULTURE AND LAND USE

The type of agriculture that may be conducted in an area is limited by factors such as soil quality, rainfall, access to irrigation water, drainage, and distance to markets. Certain types of crops and livestock are more easily grown in units of various sizes and on land with specific characteristics. This leads to a pattern of land use in the local community that reflects the efficiency of agricultural production and ownership of the land. These land use patterns in turn have important implications for local society and culture.

Subsistence farming consists of small plots of land on which farmers and their families produce what they require to live and, if possible, just enough to sell to buy other necessary items. Subsistence farming is characterized by poverty, inefficiency, and a grave risk to the community in the event of crop failure.

"Slash-and-burn" agriculture is a special type of subsistence agriculture practiced in parts of the world where communities are isolated and the soil becomes exhausted. Farmers will produce for several years until the soil quality gets to be too poor and will then move to other areas that have not been cultivated. They clear the land of forest and brush, usually by cutting small trees and bushes or burning, and then start the process over again. The land left behind sometimes recovers its fertility but, especially in the tropics, may not because of its chemical characteristics. Tropical soils (specifically, laterites) often form hard, almost impermeable surfaces after they dry out and are then difficult to put back into production.

Commercial farming is conducted on larger farms in much of the world. These may be owned by families or business owners and typically grow products to sell to the market, usually through an intermediate buyer who then sells the product to stores, distributors, or companies manufacturing food products. Sometimes farmers will take their own products to local markets and sell them directly. In many parts of the world, farmers have organized cooperatives, which are organizations that serve the function as buyers but are owned by the farmers themselves. In the developed world and in parts of the developing world, there is a very strong trend for these farms to consolidate or merge into bigger production units, often owned by partnerships or corporations. This is especially true when the

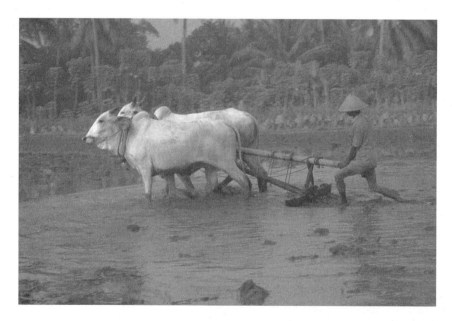

Figure 21.1 Traditional agriculture, as shown here in Indonesia. (Photograph by Brynn Bruijn, Saudi Aramco World/SAWDIA.)

local price of food is low and small farmers cannot make a sufficient profit. Commercial farming is highly dependent on financial credit. The farm owners typically borrow the money needed for planting and operating the farm against future earnings they will receive from their crops. Crop prices depend on the supply available at the time of harvest as well as what people are willing to pay and tend to be very unpredictable. If the crop yields less than the farmer borrowed, he or she incurs a debt, thus several years of low prices can threaten the business. This is why farm economics is so often an issue in the local economy, even if harvests are good and the rest of the economy is doing well.

Plantation agriculture is characterized by the production from large-scale farming units on large tracts of land, including short-rotation crops (pineapple, sugar cane) and tree crops (banana, rubber), primarily in the tropical regions of Asia, Africa, and Central and South America. Other plantation crops are tea, coffee, and palm nuts. Plantations are very large farms and need to be highly self-sufficient. Workers often live on them in camps and are relatively isolated from other communities. The plantation owners and operators must provide basic services such as sanitation and housing.

Agriculture conducted in urban areas produces food for the daily needs within cities and towns. Urban agriculture is usually conducted on a small scale by individuals and families and tends to be more closely linked to their communities and local services. Table 21.1 summarizes common specialized types of agriculture.

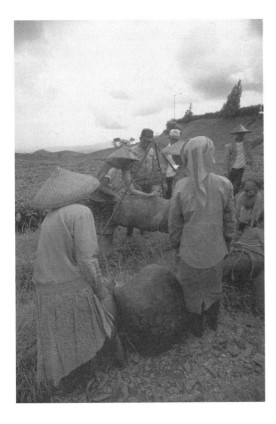

Figure 21.2 Workers on a tea plantation in Indonesia are having their bags of tea leaves weighed to determine their payment. (Photograph by Brynn Bruijn, Saudi Aramco World/ SAWDIA.)

TABLE 21.1

SPECIALIZED FARMING SYSTEMS

Farming System	Product
Aquaculture	Fish and seafood, seaweed and fodder
Horticulture	Vegetables, fruit, herbs, beverages
Floriculture	Flowers, house plants
Husbandry	Milk, eggs, meat, fur
Agroforestry	Fuel, fruits and nuts, building material
Mycoculture	Mushrooms
Sericulture	Silk
Apiculture	Honey, beeswax
Beverage crops	Grapes, palm tea, sugar cane, coffee, tea cultivation

---

Box 21.1

The Challenge of Occupational Health and Safety in Agriculture in Botswana

Agriculture is recognized as one of the three most hazardous work-related sectors causing traumatic injury worldwide. Principal risks to the health and safety of agriculture workers come from the nature of the work, the condition of tools and equipment, and exposure to chemicals or, in other words, work posture, chemical (pesticides) exposure, and machinery hazards. Because of Botswana's dependence on agriculture, particularly cattle raising, hazards found on subsistence farms and commercial farms contribute many occupational injuries.

Exposure to agrochemicals occurs in Botswana during application and storage of chemicals due to improper storage and lack of protective clothing. Exposure to infectious diseases is a big threat to the health of agricultural workers. Exposure to cattle dung during the rainy season increases the likelihood of fungal infection, particularly if workers are not provided with protective equipment and clothing. This makes the consequences of even minor injuries much worse.

Machines or equipment and tools are sources of multiple hazards. Entanglement in moving machinery may result in serious injuries or death. Under the Agrochemical Act and Factories Act, it is not a requirement to report injuries or diseases resulting from agricultural undertakings.

A National Health and Safety Policy has been proposed for Botswana. Its implementation will provide a basis for addressing health and safety matters in many workplaces, including agriculture, as well as reaffirming the government's commitment to safe working conditions.

Adapted from: Regoeng KG. Occupational health and safety: A challenge to the agriculture sector in Botswana. *African Newsletter on Occupational Health and Safety* Aug 2001;11(2):42–43.

Agriculture is closely linked to rural development and economics. Services to help farmers usually include services and advice to help farm families live better and to stabilize small rural communities on which farmers usually depend for supplies, transportation, markets, and basic services.

AGRICULTURAL WORK

Agriculture began as a way to create a stable, reliable food supply. It has been among the most successful innovations in human history, but it has also been subject to many problems. At the same time agriculture provided nutrition to farmers and their families, it created new problems. The concentration of crops in one place attracted pests and allowed crop diseases to become established. Weeds and insects destroyed the crops in the field, and mice and rats destroyed the harvest in storage. Soil was slowly impoverished and, in some places, turned the land to desert. Traditionally, farmers used manure (and sometimes human waste) to enrich the soil and sometimes left fields uncultivated, or "fallow," for a time to allow the land to regain nutrients, specifically nitrogen and phosphorus.

The fertilizer industry was started only 100 years ago. Commercial fertilizers rich in nitrogen and phosphorus could then be purchased and put onto the soil to boost its fertility. The pesticide industry developed new and effective insecticides, herbicides, and rodenticides in the 1940s and 1950s to combat pest issues. Although irrigation systems were being built 7,000 years ago, the industrial production of water pipes and electricity-powered pumps are relatively new inventions. Irrigation provided a more reliable source of water that could be controlled so that plants could be given as much as they needed on a regular basis.

Agriculture all over the world is still largely composed of family farms with only a few workers. Plantations are exceptions, as they can employ whole villages or hundreds of migrant workers on an industrial scale. In many industrialized countries, farms are increasing in size, turning agriculture into large-scale commercial production integrated with processing, marketing, and distribution in agribusiness. The mechanization of agriculture has led to a considerable decrease in manual labor and in the labor force required to operate farms.

Agricultural employees comprise half of the world's labor force. It is estimated that 1.3 billion workers are active in agricultural production. The proportion is only 5% to 10% in highly industrialized countries (Europe and North America) but is 49% worldwide with almost 60% in developing countries. Traditional farming employs all the family members from young to old. Children have always worked on the farms, primarily during the harvest period. Their contribution to the family income has been vitally important. According to International Labour Organization (ILO) estimates, the rate of economically active children (5 to 14 years old) may be up to 30% of the agricultural workforce in developing countries. Women account for 20% to 30% of the total agricultural paid employment. In some countries, like sub-Saharan Africa, women produce and market 90% of locally grown food. The situation in Asia is similar. The highest incidence of poverty is among agricultural wage laborers working in commercial agriculture, especially on plantations.

The nature of agricultural work is totally different from industrial work. It is often done in remote areas, often alone or with family members, and under all weather conditions. During busy seasons, farmers work long hours with few breaks. Children may have to help in the fields instead of going to school. Some specific characteristics of agricultural work are summarized in Table 21.2, some of which create health risks.

On family-owned or operated farms, the entire family usually does some form of farmwork. In most societies, women have traditionally taken care of cattle and milking operations, while men have worked more in the fields. Children are typically expected to do work as soon as they are able, often starting with feeding chickens and getting eggs. As a result, every member of the typical farm family is at some risk, not just the farmer. These families usually live on or close to the land they cultivate and may do some of the required maintenance work in their houses. This brings some of the hazards of agriculture into their homes. Larger operations may be able to hire workers, either full time or as they are needed during planting or harvest seasons. These workers, their families, if they have them, and the farmer's families often live together or in close proximity. Thus, agricultural hazards affect all members of the community, including children and people who are not necessarily working in the fields or with livestock.

Social factors, such as illiteracy, may also reduce the capacity of agricultural workers and their families to use preventive health measures (use of right-to-know,

TABLE 21.2

CHARACTERISTICS OF AGRICULTURAL AND INDUSTRIAL WORK

Agricultural Work	*Industrial Work*
Most of the tasks carried out in the open air, exposing the workers to climatic conditions	Most of the tasks carried out indoors, with shelter and control over the environment
Seasonal nature of the work; urgency of certain tasks to be performed at specific times	Production tends to be continuous throughout the year or driven by demand for the product
Variety of tasks to be performed by the same person	Work is specialized; one worker tends to do the same job
Working postures may be awkward and must be held for long periods of time	Worker may be able to change position and to take short breaks
Contact with the animals and plants; exposure to bites, poisoning, infections, and other health problems	Worker is generally protected against these hazards but may be exposed to industrial hazards in the workplace
Use of chemicals and biological products is common	Use of chemicals is common
Considerable distance between the living quarters and workplaces, or the home and workplace may be at the same location	Workers tend to live near jobs or where there is access to transportation
Access to emergency and other health services often poor	Workers tend to live in communities where health services are available

understanding instructions, and safety precautions) or to find medical treatment or financial compensation.

The economic environment may be one of the most potent modifying factors in relation to risk behaviors. For example, research in both South America and southeast Asia has shown that farmers' unsafe use of pesticides is largely the result of "rational" choices they make related to their economic sustainability, discounting the health consequences to themselves or their families. Therefore, the challenge to occupational health professionals is to help to change the environment so that safer methods are consistent with economic benefit perceived by farmers, for example, by facilitating technical support for safer production methods.

HEALTH HAZARDS IN AGRICULTURE

To the outsider, farmworkers seem to have an attractive life, living in the countryside in fresh air where the work itself can be almost like exercise. This positive picture of farmwork is offset by the actual increased risk of injury. Currently, agriculture is ranked as one of the most hazardous occupations, along with mining, fishing, logging, and construction. In addition, agricultural work is also associated with a variety of health risks. Farmwork may involve exposure to the physical hazards of weather, terrain, and machinery and the toxicological hazards of pesticides, fertilizers, and fuels. Biological hazards may include exposures to organic dusts. In general, farmworkers are at high risk for injuries, respiratory diseases, and certain cancers.

Characteristic health hazards and occupational diseases of agricultural work can be grouped into the following categories: traumatic injuries, respiratory diseases, toxic and neoplastic hazards, zoonotic diseases (diseases arising from contact with animals), dermatological hazards, mechanical and thermal stress, and mental health.

Box 21.2

Occupational Allergy and Asthma among Food-Processing Workers in South Africa

Occupational food allergies and asthma are diseases resulting from hypersensitivity of the immune system to food substances encountered in the work environment (see Chapter 16). The proportion of adult asthma cases attributable to occupational exposure is estimated to be 10%–15%. Worldwide, the most commonly reported causes of asthma in the workplace are agents of biological origin such as cereal flours, enzymes, natural rubber latex, laboratory animals, and some low molecular agents (isocyanates and acid anhydrides).

In South Africa, the food-processing industry (grain milling, bakery) is one of the top three industries with increasing numbers of workers with occupational allergies and asthmas. Food processing techniques such as thermal denaturation, acidification, and fermentation generate new allergens, while others such as slaughtering, cooking, gutting, grinding, milling, drying, centrifuging, and lyophilizing generate high-risk aerosol exposures to food products that are capable of causing allergic health outcomes. Occupational allergies and asthma are increasingly becoming an important health problem.

Environmental control of allergens is still the primary method of preventing the development of allergic diseases, including asthma, in the workplace. Improvements in the work environment can contribute significantly to decreasing the risk of sensitization for other, as yet unaffected, workers. It will also reduce the risk of precipitating an asthmatic attack among already sensitized workers.

Workplace strategies for controlling allergen exposures generally use a combination of approaches that include substitution of the product, engineering controls, personal protective equipment, and administrative controls. Education and training programs that inform and educate workers about the allergic health effects associated with food handling are equally important. Material safety data sheets, if adequately compiled, can be a useful adjunct to these programs, enabling workers to take the necessary precautions when working with these agents. The most widely used methods for the medical surveillance of occupational allergic respiratory diseases are questionnaires, spirometry and immunological tests, such as skin prick tests, or allergen-specific serum IgE levels. This way immunological sensitization or occupational asthma can be detected early before it becomes severe or irreversible.

Adapted from: Jeebhay, M. F. 2002. "Occupational Allergy and Asthma among Food-Processing Workers in South Africa." *African Newsletter on Occupational Health and Safety* 12: 59–62.

Traumatic Injuries

Of all the health problems facing agricultural workers today, work-related injury is the most important in both developed and developing countries (see Table 21.3). Rates of workplace injury in agriculture are among the highest of any occupational sector and may arise from different types of biomechanical hazards inherent in the agricultural production process.

The National Safety Council in the United States has estimated that in 1989 there were 1,500 deaths and 140,000 disabling injuries from farming, numbers comparable to underground mining and construction. The fatality rate for farmers has been about five times higher than that for all U.S. workers. A 1993 survey of farm injuries found the major causes to be livestock (18%), machinery (17%), and hand tools (11%). The most frequent injuries reported were sprains and strains (26%), cuts (18%), and fractures (15%). Studies of death certificates and rescue records indicate that tractors cause at least 50% of all the deaths in U.S. farming each year. Frequency of injury seems to follow the farmwork season; it is

TABLE 21.3

INJURY HAZARDS ASSOCIATED WITH AGRICULTURE

Exposures	Health Effects
Road vehicle crashes, machinery and vehicles	Fatalities, serious injuries (to adult workers, child workers, and family members)
Tractors	Crushing of the chest associated with getting pinned under an overturned tractor, with risk of strangulation/asphyxia
Augers	Severe injury leading to hypovolemia (loss of blood), sepsis, and asphyxia
Electricity	Electrocutions
Machinery and vehicles, draft animal kicks (e.g., assaults, falls)	Nonfatal injuries, infection (e.g., tetanus)
Hay balers	Friction burns, crush injuries, neurovascular disruption
Power take-offs (external power source run by tractor engines)	Skin or scalp avulsion or degloving injury, amputation, multiple blunt injuries
Corn pickers	Hand injuries (friction burns, crushing, finger amputation)

Adapted from Myers, 1998.

the highest in the summer and lowest in the winter. As work hours increased, the risk of injuries also increased. In addition to the adult workers, children are also hurt in farming. In the United States, estimates are that approximately 300 children die each year on farms, and another 23,000 sustain serious injuries. There are no figures from developing countries for comparison.

Agricultural injuries range from the simplest exposures related to working with heavy loads or with livestock (kicks, bites, shoves, and falls), to the hazards associated with the use of unprotected or poorly designed tools as well as machine injuries. For example, high rates of traumatic lacerations occur among sugar cane workers using machetes to harvest cane in the absence of leg protection. Similarly, tractor drivers without protected cabins are at risk from overhanging trees and branches, which may result in serious injuries (e.g., branches poking or thorns to the eyes). As agricultural work becomes further mechanized (which is the trend internationally), the absence of adequate safety precautions is likely to increase the risk of injury.

Climatic or organizational factors (such as piecework, seasonal urgency, long and atypical hours of work, or lack of resources to maintain equipment) may aggravate both the severity and the likelihood of the hazards and may magnify the health consequences of an injury. For example, piecework encourages workers to speed up their work rate, take shortcuts on safety precautions, or neglect protective measures. Pressure to complete certain tasks dictated by the presence or absence of rain, sunshine, and other climatic factors may impose extended periods of intensified work. Furthermore, the isolation of rural agricultural workers often results in delays in treatment or inaccessibility to adequate means of prevention (training, safe technology, maintenance support, etc.). In many rural areas, emergency services are limited and acute care facilities are poorly equipped to deal with major traumas.

Respiratory Diseases

The respiratory tract is one of the systems more commonly affected by hazardous exposures in agricultural work. Health effects that result from these exposures include grain fever, chronic bronchitis, farmer's lung, silo filler's disease, asthma, and hypersensitivity pneumonitis (see Table 21.4). (These diseases are discussed in Chapter 16.) These pulmonary diseases linked to agricultural exposures have been found in several different countries.

A febrile, flu-like illness has been described following the inhalation of agricultural dust in high concentrations. This phenomenon is likely similar to

TABLE 21.4
RESPIRATORY HAZARDS ASSOCIATED WITH AGRICULTURE

Exposures	Health Effects
Grain pollen, animal dander, fungus	Asthma and rhinitis
Antigens in grain dust and on crops, mites	Asthma
Organic dusts	Nonimmunologic asthma (grain dust asthma)
Endotoxins, glucans, mycotoxins	Mucous membrane inflammation, fever, chills, short-term illness
Insecticides, irritant dust, ammonia, grain dust (wheat, barley)	Bronchospasm, acute and chronic bronchitis
Fungal spores or thermophilic actinomycetes (a type of microorganism) released from moldy grain or hay	Hypersensitivity pneumonitis (the hypersensitivity pneumonitis associated with moldy hay is called *farmer's lung*)
Thermophilic actinomycetes: moldy sugar cane	Bagassosis
Mushroom spores	Mushroom worker's lung (a form of hypersensitivity pneumonitis)
Compost	Hypersensitivity pneumonitis
Plant debris, starch granules, molds, endotoxins, mycotoxins, fungi, enzymes	Organic dust toxic syndrome
Dust from stored grain	Grain fever
Moldy silage in silo	Silo filler's disease
Decomposition gases: ammonia, hydrogen sulphide, carbon monoxide, methane	Toxic inhalation, including acute pulmonary responses
Nitrogen dioxide from fermenting silage	Silo filler's disease, including pulmonary edema
Soil dust of arid regions, which may be contaminated with fungal spores	Mycoses (fungal diseases) such as Valley Fever (coccidiomycosis), histoplasmosis

Adapted from Myers, 1998.

other inhalation fever reactions seen with a wide variety of substances ranging from cotton and grain dust to zinc welding fumes. In agricultural settings, this disease has been called organic dust toxic syndrome (ODTS). Surveys among Swedish farmers indicate that 1 in every 100 has had febrile reactions, and grain elevator workers have reported them even more frequently. Ten percent of animal-confinement workers describe symptoms of ODTS. The data available suggest that this disorder is probably related to levels of natural chemicals that can cause fever (called *endotoxins*), which are the biologically active part of gram-negative bacterium cells or high concentrations of glucans from molds and fungi. Most individuals are able to return to work within a few days following symptomatic treatment. Although there is a clinical resemblance to hypersensitivity pneumonitis, these two diseases are substantially different, which is important in diagnosis. Hypersensitivity pneumonitis is a more serious disease.

Airway reactivity, as seen in asthma, has been associated with several different types of agricultural exposure to barn dust, particularly exposure to animal dander and mites living in feed. Other natural products causing asthmatic reactions are vegetable gums, flaxseed, castor beans, grain products, flour, orris root, papain, and tobacco dust.

BOX 21.3

Safe Use of Pesticides in Agricultural Production in Vietnam

In recent years during the implementation of an economic development program, Vietnam has moved from being a rice importing country to becoming the third-largest rice exporter in the world. However, the increasing use of pesticides and agrochemicals necessary to achieve this level of production has had environmental and human health consequences. As a result of the unsafe use and handling of hazardous pesticides, many Vietnamese farmers have been suffering from dizziness, headaches, itching, vomiting, lack of appetite, and insomnia.

To protect agricultural workers' health and ensure sustainable development in agriculture, the government of Vietnam, in collaboration with other scientific institutions, has developed and is implementing activities aimed at raising awareness of the dangerous effects of pesticides on human health and the environment. These include providing guidance on the safe handling and storage of pesticides, providing investment capital and financial support to farmers for reconstruction of irrigation systems and land enrichment, the use of personal protective equipment, and improvement of occupational safety and health in agriculture. The application of Integrated Pest Management (IPM) and use of new strains in agriculture have reduced the sums spent on agrochemicals and pesticides by one-half or even two-thirds; at the same time the health and living standard of farmers have been improved, and agricultural productivity has been enhanced as well.

Adapted from: Luong NA, Nam DQ. Safety and the sound use of pesticides in agricultural production. An important approach to the protection of human health and sustainable development in Vietnam. *Asian-Pacific Newsletter on Occupational Health and Safety* (1999;6(3):64–5.

Hypersensitivity pneumonitis is caused by repeated antigen exposures from a variety of substances. Antigens might be microorganisms from spoiled hay, grain, and silage. Hypersensitivity pneumonitis has been seen among workers from mushroom houses. Other causative agents of hypersensitivity pneumonitis are moldy malt (from barley), paprika dust, and coffee dust. Byssinosis is caused by raw cotton, flax, and hemp dusts where the main responsible component is an endotoxin (a constituent of bacterial cell walls).

Chemical Hazards

Chemical hazards encountered in agriculture include pesticides, fertilizers, oils, and many other hazardous chemicals.

Although developing countries use only slightly more than 20% of global pesticide production, more than 70% of the total burden of acute pesticide poisoning occurs there. Besides the acute toxicity of pesticides, such as organophosphates, a number of pesticides are responsible for chronic health sequelae, including neurological and respiratory effects. Specific pesticides have been implicated in increasing risks for particular cancers, and there is increasing concern for reproductive and immunological effects associated with specific pesticide exposures.

The Pesticide Manual, compiled periodically by the British Crop Protection Council, is a collection of information on almost all pesticides used worldwide, contains approximately 800 entries describing the structures and properties of active ingredients. There are more than 100 classes of pesticides, making it very difficult to generalize about the potential health hazards or other adverse health effects of pesticides. At the same time, pesticides are important agents in the prevention of several vector-borne diseases (e.g., malaria, yellow fever, onchocerciasis, or river blindness) and losses of crops and harvest. However, some pesticides pose toxic effects either of an acute (organophosphate and carbamate compounds) or long-term (organochlorine compounds, chlorophenoxy herbicides) nature. The organophosphate pesticides, which are among the most commonly used, can cause neurotoxicity. Allergic skin reactions present another type of health issue seen especially with the pyrethrins. Operators involved in handling, dispensing, and applying pesticides and post-application crop re-entry workers will be exposed to these compounds through different biological routes and to varying degrees.

Pesticide applicators may be exposed through inhalation and direct skin contact with formulations, and re-entry workers may inhale the pesticide or be dermally exposed to parent pesticides or their metabolites. Several pesticides become more toxic after application to plants: parathion converts to paraoxon, malathion to malaoxon, dithiocarbamates to ethylenethiourea, benomyl to carbendazim, and DDT to DDE. According to a rough estimate by WHO, approximately million people worldwide experience pesticide poisoning annually, and about 20,000 of the cases are fatal.

The potential for exposure to toxic gases and other compounds (pesticides, fertilizers, fuels, solvents, etc.) in agriculture is high (see Table 21.5). Toxic gases such as hydrogen sulfide and methane are released from manure in animal houses, especially at large dairy farms.

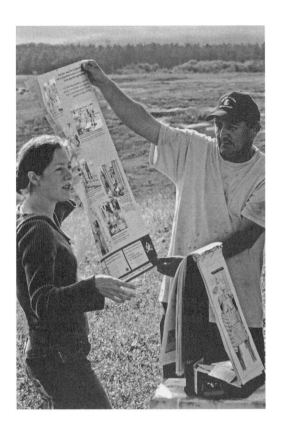

Figure 21.3 A volunteer instructor in Southern California teaches principles of pesticide and farm safety to immigrant workers in either English or Spanish, their native language. (Photograph by © Earl Dotter, all rights reserved.)

Hydrogen sulfide, a potent inhibitor of cytochrome oxidase, affects energy metabolism at the cellular level of organs with high oxygen consumption, such as the central nervous system, kidneys, and heart muscle. The typical effect of hydrogen sulfide exposure is to render the person unconscious. Inhalation can be fatal.

Ammonia vapor is a special health hazard in poultry houses and may also occur when ammonia fertilizer tanks leak. Ammonia has been reported to produce eye and skin irritation, respiratory distress accompanied by mucous membrane irritation, and coughing.

Silage, the product formed when grass or other crops are stored anaerobically (with little oxygen present) in vertical towers for the winter diet of ruminants such as cows, is a source of oxides of nitrogen, especially nitrogen dioxide. This gas may displace oxygen in a closed silo environment, thus increasing the risk of immediate unconsciousness and asphyxia. The typical outcome of silo filler's disease is the development a few hours after exposure of pulmonary edema, a condition in which the lungs fill with fluid due to inflammation and injury. This can be fatal.

In northern European countries, some formic acid-containing solutions are added to the forage to preserve silage. Formic acid, a very strong organic acid and irritator, is also a well-known irritant and is highly toxic.

Although in developed countries farmers appear to have a lower risk of cancer overall than city residents, there are some work-related hazards that increase the risk of certain cancers. Exposure to pesticides is associated with an increased risk of certain cancers among farmers. Exposure to ultraviolet light from long periods outdoors in the sun is associated with skin cancers.

Occupational Safety and Health in Agriculture

Occupational safety and health professionals face particular challenges in agriculture. Farms are usually far away from cities and may be remote from health-care services.

Many countries have recognized that improving conditions on farms and in rural areas is an important measure to ensure agricultural productivity as well as the health of rural populations. To keep sustainable growth in food production means that the basic needs of agriculture have to be met by encouraging farmers and their families to improve their working conditions and the municipalities to organize health services to rural areas. In addition, knowledge of the special features of occupational safety and health issues pertaining to agriculture must be taught in technical and medical schools. Governments, working with and through international agencies (e.g., ILO, WHO), have many reasons to be committed to occupational and environmental health in agriculture and to the economic and social development of rural communities.

Table 21.5 provides an overview of occupational health and safety issues in different agricultural settings.

Ill health High levels of existing illness, or *comorbidity*, among rural agricultural workers and their families may increase their risk from workplace exposures. Undernutrition, anemia, high levels of alcohol consumption, high rates of violence due to conflict, concomitant chronic illness (such as TB or HIV/AIDS) are risk factors increased in many rural agricultural regions around the world and may increase the risk of work-related injury or illness arising from agricultural exposures. For example, undernutrition in adult farm workers in South Africa has been shown to be associated with both poorer vibration sense, an early marker of

TABLE 21.5

TOXIC AND NEOPLASTIC HAZARDS IN AGRICULTURE

Exposures	Possible Health Effects
Manure gases, solvents, fumes	Acute intoxication, long-term toxicity
Pesticides; organophosphates, carbamates	Neurotoxicity, acute poisoning
Phenoxyacetic acids	Increased risk for certain cancers (non-Hodgkin's lymphoma)
Bipyridyl herbicides; paraquat, diquat	Severe lung injury
Other pesticides, fumigants	Various poisoning syndromes
Solar radiation	Skin cancer

Adapted from Myers, 1998.

neurobehavioral impairment, and increased oxygen desaturation, a marker of subclinical lung impairment resulting in oxygen deficiency.

Rural Development

Most agriculture takes place in rural communities, although urban agriculture is increasing in major cities. The agricultural economy and development patterns of rural areas are therefore intimately linked. Among the development issues faced by rural agriculture is how to get goods to market, how to cope with the labor surplus introduced by more efficient agriculture, how to maintain communities in the face of out-migration, and how to maintain essential services in a countryside that is often depopulated due to migration of young people to urban areas in search of jobs.

Rural communities undergoing development must deal with realities of time and space that are different from those of urban communities. In rural areas, distances between suppliers and consumers are greater, transportation takes longer, and the density of population is much less than in a city, so there is less efficiency in conducting business. Because the density of population is lower and usually more evenly distributed than in an urban area, it is often more practical to do business by bringing people together at a particular time rather than in a particular place. This is the basis for the traditional marketplace, where people would come on a special day to buy and sell goods and to conduct their personal business. Similarly, fairs, festivals, and expositions accomplish the same purpose. Many cities actually began as permanent settlements that grew on the sites for such markets and fairs. Prices for local commodities and land (except in agriculturally rich areas) tend to be low in rural areas compared to cities, but the cost of construction and transportation can be much higher.

The economy of most rural areas is based on agriculture and resource industries, such as mining, forestry, and fishing. Agricultural commodities and fishing may help to sustain the community, but most rural areas survive economically by selling these commodities or trading for the goods they need. Because commodities produced in the rural area must be sold or traded, rural areas tend to be very susceptible to changes in prices. If the demand for their commodity drops, prices may fall abruptly, as has often been the case for crops such as coffee or cacao. This means that rural areas are often highly dependent for their prosperity on goods that have fluctuating prices, and this leads to economic instability. Diversification of the rural economy has therefore been a goal in many countries. Where the density permits, some limited manufacturing can be supported, as with township industries in China where the rural districts are much more densely populated than in most countries. In developed economies, industries based on information services are now increasingly common in rural districts because improved communications makes it easier to live farther away from customers.

In developing countries, rural areas are often less developed than the local cities. The infrastructure is often relatively poor because investment is less productive in less dense settlements and the area to be serviced is much greater. Rural poverty is a common problem, aggravated if the rural area is remote from industries that could provide employment or if agriculture is weak or commodities are unstable. Land ownership is an important issue in agricultural communities and often lies at one of two extremes: widespread ownership of small plots of land that are too small to be economically productive or concentrated ownership of very large areas of land in the hands of a few people or families. Concentrated ownership is often associated with social unrest, exploitive labor practices, and overreliance on cash crops that are dependent on commodity prices. The tension between landowners and a class of resident farmers who farm the land and are required to pay rent is often at the basis of social unrest in such societies.

The economy in rural areas tends to be seasonal. Crops are planted, tended, and harvested according to the time of year and weather, and fishing may occur only during certain times of the year. Many rural residents therefore manage by making their money in mining or industry or crafts during the "off-season" and farming or fishing when they can. As a result, a "farmer" in a rural area may be more accurately described as someone who does many jobs, among them farming during the growing season.

Increasingly, globalization and high-speed transport has changed agriculture and rural development by creating opportunities for export worldwide. For example, in Colombia flowers are grown year-round to be flown to North America and Europe.

Socially, rural areas tend to be conservative and traditional. Families, clans, and neighbors are very important when there are few social institutions that can

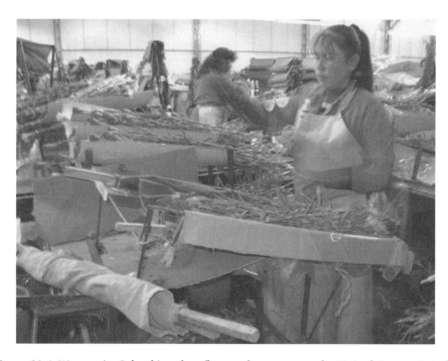

Figure 21.4 Women in Colombia select flowers for export to the United States, Canada, and Europe. (Photograph by Julietta Rodríguez Guzmán, Universidad El Bosque, Colombia.)

guarantee security and when communities are small. This conservatism is not absolute, and the influence of modern communications and transportation has clearly reduced the isolation of many rural areas. Likewise, the need to pay attention to commodity prices has made many rural residents experts on the operation of international markets. Overall, however, rural areas tend to be places where traditional values are held for a long time and where change is resisted. Partly as a consequence, the more adventurous of rural young people often leave the area to try their luck or to find opportunity in cities.

Environmental protection has a mixed meaning for rural areas. To the extent that environmental protection preserves the advantages of rural life and makes life in villages and isolated communities safer, it is often welcomed. However, environmental protection may be perceived as threatening to a community if it changes farming practices, removes resources from economic use, or interferes with the construction or development of infrastructure. Villagers who make their money, representing their entire disposable income, during a certain season— from, for example, wood-cutting or catching fish or harvesting a crop—may not accept that it is necessary to preserve the forest, reduce the catch, or save the soil. For them it may be a stark choice between the future they wish to have and having a future at all.

22

OCCUPATIONAL HEALTH AND SAFETY IN SMALL ENTERPRISES

Jeffrey Spickett and E. Wallis-Long

Small businesses are essential to the economy in every country and often account for more than 90% of businesses. For example, United Kingdom statistics indicate that small businesses account for 99% of private-sector businesses and 57% of total employment, which is similar to many other countries, including Australia (Health and Safety Commission 2000). Small businesses may include retail outlets, manufacturers, food outlets, workshops, builders, primary industry workers, health workers, offices, and professionals. A small business is generally defined as either a small nonmanufacturing business having 20 or fewer employees or a small manufacturing business of 100 or fewer employees. If a business has fewer than five employees, it is considered a "micro" business and in some countries, such as the United Kingdom, is dealt with differently under occupational health and safety law. Recent research indicates that many small businesses have neither the resources nor the time and ability to meet occupational health and safety requirements, but with the accident and injury rate at a higher level than medium and large businesses, a change in the culture of small businesses has to occur to lower the incidence of disease and injury. This chapter discusses the features of small business that have implications for occupational health and safety.

CHARACTERISTICS OF SMALL BUSINESS

Small businesses are usually managed by only one or two decision makers, frequently the owners, who often have received no substantial tertiary education or managerial training, with many of their employees having attained only secondary education or undertaken an apprenticeship. Employees are often family, friends, or personally recommended individuals. Partly associated with this practice is that previous work history, including any workers' compensation claims, may be known to the employer, and it is hoped that both loyalty to the employer and subsequent rewards to both parties will be of importance to the success of the business.

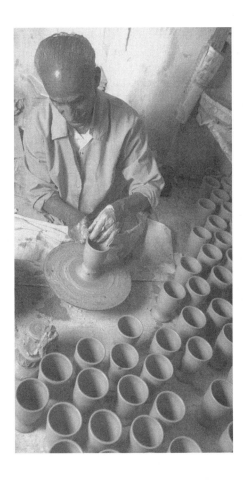

Figure 22.1 An example of a very small enterprise: a potter makes drinking cups in Palestine. (Photograph by Bill Lyons, Saudi Aramco World/SAWDIA.)

The culture and social norms of a small business mean that the working day is long, hard, and overly demanding, leaving insufficient time for anything that does not increase the economic well-being of the company. Any spending, either of time or money, on issues such as occupational health and safety is not seen as advantageous, especially as injuries from working at home and long-term health problems are often incorrectly seen as not being work-related.

Small businesses usually have very limited financial resources, with most owners concentrating on turnover and profit to ensure continuity of their business. Business time is therefore devoted to activities directly related to production and profit rather than paperwork and other regulatory activities. This results in a shortage of time for managers to consult with employees on issues including health and safety, with administrative matters tending to relate more to taxation and other governmental regulatory matters.

The business knowledge level of the workers in any small business is usually limited to the requirements of the actual business, e.g., car mechanics in garages, salespersons in shops, and so on. Management skills may be lacking, and time and money may not be available for additional staff training. The decision maker will be aware of some regulatory matters but will depend upon an outside person to advise the business on such requirements, usually the business's accountant or bank manager. It is often the accountant that the owner will turn to for help concerning occupational health and safety issues—and that is usually limited to workers' compensation. More often than not, a small business will only be able to afford an accountant from a small firm, and the accountant may be limited in his or her knowledge. Consequently, the requirements for duty of care, risk management, etc., are overlooked, with workers' compensation and taxation requirements taking prime position.

HEALTH AND SAFETY AWARENESS

The level of awareness of occupational health and safety is still low for the majority of businesses in relation to both costs/benefits and legislative requirements, with most business owners being concerned only about workers' compensation payouts. There is often a lack of knowledge regarding issues such as owners' legal duty of care, hazard assessment, safe procedures at work, consultation, training, and provision of personal protective equipment and clothing.

Occupational health and safety awareness does differ greatly between businesses; the larger of the small businesses are usually the most aware. The type of business also has some bearing on awareness; in businesses where employees have undertaken an apprenticeship somewhere other than their present workplace (motor mechanics, carpenters, electricians), there will be greater awareness

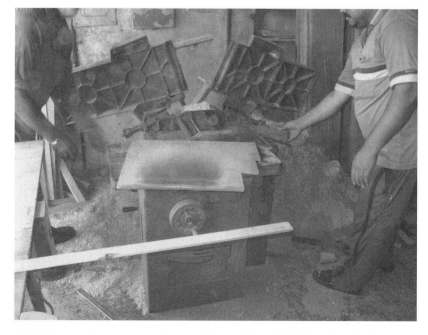

Figure 22.2 Heavy dust exposure in a small woodshop illustrates the challenges of small enterprises. (Photograph by Seifeddin Ballal, King Faisal University, Saudi Arabia.)

about health and safety issues. If employees are trade union members, there will certainly be a much higher awareness level of occupational health and safety leading to improved awareness for that business. Though very few small businesses have trade union members, more may have ex-union members.

Formal consultation on any matter between the decision makers of a small business and the employees is rare. It is more likely to revolve around a chat over a meal break, where health and safety issues may be raised in passing. No formal consultations occur in many small businesses, as time is money, and getting the job completed takes all the working day. Decision makers see time on consultation as precious time wasted.

While the occupational health and safety laws and regulations are a requirement for all businesses, the appropriate regulatory bodies do not have sufficient resources to regularly visit small businesses to enforce rules or offer guidance and assistance. Most businesses will never be inspected unless there is a serious accident that is referred to the regulatory body. Many small businesses are not even aware of their requirement to report serious injuries, which in turn leads to the publication of unreliable injury statistics. Statistics consequently indicate that only a small percentage of businesses will be inspected at most once over a 5-year period, even in a rich country like Australia.

Many small businesses are struggling to remain viable, and any spare time during the working day tends to be devoted to completing paperwork for the many government regulations that affect a business, usually taxation and other similar regulations. Occupational health and safety regulations are a long way down on the list of priorities, if they make the list at all. Current bureaucracy requirements have alienated many small business owners, and therefore they will undertake only what is necessary—usually paperwork that has to be submitted periodically to a government department to avoid a financial penalty.

COMPLIANCE WITH REGULATIONS

Small-business compliance with the occupational health and safety legal requirements depends upon a number of elements.

- Access to financial, time, and knowledge resources—If the business has sufficient funds to devote to health and safety (by way of hard-earned profits, a reduction in workers' compensation insurance premiums, government grants, bank loans, etc.), then a company may well increase its compliance. If occupational health and safety legislative requirements are easy to understand through Internet access or mentoring or assistance from larger companies or trade associations, then compliance will become part of the business.
- Training and industry experience—Apprenticeship training or previous work from a larger industry will increase compliance, as the knowledge and awareness are likely to have been learned as part of the training program. Financial constraints may mean that the compliance is not 100%, but at least a duty of care and risk assessments are likely to be carried over into the smaller workplace, yielding good, safe work practices.

- Mentoring and product provider safety advice assistance—Many large companies will offer assistance to small businesses with whom they have a contractual relationship to ensure that their partners' occupational health, safety, and environmental compliance is the same as their own, especially if working on government contracts or where union membership is high. Companies that supply products to small retailers, such as hardware stores, may provide training to ensure that their products are sold with the correct health and safety information, such as materials safety data sheets, use of personal protective equipment, and other safety practices. This knowledge flows to other areas of small businesses, increasing their health and safety knowledge and compliance.
- Trade associations, peak bodies, and other business councils—If a small business is a member of a trade association, chamber of commerce, or has a "peak body" to refer to, compliance is often greater because access to the necessary information will be more readily accessible, and members will be made aware of their obligations on a regular basis. A peak body is an advocacy coalition, consisting mostly of other organizations, often with union participation.
- Management skills and systems—Where decision makers hold tertiary education qualifications or a quality assurance system is in place, compliance will be higher. A safety management system that has good policies and procedures, risk management, and safe work systems will result in a high duty of care.

A good relationship between the small business and the occupational health and safety regulatory agency will make a very great difference to the occupational health and safety standards of that business and ensure better compliance.

RELATIONSHIPS WITH REGULATORY AGENCIES

Many small businesses view their country's occupational health and safety regulatory agency as an enforcement agency that seeks only to find violations and punish them, not as an advisory body that exists to help them. This is understandable because usually whenever they are visited by the agency, it is due to an incident that ultimately leads to a citation and a penalty. There may also be some confusion as to the role of the agency and the difference between enforcement and injury compensation. Most small businesses find occupational health and safety regulations very confusing, complex, and inflexible and believe that they apply more to large business. Small businesses also believe that they have not been consulted by government in the formation of the legal requirements and that the culture of small business has not been accommodated when drafting the regulations.

Surveys have indicated that many small businesses are often not sure as to which government agency they should contact for assistance, and they complain that it is not easy to contact the agency's representatives directly. But for those small businesses that do have regular contact with the agency, and where a good relationship has formed, the advice and assistance offered has greatly improved their commitment to good health and safety practices.

Most occupational health and safety regulatory bodies are now beginning to consider the culture and requirements of small enterprises, and many new initiatives are being put in place to target them. Free advice is always welcome. Thus, most agencies now produce industry- and business-specific pamphlets to assist in the recognition of hazards related to specific industries and offer suggestions as to mitigating strategies. This has enabled small businesses to understand the regulations that are unique to their industry and has led to increased compliance and lower incident rates. There is some evidence that the promotion of written information like this is not very effective, however.

ADVISORS AND SOURCES OF HELP

Small-business owners and managers frequently turn to outside businesses to advise and assist them with occupational health and safety requirements. Surveys have shown that, in most cases, the businesses' chartered accountants are the primary advisors on many matters including health and safety.

More small businesses are turning to specific occupational health and safety consultants for assistance in setting up a suitable safety management system for their business. While the service offered may be good, it is often quite generic, as the consultant may not have specific industry knowledge. At the end of the consultation process, the new safety management system may wind up sitting on a shelf in the business owners' office—never to be looked at again—but the owners have a system in place that meets their legal obligations, though it is not much of a benefit for employee safety if it is never implemented.

In many countries, the use of independent private providers is an innovation that is becoming increasingly successful. These are companies providing services under contract to a group of small firms in a specific geographical area with multidisciplinary teams to provide a total occupational health and safety service plan, from policies and procedures to injury management and rehabilitation. A recognized and well-documented historical example of such a success is a provider that was set up as a demonstration project in Slough, United Kingdom, to service a major industrial estate comprising large and small businesses. (Herford 1950) This service allows for the provision of permanent staff on site working alongside the business's own health and safety staff in a large company, and periodic provision of specific services to the smaller businesses (Health and Safety Commission 2000). Similar arrangements have been in place in some areas in South Korea where there is a concentration of small businesses.

Many trade associations, chambers of commerce, and other industry groups are now providing literature aimed at assisting small businesses to comply with regulations. Many of these groups also offer seminars and training, but these courses cost money and necessitate time away from work to attend, which is often not a viable option for very small businesses. Franchised businesses, however, will usually have excellent assistance from the franchiser, who supplies very specific safety manuals and a great deal of ongoing oversight to ensure that all legal obligations are maintained.

Easy access to free information is primary. The information should include industry-specific guidelines with policy and pro forma procedures to enable small businesses to understand their legal requirements and to offer the best way of managing their businesses' safety and health. This information needs to be in plain language and concise; the advice must be practical, supportive, and not dictatorial. There should be an easy format for businesses to follow in order to undertake risk assessments in their specific industry, with hazard control information that is practical and applicable to the size of the business. All personal protective equipment and clothing should be illustrated to give a very clear picture of what is required. Telephone help lines would be an easy option to help many busy small businesses.

Increased Internet access and online courses would benefit many small businesses, and media coverage of success stories should be more prominent. Trade associations should be encouraged to include an occupational health and safety section in their newsletters and outreach materials. Computer software is now readily available at a reasonable cost to enable small businesses to better manage occupational health and safety issues.

Occupational health and safety education should commence in grades 11 and 12—it would then become part of the essential education of preparing students for the workforce. All tertiary or higher education courses should include a health and safety component, especially for those students undertaking management, engineering, physical and chemical science, agriculture, mining, health studies, industry, building, hairdressing, and hospitality apprenticeships. Training and seminars should be made available at times more suitable to small businesses, such as in the evening or off-season, to ensure the best participation.

Accountants, bankers, lawyers, and other small business advisors must increase their knowledge of health and safety issues, with larger companies offering a specialist service. Increased mentoring and sharing facilities and personnel by larger companies would benefit many smaller businesses, especially those in a contractual relationship Occupational health and safety information and advice could be given to a new small business when it commences registration procedures, which would ensure that every small business became aware of its obligations prior to starting up (Howell 1998).

One strategy is to build on the successful plans that are currently in place by providing streamlined occupational health and safety services in areas where many smaller businesses are grouped together, such as the Slough model referenced above. The United Kingdom's Health and Safety Executive has also set up a Good Neighbor Scheme where larger companies assist their small contractors, suppliers, and neighboring businesses (Health and Safety Commission 2000). Finland, a country well advanced in occupational health and safety practices, is often praised for their excellent model in occupational health support, which is provided to employers by municipal, multidisciplinary, and primary care centers (Health and Safety Commission 2000).

Incentives to improve occupational health and safety awareness and increase safe work practices could be offered by insurance premium reductions, increased bank loans, and possibly increased tax relief Equality in contract tendering would increase occupational health and safety awareness if all goods and services contracts contained an occupational health and safety clause. Currently, small businesses that endeavor to comply with such requirements feel that they are financially penalized if their tender price is higher than noncomplying bidding businesses.

TRENDS IN VARIOUS COUNTRIES

It is now recognized that small businesses require substantial assistance to increase occupational health and safety awareness, improve workplace safety, and ensure that all workers remain healthy. Recent advancements in some countries are listed below.

United States

- The United States Occupational Safety and Health Administration (OSHA) in 1997 published a *Small Entity Compliance Guide*.
- The Small Business Regulatory Enforcement Fairness Act (1996) requires OSHA to consult with small business employers whenever a new regulation is introduced that will have a significant economic effect on their business.
- Voluntary Protection Program: Large companies have gone beyond the standard legal requirements for occupational health and safety and are using their expertise to mentor and assist smaller companies to improve the health and safety in their workplaces.

United Kingdom

- Free guidance for small firms entitled *Stating Your Business*, which contains a model health and safety policy and notes on how to set up a suitable safety management system.
- Safety Information Centers: Voluntary bodies offering assistance to small businesses to manage their health and safety issues effectively.

Europe

- Optimum Model: Special regulations for small- and medium-sized enterprises have recently been introduced in a number of European countries.

Finland

- Finland offers up to a 50% cost reimbursement through national health insurance if employers meet selected criteria for competence and worker consultation to comply with the country's occupational health and safety legal obligations.
- Small Workplace Program.

Hong Kong

- The Hong Kong Occupational Safety and Health Council has produced a Safety and Health Management Do-It-Yourself Kit for Small and Medium Enterprises containing a video, several CDs, a user manual, and a compact booklet directed at small businesses specifying safety legislation and the Council's work divisions.

Australia

- The Australian Chamber of Commerce and Industry has produced a publication, *Small Business Safety Solutions*, in order to improve the health and safety commitment in small businesses. Each state in Australia has its own occupational health and safety legislation, and every state's regulatory agency is currently promoting occupational health and safety awareness in small business.

BOX 22.1

The Informal Sector

The term "informal sector" was first used in the 1970s to describe that part of the economy that is not visible in economic statistics, organized for long-term economic activity, or recognized by government. The informal sector includes barter, street and traditional marketplace retail vendors, odd jobs and casual labor, mutual assistance (such as loans between friends or neighbors), and irregular services, such as providing local transportation. The informal sector is not restricted to the poor: informal transactions occur frequently among the rich, but the poor are much more often dependent on them for income. Some economists include criminal activities in the definition of the informal sector, but others do not and make a distinction, although many informal economic activities are illegal because they are almost always conducted without taxation or regulation.

Economic activities in the informal sector are very diverse but have common features: they are labor intensive and most of the workforce is self-employed. Many informal transactions and activities take place within or involving the family. Children often accompany parents to the workplace. Many workers in the informal sector are children of school age.

The informal sector is much larger than the formal economy in some countries and is estimated to employ from 30% to 80% of the workforce in many, probably most, countries. Many political leaders and economists refer to small enterprises and the informal economy as "engines of growth" and actively encourage their development, such as Mexico.

"Undocumented work" is performed by workers who agree to work "off the books," for cash or barter for "in-kind" goods or services. There is no permanent place of employment, no guarantee of employment security, and no fixed or dependable wage. Wage levels are usually low and the hours worked can be very long; highly paying

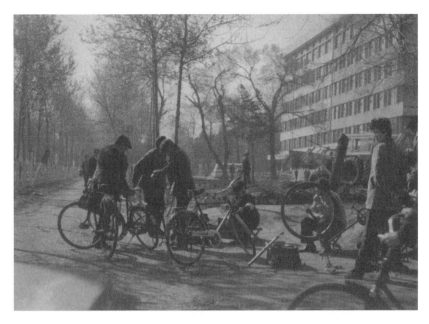

Figure 22.3 An example of an informal enterprise, a bicycle repair business on the street in Harbin, Helongjiang (China) in 1987. (Photograph by Tee L. Guidotti, University of Alberta.)

informal jobs tend to be criminal or at best one-off opportunities. Usually, such earnings are not reported to authorities and therefore escape taxation and regulation. However, the absence of any contractual employer-employee relationship places the workers at risk because they have no legal protection, they are not covered by workers' compensation, they do not earn social insurance or security benefits, and they are not visible to occupational health and safety regulation. In a dispute, the worker has no way to take legal action or to force compensation from an employer, supplier, or partner.

Informal work is often part-time and episodic, such as housekeeping, in which the worker may divide time among several customers during the week. It sometimes involves live-in arrangements, particularly for nannies, domestic help, and child care. These jobs often involve immigrant workers from poorer countries, some of whom may be imported for their labor illegally and because of their irregular legal status may lack protection from harassment, physical abuse, and exploitation.

"Moonlighting" is work done after employment hours by a worker who has a regular job.

Traders, street vendors, and "hawkers" selling in outdoor markets are an especially large group of informal workers. This type of work is often undertaken without adequate shelter, without access to toilets or clean water, and near streets with heavy traffic.

Scavenging is a common informal activity in developing countries, in which scavengers, often women and children, sort through rubbish and garbage to find items that can be used, sold, or burned as fuel. Recyclable material, such as aluminum or copper, is particularly prized because it has a ready market and high value. Scavenging is often done by families who live near or even in the rubbish dumps, where they are exposed to public health hazards in an unsanitary environment and often smoke from garbage fires. Injuries are common, and sometimes scavengers who have been digging are buried when a mound of rubbish collapses on them. Similar scavenging sometimes takes place around abandoned mines, in search of lower-quality ore that might have been left behind; such sites are extremely dangerous.

Child labor is a particular problem in these informal retail activities, scavenging, and in certain types of low-value manufacturing, such as rugs and brick making. Children engaged in this type of work miss school and therefore the opportunities that an education can provide to escape this life. They are often forced to carry heavy loads or perform physical tasks that their young bodies cannot handle without injury or disability. They are also vulnerable to abuse.

"Home work," "piece work," and "out work" is undertaken by home-based workers who make things in their own home for an employer. The home-based worker either makes and sells the finished piece to the employer or assembles the finished piece from supplies provided by the employer. The amount paid to the workers is based on a fixed price for each finished piece. This is attractive to employers because it reduces their overhead cost and shifts it to the worker. Because the employer has no investment in a plant, production is very flexible and can be increased, reduced, or even shut down very quickly. Workers may see piece work as initially advantageous because it does not require travel to work, allows highly flexible hours, and permits the worker to stay at home to care for children or dependents, which is why it is particularly attractive to women. However, home workers often encounter unexpected or rapid reductions in the price they get for their work or demands for increasing production to maintain the same income level. Some home work involves occupational hazards that are then brought into the home and may expose children and other family members.

Some countries are attempting to regulate home work by requiring employers to obtain a license before they are permitted to engage home workers and to keep records that can be inspected by the authorities. Thailand documented its home work sector in a survey published in 1999 and found approximately 311,790 exclusively home workers and another 644,038 homemakers who were also self-employed in the country, 54% of whom worked more than 250 days per year and 71% of whom worked 7 to 10 hours per day. They made at least 344 distinct products, including dresses, shoes, belts, purses, artificial flowers, wigs, fishing nets, ceramics, wood items, crafts, and foods. Home-base industries included weaving, metal-working, gemstone cutting, and woodworking, all of which may involve some hazards in the home. Documented problems included lack of ventilation, high temperatures, unsafe machinery, lack of personal protective equipment, inadequate lighting, exposure to toxic chemicals and dusts, and many ergonomic problems ranging from equipment to awkward seating arrangements. At the time, home workers were not covered under Thai labor law and therefore had no protection with respect to wages, working hours, employment security, occupational health and safety, and welfare.

The informal sector is often uniquely vulnerable to economic downturn. Globalization has brought changing international tastes and fashion into the local village and home, where home workers and sometimes child laborers make consumer products for export. Suppliers, frequently making products for major companies with international brands, prefer home work because of its flexibility. However, when tastes change or the world economy slows down, there may be a disproportionate loss of jobs and reduced earnings among home workers.

For all these reasons, it is much more difficult to provide effective occupational health services to the informal sector than to organized small enterprises, which itself is a much more difficult challenge than large enterprises. These problems are urgent because so many families and the economies of so many countries depend on the informal sector. The International Labour Organization, the World Health Organization, and the Scientific Committee on Small Enterprises and the Informal Sector of the International Commission on Occupational Health (a non-governmental organization) have drawn attention to these issues and the need for programs on a national level. Particularly high priorities are:

- uniform definitions and criteria so that different governmental organizations can exchange information
- research, so that the magnitude and complexity of the informal sector can be documented and understood
- formulation of effective models for delivering occupational health services
- more attention to the informal sector in education and training in occupational health and safety
- recognition of the informal sector's importance in job creation
- allocation of a share of attention and assets to the informal sector proportionate to its importance in every national economy

Solutions are possible, however, and some of them are very easy. Adjusting fluorescent lighting to meet the needs of the task, for example, costs very little and improves productivity. One small furniture manufacturing enterprise greatly improved the lighting in its factory by making an improvised skylight in its galvanized iron roof with clear polyethylene sheets, which the workers were able to make themselves cheaply and quickly.

The International Labour Organization has launched an initiative known as WISE (Work Improvement in Small Enterprises) emphasizing practical solutions for common problems in small and informal enterprises. In one early success in a garment factory that had many ergonomic and safety problems, both productivity and risk of injury improved when the workplace was fitted with improvised platforms to put the work at an appropriate height and backrests for the workers, which were made comfortable with cushions made from scraps from the factory. Evaluation by professional ergonomists confirmed that the energy requirements and injury risk experienced by the workers were much reduced.

Other practical small-scale improvements, easily achieved with little cost in time and materials, include work organization, organized transportation, worker training, education on occupational hazards, improved lighting, more sanitary kitchens and toilets, better organization of child care, and local food preparation with better nutrition.

Contributed by Wai-On Phoon.

23

THE WORKER

Tee L. Guidotti

An understanding of the worker is essential to understanding health in the workplace. In occupational health, engagement in work is what defines a worker, not social class or status or how the money is earned. A "worker" may be a professional with high status in the community or someone who of necessity works in a job that other people do not want. Some workers are temporarily out of work, and others are permanently unemployed, but they have worked at one time and usually expect to work again. This chapter discusses social issues affecting workers and special problems faced by particular groups of workers.

It is difficult to think about workers, as such, without relying on stereotypes. Social theorists usually see workers as an abstract class of people, mostly concerned with their lives and passively shaped by media, education, and class identification but sometimes allowing themselves to be organized into mass movements. Economists visualize the workforce as a vast, undifferentiated, predominantly male reservoir of labor, consisting of individual units (workers) who should be more mobile than they are and who usually demand too much money for their work. Management often sees workers as individuals with or without talent, motivation, and problems; the workforce as a whole is typically seen as consisting of numerous abstract categories defined by occupational or skill level or role in production, or organized into bargaining groups. Labor unions see workers as the bedrock supporting the rest of society and think of the workforce as a collection of organized trades and occupations. In the business model, a worker is defined as someone who is paid an hourly wage, as opposed to an executive who is paid a salary in monthly installments. People from more advantaged social classes may see workers as belonging to "the masses," a large population defined by the capacity to do necessary work and consisting of people without visible individual characteristics, except for the few they happen to meet. People from less advantaged social classes, and those who advocate for their interests, may see workers as heroes, supporting society without recognition or appreciation and accumulating grievances over injuries at the hands of their employers. Each of these points of view may contain some truth, but they all distort reality.

The problem is that these points of view deal in generalizations and ignore the great diversity and individualism among workers. Generalizations on the basis of social class, education, occupation, and so forth mislead more often than they provide guidance. Above all, workers are people and their involvement in work is a role that they play, not the sum of the meaning or the value of their lives. Workers are also family members, members of a community, adherents of particular beliefs, and consumers in an interconnected economy, who must purchase, with money earned from their employment, what others produce through their work. They have roots in a particular community, whether or not they travel, and they have connections with the world that have little or nothing to do with their jobs.

The occupational health professional regularly deals with workers on two levels, as individuals and as groups. It helps to be explicitly aware of these two levels in one's thinking.

Individual workers come with group characteristics, such as ethnicity, but every worker represents a highly individual combination of group, family, and social characteristics, each of which may or may not predict or influence his or her personality or lifestyle. To treat individual workers as members of "the masses," a vast, undifferentiated (without distinct characteristics) or amorphous (without shape or structure) workforce characterized by group averages is therefore to miss their real needs and the determinants of their health.

Groups of workers may be organized or unorganized. Unorganized workers are not represented by a formal organization representing their interests. *Organized labor* refers to labor unions, which exist to protect the interests of their members and to engage management in negotiations over wages, hours, and working conditions, including occupational health. Unions are usually organized as *locals* (local chapters) of national unions, and several unions may be *confederated* into larger national organizations or *federations* with a common policy. However, some unions represent only workers in a particular workplace or for a particular employer. The workers' representative in a particular workplace is called the *shop steward*.

In some countries, workers play a central role in addressing their own occupational health and safety. In Canada, for example, provinces require *joint health and safety management committees*, which hold mandatory meetings to review safety performance and the management of occupational hazards. In Germany, the model of worker participation in corporate governance through work councils and supervisory boards gives workers a direct and powerful voice in health and safety issues. However, in all countries with contemporary labor legislation, the employer is held ultimately responsible for health and safety in the workplace.

It is useful to make certain distinctions in describing the patterns of employment that are characteristic of certain jobs and the workers that fill them. *Skilled work* is work that requires training. This training may be formal, through education; it may take place in the form of an *apprenticeship*, in which an older and more experienced worker (sometimes called a *master*) teaches a new worker (the *apprentice)* until he or she attains a certain level of skill (and is then sometimes called a *journeyman*); or it may take place informally through experience, usually on the job. *Unskilled work* is work that does not require training, experience, or capacity

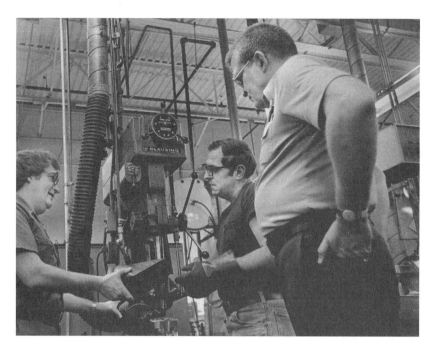

Figure 23.1 A discussion among workers on the shop floor of a factory in the United States. (Photograph by © Earl Dotter, all rights reserved.)

beyond physical ability, such as a laborer who carries boxes and unloads trucks. *Casual labor* is unskilled work that is done on a daily, as-needed basis without long-term contract or commitment from the employer. *Informal work* is work that is irregular, usually occasional, and is conducted outside the wage economy, such as street vendors, farmers' markets, shoeshine workers, and bicycle repair on the street. Typically, such work is poorly paid, no records are kept, income is not declared for taxes, and activity in the informal economy does not show up in government statistics. The *underground economy* is also unrecorded but consists of undeclared, untaxed, or illegal activities, including black-market money changing, prostitution, and drug dealing. Some authors consider the underground economy to be a subset of the informal economy.

An *occupation* is an activity that individuals perform to earn a living, usually to earn money to support themselves and their family if they have one. A *usual occupation* is what a worker does most of the time to earn a living. A *career* is what a skilled or professional worker does over a long period of time, often a lifetime, with the expectation of improvement or advancement. *Trades* are occupations that are learned through apprenticeship and that are usually practiced on different projects for different employers and not necessarily for a single employer in a single location. Construction trades, for example, include electricians, plumbers, carpenters, and tile setters, the first two of which are usually subject to state regulation to protect their clients. A *job* can mean any occupation, but it sometimes means a particular task and sometimes an occupation in which the person

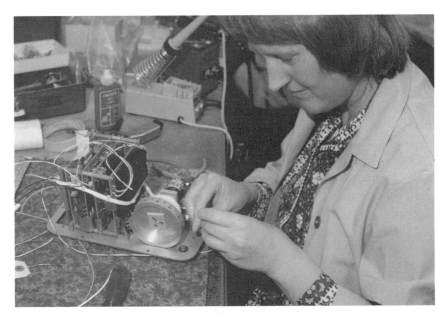

Figure 23.2 A skilled electronics assembly worker assembles components in Nevada in 1977, work that is often done today by robots but at that time seemed irreplaceable and secure. (Photograph courtesy of Saudi Aramco World/SAWDIA.)

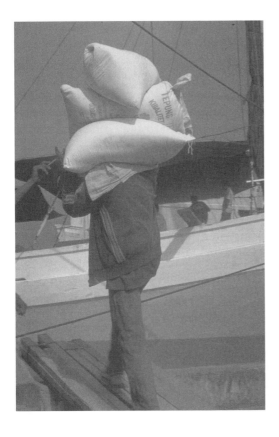

Figure 23.3 Laborer carrying bags of rice in Indonesia, unskilled work that is hard, poorly paid, and insecure. (Photograph by Bryn Bruijn, Saudi Aramco World/SAWDIA.)

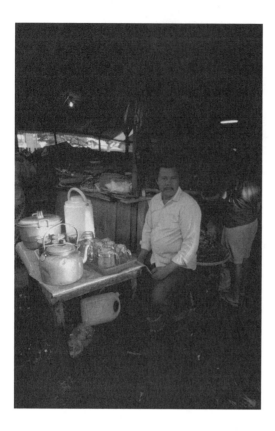

Figure 23.4 A food seller sells flavored rice from a pushcart in Indonesia, an example of informal work. (Photograph by Brynn Bruijn, Saudi Aramco World/SAWDIA.)

works for an hourly wage. A *profession* is a skilled occupation that requires education, is more or less self-regulated, and, in theory, improves itself in knowledge and technique over time. The traditional professions in Europe were medicine, law, and the clergy. Now the term is used to include architects, scientists, administrators, and many other occupations that require education and standardized qualifications.

In English-speaking countries, especially in North America, the term *blue collar* is used to describe workers in skilled occupations who work with their hands, and the term *white collar* is used to describe workers in offices and occupations where most of the work is mental or involves paperwork. By extension, *pink collar* is sometimes used to refer to jobs that in those countries were traditionally performed by women, such as secretaries, nurses, and elementary school teachers.

OUTREACH PROGRAMS

Designing an outreach program to target a particular group that has special needs or faces particular obstacles requires sensitivity to the community's culture, predominant beliefs, language, and means of communication. Outreach programs may be generally educational, may raise community awareness of a specific problem, or may provide services. They are intended to change behavior, however. In occupational health, they are most common in situations where an employer, the government, or a non-governmental organization is trying to improve conditions for a group of workers.

Designing programs to meet the needs of workers as a group absolutely requires attention to group characteristics, but it is important to retain enough flexibility to accommodate individual needs.

Some of the characteristics of any group of workers that are important to keep in mind when designing programs follow.

Race, ethnicity, and degree of assimilation. Programs may become more attractive to or identified in one socially and culturally defined group than another, and there are often cultural barriers to participation in health-related programs. Immigrant groups are often particularly difficult to reach through programs designed for the majority culture and respond better to programs in their own language and communications from their own leaders.

Immigration status. In many countries, such as Saudi Arabia and Germany, large populations of immigrant (expatriate) workers are an important part of the national workforce. They often perform work that residents will not do or for which there are not enough workers in the national labor pool. Often, their wages are sent home and become important sources of support for their home communities and countries. However, while they are in the host country, they are often isolated and have to overcome many obstacles. This is even more true for workers who are in the country without documentation, as illegal immigrants.

Language and literacy. For many groups of workers, the standard national language is not the major means of expression. Literacy in the national language or even in a mother tongue may be weak in some groups. For example, in remote and often impoverished places in Peru, many native workers do not speak Spanish well and may not be able to write in Quechua, their native language.

Urbanization. Workers who have been born into or have become accustomed to city life and urban cultures may respond quite differently than those who are accustomed to rural values. In countries such as South Africa and Zambia, for example, programs to educate workers about the risk of HIV/AIDS are different for the urban residents, miners (who are urbanized workers who live in employer-sponsored communities while they are working), and rural residents.

Community identification. Neighborhood boundaries may be invisible to outsiders but constitute psychologically perceived barriers when they must be crossed by members of a social group with close community identification, regardless of the actual distance. In Africa, residents of informal communities may consider themselves very different from townspeople who live in organized communities.

Social organization. Certain trades, jobs, and employers rank higher in status in the community than others. For example, among the construction trades in North America, status is largely based on the technical complexity of the work. Electricians are usually considered to have the most prestige, followed by plumbers and carpenters, and then by drywall installers or bricklayers.

Social status. Outside the plant gate, status in the social organization of the community may be entirely different than the hierarchy seen inside a plant. The relative status of a factory worker, foreman, supervisor, and manager (in ascending level of status in the workplace) may break down in their own community, where the factory worker may be an official in his or her church, the foreman may be the head of his very large family, the supervisor may consider running for mayor of the village, and the manager may have a bad reputation. Likewise, in Africa a worker may often hold status in his tribe or clan that places him (usually male) in a superior social position to his supervisor at work.

Religion. In certain communities, prevailing religious sentiments may require that certain food preferences or days of observance be respected by management. For example, religious holidays may require time off for observant workers, even if the holiday is not observed by the predominant religion of the community.

Educational level. In some communities, formal education may be highly valued, as it has been traditionally in Chinese culture. In others, formal education may be less highly valued than skills, trades, and the wisdom of experience. For example, the Masai people of Kenya are renowned as warriors and for their skill in raising cattle. Traditionally, they have valued this skill, and their independence, more highly than formal education. Because their pastoral lifestyle has been very successful, the community's priority was placed on traditional education rather than school. Only recently have large numbers of Masai children, especially girls, left their tightly organized communities to participate in formal education.

Standard of living. Workers accustomed to a middle-class lifestyle may fiercely resist downward wage adjustments and may go into debt to maintain their living conditions and social status. For example, in North America many workers ran up large credit card debts in order to maintain their lifestyles for as long as they could after the software industry laid them off, on the expectation that their period of unemployment would be brief. On the other hand, the recent recession from the beginning in 2008 and afterward clearly looked like it would be worse and so it was associated with a reluctance to spend money by people who instead wanted to save in order to protect themselves. This reluctance to spend caused a sharp dip in spending that complicated economic recovery.

Social class. Quite apart from income and education, self-perceived social class is as important a determinant of lifestyle and attitudes as income. Awareness of social class was historically a particularly strong characteristic of British culture, among many others, and its effects can be seen in speech patterns, fashion, and choice of careers. However, as in many countries, the United Kingdom is experiencing a blurring of social classes and this feature, while still very important, is less of a limiting factor for young people than it once was. In India the caste system still exerts a strong influence on social interactions.

Family ties. Certain behaviors, especially those associated with taking risks, are strongly associated with a sense of responsibility and social stability. For example, in traditional societies, the firstborn son of a man who is leader of the family is naturally expected to take over. In parts of Africa, the brother of a man who dies is expected to support and even marry the widow, in order to ensure that family is taken care of.

Legal status. Illegal immigrants, or "undocumented" workers, are very prevalent in some industries in certain regions of the United States, particularly the Southwestern states. These workers may be very reluctant to participate in any activity requiring personal identification.

Health trends in the local community. Tuberculosis, hepatitis B, dental problems, intestinal parasites, side effects of traditional medications or treatments, and anemias of various causes, among other disorders, are more common in many disadvantaged communities. Disease and disability are almost always more common in less affluent communities compared to those with a higher income. Communicable diseases may require special attention to protect the health of other workers.

The complexity of the interaction of these factors becomes apparent when one considers the examples in Box 23.1.

Input from people who are part of and know the community is essential. One good way of doing this is to organize committees or panels of worker representatives to react to proposals and to suggest modifications. A much less effective way to obtain input is to ask one particular individual to serve as a permanent advisor, because that person may not be representative of the community in the first place, will cease to be representative as soon as he or she is singled out, and will become less representative the more he or she is consulted. Community representatives often have personal interests in the community, such as family obligations or tribal rivalries, that are separate and not necessarily in line with the interests of the rest of the community. Perhaps the best way to proceed is to turn the design of the outreach aspects of the program over to members of the target group itself but to retain control over the message itself.

BOX 23.1

Programs for Worker Health Protection or Health Promotion

Outreach programs are targeted to a particular group of people and are intended to meet their particular needs. The following are hypothetical examples of outreach programs for the protection and promotion (see Chapter 18) of the health of workers, based on cases in particular communities in North America in the 1980s and 1990s.

Example 1

White, mostly high-school-educated, blue collar workers in a medium-sized Appalachian town were recruited to work for a Japanese-owned automotive assembly plant. How will they respond to a corporate fitness and health promotion program? These programs are very important in Japanese corporations as a way by which workers and management forge a common bond. Will they work in an individualistic society such as the United States?

The Japanese managers found that although American workers appreciated the fitness programs, they were not inclined to identify with the company to the same degree as Japanese workers. The programs in the U.S. therefore emphasized personal health and fitness rather than company loyalty.

Example 2

Recent Philippine immigrants in California, mostly women with a middle-school education who speak heavily accented but fluent English, work in a medical instruments assembly plant requiring tight control over product quality and sources of contamination. How will they react when a newly arrived sister in a well-known family is found to have tuberculosis and management wishes to have everyone in the workplace screened? Will disclosure of her condition be considered an invasion of privacy or an insult to the community?

Although the company was worried about offending the workers, the workers were actually concerned enough about their own health risk that they wanted to be tested.

Example 3

A small hospital in Toronto employed primarily Portuguese and Italian workers from immigrant families, now well-established but still not completely assimilated. What will be their response to an employee assistance program? Will they ask for help and provide sensitive information to someone outside their community? Would they prefer to deal with members of their own community when they have personal problems?

The workers were very reluctant to trust the employer's program. They preferred to deal with their own institutions, such as churches and social organizations.

Example 4

Hispanic workers, mostly from Central America, make up a very large percentage of the construction workers in Washington, DC. Their risk of serious injury and even death on the job is much higher than that of native-born residents. What outreach programs would help to reduce this risk and improve the situation?

Programs oriented toward young men with families seemed to be most successful, delivered through social service agencies and churches. Employers were also made aware of the problem through local government activities.

There is no single correct solution to any of these examples, but in every case the program in question must be analyzed from the point of view of the workers, not just from the point of view of management.

WOMEN IN THE WORKPLACE

Women work for the same reasons as men, and their motivations are as simple and practical as are the motivations for men. They need the economic support for themselves or their families. They may also wish to develop personal careers and/or to pursue professional goals.

In many societies, women, especially in certain social classes, are not allowed to work outside the home. Educational opportunities may also be restricted for women in those societies. In other societies, women may participate as fully as men in the workforce, taking any job and rising as high as their ability will carry them. In any society, however, the experience of women who work is different

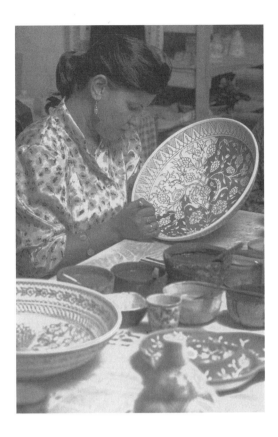

Figure 23.5 A skilled artisan paints intricate designs on pottery in a family-owned workshop in Palestine. (Photograph by Bill Lyons, Saudi Aramco World/SAWDIA.)

from that of men and is shaped by certain social and biological differences. These include the following.

Social expectations. In most societies, the woman's community and family have different expectations for women than for men. The woman is expected to take care of the home and the men to earn a living. In many countries, this division of labor broke down in the 1980s and 1990s, when social attitudes changed and two incomes became the norm for many families.

Gender roles. In most societies, little girls are brought up differently than little boys. The girls are usually taught to play house and the boys are taught to hunt or play sports. These differences carry over in adult life. Certain jobs are traditionally considered to be women's work (e.g., nurse, secretary, and elementary school teacher). These gender roles do not always make sense—in North America, women usually serve at tables (waitresses) in restaurants that are not expensive, and men usually serve at tables (waiters) in expensive restaurants, but both can do the same job equally well.

Wages. In general, jobs traditionally associated with women are lower paid than jobs traditionally associated with men. This is partly because those jobs are often in supporting roles (such as librarians) or in helping professions (such as nurses), which pay less. In many countries, women are paid less to do the same job, regardless of qualifications. This is usually justified by claiming that men are more likely to be the principal wage earners in the family or that women are more likely to take time off to raise a family, but the effect is to discriminate against women.

Biological factors. There are only a few biological factors that make a difference in the ability of women to do work compared to men: one of them is relative strength. Although individual women may be as strong as or stronger than the average man, the average woman has less upper body strength and is therefore less likely to be able to perform certain jobs. There are certainly women firefighters and miners around the world, but there are many fewer of them than men, in part because of the strength difference.

Pregnancy. Because women give birth and men do not, women often must make adjustments in their career for pregnancy and to care for children. Even in Sweden, which has generous allowances for parental leave, mothers take much more time off for child care than fathers. Many countries have legislation mandating allowance for maternity leave, particularly in Europe, and guarantees of return to the same or similar jobs.

Education. Some societies do not place a high value on education for women, while others do. In the United States, it was once uncommon for women to become medical doctors. Today, over half of students training to be physicians are women. This has been true for many years in some other countries, such as Russia.

Mentorship. Because there are few women in positions of business leadership in some countries, it is difficult for women to look up to successful role models and to get good advice and practical help on problems that are unique to women. As a result, fewer women make it to the top, continuing the cycle of fewer female role models in business.

Family and home responsibilities. When women have a career, they usually continue to provide a disproportionate share of support for their families than men, even when men try to help. In North America, the most recent trend is that women are increasingly providing care for the elderly who live with them at home in addition to caring for their own children, even when they work full-time.

Mobility. Because of family ties, safety concerns, and social expectations regarding marriage, women are less likely to move or emigrate to seek jobs. In many traditional societies, there are restrictions on how women may travel. In some countries in the Middle East, for example, women cannot drive and cannot ride in cars with men to whom they are not related. This makes it difficult to work outside the home.

These factors act together to the disadvantage of women. For example, women who enter an occupation where men and women are equally represented may find that over time they fall behind the men in income and seniority because they need to take more time off for child care and family. Many jobs traditionally held by women are exacting, monotonous, and dead-end in career potential. Women deal more often than men with conflicts about time management, child care, and expectations for themselves and others.

Occupational inequality also exists because a woman's traditional reproductive and maternal roles cause some employers to expect a lack of continuity in pursuing a career. Hiring women may be discouraged because of fears that employees will quit or take time off to rear children or pursue family responsibilities. This attitude becomes a self-fulfilling prophecy when employers are reluctant to risk hiring women for positions that require a substantial commitment and time investment from the employee. Women may become concentrated in less meaningful positions. Women who work in occupations generally considered appropriate for men may enjoy increased earnings but often do encounter some discrimination on the job. For example, in North America, women college professors in math and science earn more than women in traditionally "female" disciplines, such as the humanities, but earn less than their male counterparts, often because they lose seniority in their department because of time taken for pregnancy and child care.

Concern over the occupational health aspects of increasing numbers of women in the workplace has centered on three main issues:

- health risks during pregnancy, both to the mother and the fetus
- relative capacity of women to perform certain types of work
- vulnerability of women to certain types of exposure and health risks

However, the occupational health issues of women can be overemphasized as well. Concern over the effects of work on women during pregnancy has sometimes had the effect of excluding women from jobs, reducing their earning potential, limiting their ability to provide for their families, and closing opportunities in their personal and professional growth. As well, managers often consider women to be poor employment risks because marriage and relocation or pregnancy might cause them to leave, to reduce their productivity, or to show less serious interest in building a career. Employers who understand the problem and appreciate the potential of their women workers make the organization of work more flexible in order to accommodate their needs.

General health precautions that apply during pregnancy depend on the individual woman. In general, it is advisable to avoid excessively tiring work, heat, prolonged standing, and heavy lifting during the last weeks of pregnancy, but unless there are complications or other medical reasons, pregnant women can perform essentially any of the duties that would be required of them before pregnancy. There is no basis for the common practice of asking women to leave their job in the fifth or sixth month whether or not there is potential for harm to the mother or fetus.

Chapter 16 discusses reproductive health risks. Exposures that may be dangerous during pregnancy to a child-bearing woman, such as lead and solvents, may also be cumulatively dangerous over a longer period of time to a male or nonpregnant female worker. The principle to be followed is to control the hazard rather than to exclude the worker (see Chapter 12) in order to create a safe working environment for everyone.

The relative capacity of women to do work compared to men is properly an issue of fitness to work (see Chapter 17). As noted above in the example of firefighters and miners, some women are able to do work requiring upper body strength as well or better than men, but most cannot. In most traditional societies women do very strenuous work in the fields and home. The capacity for hard physical labor is highly individual. Ballet dancers are highly trained athletes, for example, with remarkable stamina, and most professional female ballet dancers probably match or exceed the fitness of most male football athletes. It is often said that women are better at fine, detailed work than men and have greater manual dexterity, which has led, for example, to employment opportunities in electronic assembly plants in northern Mexico. However, in many societies, such as Pakistan, it is the men who weave rugs or make jewelry, with great delicacy and precision.

Women who are healthy and fully mature are not significantly more susceptible to toxic exposures than men. What examples there are of differences in susceptibility tend to involve reproductive health effects.

BOX 23.2

The Informal Sector: Making Charcoal in Zambia

Making charcoal is an important economic activity in Zambia, as it is throughout southern Africa, but this activity does not appear in most economic statistics. It is an activity of the informal sector, conducted by individuals, families, and small groups of primarily young men. Unfortunately, this activity is very destructive and is a root cause of serious ecological problems in the countries where it is practiced.

Charcoal is made by heating wood until it is converted to almost pure carbon and thus is a lightweight fuel that is more efficient to burn than wood. It is mostly used for heating and cooking in informal settlements, which are poor and have inadequate or irregular public services such as electricity, transportation, or running water.

The first step is to locate a source of wood as close as possible to a roadway but far enough away that nobody will try to stop this activity. Unfortunately, in the central part of Zambia, much of the forest and tree cover has already been cut down, a process called *deforestation*. Deforestation has caused severe environmental problems throughout Africa. The remaining trees are needed for shade and for protection against erosion and flooding. However, due to a shortage of wood the trees continue to be cut down. Because the people who do the cutting have only hand tools, they cannot chop thorough the trunk of a large tree, so they cut off the branches. The result is destruction of an entire tree for the wood of a few large branches.

The branches are partially buried and a fire is started over them. These fires are hard to control. Smoke blows in the direction of the wind and sparks fly and may set off brush fires. The heat from the fire chars the wood without burning it and turns it into charcoal. The fire has to be kept hot enough to char the wood, but the buried wood cannot be allowed to catch fire because then the wood would burn instead of creating charcoal. This is very dangerous, and the charcoal makers have to work in smoke and around intense heat.

When the fire cools down, the charcoal makers dig out the new charcoal and chop it into pieces. The charcoal pieces are wrapped in plastic or paper to make large bundles. These bundles are then brought to the side of a nearby road and sold. Anyone who has transportation can buy bundles for approximately K5,000 each (Zambian kwacha) or approximately one euro or one U.S. dollar. Some charcoal makers have their own transportation, but it is not unusual to arrange for transportation of charcoal in trucks or cars that are going between cities for other purposes. Sometimes this use of the vehicle is unauthorized, and the owner of the vehicle is unaware of the additional load.

The bundles represent a wholesale commodity, bought and transported in large quantities. The charcoal is sold as a retail commodity, a small amount at a time, to families for household heating and cooking. Once the bundle is brought into a community, it is broken down into more than a hundred smaller packets for distribution. Several packets at a time are then sold to a retailer. Each retailer takes their packets to their marketplace stall or to their home for sale to their neighbors and village customers for a few kwacha each. Because the people who use charcoal for fuel are mostly poor, they can afford to buy only one or, at most, a few packets at a time, as they would not want to risk wasting it or having it stolen if they kept bigger quantities at home.

The entire system depends on a steady stream of charcoal being supplied by this informal mechanism. No records are kept and no taxes are paid, but charcoal is an essential product for millions of Africans. Unfortunately, it has also been a powerful cause of deforestation, air pollution, and injuries. This is clearly not a sustainable economic activity and is very destructive to the environment, but it supports many people and supplies many more with needed fuel.

Prepared by Tee L. Guidotti

UNEMPLOYMENT

Perhaps the ultimate paradox is that occupational health professionals should be concerned with unemployment. There are real consequences to leaving an occupation, and occupational health professions should be aware of them.

There are several different terms that may apply when a worker leaves work. If a worker is removed against his or her will, that worker is said to have been *fired*. If the worker is released from employment because the employer is reducing the workforce, usually to save money, the worker is said to have been *laid off*, or *furloughed*. If a worker cannot find another job in the short term, he or she is said to be *out of work*, but if this condition lasts for more than a few weeks, he or she is said to be *unemployed*. *Unemployment rates* are calculated by government statistical agencies that count the number of people who are actively seeking work but cannot find it. People who stop seeking work are usually not counted.

Many countries have systems of *unemployment insurance*. While they are working, workers and their employers pay a small amount into a fund. When the worker is laid off, the fund pays out money to partially replace the lost wages to support the worker until he or she can find another job. Most systems put a limit on the period that unemployment insurance can be collected, and many require that the worker actively search for a new job while collecting the benefits. Although it is primarily intended to support wage earners during periods of layoff, unemployment insurance is also heavily used in the countries where it is offered to seasonal workers, who use it as a cushion. For example, fishermen and agricultural workers may earn most of their money during a particular season, and work may not be available in their communities during the "off-season." Unemployment insurance is used as a bridge to provide a minimum income during those times. During times of recession, it is also an economic counterweight, keeping money flowing through the economy when employment is weak.

Employees who are laid off and workers who cannot find jobs have psychological as well as material needs. Workers remain socially and psychologically identified with their occupation, employers, workplaces, and fellow workers whether working or not. To be laid off is very stressful psychologically.

Good research strongly links unemployment with adverse health effects related to psychological adjustment, migration, loss of support from social networks, self-perception of health status, and, in the United States, loss of health insurance. These studies show that unemployed workers are at greater risk than employed workers for dying earlier, substance abuse (particularly alcohol), family violence, and depression.

Some employers provide special services to workers who will be laid off. These may include:

- counseling, to reduce the psychological impact
- relocation or repatriation, to go home if the worker relocated to take the job
- placement services, to work with the worker to find another job
- benefits, which may include continuation of health insurance in countries where this is paid for by the employer directly; these benefits are continued for a limited time on the assumption that the worker will find other work before the period expires

A worker remains a worker in a social sense, whether employed or laid off. Thus, unemployment is one of the most significant determinants of health, even though it is not a typical work-related hazard.

24

COMMON OCCUPATIONS

Fu Hua, Tee L. Guidotti, and Kari Lindström

This chapter discusses the occupational hazards and health risks within small businesses, technical or office support services, and public services. These enterprises do not necessarily fall into the classical definition of industries, but they exist in all communities and have risks and health outcomes that need to be addressed. This chapter discusses the occupational health issues within key sectors of economic activity.

ARTISTS

Artists often work alone or in small groups outside formal workplaces, making them difficult to access through more formal mechanisms. Artists often work without knowing their risks or taking adequate precautions. Art studios may lack adequate ventilation or safety measures to prevent exposure to the many hazards described below. These risks described below apply equally to artists, art teachers, and art students. Performing artists, such as musicians and dancers, have a high risk of musculoskeletal injuries and behavioral disorders.

Graphic Arts

Graphic artists are often exposed to hazardous chemicals. Their families may also be exposed to these chemical if the artists work at home. They often use organic solvents. For many years, benzene was a serious hazard for printmakers and silk-screen artists, and even today there are high levels of exposure to solvents used in silk-screening and print-making, with the possible risk of neuropathy. Acids are used in etching and preparing stones for lithography.

Sculptors

For sculptors, flying marble chips have been a well-known hazard historically; Michelangelo was nearly blinded in one eye from such an incident. Today, most stone sculptors wear eye protection and gloves. Metal sculptors share the hazards of welders and foundry workers and, if they do spray painting, they may be exposed to organic solvents, such as toluene. Production of plastic and epoxy-fiberglass sculptures involves the risks found in plastics fabrication.

Decorative Arts

The decorative arts have some of the highest levels of health risks. Ceramic artists use high silica-containing clay, and some clays contain fibrous silicates, such as asbestos or zeolites. Kiln firings may produce high levels of nitrogen and sulfur oxides. Lead, cobalt, manganese, and other metal-containing glazes contain toxins that can lead to metal fume fever and chronic toxicity, especially in producing raku. Lead poisoning is a risk in stained glass making and in crystal shaping. Jewelry making and cloisonné (a method of applying enamel to a metal base) carry a risk of lead exposure from soldering and preparation of the glaze. A common and dangerous habit of "pointing" (putting the tip of brushes into the mouth to get a fine point) may lead to ingestion of toxic materials.

Textile Arts

Textile arts have been associated with many toxic exposures. Aniline dyes are associated with skin problems and cancer risk. Fiber and irritant dusts are associated with respiratory problems. Chromium in certain dyes leads to allergic sensitivity. Some textile artists who work with raw wool or horsehair may even be at risk for anthrax, since spores cling to untreated fibers. More commonly today, however, is repetitive strain injury, which is particularly associated with carpet weaving and other non-mechanized knotting and weaving operations. Cyanotype, a technique for transferring images from a photographic negative to cloth, uses ferricyanide, with possible emissions of free hydrogen cyanide gas in the presence of heat, ultraviolet radiation, or acid.

Performing Arts

In general, performers are most at risk of performance anxiety, electrical hazards from lighting, traumatic injuries involving stage or other rigging, and fire hazards from special effects. Performers are under considerable stress, particularly when they are famous, and thus may be at risk for alcohol and drug abuse and stress-related psychological problems.

Actors may experience skin irritation and allergies from theater makeup as well as injuries from falls, stunts, and other risky performance requirements. Because of the emphasis placed on their appearance, actors are more likely than other artists to undergo cosmetic surgery and to expose themselves to the risk of complications from the surgery.

Dancers are at risk of repetitive strain injuries, acute strains and sprains, and stress fractures. These risks can be prevented by sufficient warm-ups and by ensuring adequate rest periods. The physical stereotype of the tall, thin dancer capable of performing extreme feats of strength has led to very unhealthy training practices that are now beginning to change. The traditional life of a ballet dancer, with its emphasis on being thin and very strong, is associated with eating disorders (anorexia and bulimia) and amenorrhea (loss of menstrual period), which is a physiological response to strenuous exercise in girls and young women and to an abnormally low proportion of body fat (seen in many professional dancers). Amenorrhea carries with it an increased future risk of osteoporosis, or thinning of bones, in older age.

Musicians are at particular risk for work-related musculoskeletal disorders, with 75% estimated to have experienced at least one such injury while playing their instruments. Back and neck pain is common among pianists, cellists, and harpists due to their respective body positions while performing. Musculoskeletal disorders due to repetitive strain injuries are seen in players of string and woodwind instruments, particularly as hand injuries due to overuse in practicing. Good technique and, occasionally, minor adjustments to the instrument (such as moving a finger rest) may reduce the risk. Wind instrument players, especially brass, may also experience barotrauma to the middle ear, while noise-induced hearing loss is a common problem among orchestral and rock musicians and singers.

Singers may experience voice overuse. Singing with respiratory infections or acute strain may lead to permanent voice changes or vocal polyps. Artificial smoke on stage, stage dust, and respiratory tract infections infections can all affect voice quality.

The technical crew also faces occupational risks, including those chemical hazards from materials used in performances, such as paints, dyes, solvents, polyurethane, and polyester resins. Movie and stage sets are one-of-a-kind artistic creations that require the use of many chemicals. The set construction crew, lighting crew, sound technicians, and other backstage personnel or the camera crew on a movie set work in small groups on one production until it is completed. Their occupational health problems are therefore similar to those of workers in a trade

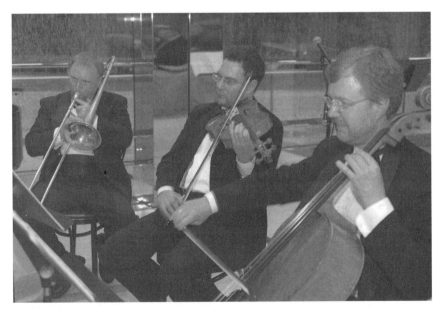

Figure 24.1 Musicians have many ergonomic challenges, and half or more experience repetitive strain injury at some time in their careers. String players, especially violinists, are at high risk for carpal tunnel syndrome. Horn players often have sinus and throat problems due to pressure, muscle spasms around the mouth, and shoulder pain. Trombone players have the greatest frequency of musculoskeletal problems. (Photograph by Barbara Tyroler, courtesy of Donna Marie Artuso.)

or in a small enterprise rather than workers in a large-scale plant or factory, even though they may work for a large theater or studio.

CONSTRUCTION

Construction is a constant among industries all over the world: every society needs workers who build and maintain structures. These structures may be houses, factories, office buildings, or civil engineering structures such as dams, roads, and bridges. Residential and commercial building construction is the most uniform and widespread construction activity and will be emphasized in this section.

As an industry sector, construction has a high overall rate of injuries and particularly fatalities in most countries. This is only partly due to the intrinsic hazards of construction, which include excavation and trenching, heavy equipment, falls from height, dangerous power tools (such as nail guns), high-voltage electricity, noise, and numerous ergonomic hazards. The high risk of construction work in many countries is also due to work organization and the heavy use of immigrant or expatriate workers who, unless trained for the job including safety, may lack the trade skill, experience, education, and language skills to protect themselves. Because construction workers usually follow the work from job to job, they may not stay with any one employer for long, and their training and welfare is often neglected.

Construction projects range from very small, as in the case of renovating a kitchen or bathroom, to very large, such as the construction of a huge building or complex infrastructure project. Likewise, builders may range from small enterprises doing home repairs to highly organized and sophisticated global enterprises with the capacity to engineer and construct highly complicated projects and to manage all design and construction aspects of the project. Every construction project, beyond a simple maintenance or repair project, is ultimately a collaboration between the owner, the contractor, subcontractors and suppliers, the workforce both skilled and unskilled, the source of financing, and government regulators with jurisdiction over the project who issue permits and inspect for compliance and safety.

There must be plans and specifications for the structure or renovation, designed by an architectural and engineering team to ensure that the structure and associated building systems that support it are safe for occupancy and practical. The actual builder is usually a contractor, which can be an individual or a firm, charged with developing the sequence of construction activities and maintaining a project schedule organized by trade, activity, and duration. For example, the foundation of a house must be prepared (poured if cement) and framed with wood or steel, followed by close-in of the exterior walls and installation of the roof. Rough-in plumbing, electrical systems, and ventilation have to be completed prior to close-in of interior walls and completion of all finishes. During the course of construction and upon completion, various inspections by government inspectors are required to confirm that it follows regulations in the building code and is safe for occupancy. These inspections require the contractor or builder to conform to local laws and regulation for the safety and durability of buildings, which are called building codes.

There are many project delivery methods available to owners or developers today. On many commercial construction projects the delivery method follows the formula "design—bid—build," which refers to a logical sequence of steps: an architect retained by the owner designs the project plans and specifications, solicits bids (proposals to construct the project for a certain, fixed price) from various contractors, and then selects the contractor. The owner frequently chooses the lowest-cost bid from a qualified contractor but may choose the bid with the best features (e.g., shorter construction duration but at greater cost). The contractor then assembles and mobilizes a team of subcontractors and suppliers to construct the job. Although contracting companies have formulas to calculate and estimate the cost of building a typical structure, bidding is an imprecise art and may be distorted by business tactics such as efforts to get a contract by bidding less than the probable cost (underbidding), which usually results in change orders and cost overruns and may result in delays as well as claims. Contractor selection and contract management are therefore central issues in all large and many small construction projects. Projects that are underbid or that are under time pressure because of delays are much more likely to have safety and health problems because the work is often compressed into shorter time frames, rushed, poorly performed, and substandard materials may be used.

Modern construction methods and materials have dramatically changed the characteristics of large buildings. Large buildings today are structural steel skeletons on which the exterior building walls hang as if draped over the frame; they are even called "skins." Increasing interest in energy efficiency in the 1970s and 1980s tried to achieve tighter skins, less ventilation and more recirculation, sealed windows, and better insulation. The effects of these changes in construction, while positive in terms of energy efficiency, led to many buildings of that era having problems with retained moisture (and, somewhat later as buildings got tighter, condensation), poor indoor air quality, and uncomfortable working environments. Over the last decade or so, many of these problems have been addressed by more advanced building science techniques that combine concern for improved building envelope performance, energy efficiency, and an optimum human environment, and there are now several recognized certification programs that classify and reward buildings built to standards of sustainable quality. Indoor environmental quality is also affected by activities in the building (such as cooking), by maintenance, and by occupancy (how many people the building houses and the dynamics of what happens to buildings when they are occupied).

Skilled construction work is organized by trades, each of which has a characteristic profile of hazards. The hazard profile sometimes overlaps when tradespersons (the gender-neutral term is preferable, but "tradesman" is still in common use) work next to one another and are subject to the same exposures.

Heavy equipment operators are workers who operate backhoes, bulldozers, earth-moving equipment, and other machines that are used to excavate and to change the land contour. Crane operators are required to be highly skilled: imbalance in the crane can lead to catastrophic failure and collapse, and poor placement of the load can lead to fatal injuries.

Electricians usually specialize in residential wiring, commercial wiring, industrial wiring, or high voltage with increasing levels of complexity. The principal risk, of course, is electrocution, which is greatest when the electrician "works live" on wires that are "hot," or carrying current. This is common practice in high-voltage situations where the current cannot be readily turned off but should be done only when absolutely unavoidable. There are also many ergonomic hazards because electricians use a variety of hand tools and frequently work in tight spaces. Electricians in most countries are highly trained and must pass an examination to prove that they are qualified and can work safely and competently.

Plumbers install and maintain pipes and fixtures in systems for potable water (drinking water), storm water, sanitary sewage (sometimes called blackwater and always treated as contaminated), and drainage water (sometimes called gray water and assumed to be significantly contaminated and therefore kept strictly separate from potable water, but increasingly often managed separately from blackwater and sometimes reused or recycled). In addition to handling the hardware of the plumbing system, the plumber must be aware of numerous complications, including pressure relationships that could result in backflow, leaks, and inadvertent interconnections that could contaminate drinking water. Piping is a more general term for laying pipe and includes piping systems for fuel gas, process chemicals (for example, in a chemical plant or oil refinery), and air delivery. Pipefitters maintain piping systems in industry and commercial buildings. Pipes may be made from many materials: conventional residential water pipes (lines) have been made from wood, lead, cast iron, copper, polyvinyl chloride, and a variety of other materials over the years. Historically, the characteristic disease of plumbers was lead poisoning, as a result of using lead-containing solder, joints, and caulking to join lead or copper lines. The word *plumber* is even derived from the Latin word for lead (*plumbum*).

Carpenters work with wood (or light-gauge metal today) and are primarily responsible in residential construction for work in wood (or metal), including framing, building structural elements, and creating the fine finish details of a wooden structure, such as molding, window casings, and ornamental work in interiors. Cabinetmakers are a type of woodworker who specializes in shelves and cabinets and other products that are usually made in a shop and installed in the house late in construction. There are many opportunities for injury in these occupations and many ergonomic hazards. The principal biological or chemical hazard is from wood dust and the solvents used in finishing and painting cabinets. Framers construct the frame of the house or forms into which concrete is poured. Framing is also done with metal studs.

Ironworkers place steel and other structural or ornamental metalwork generally in conjunction with crane operations. The occupation often involves working at heights, requiring fall protection, and carries obvious ergonomic hazards and risk of injury.

Masons are skilled craftspersons who work in stone. Since ancient times, the craft has had great prestige but carried a risk of silicosis and injury. Cement masons, also called cement finishers, mix and pour cement, the common building material consisting of crushed and calcined (heat-transformed) limestone, which when combined with aggregate is called concrete. Cement is irritating to skin and mucous membranes, and the chromium in it may cause skin allergies and tiny skin ulcers.

Bricklayers lay brick and apply mortar between them for adhesion and to seal gaps. They repeatedly lift a great deal of weight and so are at risk for sprains and strains and repetitive strain injury. Hod carrier is an unskilled job involving bringing bricks to the bricklayer in a box-like device called a hod that is carried over the shoulder. In many countries bricks are now carried by machinery, not people.

Glaziers install and replace glass. In addition to the obvious hazards of injury from handling glass, some glaziers have experienced lead toxicity in the past because their job required them to remove putty that contained lead from windows.

Plasterers apply plaster to walls, a job involving repeated movement of the arm and ergonomic hazards, but this form of construction has been replaced in many settings by the use of drywall, prefabricated sheets of gypsum that are nailed or otherwise attached to the frame for interior walls and dividers between rooms. Ornamental plastering is considered a highly skilled trade and is often encountered in restoration work in historical buildings.

Roofing is a specialized trade involving construction and maintenance of a weatherproof skin on top of a building, which often involves application of asphalt and therefore exposure to polycyclic aromatic hydrocarbons. The principal physical hazard, obviously, is fall from heights.

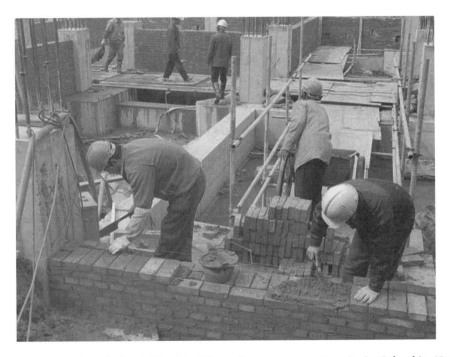

Figure 24.2 Workers laying brick to build a wall on a construction site in Colombia. Note that the workers in the back are walking across sheets of plywood that do not appear to be secured. (Photograph by Julietta Rodríguez Guzmán, Universidad El Bosque, Colombia.)

Insulation workers apply insulation between interior and exterior walls, and elsewhere where needed, for thermal efficiency and for fireproofing. Historically, insulation workers were heavily exposed to asbestos and therefore at high risk of lung cancer and other respiratory diseases. Substitute materials, such as fibrous glass, rock wool, and synthetic vitreous fibers, carry a much lower, but not negligible risk, making this still a relatively high-risk occupation in the construction sector.

Heating, ventilation, and air conditioning (HVAC) workers install the equipment, ducting, plenums (chambers that guide air movement), and registers (grates that cover air vents) that move air around a building. Their work involves cutting and shaping sheet metal, with associated ergonomic and injury hazards.

Unskilled laborers face many safety hazards on construction sites, but trenching deserves special mention. A trench is a long hole in the ground and is usually dug using a backhoe, sometimes by hand. The walls of all deep trenches are unstable because the dirt on the sides of the trench may easily collapse and fall in, depending on soil conditions and moisture. When this happens, any worker who is in the trench is buried and may suffocate, even if his head is not buried, because the weight of the soil on the upper body makes it impossible to breathe. Trenching accidents are often fatal. For this reason, building and safety codes mandate that the walls of trenches of more than a specified depth have sloped walls to widen the top of the trench or be restrained (shored) with timber or metal shoring boxes before any worker can enter the trench.

OFFICE WORKERS

While office workers do face risks, they are low in comparison to most other types of occupations. The growth in office work makes the risks worth noting, however. Building-associated illnesses include asthma, hypersensitivity pneumonitis, inhalation fever, and infection. Intensified job demands may induce stress, and ergonomic problems may lead to back strain and repetitive strain injury. Computers, and their video display terminals (VDTs), have been associated with visual dysfunction and ergonomic problems (see Chapter 7).

Photocopying machines may emit small quantities of ozone that can reach irritating levels in a confined space. The carbon black used in toner, the suspension of particles that make the image, has been extensively studied and does not appear to be hazardous. Methanol released from spirit duplicators was once common and used to result in blurred vision, headache, and nausea, while heat-activated photocopiers have been associated with a hypersensitivity angiitis. Both have been replaced by modern photocopiers that emit small amounts of ozone but are otherwise unremarkable.

PUBLIC SAFETY PERSONNEL

Public safety personnel rescue or otherwise protect others who are not able to save or protect themselves. If the risk is acceptable, their secondary objective is to protect property from destruction or damage, but not at the expense of their own safety. Public safety personnel allow themselves to be exposed to hazards that are unusual for anyone else in the community and that would not be tolerated in other occupations. For this reason, workers in these occupations often have special dedicated medical services and compensation arrangements.

Public safety occupations primarily include:

- police
- firefighters
- emergency medical service (EMS) personnel

Other, specialized public safety personnel face hazards that are predictable from their responsibilities and the equipment they use. For example, the risk profile of hazardous materials (hazmat) responders is determined by the chemicals in which they come into contact and the heat stress that often results from the protective suits they wear.

The occupational hazards faced by public safety personnel include the same hazards that threaten the victims they are trying to help. Although each of the occupations that constitute public safety personnel has its own set of hazards, risks, and traditions, public safety personnel share several features in common:

- long periods of relative quiet or routine, even boredom, interrupted abruptly by periods of intense and stressful activity

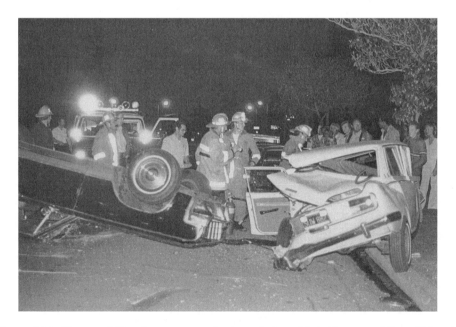

Figure 24.3 Many public safety personnel responded to this bad automobile collision in California in the 1950s: firefighters, police, and ambulance attendants, the forerunners of today's EMS technicians. (Historical photograph from the collection of Tee L. Guidotti.)

- psychological stress due to an awareness of personal danger and the urgency of their mission
- psychological stress due to a strong sense of responsibility for the well-being of others who depend on them and high expectations for performance
- a strong ethic of teamwork and camaraderie, which adds to their resilience under stress
- a rigid hierarchy or "chain of command"

Firefighters

Of all public safety occupations, firefighting probably experiences the greatest diversity of hazards. This is especially true when firefighting positions are combined with emergency medical services (discussed later). Firefighting also may require extreme work effort, under conditions close to the limits of human tolerance. Fitness for duty is therefore a major issue in the fire service.

There is rotation among the active firefighting jobs in each team or platoon, and a regular transfer of personnel between fire halls. Firefighters may also have special rank and duties. "Captains" accompany and direct the crews but are still actively involved in fighting the fire on site. Fire "chiefs" are the heads of the fire service and are called out only in the worst fires. Individual firefighters may still experience unusual exposures in particular incidents, of course. Small communities often depend upon volunteer, or paid-on-call, firefighters, either for full staffing or to assist a skeleton force of full-paid regulars.

Urban fires require tight containment to prevent spread to adjacent structures. The basic strategy is to keep the fire confined on the property and to the structure and to shrink the size of the fire.

Knockdown is the phase of firefighting in which the flames are brought under control. Water is laid onto the fire at the highest possible point to contain the spread of the fire and to cool the fire at its hottest point. This is usually accomplished by dispatching at least two pumpers to lay water on the fire, from the front and rear, as well as ladder trucks to allow firefighters to climb over the fire and to lay water on from above. As the fire is brought under control, it is extinguished from the periphery to the center.

Another strategy is to cut or chop holes to ventilate smoke and to promote more rapid and complete combustion at the base of the fire to prevent combustible gases from rising and igniting.

The structure must then be inspected to ensure that no burning embers are present that might restart the fire. This phase is called "overhaul," and it is associated with the greatest hazard from inhalation of toxic, partially combusted gases, some of which are absorbed into concrete (which acts like a sponge) and released as it cools. Many firefighters, especially in the past, are tempted to remove their respiratory protection at this point and even to smoke after the exertion of knockdown.

Because of the organization of modern firefighting, key tasks to which firefighters are assigned at the scene of a major structural fire are likely to include dragging hose, laying on water, ventilation (by breaking windows or chopping holes with an axe), climbing ladder, and rescue or salvage. Climbing the ladder with hose, especially using protective equipment, is exceptionally strenuous.

Fires in sparsely populated areas often involve brush, trees, or temporary structures. Here the emphasis is on containment in a broad area, cutting fire-breaks to block the spread of a fire, setting backfires to burn off fuel in a controlled manner before the fire reaches a critical position, and preserving structures where possible. Forest fires are particularly dangerous under conditions of shifting wind, and firefighters can be trapped if the effort is not well coordinated.

Some fire departments have compiled computerized databases on structures, materials, and potential hazards likely to be encountered in the district. Quick access to these databases assists the crew in responding to known hazards and to anticipate possibly dangerous situations. Fire services have also placed increasing emphasis on prevention in recent years and on criminal investigation in suspected cases of arson.

There are many physical dangers in firefighting that can lead to serious injury. Walls, ceilings, and floors may collapse abruptly and trap firefighters or cause them to fall from a height. Exposed wires may present a risk of electrocution. The structure that a firefighter enters is not only on fire but often weakened structurally. This is a particular problem with roofs, which may collapse on top of the firefighter.

Injuries associated with firefighting are predictable and often serious: burns, falls, and being struck by falling objects. Firefighters have a high rate of fatal injuries from these causes. Falls tend to be associated with ladder work, assignment to truck companies, and use of self-contained breathing apparatus, which unfortunately is heavy and awkward. Injuries can be minimized by intensive training, job experience, strict pre-placement evaluations, and physical fitness.

Firefighters exert themselves to maximal levels while fighting fires. The metabolic demands of coping with retained body heat, heat from the fire, and fluid loss through sweating add to the demands of physical exertion. Aerial ladder climbing, dragging hose, carrying the traveling ladder, victim rescue, and raising the ladder are among the most strenuous tasks, in declining order of energy demand. The most demanding activity is building search and victim rescue, followed by exterior firefighting, and serving as crew captain (directing the firefighting, usually at some distance from the fire). Other demanding tasks, in decreasing order of energy costs, are climbing ladders, dragging hose, carrying a traveling ladder, and raising a ladder.

During firefighting, core body temperature and heart rate increase slightly in response to work in preparation for entry, then both increase more as a result of environmental heat exposure, and subsequently increase more steeply as a result of high workloads under conditions of heat stress. Over 20 to 25 minutes, the usual length of time allowed for interior work by the self-contained breathing apparatus (SCBA) used by firefighters, the physiological stress remains within limits tolerable by a healthy individual. However, in extended firefighting involving many re-entries, there is often insufficient time between SCBA air bottle changes to cool off, leading to a cumulative rise in core temperature and an increasing risk of heat stress (see Chapter 9). That is why firefighters are required to take rest periods during long, intense fires.

Firefighting carries a high risk of burns, not surprisingly, especially jobs involving early entry and close-in firefighting, such as holding the nozzle. However, standard turnout gear is very effective in minimizing the risk of burns. Serious burn injuries are more commonly associated with basement fires, recent injury before the incident, and inadequate training. Flashovers are explosive eruptions of flame in a confined space that occur as a result of the sudden ignition of flammable gas products that are driven out of burning or hot materials when they combine with superheated air. Fire situations that lead to flashovers may engulf the firefighter or cut off escape routes.

Hot air by itself is not usually a great hazard to the firefighter. Dry air does not have much capacity to retain heat. Steam or hot wet air can cause serious burns because much more heat energy can be stored in water vapor than in dry air. Fortunately, steam burns are not common. Radiant heat is often intense in a fire situation. Burns may occur from radiant heat alone. Heat stress is compounded by the insulating properties of the protective clothing and by physical exertion, which result in heat production within the body. Heat may result in heat stress, with the risk of dehydration, heat stroke, and cardiovascular collapse.

Although there is no conclusive evidence for an increased risk of death overall from heart disease among firefighters, this is widely assumed and is the basis for presumption for compensation in many jurisdictions. If a firefighter has a heart attack during or within a day after a fire, it is normally considered work-related.

Over 50% of fire-related fatalities are the result of exposure to smoke, rather than burns. One of the major contributing factors to mortality and morbidity in fires is inadequate oxygen in the atmosphere. The constituents of smoke, singly and in combination, are also toxic, especially carbon monoxide and cyanide. Polymeric plastic materials in building construction and furnishings pose particular hazards because they combust into toxic products. Firefighters may be exposed to nitrogen dioxide, sulfur dioxide, hydrogen chloride, aldehydes, and organic compounds such as benzene, depending on the material involved in the fire. The composition and therefore toxicity of smoke depends on the fuel, the heat of the fire, and how much oxygen is available for combustion. Sometimes firefighters encounter unusual hazards during fires, such as pesticides, volatile chemicals, and the fumes of burning plastics.

Firefighters on duty have sustained psychological stress while on duty, in anticipation of an alarm. At the sound of an alarm, a firefighter experiences heightened stress because of the inherent unpredictability of the situation he or she is about to encounter. The most stressful event of all is the death of a victim during an attempted rescue, especially if the victim is a child.

The introduction of SCBA and other protective equipment within the last 20 years has created a much safer working environment for the firefighter. However, the added weight of the equipment increases the physical exertion required and may throw the firefighter off balance in some situations. The firefighter's typical turnout gear may weigh 23 kg (51 pounds) and imposes a high energy cost. The protective clothing also becomes much heavier when it gets wet.

Firefighters are as or somewhat more fit than the general adult (male) population. In recent years, more women have applied to be firefighters and this has caused a re-evaluation of performance tests and studies comparing the characteristics. The general conclusion of these studies is that women who can perform the job can perform as well as men, but fewer women have the capacity than men, especially with respect to upper body strength.

Law Enforcement

Police services maintain order and conduct criminal investigations. Corrections officers maintain order in prisons. Security guards and protection services monitor and protect the occupants of buildings and the property inside. Bodyguards travel with an individual who is a potentially an object of attack or kidnapping and protect their person. In recent years, these law enforcement officers (commonly called "LEOs") and protective services have increasingly adopted common standards for fitness for duty but there is still great variability.

Police are subject to the obvious hazards of violence. However, they are also at a high risk for motor vehicle accidents and other trauma. In the course of their work they have occasional contact with blood-borne pathogens and other body fluids (see Chapters 10 and 20).

Police work is physically demanding for short periods, as when trying to apprehend a suspect, and presents many ergonomic problems, particularly when trying to restrain someone.

Some studies suggest that police are at greater risk of cardiovascular disease than the general population.

Police work is highly stressful. In some countries, such as the United States, police have a higher rate of suicide and depression than other occupations. In other, similar countries, such as Canada, they do not. The difference may have to do with how the police are perceived and therefore treated by the public and on social conditions.

Much of the stress seems to be tied to the context and culture of policing. The psychological and social world of police is more complicated than the threat of physical violence. Because of the high potential for abuse and misuse of force, society in general has imposed strict limitations on how force is used, especially toward civilians. Police are watched more closely than other emergency and security personnel to ensure that they use their monopoly on force correctly. This sometimes leads to stress and the perception by police officers that they are not trusted by the people they are trying to protect.

Shift work also contributes to stress (see Chapter 11). Sexual harassment has been a frequent problem for women in the police, which has been a male-dominated occupation in all countries.

The demand for quick response to critical events and high danger levels in police work generate psychological stress. Police have been found to suffer from high levels of post-traumatic stress symptoms, with symptoms of personal stress (introversion, emotional exhaustion, acute hyper arousal), difficulties with the work organization response (insufficient time given to come to terms with the trauma, dissatisfaction with the job and organizational support, insecure job future), and lack of social support.

Police officers experience musculoskeletal problems from long hours of driving, particularly low back pain.

Traffic police are exposed to traffic noise, chemicals from vehicle exhausts, and ergonomic problems from standing for long periods of time.

Emergency Medical Technicians

Emergency medical technicians (EMTs) go by various names in different places, often emergency medical services (EMS) workers and paramedics (which in some places implies a higher level of training). They are specially trained health-care workers who respond quickly when a person is injured or acutely ill, assess the situation to determine how urgent the problem is, determine what immediate intervention is required (often with consultation to a backup physician), provide enough immediate pre-hospital treatment to stabilize the patient for transport, and bring the patient to a hospital for definitive care. EMTs follow medical directives that cover common health emergencies and can call on a physician who can provide additional guidance if needed.

The occupation of EMT grew out of ambulance attendants and became organized in the 1960s as municipal governments took over responsibility for maintaining ambulance services from hospitals. EMS is often combined into an emergency services department with the fire service on the municipal level.

EMTs deal with all types of medical problems in all types of situations. They are at risk of acquiring communicable diseases from their patients. Like other health-care occupations, there is a risk of being exposed to blood-borne pathogens (see Chapter 20).

The greatest risk of EMT work, however, is injury. The fatality rate for EMS workers in large cities approaches that of firefighters. Serious injuries may result from motor vehicle accidents, from being thrown around inside a cramped ambulance with many safety hazards inside while attending to a patient's needs, or from being hit by loose objects, such as oxygen tanks, inside the ambulance.

Ergonomic problems resulting in injuries may also occur when trying to move an unconscious or uncooperative patient, particularly if the patient is obese.

Intentional injury is another risk for EMTs, as it is for police. Some of the sick or injured patients may be hostile, delirious, or mentally deranged and may attack the EMT who is trying to help them.

EMS work is very stressful by nature, and many workers drop out to do other jobs after a few years in EMS. EMT jobs also involve shift work (see Chapter 11).

SERVICE AND RETAIL WORKERS

Workers in service industries perform a task or do something for the client or customer rather than make something or manufacture a product. Service work is characterized by many brief personally superficial contacts with clients and patients which may be short or long-lasting and intensive, as well as transient relationships with coworkers. These contacts can be neutral or either positively or negatively emotionally loaded.

Both the occupation and type of organization where health-care personnel are working determine the occupational safety and health problems affecting them.

The main occupational health and safety problems in service work are 1) ergonomic problems leading to musculoskeletal symptoms, and 2) psychosocial problems leading to stress symptoms (distress). In addition, physical violence, chemical and physical exposures, and microbiological hazards occur that are characteristic of the individual service or task.

Psychosocial problems can be found in every kind of work but are a particular problem in service work. Service providers often face time pressure, low job control, or low challenges of work (see Chapter 11). Social relations among workers and supervisors are other areas of potential psychosocial stressors. Interpersonal conflicts, mental violence, and poor supervisory practices are part of the problem. In addition, social relations in the service sector are of two kinds: relations among coworkers and relations to supervisors and customers. Uncertainty and unexpected changes can be important causes of job pressure. A resolution to these problems usually requires special efforts by employees to find balance between work and family roles at the individual level, especially as the majority of employees in this sector are women.

Profile of Service and Retail Workers

This section uses as examples two main groups of service workers, health care and retail shop workers. However, the principles apply widely to service workers in various industries. Retail workers share the same characteristics.

The hazards characteristic of the health-care sector are discussed in detail in Chapter 20. Health-care workers are a rather heterogeneous group including physicians, nurses with various levels of qualification, laboratory personnel, housekeeping and maintenance personnel, and administrative and office employees. The focus here is on those occupational groups that are in close or direct contact with patients. The organizational settings vary from primary health care to various sectors of specialized health care, with their own hazards. Long-term health-care provision for elderly people and their home care has greatly expanded the burden of providing health care and the responsibilities of the social welfare sector rather than just that of the health-care sector alone.

The main function of retail trade is selling goods to individual customers, whereas in wholesale the customers are retail shops and large chain stores. Restaurant and hotel trade also provides services similar to those of retail trade. Retail trade occupations include salesperson, shop clerk, supervisor, manager, cashier, and warehouse/storage room worker.

In retail trade, workplaces show a great difference between developing and industrialized countries. Large chain stores are common in most industrialized countries. There are, however, many differences between countries with different cultures in how retail trade is organized. In developing countries, retail traders very often operate in open markets and on streets.

The main occupational health and well-being problems among service employees are job dissatisfaction, lowered mental well-being, and musculoskeletal symptoms and illnesses. Some groups of employees also suffer from health problems caused by physical, chemical, and microbiological factors. Occupational injuries are also common in some service occupations.

Ergonomic and Musculoskeletal Problems

Ergonomic problems in service work are disproportionately associated with lifting and carrying heavy burdens as well as difficult working positions and monotonous repetitive movements (see Chapter 7).

There are physically heavy jobs both in health care and retail trade sectors. Ergonomic problems are related to direct patient care and work in supporting services, such as maintenance and housekeeping.

Ergonomic problems in health care are often due to lack of space, difficult maneuvers in lifting patients, and inadequate furniture layout. Health-care workers have to stand for long periods of time during their workdays. Lifting of patients is physically heavy, especially in hospitals with chronic and elderly patients. Heavy lifts can cause traumas and low back pain. The prevalence of nurses suffering from low back pain varies between institutions and countries (ranging from 24%–51%). Nurses in direct patient care are at the greatest risk for low back pain. Nurses usually suffer from low back pain that is related to the lifting of patients. During the first year of employment, the major risk factors for back injuries have been found to be poor patient-handling skills and heavy workloads. Higher rates of premature births have also been reported in association with heavy lifting.

Therefore, personnel should have adequate ergonomic training to manage lifting as well as have access to proper equipment for patient lifting. Sometimes lifting equipment is available, but it is not used at all because the personnel has not been trained or are not motivated to use it. Having a qualified person in each work unit responsible for training helps maintain motivation to use the equipment in the proper way.

In retail shops, the increase in heavy lifting and moving has been related to recent developments in logistics and transport of products from warehouse to shop. The cartons are becoming bigger and heavier, and the shortage of space and lifting equipment is a problem when trucks are unloaded and cartons are moved about in the storage room. These problems are associated with back pain. Supervisors and clerks in bigger retail shops have reported frequent heavy lifting.

Heavy lifting has not been studied as extensively in retail shops as in hospitals. In retail trade, however, sitting position and repetitive hand and arm movements are the main problems leading to musculoskeletal pain.

Both in retail trade as well as service, social and welfare sectors, the use of computers and VDT by service personnel is seldom prolonged, although it may be frequent. They are mainly used by supervisors as well as administrative and office personnel. It has been shown that intensive VDT use as well as frequent disturbances, long delays, and interruptions in data processing systems are associated to psychosocial stress symptoms in client service among insurance and bank employees.

Frequent keypad pounding and other repetitive tasks requiring hand movements are risk factors for upper limb symptoms and conditions such as tendinitis, carpal tunnel syndrome, tenosynovitis, etc. However, devices to avoid keyboard use introduce their own issues. Shop cashiers continuously use bar code readers, suffering from pain in the wrists and arms. Bar code readers with a fixed scanner easily cause arm and wrist symptoms. Also, long periods in the standing or sitting position can be a risk factor for low back pain.

Psychosocial Stressors

Psychosocial stressors at work are related to the individual's job, collaboration, and workplace social relations as well as organizational practices and changes. Client/customer relations in service work are potential motivating factors but also a source of strain (see Chapter 11). In providing services, the pace of work is usually geared to client or customer demands and is out of the control of the worker, especially in customer-service occupations such as sales.

Organizational and management practices influence the entire workforce, and during changes, especially structural changes such as downsizing, restructuring affects everybody. Just and fair leadership is one of the key elements of job satisfaction, in addition to sufficient challenges and personal development opportunities. Downsizing in an organization as well as experienced organizational and management injustices have been found to increase sickness absenteeism and strain symptoms.

Group work and teamwork in health care usually translate into positive social relations, whereas poor relations among coworkers can be a source of stress. High-quality teamwork is also the basis of high-quality patient care. In retail shops, social relations among personnel are scarce, and having to work alone may be a problem, especially in small shops, without social support and with an increased risk for physical violence.

According to the job demand-control model, an individual's good control of his or her work situation and opportunities to develop skills can be a buffer against stress induced by time pressure. Social support from coworkers and supervisors also seems to have a buffering effect. The main stressors in service work today are irregular working hours, time pressure, and unlimited work. When the weekly working hours are too high or irregular, balance between work and private-life duties is hard to achieve. Flexibility of working hours and work contracts are common in the service sector. The individual can also have too much freedom in the choice of work hours and duties. This easily leads to too many commitments and parallel tasks and is especially true of women when they have young children. This has been shown in retail shop cashiers who have repetitive physical work and young children at home.

It is common that people suffer from increased fatigue and exhaustion in such situations. Burnout has been closely studied in health-care personnel. It is characterized by a syndrome of emotional exhaustion, cynicism, and decreased professional competence. Psychosocial stressors in service work are usually associated with an overflow of patients and clients. Employee-patient, employee-client, and employer-client relationships/interaction can be rewarding but also burdensome. Continuous negative emotionally loaded situations are stressful and may expose employees to burnout.

Job redesign and optimizing the workload (e.g., number of patients received each day) may help people suffering from exhaustion and burnout symptoms.

Burnout interventions based on relaxation and discussion group methods have been successful in some cases, but not always. If the individual suffers from severe burnout, his or her work and life situation should be carefully analyzed, and an individualized plan should be prepared for the person. It usually takes a long time to recover from burnout.

Dealing with customers in retail shops can have both negative and positive effects but the two parties are usually focused on a financial transaction, not emotion. In health care, the relatives of patients can also cause stress because the interaction is usually emotionally charged. For a nurse, hospital patients or elderly people in nursing homes involve long-lasting contacts. When a nurse has to work faster in a social situation when seeing that a patient needs social inter-action, this can be a strain. Frequent interruptions in work during a shift can also be burdensome. Involvement in several patients' problems within a short time is emotionally demanding.

Violence

Violence is an ever-present threat in modern society. Bank personnel have been exposed to acts of violence and know that they face a threat of robbery. Health-care workers, especially those working in psychiatric health care and emergency units, may experience physical violence by patients. Rarely, workers may become violent against coworkers within their workplace, as in well-publicized incidents involving postal workers or disgruntled employees who have been recently fired, laid off, or disciplined. All workers face the possibility of mental violence, which can be as destructive and threatening.

Acts of violence are traumatic for the victims, who may or may not benefit from what is known as *debriefing* after the event. The purpose of debriefing is to prevent post-traumatic stress symptoms, characterized by recurrent thoughts, intrusive memories, sleep disorders, and anxiety, which can be disabling. Many companies have set practices for handling these situations to avoid violence and helping affected employees. Other authorities are skeptical of mandatory or routine debrief-ing and suggest that workers who have experienced traumatic events should have access to counseling and support when they feel ready to talk about it.

Physical violence against service personnel in retail shops is increasing. People working in small shops, especially, working alone late evenings are exposed to threats of physical violence or violent acts. One distinct group of perpetrators con-sists of drug addicts robbing shops for money.

Mental violence or bullying occurs among staff members or between staff and supervisors. The prevalence of mental violence or bullying is about 3%–8% at workplaces, and in health care in particular it has been somewhat higher than in other sectors. Bullying is usually defined as a negative act toward a colleague or a supervisor that is prolonged and sustained, that has lasted for at least half a year. Mental violence refers to social isolation or exclusion, devaluation of a worker's performance and efforts, threats, or other similar action causing the worker to feel worn down or frustrated. One single negative event between two people is not classified as bullying.

Bullies often target people with vulnerabilities, physical or psychological, or people who are different from others due to appearance, ethnicity, or sexual preference. This often has the effect of isolating the victim, causing a sense of shame and self-blame. They may also intimidate other workers, discouraging other members of the workplace community from defending or supporting their victims.

Bullying cases are difficult to manage. Usually, an outside consultant is needed to help the victim and his/her work group to solve the problem. There may be privacy issues that preclude making the case public, and it may be difficult to make other people believe and appreciate what has happened. Because the bullying may have continued for a long time, it also takes a long time to help the affected people. The health effects of prolonged bullying are severe: depressive symptoms, prolonged sickness absenteeism, and even suicide. Help can be obtained from occupational health personnel or outside consultants specialized in handling these problem situations.

Shift Work

Hospital work often involves working night shifts. Night shift is a burden to the circadian rhythm. Work schedules and shifts can be planned ergonomically to avoid or reduce physical and mental fatigue and sleep problems. The social aspect of the shift system is also important because employees have to balance their work, private and family life, and duties. (Shift work is discussed in detail in Chapter 11.)

In retail trade, temporary or short employment contracts and various forms of "flexibility" are common. This means higher demands for organizing and dividing work among individuals. Extra measures are needed to maintain links between staff members who may seldom see and meet each other. Working hour arrangements should be adapted to the life of the employee as a whole in an effort to avoid adverse social and health effects.

In health care, night shift work usually means responsibility for a large number of patients for each nurse. Various systems have been used in planning shift work schedules, numbers of shift hours, and the rotation of the system forward or backward. This creates a demand for participatory designing of the work organization and shift systems. Trials using shorter daily working hours have shown favorable results in hospital work.

Special Hazards

Depending on the country and type of retail trade work, some workers are exposed to hazardous chemicals such as cleaning agents. Chemical safety information should be provided for those handling chemical materials in warehouses, storage rooms, and shops. Pesticides and formaldehydes are used in shops to keep vermin away from rooms and textile products.

Occupational hygiene assessments are helpful for working environments where physical, biological, and chemical exposures occur. However, such services are rarely available at reasonable cost for small enterprises, which dominate the service sector.

Psychosocial and organizational factors are more difficult to monitor. The easiest solution is a questionnaire survey among all employees or employees from certain departments. Standardized questionnaires provide certain reference values for evaluation of individual workplaces. More important, however, is to follow a situation longitudinally and be aware of changes in workers' perceptions of their work and organizational factors and job satisfaction. The questionnaire results should be given as feedback at the group level to employees. Again based on group discussion and interpretation of the results, a participatory approach to developing an action plan and carrying out it is usually the best strategy. However, this procedure usually requires experts trained to carry out the survey feedback process and to support the follow-up of the intervention process.

TRANSPORT WORKERS

Drivers are exposed to a variety of physical, chemical, and psychological hazards (see Box 24.1 below). Vibration, and the changes it produces in intra-abdominal pressure, is a plausible cause for many disorders reported by drivers: hypertension, bone and joint disorders, venous damage, abdominal hernia, colitis, peptic ulcer, diverticulosis, esophageal reflux, hemorrhoids, varicose veins, and prostatitis. Drivers and garage workers can be exposed to vehicle exhaust fumes. Drivers have a higher prevalence of musculoskeletal disorders, headache, and gastrointestinal disorders. They also report low job satisfaction and alienation from their organizations.

TABLE 1

MAJOR OCCUPATIONAL HAZARDS ENCOUNTERED IN THE SERVICE SECTOR

Occupational Hazard	Effect on Health	Intervention and Prevention
• Lifting, moving of patients, material handling, etc.	• Low back pain, injuries	• Lifting equipment, training of lifting skills
• Repetitive hand movements	• Tendinitis, carpal tunnel syndrome	• Ergonomic design of tools, work breaks
• Time pressure, low control	• Strain symptoms, burnout	• Job redesign, participatory planning, individual support
• Poor supervisory and organizational practices	• Increased absenteeism, lowered satisfaction and well-being	• Improved flow of information, joint discussions
• Mental violence	• Depression, suicide	• External consultation, individual social support
• Physical violence	• Post-traumatic symptoms, fear, anxiety, injuries	• Preventive structural changes at the workplace, debriefing
• Shift work and work schedules	• Work/private life imbalance strain symptoms, limited social relations	• Ergonomic and social work shift planning
• Chemical and biological hazards	• Irritation, sensitization	• Safety training, protective equipment, proper ventilation

The increased risk of back pain in transit workers results from complex factors, including posture, vibration, transmitted road shocks, muscular effort, repetitive motion, and psychological perception. Duration of employment does not seem to be a strong risk factor, suggesting that the stresses producing back pain act early. Rapid heart rate and signs of cardiac stress in drivers also suggest that driving confers some degree of stress. Experienced and older drivers did not show an increase in circulating catecholamines, an adaptive mechanism to enhance performance under stress, but drivers with higher rates of absence from work had disproportionately greater neuroendocrine responses, suggesting that absence is associated with greater stress. One clinical indication of stress among drivers is the higher prevalence of insomnia found among this group compared to other occupations results from complex factors, including posture, vibration, transmitted road shocks, muscular effort, repetitive motion, and psychological perception. Duration of employment does not seem to be a strong risk factor, suggesting that the stresses producing back pain act early. Rapid heart rate and signs of cardiac stress in drivers also suggest that driving confers some degree of stress. Experienced and older drivers did not show an increase in circulating catecholamines, an adaptive mechanism to enhance performance under stress, but drivers with higher rates of absence from work had disproportionately greater neuroendocrine responses, suggesting that absence is associated with greater stress. One clinical indication of stress among drivers is the higher prevalence of insomnia found among this group compared to other occupations. Studies in China have found that 18.9% of drivers experience insomnia compared to 9.1% among construction workers.

Box 24.1 describes the occupational health problems of truck drivers, one particular group of transport workers.

Box 24.1

Truck Drivers

Truck drivers may experience a variety of health problems. Here is one example.

Mr. M is a 45-year-old truck driver and picker operator who injured his back on January 30, when steadying a bundle of 200-pound pipes while they were unloaded from a truck. He continued working 50–70 hours weekly after the incident despite continued pain. In April, his back pain increased after changing tires. Light-work duties were provided by his employer. He was referred for evaluation by an occupational health service.

Physical examination revealed no neurological deficit (symptoms of nerve damage). Lumbar flexion (the angle at which the lower spine could bend forward) was 45 degrees. Lumbar extension (backward) was limited to 10 degrees and his pain increased.

Lumbar spine X-rays and an MRI showed L5 extensive lumbar spondylosis (indicating that the bones at the bottom of the spinal column, or vertebrae, were slipping). A bone scan showed focal abnormal uptake of radioactive tracer in the left L4-5 facet joint area (evidence of inflammation between two vertebrae).

The diagnosis was osteoarthritis of the lumbar spine with left L5 facet joint arthropathy. This is a form of damage to the joint and bony structures that is caused by repeated heavy lifting. The one incident unloading the pipe did not cause it; it must have been present before, but the load of the pipe would have placed stress on the joint and made his back sore. The condition is unlikely to cause a serious problem besides pain.

Treatment involved anti-inflammatory medications and a multidisciplinary treatment program. Mr. M returned to his truck driving job in July.

Here is what truck drivers have said about their own health to an occupational physician:

"I have been driving in Canada for 28 years. Starting from the top, I have thinning gray hair (stress). My hearing is about 30% less than it should be (from 28 years of sitting in cabs of super-charged and/or turbo-charged 300 HP diesel trucks). My shoulders and elbows have bursitis and tendinitis from steering and shifting these damn things every day. My stomach hangs over my belt from eating fast food at odd hours. My back is wrecked from lifting millions of pounds over the last 28 years, as well as my knees and legs."

"I've 30 years' experience, in the U.S., mostly with a nationwide common carrier. I've observed the following: 1) upset sleeping and eating; 2) poor nutrition; 3) lack of exercise; 4) inhaling noxious gases, from your own vehicle and from others, worse in heavy, slow traffic and traffic jams; 5) rough riding tractors, causing spinal problems; 6) 70- to 100-hour workweeks, 50 weeks a year, for many years; 7) eight-hour layovers in noisy environments, causing poor sleep and inadequate rest; 8) being away from home and the ensuing family problems; and 9) high divorce rates from women who can't handle number 8."

Truck drivers in North America have more job-related injuries and illnesses than the average for other workers. In addition to driving trucks, other tasks include putting on tire chains, changing tires, loading and unloading heavy cargo, coupling and uncoupling trailers, cargo inspection, and cargo adjustment. Truck drivers have more degenerative spine changes than is seen in other occupations.

Truckers spend many hours daily in a seated position. They must control a large steering wheel by assuming a rigid upright position. This position is ergonomically incorrect and causes discomfort in the neck, back, and limbs.

Vibration, in combination with lifting, contributes to back, neck, and shoulder pain. Vibration has effects on the digestive system and may contribute to hemorrhoids and ulcers.

Cabs of older trucks reach 90 dBA noise levels, which is above the 85 dBA action level at which hearing protection is recommended. With highway noises, drivers may be exposed to 110 dBA at times. Noise more than 90 dBA can affect speech comprehension, even in a person with normal hearing. Horns and sirens may be difficult to hear.

Lifestyle risk factors also complicate the health of truck drivers. Truck drivers tend to eat meals hurriedly and irregularly because they take so many of their meals on the road. Meals are often low in nutritional value. They are away from home for prolonged periods and find it difficult to exercise. Physical fitness deteriorates with prolonged sitting. Almost 90% of drivers in North America rarely exercise, and about 75% are overweight. On their travels, there are numerous opportunities and incentives to drink alcohol and engage in unsafe sexual behavior.

Motor vehicle-related injuries are usually related to excessive speed, following too close, or making unsafe lane changes. Fatigue was the main cause of 67% of truck accidents. Equipment problems cause another 12% of truck accidents. Defective brakes have been found in 30%–40% of trucks in North America. Defective tires, steering components, and towing connections are other factors contributing to accidents.

Driving is stressful because high vigilance is required for long periods of time. Truck driving requires constant vision and hearing with high mental alertness. Driving at dusk or at night, in adverse weather, in heavy traffic, on poor roads, or on mountainous roads increases stress. Further stress is caused by schedule shifting, irregular work/rest cycles, irregular mealtimes, poor nutrition, sleep deprivation, unsatisfactory sleeping accommodations, delays in departure, traffic problems, prolonged driving, monotony, and economic pressures. Frustration, delays, and schedule changes can cause anxiety. Poor work, family, and social relationships and economic pressures contribute to stress.

Insomnia is related to shift work stress and poor sleeping conditions. Drivers average only 4.8 hours of sleep during an 8-hour rest period. Driving schedules are not conducive to family or social life. Drivers may be on the road for weeks before seeing their families. Prolonged times away from home may contribute to divorce. Wife–husband driving teams manage to avoid the problem of separation but at the cost of both being away from home for long periods.

Long work hours may contribute to social isolation. Some trucking accidents have occurred after drivers experienced domestic conflicts, separation, divorce, or serious health problems in the family. Drivers are often away from family, friends, and other sources of social support for long periods, which may aggravate domestic problems. However, electronic communications, such as cell phones and the Internet, enable truckers to keep in touch with their friends and family better than in the past.

Truck driving is not well paid. Minimal hourly wages require the truck driver to put in long hours of work to make a living. The tight schedules and economic pressures force drivers to drive for long periods of time with insufficient sleep. Drivers often drive for longer than the law or regulations allow. In one investigation, 20% of truckers drove more hours than permitted by regulations. This contributes to drug and alcohol abuse, particularly when drivers drink lots of coffee (for the caffeine), smoke (for the nicotine), and take drugs to stay awake and then need alcohol or other drugs to get to sleep. More than 50% of truck drivers smoke 1–2 packs of cigarettes per day. Approximately 25% of drivers may have a problem with alcohol, as indicated by some studies.

Even in developed countries, truck driving is not an easy occupation and is associated with many occupational health problems.

Box contributed by Harold Hoffman, MD.

Drivers are also exposed to shift work, associated with sleep disturbances, eating and digestive disorders, and social adjustment problems. Studies from England in the 1950s showed that drivers have more frequent and severe angina than those in other occupations, while other studies show elevated risk factors for cardiovascular disease, including serum cholesterol, hypertension, smoking, and indices of stress. Bus drivers have also shown an overall excess mortality from lung cancer on the order of 50% to 200% in a number of studies.

In addition, transport workers of many classes are considered safety-sensitive workers and must pass regular examinations and comply with regulations to ensure that they are medically fit to operate vehicles safely. (This topic is explored further in Chapter 19.)

WASTE HANDLERS

Solid waste collectors and handlers suffer from a high number of occupational injuries. They also suffer skin disorders, exposure to dust and other inhalable particles from landfill sites, and exposure to bacteria, particularly from municipal solid waste on warm, windy summer days. A well-operated sanitary landfill should avoid these problems, but in many countries open garbage dumps are still used. Scavengers in dumps are exposed to the same hazards.

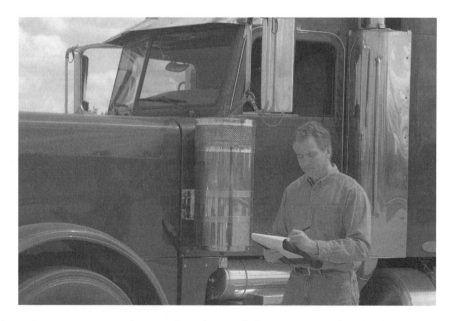

Figure 24.4 Transport workers, such as this truck driver, are considered to be "safety-sensitive personnel" in some countries and are required to pass regular medical examinations to ensure that they can operate their vehicles safely. (Photograph by Big Wind Media, iStockphoto.)

Sewage workers, who operate municipal wastewater plants, may be at risk from the infectious agents found in the sewage. These may include viruses that cause diarrhea and hepatitis.

Rats often infest garbage dumps and sewers. They may carry leptospirosis, a bacterial disease that causes a form of hepatitis. Exposure to leptospirosis usually occurs when workers come into contact with rat urine.

WELDING

A welder performs many tasks in addition to welding to shape and finish metal. Welders experience hazards found in most workshops—noise, dust, metal waste objects, lifting heavy objects, and flying metal shards from grinding. Welding exposes workers to potentially toxic gases, dusts, infrared irradiation, ultraviolet irradiation, and extremes of temperature. Welders can experience welder's "flash," an intensely painful but self-limited conjunctivitis from exposure to intense ultraviolet light from the welding arc. This generally occurs due to exposure from the side or by reflection off of a white surface. Infrared exposure is more insidious, and repeated exposure without protection can lead to a risk of cataracts. As a result of lifting heavy metal objects, many welders also suffer from chronic shoulder and upper back problems.

Toxic fume exposure arises from the welding technique used. Cold steel welding, the most common form, presents the hazards given above and some exposure to nitrogen dioxide and particulate matter. Stainless steel welding has higher fume levels and a potential for exposure to the carcinogenic and systemically toxic

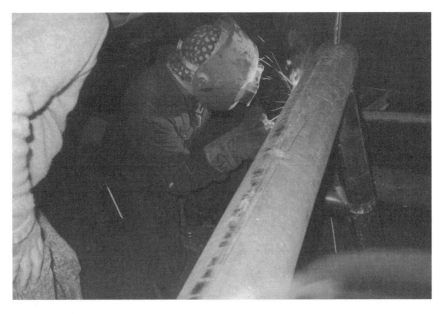

Figure 24.5 Arc welder welding a pipestand in Alberta (Canada) for use in an oilfield. (Photograph by Tee L. Guidotti, University of Alberta.)

metals, nickel and hexavalent chromate. Aluminum welding, which is technically difficult, presents a risk of ozone exposure.

Manual metal arc welding, in widespread use, has effective measures for fume control (lower power levels, shorter arc length, reduced sputter through the pulsating MAG technique, and local ventilation). Electron beam and laser welding present hazards (ionizing radiation, infrared and visible laser light, respectively) but are more amenable to containment and automation. Other toxic fumes that can arise from welding include oxides of nitrogen, ozone, phosgene, copper, lead, zinc, arsenic, silica, asbestos, fiberglass, magnesium, manganese, polycyclic aromatic hydrocarbons (especially in tank and pipeline welding, and fluorides.

While new technologies are changing exposures (e.g., aluminum or stainless steel MIG welding produces considerable ozone), there is increasingly efficient protective equipment (e.g., low-pressure, high-volume exhaust fans), and welding is becoming more automated. Establishing more stringent exposure standards, and particularly process-specific performance standards, drives development of control technology and protects against other hazards yet to be identified or newly emergent. Primary prevention methods—ventilation and modification of the process (different rods, minimum power, and shorter arc length)—are more effective than personal protection.

Arc welders' pneumoconiosis has been recognized since 1936. This specific occupational lung disease is associated with a dramatic chest X-ray often showing

---

Box 24.2

Hazards Faced by Police in Hefei, China

The occupational health of police is affected by more than stress. Noise, carbon monoxide, and lead exposure may also cause health problems.

In Hefei, China, traffic police were found to be exposed to an average noise level of 84.63 dBA for 70% of their working time, with associated noise-induced hearing loss and metabolic problems.

Concentrations of carboxyhemoglobin (COHb) among traffic police have been found to be significantly increased.

Leaded gasoline is used in motor vehicles in China. In countries where leaded gasoline is used, blood lead levels in traffic police are also higher than those levels among the general police.

The concentration of the vehicle exhaust at traffic lights is often higher because that is where vehicles stop and start. Concentrations of the amount of carbon monoxide (carboxyhemoglobin, or COHb) and lead (blood lead, Pb) in the blood were measured among traffic police and general police in Heifei. They were both found to be significantly increased compared to general police and the general population, and the elevations were related to work shifts.

Contributed by Fu Hua, Ph.D.

---

what is called siderosis, which has virtually disappeared in developed countries. The metal in the dust causes a very visible pneumoconiosis. Fortunately, this disease is not serious and is compatible with normal health and life expectancy despite the alarming appearance of the chest X-ray.

Pulmonary function abnormalities appear to be associated with a history of chronic bronchitis among welders and probably also with smoking history. X-ray readings give a less definitive diagnosis, and X-ray opacities in the lung do not predict the level of lung function impairment from welding fumes.

25

OCCUPATIONAL HEALTH AND ECONOMIC DEVELOPMENT

Tee L. Guidotti

"The seven social sins [are] politics without principle, wealth without work, commerce without morality, pleasure without conscience, education without character, science without humanity, and worship without sacrifice."
—Mohandas Gandhi

All countries are, in a sense, developing countries. There are countries that are in transition from traditional, locally grounded subsistence economies to post-industrialized trading societies, from "less developed" or "developing" to "developed" or "industrialized" economies, and from developed economies to the economies of the future, which are based less on the value added by manufacturing than on information and services. Every country in the world is experiencing its own economic transition and is evolving into another form.

The role of occupational health in economic development is not obvious. For this reason, occupational health usually is left out of development plans for emerging economies. This is a mistake. Occupational health is especially important in economic development for the following reasons.

- Protecting the health of workers protects families from catastrophic loss of income and resulting poverty, making it a very cost-effective form of social insurance.
- Workers are the most economically productive sector of society, thus protecting their health is a way of protecting productivity.
- Occupational health services, in the form of clinical facilities and preventive services for workers and their dependents, are usually the foundation for later systems of social security and health care as a society develops economically.
- Both hazard control and health-care costs are low at the beginning of the development cycle and increase dramatically once industrialization has been achieved. A small initial investment in protecting the health of workers may thus prevent a huge drain on the economy later by reducing the burden of disability and occupational disorders.

- Effective occupational health protection protects the relationship between workers and employers, which can become very strained if workers believe that they are being exploited and that their lives are not valued.
- Occupational health protection promotes equity in society and prevents the creation of an underclass of injured workers and their families, who are excluded from society.

These factors are often overlooked by economic planners. This appears to be less the result of prevailing economic theory than of attitudes and unexamined assumptions. Most development economists assume or accept the proposition that occupational health is a late addition to development and should normally be undertaken once the economy is strong enough to absorb the additional expense. The theory is that rapid industrialization requires investment in production first and that once wealth is created, it can be invested in social goods such as improved health, worker protection, and protecting the environment. So these social goods are generally considered to be *amenities*, satisfying but not essential. This is wrong.

Occupational health is generally considered by economists to be a consumptive expensive, one that consumes resources but does not lead to increased production or a tangible return on investment. However, this model of development is obsolete. It is now understood that health, worker protection, and environmental quality are also inputs into the economy and that they create wealth as well as consuming it.

Economic development that excludes protection of workers' health (as well as environmental protection and community health) tends to fail or to experience serious disruptions. There are many examples:

- The European and American "Industrial Revolution" of the early and middle 1800s, respectively, brought a crisis in occupational health and working conditions, with massive social unrest and conflict that forced the adoption of the first laws on factory inspection, child labor, and public health.
- The later stages of industrialization in Germany, the United Kingdom, and the United States gave rise to the belief that industrial workers were being exploited and treated as dispensable commodities (occupational injuries were only one part of this picture). This was one political factor that led to acceptance of the theories of Marxism and the rise of the political movement that later became Soviet communism.
- In the United States and the United Kingdom, the exposure of workers to asbestos in the 1900s created an enormous liability for medical care, lost wages, and death benefits that caused a crisis and resulted in many companies declaring bankruptcy (a judicial procedure by which most debts owed by a person or company are extinguished or reduced to the value of its assets and the debtor is relieved of further liability for those debts).
- The globalization of the manufacturing economy has resulted in the export of numerous hazards in industry to countries poorly equipped to control them. This has been a major argument used against globalization by people who do not believe that freer trade brings benefits at the community level.

- In Ukraine, the health and safety of coal miners is one of the most volatile and persistent political issues, due to high levels of injury and the importance of these workers to the economy. The same was true in the United States in the eastern region known as Appalachia.

The importance of worker protection has been recognized as a major obstacle to economic development by the governments of some countries, such as the People's Republic of China. China, due to its rapid industrialization, has faced an occupational health problem of huge proportions, sufficient to be given priority by the Ministry of Health as a national public health problem.

STRATEGIES FOR ECONOMIC DEVELOPMENT

Economic development is not easy. Economic and social development may destroy as much as it creates, and its path is often unpredictable. Economic development transforms what is traditional into something new and sometimes disturbing. The issues that development brings to less developed societies reflect the extent of destruction and the new problems being created. During the transition much is lost, much is gained, and much must be rebuilt in a structure that makes sense to the culture. However, the option of not developing is seldom viable. Traditional societies may or may not have a strong sense of community and deeply held values, but they always find it hard to sustain themselves against the pressure of change around them.

Because occupational health reflects many ethical and human rights elements, it is in many ways an indicator of progress in maintaining a civil society in the face of economic change. Occupational health reflects the value placed on the worker and on income security for the worker's family. The priority put on occupational health in society, and indicators of its performance in protecting workers' health, reflects that society's internal strength, values, and capacity to manage the difficult economic transitions it must undertake.

Societies are faced with a paradox: to develop economically and to secure a future for their people that is more attractive and humane than the present, they must destroy much of the society on which their system is based and risk the culture of their people in the transition. The transition from a traditional to an industrial economy is messy, inefficient, dangerous, destabilizing, and sometimes cruel. It involves the destruction or subordination of traditional institutions and cultural norms to support a social and economic structure that is usually much larger, much more institutionalized, and much less sensitive to the needs of the individual at the local level. However, the new structure that results may be also more economically stable, less tolerant of minor and debilitating inter-group conflict, more equitable in the distribution of its benefits, and more economically secure overall for its members. Before this can be achieved by a traditional society, there must be a successful transition to a society with effectively functioning institutions, social cohesiveness, access to technology, and access to information. How a society manages this transition is a test of how strong it was in the first place and how resilient its institutions are.

Broadly speaking, there are two transitions inherent in the stages of development that are commonly recognized by economists. The first is the passage from traditional economies to industrial economies. The second is the transition from industrial economies to sustainable economies, in which the core economic activities are based to the greatest extent possible on renewable or recyclable resources, and the environmental impact of economic activity is within the carrying capacity of the ecosystem. As the developed world comes to grips with the reality that it, too, is undergoing transition, the experience of the developing world takes on more universal relevance. This second transition may lead to a sustainable model of development that balances renewable resources with economic demand and that places minimal pressure on nonrenewable resources and environmental quality. The form and structure of such a sustainable society is still being worked out.

Countries use various strategies for economic development. Among the more common in recent years have been the following:

- Socialism and state direction, in which the means of production are owned or controlled by the state and economic development is centrally planned. The collapse of the Soviet Union and the absorption of its allies into market-based systems have greatly reduced the number of countries following this strategy.
- Market-driven development, in which markets respond to supply and demand, and demand is used whenever possible to set prices, distribute goods, and direct new investment.
- Export-driven development, in which countries achieve industrialization quickly by producing in excess of their domestic capacity to absorb the supply, export the excess, and finance the cost of their development by earning export revenues.
- Mixed economies, in which elements of state direction, public (although not necessarily state) collective control, and markets are used selectively.
- Self-sufficiency, in which countries try to produce as much as they can from within their own borders using their own resources. The inefficiencies of this system have limited its application to small and isolated economies.
- Mercantilism, in which one country directs or controls the development of others. This economic theory was the underpinning of the now-discredited system of colonialism.

Occupational health is more easily managed in systems that have a strong public component to their economic direction, but the benefits of effective occupational health are as important in market-driven economies as in mixed economies. Gains on productivity, population health, income security, and social equity are as great.

Occupational health protection is generally counted by employers as a *consumptive cost*, a cost that is incurred by the employer for little or no direct anticipated gain. From an occupational health and safety perspective, it is more accurately considered as an *investment*, an expenditure that is made with the anticipation of a future benefit. Employers often take the view that if they pay for increased worker protection, they will not benefit because the worker will take another job elsewhere, the gains will not be seen until later in the worker's life, and the company may not even be in business to see the benefit. The benefit is often difficult to quantify because it is expressed in terms of disability and health problems that have been avoided, not a tangible return on investment. Employers may then take the view that because their role in the economy is to create wealth and not to distribute benefits, it is not their job to protect the health of workers. Obviously, this point of view ignores the ethical and social benefits of worker protection. However, it is an attitude that one encounters often, particularly in small and medium-sized enterprises that are struggling to compete.

OCCUPATIONAL HEALTH IN THE DEVELOPMENT CYCLE

Economists often speak of the economic development cycle, which is the theory that economies begin with an emphasis on traditional activities to meet personal and family needs, or subsistence agriculture (see Chapter 21), move through more organized rural and agricultural activity, which is called an *agrarian* economy, and then, in a substantial economic transition, move toward the production of more valuable commodities and finally manufactured products and services, yielding an excess of revenue over cost. This excess value is invested back in the economy as capital as it becomes available, creating more capacity and infrastructure, such as transportation, communication, and energy sources. Over time the economy becomes richer, more diversified, and emphasizes adding value with every economic activity rather than meeting basic needs. This ideal has indeed occurred in many countries. In others, the economy may get stuck or there may be internal obstacles that distort growth, such as poor management, corruption, or barriers to trade and the movement of goods.

On a national level, it is tempting for development economists to defer making the investment in occupational health on the grounds that occupational health is primarily an investment in population health and should not be undertaken until the economy is strong enough to absorb the additional expense. However, the amenities of improved health and worker protection are essential to development and stability: they are what people look to as evidence that their lives are getting better. Without such improvements, and sharing the wealth, workers feel that they have no stake in the economy and that there is nothing in it for them. The prevailing attitude in this approach is that one generation must accept the "pain" of rapid development, with all its unfairness and risk, so that the next generation can prosper.

The economic strategy of development that has been generally adopted by the "tiger" economies of Southeast Asia (including the biggest tiger of them all, China) implicitly emphasized taking all the pain in one generation, to get through the process as quickly as possible until the economy was sufficiently strong to support social programs and welfare. The generation of workers of the 1980s was expected to shoulder an immense burden while the country developed. The economic burden of occupational disease in a more affluent China now falls on workers who expect a better future, whose life expectancy is longer, and whose expectations of a quality of life are higher. In China, parents today naturally expect a better life for their children, and this is already a powerful force for social change.

In practice, this meant that certain economies that underwent rapid development concentrated the burden of exposure to occupational hazards onto a cohort of workers that already had a limited life expectancy because of other social conditions and determinants of disease. For these workers, the risk of occupational disease competed with the risk of other health outcomes that shortened life expectancy. However, the accumulated burden of disability from work-related disorders and the secondary deprivation from income insecurity that results from disability is a huge and destabilizing burden on society, as demonstrated in Chapter 29.

COST OF HEALTH CARE

In developing countries, the cost of health care for injured workers is generally low, but the enterprises that provide employment are often undercapitalized and find it difficult to invest in occupational health protection. Although the costs of providing health care and occupational health protection are minimal on an international scale of value, they may be perceived as high as a proportion of the cost of production and in light of the capital invested in the enterprise, particularly if an employer is in a competitive international market.

Because the cost of occupational injuries and illness is low early in the development cycle, this makes it easy for employers to ignore the issue. Given that many such jobs require low skill levels and employment is often *casual*, meaning that workers are hired without paperwork for short periods on an as-needed basis, there is little incentive to protect workers or to take care of them when they are injured.

The World Health Organization is strongly committed to the concept of "Basic Occupational Health Services," by which it means, in part, the provision through the primary health-care system of the most basic services to workers and employers in protecting occupational health and treating injured workers. The primary health-care system, where it functions, must accept this burden because the great majority of all new enterprises in developing economies (and, in fact, in developed economies) are small and medium-sized enterprises that cannot support their own health-care system or occupational health specialists.

However, as the economy develops, the cost of health care soon rises. A high level of occupational injury and illness thus inflates health-care costs throughout the health-care system. When disability pension programs are added, the cost becomes much greater because injured workers tend to be younger than the general population with disabilities. In the absence of disability pensions, families may be thrown into poverty by the injury of the "breadwinner" who is supporting them. Thus, a high rate of injuries and illness may plant a time bomb in health-care costs, either by inflating costs in the near future or creating a dispossessed underclass that missed out on social equity, with the attendant possibility of social unrest.

It is tempting to draw lessons from one point in the history of developed countries to developing countries at what appears to be a similar point. However, this is as often misleading as instructive. Economists and decision makers know much more today and have access to much more information. It is not necessary to repeat mistakes of the past. The world is also much more complex today at the village level than it was at the time of the European Industrial Revolution, when technological change took place against the background of a static agrarian society. Moreover, developing communities today are often much more in touch with global communications and can access information about their economic prospects, political events, and their health. This may change their behavior (or not—it may reinforce resistance to change) and introduce new, confounding health issues, such as changes in diet, smoking habits, health care, and demographics.

A MODEL OF ECONOMIC DEVELOPMENT

In order to understand the place of occupational health in economic development, it is useful to build a model of development from first principles. There are three primary issues that will be building blocks for the model itself. It is easy to dismiss the complexity of these relationships with the belief that "everything is connected to everything else," but while demonstrably true, this belief is also limiting in dismissing the most important aspect of these relationships: they are highly structured, but not in simple ways. Rather, one issue tends to "drive" another and in turn to be driven by others.

Some of the most important elements of the development process, and an idea of its complexity, are shown in a diagram that will be built in a series of steps in this section. The first step in building the diagram is to define the initial, essential elements (shown in Figure 25.1). These initial elements are:

- human rights
- population/resource imbalance
- urbanization

Other elements will be added as the model is built. These three and the later elements of the model are linked, and affect one another in specific ways that will be illustrated by arrows. The direction of the arrow is what is important: it shows that one factor tends to "drive" another factor, meaning that it pushes the second factor forward. The model is organized to place human rights on the left and social and cultural institutions on the right, and to place population/resource imbalance, environmental, and occupational effects on top and individual and cultural effects on the bottom, in concentric rings as the model is developed. Obviously, each element affects many more elements than will be shown, and the relationships are much more complicated, but it is necessary to keep the model relatively simple for learning purposes.

Figure 25.2 represents this central axis of a model of economic development, with arrows in direct relationships. The central issues of human rights, population/ resources, and urbanization are linked and are critical driving factors for the rest

| Human rights | Population / Resource imbalance | Urbanization |

Figure 25.1 The core elements in the model of economic development reflect the stability of civil society and material security.

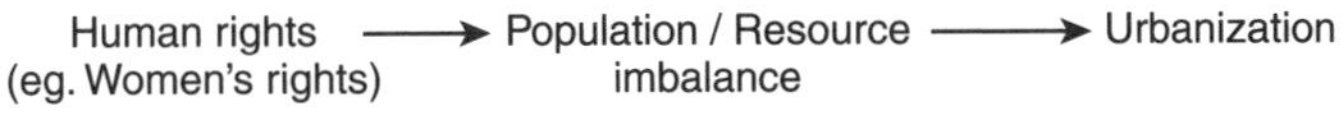

Human rights   ⟶   Population / Resource   ⟶   Urbanization
(eg. Women's rights)   imbalance

Figure 25.2 The relationship among these core elements goes in one direction during successful development.

of the model. While inextricably linked, the three may also respond to other factors not represented on the diagram. They each have their own dynamics in a given society; the specific economic patterns of China, for example, are very different from Latin America, which is very different from Africa. However, the underlying elements and their relationships are similar.

"Human rights" is a shorthand term for a broad range of values and concepts of individual worth in a society. From the work of Amartya Sen and other scholars of development, a fundamental principle is that economic development is connected to social development and that both involve the capacity of individuals to function in social roles in their community. At any point in time, a society has certain norms of behavior with respect to what is and what is not permitted, the appropriate penalties for infractions of this code of behavior, and expectations for the role of people in the society. Human rights are not simply a matter of personal political freedoms, but a complicated set of behaviors and responses. Human rights affect the individual members of society and their capacity to live their lives and play their social roles, the political system, the economic system, hierarchy in the society (in an anthropological sense), gender and race relationships, and the specific history of ideas that have been discussed, disputed, and resolved in the past and currently. Human rights is therefore a cluster of values and relationships that reflect the place, limits, and norms of behavior acting on the life of an individual resident in that society. One set of human rights concerns of particular importance as a development issue is women's issues (discussed below).

Population and resource issues are taken together as a single fundamental relationship. The effect of a country's population on its wealth and stability is not a simple relationship. In general, the impact of population depends on the level of demand and the distribution of consumption in the society and the demand for goods that require resources. However, demand for local resources is not just a matter of income. Impoverished populations may place great demands on local resources out of desperation, such as deforestation and overly intensive agriculture. The issue is one of an imbalance between the human population and the resources available to sustain it without degrading the environment or exhausting the alternatives to the extent that society is impaired. The problem of population and resource imbalance is driven to a considerable degree by issues of human rights. Rights to education, to economic security, and to the participation in public society of women have profound but indirect shaping influences on the population structure by increasing the ability of women to make reproductive decisions. Education and changing cultural values shape the ability of both men and women to accept such decisions.

The resource side of the population/resource imbalance is affected in part by productivity, reflecting the application of technology and the efficiency of work in the society, factors which are in turn affected by urbanization (discussed below) but can be understood as a social transformation involving growth in population centers, more extensive infrastructure, and modernization of social and family relationships. Population/resource imbalance drives urbanization in part by creating demographic trends that accelerate the growth of urban centers and that increase the size of communities on the periphery. Urbanization also provides an infrastructure and access to technology that changes the use of resources: energy resources may be used more efficiently, transportation may make it possible to sell excess crops, and water may become more accessible. This changes the relationship between the population and the resource base, usually making it possible to support more people but increasing the total pressure on the environment as more people are added to the community.

The last key factor placed at the center of the model is urbanization. This, and the contrast with rural life, is the subject of the following section.

URBANIZATION AND THE SHIFT FROM RURAL LIFE

Urbanization means more than the growth of cities. Urbanization also means the reorganization of society from an essentially modular, or village, structure in which the connections are relatively few, low in capacity, and restricted in scope to a wide network in which the connections are open, high in capacity, and virtually unlimited. Urbanization carries with it access to technology, communications, ideology, political influence, wages, and the increased level of personal and institutional interactions that drive social development. It also carries with it crowding, the risk of cultural alienation, and the forcing of new hierarchies that through inequality may impede distribution of the benefits of urbanization.

Rural areas change as well with urbanization. In the countryside, and in remote areas served by improved transportation and communications linkages, there may be rapid incorporation of urban habits, lifestyles, tastes, and ideas into the local milieu. In rural areas, distances between suppliers and consumers are

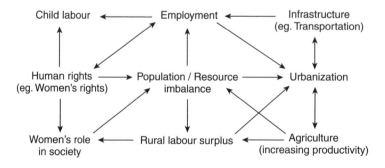

Figure 25.3 The next ring of relationships deals with infrastructure and human capacity.

greater, transportation takes longer, and the density of population and therefore potential interactions among parties is much less than in a city, so there is less efficiency in conducting business. Because the density of population is lower and usually more evenly distributed than in an urban area, it is often more practical in rural areas to do business by bringing people together at a particular time rather than in a particular place. This is the basis for the traditional weekly market. Prices for local commodities and land (except in agriculturally rich areas) tend to be low in rural areas compared to cities, but the cost of construction and transportation can be much higher.

The economy of most rural areas is based on agriculture and resource industries, such as mining, forestry, oil and gas development, and fishing. Most rural areas survive economically by selling these commodities and trading for the goods they need; however, for these reasons, rural areas also tend to be very susceptible to changes in prices. If the demand for the commodity drops, prices may fall abruptly, as has often been the case for crops such as coffee or cacao. This means that rural areas are often highly dependent for their prosperity on goods that have fluctuating prices, and this leads to economic instability. Diversification of the rural economy has been a goal in many countries. Urbanization involves the diversification of opportunity as well as an increase in the local population, which makes it possible to hire labor cheaply and efficiently for bigger enterprises.

In developing countries, rural areas are usually less developed than the local cities, and as a result the quality of life may suffer. The infrastructure is often poor because investment is less productive in less dense settlements and the area to be serviced is much greater imposing greater transactional costs. Rural poverty is a common problem, aggravated if the rural area is remote from industries that could provide employment or if agriculture is weak or commodities are unstable. Land ownership is an important issue in agricultural communities and often lies at one of two extremes: widespread ownership of small plots of land that are too small to be economically productive or concentrated ownership of very large areas of land in the hands of a few people or families. Concentrated ownership is often associated with social unrest, exploitive labor practices, and overreliance on cash crops that are dependent on commodity prices. The tension between landowners and a class of resident farmers who farm the land and are required to pay rent is often at the basis of social unrest in such societies. (See Chapter 21.)

The economy in rural areas is usually seasonal. Crops are planted, grown, and harvested at specific times of year. Fishing may occur only during certain months. Therefore, many rural residents manage by making their primary income in mining or industry or crafts during the "off-season" and farming or fishing when they can. As a result, a "farmer" in a rural area may be more accurately described as someone who does many jobs, among them farming during the agricultural season.

Socially, rural areas tend to be conservative and traditional. Families, clans, and neighbors are particularly important when there are few social institutions that can guarantee security and when communities are small. However, the influence of modern communications and transportation has clearly reduced the isolation and conservatism of many rural areas, particularly those close to highways or where there has been a return of migrant workers who have had experiences with the wider world. Similarly, the need to pay attention to commodity prices has made many rural residents experts on the operation of international markets and have made some heavy users of the internet and other information technology. The impact of cell phones, for example, has been felt very strongly in rural and fishing markets as farmers and fisherman are able to find out the current price even while at sea before they arrive at port and the market. Overall, however, rural areas tend to be places where traditional values are held for a long time and where social change is resisted. Partly as a consequence, the more adventurous of rural young people often leave the area to try their luck or to find opportunity in cities.

THE NEXT LEVEL OF RELATIONSHIPS

The next set of relationships, shown in Figure 25.3, builds on the basic axis of human rights → population/resource imbalance → urbanization by incorporating six additional social processes.

- Women's role in society. When women are empowered to take a public role, obtain an education, participate in family decisions, and have control over some money, traditional societies begin to change.
- Child labor is related to family earning power, occupational health risk, and lost opportunities for children to be educated, as well as increased risk of abuse to the child.
- Employment opportunities in the wage economy draw people away from rural areas and agriculture. Being paid a wage by an employer for a regular job is very different from farming or seasonal agricultural work. The availability of

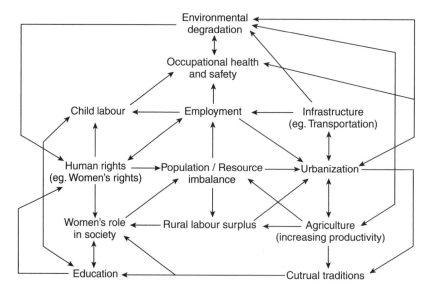

Figure 25.4 Occupational health and safety and environmental impact come into play as infrastructure becomes stressed.

cash moves the process of urbanization forward as young workers are able to buy things they want and create a market for consumer goods.

- A rural labor surplus typically results from decreased mortality in rural areas, mostly from clean water, better nutrition, and health care at a time before birth rates fall. Because they are not needed in agriculture due to increasing productivity, young people migrate to the nearest cities or to secondary towns.
- Increasing productivity of agriculture due to improved agricultural practices (agronomy) typically provides villagers with more cash and better nutrition and may provide the capital required for small enterprises.
- Improved infrastructure makes an economic transformation practical by allowing goods to come to market at a reasonable cost, transporting people to their jobs, and making it practical to have larger cities and towns.

Women's issues require more detailed discussion. In most traditional societies, women have been marginalized in public life and have had limited influence on important community and family decisions. This is not absolute: in many societies women make the decisions involving family and home even though their public role is restricted. Men typically have made the "important" decisions and have dominated organized economic life, especially at the village level, although in many traditional societies women do the farming, buy for the household, and may sell small items and animals. When women are empowered to play a role in public, for example, on village councils or in lending circles (where groups of women borrow money for small enterprises such as raising animals), the social order is changed. Women in these societies gain some control over money, become informed about events, and acquire authority. They create the leverage to make or influence decisions. Within the family, these decisions may involve whether to educate children or what business to engage in. As time goes on, this may bring higher expectations for educational attainment. Men, who in most traditional societies are accustomed to making the major decisions, are given the opportunity to learn to negotiate and to rethink the value of education for children, both sons and daughters. Eventually, the presence of strong women as role models in politics and business helps both sons and daughters to adopt new attitudes and to achieve more that is within their capacity. Gender equality shows a strong correlation with economic development.

Child labor is a great concern for occupational health and safety professionals because young bodies are more susceptible to hazards, and children injured at a young age may be disabled for life. Many families in some developing countries depend on the income from children to support the household. Children are also valued in some occupations for their small size and dexterity (for example, in rug weaving). As a result, there is great resistance in some societies to end the practice. However, it is generally understood by everyone that full-time work by children deprives them of an education and the ability to improve their lives in the future. The worst forms of child labor include severe abuse and child prostitution. The absence of parental supervision when children are sent away from their homes increases the risk of abuse and that decisions on education and discipline will be made against the child's interest.

The other factors involve employment opportunities and the means to create or expand them. One way to think about the importance of the other factors is to consider what happens when they fail. For example, if the infrastructure fails, the living conditions in crowded cities get worse and the cost of economic transactions rises sharply. If traffic congestion chokes the city, this makes getting to work and getting goods to market more costly, in terms of time, fuel, and vehicle maintenance. If agriculture fails, it leads to a crisis not only in the countryside (where people usually can grow enough to live) but also in the towns that depend on agricultural commodities for their economy. If agriculture becomes so much more productive that fewer farm workers are needed, those who cannot find jobs will often migrate to the cities and towns. Even if people cannot find jobs in the city, they usually stay anyway with the hope that they will eventually do better. The crowding that results creates informal settlements and substandard communities that lack basic infrastructure, such as piped water, sanitation, and law enforcement.

ADDITIONAL LEVELS OF RELATIONSHIPS

The next "ring" of factors, shown in Figure 25.4, builds on these fundamental economic and social relationships and relates them to a set of consequences that have secondary and feedback effects. At the top and at the bottom of the diagram, two new outcomes are introduced:

- environmental degradation
- occupational health and safety
- cultural traditions
- education

Environmental degradation and occupational health and safety problems are predictable consequences of the urbanization process in the absence of controls or a mature civic culture. Environmental degradation is not exclusively a consequence of development, of course. Clean water is critical for health protection, and control of contamination by human wastes is the most critical element of all. Air pollution, in general, is more closely tied to the urbanization process and represents a particular level of development of infrastructure, usually reflecting the number of cars and trucks on the road.

The most obvious impact of environmental degradation is illustrated by the severe air and water pollution encountered in many of the world's new megacities. However, environmental degradation is a cluster of issues that reflects potential adverse effects on health, reduction of biodiversity and habitat (trading short-term economic gain for long-term destruction of potentially renewable resources), depletion of nonrenewable resources, limitations on future land use, risks to agricultural productivity and food supply, and diminished appeal for tourism, trade, and quality of life. Environmental degradation limits both personal opportunities in the society and future economic options, and when very severe may restrict economic productivity. However, environmental degradation usually acts in more subtle ways. At extremes of pollution, as observed in some of the formerly socialist countries, it may be associated with health effects sufficiently severe to be visible as an economic factor. Most of the time, however, the effect is more insidious, by increasing the risk of adverse outcomes, reducing sustainability, and closing off future options.

Occupational health and safety is rarely considered to be a separate factor, but should be. It reflects the risk of injury and illness in the most productive segment of the population during development. Occupational health and safety issues relate directly to productivity and to income security, which are important determinants of health in an economically critical and productive segment of the population. It also reflects some of the same behaviors and controls that operate for environmental degradation. Poor performance in occupational health and safety is likely to reflect poor performance generally in environmental protection and management of human resources.

Cultural traditions may be eroded by the urbanization process and by the increasingly productive agricultural sector, which may result in the disintegration of patterns of social organization based on shared work and the regular need for field labor. Education, on the other hand, may either preserve or undermine traditional culture, often doing both simultaneously. Children and young adults can be taught about their culture, history, and politics, while being exposed to ideas from other cultures and to different points of view.

HEALTH OUTCOMES

With the basic development model now connected to environmental indicators and to occupational health and safety, one may take the final step of incorporating a variety of health-related outcomes, in Figure 25.5. These outcomes may reflect illness, disability, and invalidism. The outcomes may be largely socially defined by the expected role of the person in a community. Whether a given condition is recognized as disabling or not is often culturally determined and reflects whether the individual works for a wage, whether others can take care of him or her, if need be, and what his or her role is in the family.

- Population health status reflects the health of the population on average or overall for the community as a whole, as reflected by the frequency of public health problems and the level of health by various indicators related to personal risk and behavior, and how these health indicators are distributed.
- Access to health is part of infrastructure development and reflects urbanization. Medical care and healthcare in general is often predominantly private in developing countries, with effectively limited public access to hospitals and practitioners that are often overcrowded and sometimes of lesser quality. Preventive health services are often public and have a large impact on public health, driving population health status with protective interventions such as immunization. Public and preventive health services have a demonstrable impact on a community-wide level in reducing the burden of disease and therefore has a direct effect on population health status. Medical treatment, on the

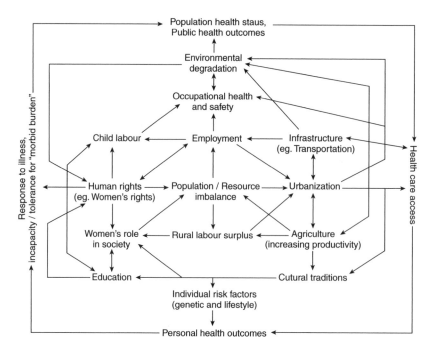

Figure 25.5 The cultural response to illness, access to health care, and the meaning of inca-pacity in a particular society all condition the effects of economic development on individual and population health.

other hand, drives population health status only indirectly, by influencing personal health outcomes in the individual case, one patient at a time.

- Personal health outcomes are individual illnesses or injuries and result from the interplay of the causes of the injury or illness and the risk factors present in the individual. For example, heart disease is more likely in people who smoke and who have a family history of heart disease. Population health factors such as cholesterol in the diet are important for the population as a whole but may or may not be important for the individual. Once a person has a heart attack, it is a personal illness with specific implications for that one person. Treatment and rehabilitation of cases on an individual basis have less effect on the population health status as a whole because the individual's experience averages out in the greater numbers.
- The "response to illness" term reflects how people deal with injury or illness in their lives and the extent to which it interferes with their lives and the security of their families.

This part of the model is a departure from most models, which interpret population health measures as just the aggregate of personal health characteristics in the population. In this model, the measures of population health status are assumed to represent the risk of ill health for the majority of people and the current state of ill health for a minority of sick people at any one time who need access to health care. The total illness burden on society is translated into a population health level that is modified by the process by which society defines illness and chooses to accept or to act to prevent a burden of illness.

If a society is accustomed to a high frequency of endemic disease, it may still be perfectly functional and its overall health indicators may still be relatively favorable, despite the high personal risk of disease. It could be argued that until the recent decline in mortality from cardiovascular disease, this was the situation in much of North America and Western Europe. High frequencies of death from myocardial infarction and stroke were part of life for many people, but on a population basis the indicators of health and longevity appeared favorable compared to the past. The mortality from heart disease, while increasing at that time, did not keep people from living longer lives than previous generations.

There is a general pattern in the public health issues associated with economic development. Early on, the public health agenda is dominated by water availability and quality. Diarrheal disease is a particularly common health issue, and access to clean water is the major development strategy for environmental health.

With economic development, other environmental issues assume greater priority and occupational health becomes a more visible threat to productivity and personal security. Access to health care and the rising cost of health care become more obviously problems for the country as well as the individual.

How people respond to their illness is conditioned by what society expects them to do. In the past, a heart attack was considered in many societies to be the

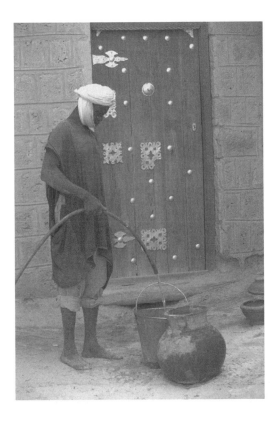

Figure 25.6 In developing countries, obtaining clean water is usually a major problem, seen here in Timbuktu, Mali. (Photograph by Lorraine Chittock, Saudi Aramco World/SAWDIA.)

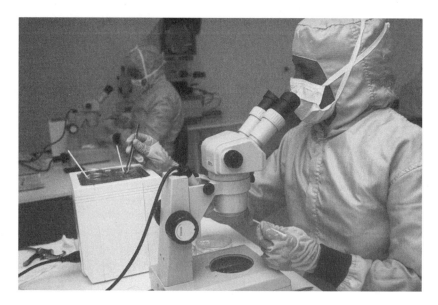

Figure 25.7 These workers in Asmara, Eritrea, are making implantable lenses for use in cataract operations, for export. (Photograph by Lorraine Chittock, Saudi Aramco World/ SAWDIA.)

end of a person's productive life; people who had suffered one heart attack lived out their lives in fear that they would die if they had another. Now, with improved medical care, but also because of social attitudes more attuned to rehabilitation, people fully expect to return to work after a heart attack and to live for many years.

The implications of an illness, injury, or disability are different at different levels of development and personal wealth. Table 25.1 suggests what it may mean to be sick or disabled under various economic circumstances.

TABLE 25.1

IMPLICATIONS OF ILLNESS ASSOCIATED WITH LEVELS OF DEVELOPMENT

Economic State	Characteristics of Sick Role in Acute Illness	Characteristics of Sick Role in Chronic Illness
Destitution, dependence	Desperation	Lost hope
Subsistence	Dependence on family	Desperation; survival insecure
Essential needs met	Potential drop to subsistence or destitution; loss of property, income, and status	Permanent loss of property, income, and status; survival insecure
Essentials met and marginal disposable income (i.e., no savings)	Potential drop to subsistence or destitution; loss of amenity, security, and future prospects	Insecurity of status and reduced capacity to cope in future (i.e., new vulnerability)
Essentials met, comfortable disposable income (little savings)	Possible drop to subsistence level and destitution depending on savings, loss of fundamental choices (such as where to live and how), potential for recovery	Insecurity of social role and capacity to restore status quo, permanent loss of fundamental choices (such as where to live and how)
Moderate wealth, no safety net	Possible economic insecurity, threat of loss of fundamental choices, capacity to recover if limited	Loss of autonomy, depletion of personal property, capacity to restore status quo ante reduced, social role may or may not be reduced
Moderate wealth with safety net	Possible economic insecurity but not destitution, loss of choices in lifestyle	Economic and social dependency, reduced expectations
Affluence	Concern for accumulated wealth, loss of future choices within lifestyle	Focus on personal implications and subjective meaning of illness

26

COVENANTS IN OCCUPATIONAL HEALTH

Igor Fedotov

The right to a safe and healthy work environment is a fundamental human right. This right is an integral part of the humanization of work and a basic requirement for the achievement of social justice. It is incorporated in international law and embedded in international treaties. This legal framework is administered by an international structure in which the lead organization is the International Labour Organization, which will be described in detail below.

The legal foundation for a right to a safe and healthy work environment is laid out in three major international treaties agreed upon by the nations of the world regarding occupational health and safety:

- "Protection of the worker against sickness, disease and injury arising out of his employment."
  (Preamble, International Labour Organization Constitution, 1919)
- "Everyone has the right to work, to free choice of employment, to just and favourable conditions of work and to protection against unemployment."
  (Article 23, Extracts, Universal Declaration on Human Rights, United Nations, 1948)
- "Covenant recognises the right of everyone to enjoyment of just and favourable conditions of work which ensure safe and healthy working conditions."
  (Article 7, International Covenant on Economic, Social and Cultural Rights, United Nations, 1976)

THE INTERNATIONAL LABOUR ORGANIZATION

In the United Nations system, two specialized agencies are directly concerned with occupational health taken as a whole: the International Labour Organization (ILO) and the World Health Organization (WHO). The ILO was set up in 1919 to bring governments, employers, and trade unions together for unified action to promote social justice and better working and living conditions everywhere. In 1946, the ILO became the first specialized agency of the United Nations. The ILO has a unique tripartite (three-part) structure with workers and employers participating as equal partners with governments. In 1969, the Organization was awarded the Nobel Peace Prize. The ILO is composed of a general assembly that meets yearly, the International Labour Conference, which adopts Conventions and Recommendations; an executive council; the Governing Body; and a permanent Secretariat, the International Labour Office, based in Geneva, Switzerland. The protection of workers from hazards arising from their employment is one of the major tasks assigned to the ILO in the Preamble to its Constitution. The ILO mandate in occupational health is intended to guarantee that:

- Work is carried out in a safe and healthy work environment.
- Working conditions are consistent with workers' well-being and human dignity.
- Work should offer real possibilities for personal achievement, self-fulfillment, and service to society.

One of the key functions of the ILO is its standard-setting activities. The ILO formulates international labor standards in the form of Conventions and Recommendations. As of May 2008, the ILO has produced 188 Conventions and 199 Recommendations with approximately 30 of them dealing directly with occupational health and safety. Together, all these international instruments (Conventions and Recommendations) comprise the International Labour Code.

The ILO Conventions are international treaties that are subject to ratification by national parliaments. Ratification means that the nation accepts a Convention as a treaty, adheres to it in its national legislation, and brings domestic law and practice into conformity with the provisions of the ratified Convention. Recommendations are not subject to ratification. They usually accompany Conventions and provide guidance for the most efficient ways to apply the provisions of the Conventions. Recommendations are detailed standards that serve as guidelines for nations in their legislative decisions, policy, and practice. Both instruments are flexible enough to address a large variety of local occupational health and safety conditions and practices. Each is crafted to have the following features:

- Universality: Wide-ranging consideration of diverse national occupational health practices goes into their preparation and framing, representing widely accepted goals for national action that all countries can follow.
- Flexibility: Drafted in a spirit of realism and effectiveness, aimed at protecting workers' health and life, and universally applicable.
- Viability: Elaborated in the tripartite environment, the decision to ratify a Convention is the sovereign will of independent states.
- Adaptability: Continually revised and updated to adapt to rapidly changing working conditions and environments.

BOX 26.1

The International Code of Ethics for Occupational Health Professionals

The world standard in ethics for occupational health is the International Code of Ethics for Occupational Health Professionals of the International Commission on Occupational Health, as revised in 2002. The International Commission on Occupational Health (ICOH) is the international organization for occupational health professionals, founded in 1906 and recognized as a non-governmental organization by the United Nations. The code is available on the Internet at http://www.icohweb. org/core_docs/code_ethics_eng.pdf. This code should be read and understood by all occupational health professionals.

This is a universal code of ethics for the occupational health professions, whether they are professionals with established codes, such as physicians, nurses, safety professionals, and hygienists, or occupational health workers without professional standing. It applies to any person who has accepted a position dealing with the health and safety of workers. Much of the Code is based on ILO covenants and conventions and national codes of ethics. In some countries, it is recognized as the standard against which occupational health professionals would be judged in legal or professional disciplinary actions.

Occupational health issues often present ethical challenges. The context of the issues are often complex, there are sensitive issues of confidentiality, and many occupational health professionals have a dual responsibility to the worker (as guardian of their health) and the employer (as an employee and/or a regulator). In occupational medicine, there is an additional source of confusion because sometimes the worker is a patient and sometimes no physician-patient relationship exists, as when a physician is evaluating a claim. In such situations, standards of ethics are even more important to guide the professional and to defend his or her actions against pressures to compromise or to bend the rules.

The ICOH Code reflects a shared set of values that apply to all aspects of occupational health and that emphasize fair treatment for the worker. The existence of a single code for all occupational health professions avoids confusion and exploitation that would result from differences in rules among different occupational health professions. For example, if occupational medicine, occupational health nursing, and office staff followed different rules on confidentiality and privacy, managers who had no business obtaining confidential medical information on a person could simply ask for it from someone else in the same office.

However, the ICOH Code does not substitute for established ethical codes in the professions, such as medical ethics and nursing ethics. Rather, it complements them and fills in the gaps where they do not apply.

Principles of the ICOH Code of Ethics

The Code begins with an introduction that explains its history and significance. Then, three paragraphs outline the basic principles of the ICOH Code of Ethics, on which the full code is based. These paragraphs are reproduced below in their entirety.

The purpose of occupational health is to serve the health and social well-being of the workers individually and collectively. Occupational health practice must be performed according to the highest professional standards and ethical principles. Occupational health professionals must contribute to environmental and community health.

The duties of occupational health professionals include protecting the life and health of the worker, respecting human dignity and promoting the highest ethical principles in occupational health policies and programmes. Integrity in professional conduct, impartiality and the protection of the confidentiality of health data and of the privacy of the workers are part of these duties.

Occupational health professionals are experts who must enjoy full professional independence in the execution of their functions. They must acquire and maintain the competence necessary for their duties and require conditions which allow them to carry out their tasks according to good practice and professional ethics.

There follows a section on "Duties and obligations of occupational health professionals" with 26 specific items. The entire Code is extensively referenced.

Summary of the "Duties and Obligations" Section

The language of the Code is not always clear, and it is rather long. For these reasons, it is described here by an interpretive summary. This summary is not a definitive legal or ethical interpretation, however. All occupational health professionals should read the Code for themselves, on the ICOH Web site, and think it through carefully.

Occupational health professionals are defined by their role, not by credentials or formal titles. Anyone with responsibility for workers' health has a duty to protect and promote workers' health and a commitment to a safe and healthy workplace. Occupational health professionals should practice at the highest level of their profession and training and know themselves whether their work is adequate, competent, and sufficiently well supported to be effective. This requires that an effort be made to see the actual workplace and to talk to workers, outside of clinic as well as in, in order to better understand the reality of the workplace.

The highest goal of occupational health practice is protection and prevention. A safe and healthy workplace is fundamentally the responsibility of the employer. Protection of the worker should not be delayed or wait for the perfect solution. A hazard should be corrected now, even if is only a partial solution.

Protection of workers' health is primary but not absolute. There are also legitimate balances between the interests of workers and employers and between individual and collective interests (such as safety-sensitive positions). There is a balance among the interests of the parties in occupational health, and this balance is legitimate, not an ethical compromise. Conflicts of interest (such as between workers and employers) should be resolved objectively and professionally.

The occupational health professional is required to document issues and solutions, to be transparent in all dealings, and to communicate clearly to all parties. In particular, the occupational health professional is expected to use judgment. (Several provisions of the Code involve balancing rights, requiring the occupational health professional to weigh serious issues.)

Occupational health professionals should be independent, free to give advice, adequately provided with resources, and allowed to practice according to the highest professional standards. Occupational health has a moral dimension. If these conditions are not met, the occupational health professional has to consider whether he or she wishes to be part of the employer's organization.

The workplace should be changed, working conditions should be safe and healthful, and work should be adapted to the worker rather than the other way around. Hazards should be controlled rather than workers selected for their ability to work around the hazard.

Discrimination is not acceptable.

Occupational health professionals should assist workers in obtaining and maintaining employment, including the disabled. The purpose of occupational health is to make work safe and accessible to the worker, not to screen out workers to make hiring decisions easier or to select only those who are super-fit. Fitness-for-duty evaluations, in particular, are intended to ensure that a worker can do the job to which they will be assigned, safely and adequately, not to screen out persons with disabilities. Disability is a condition of mismatch between the person's ability and the environment ("you have certain capabilities that fit this task at work and not another task at work—how important is the task?"). Disability is not a category of person ("the disabled" as a special group) or a label on a person ("you are a disabled person").

Workers have rights. Workers should be represented in decisions that are made for their protection. (This is not the norm in many countries.) Workers must be allowed to opt out of periodic health surveillance and other studies unless required by law or regulation or in the work contract. Much of occupational health practice is governed by law and regulation and by various International Labour Organization conventions and recommendations that are binding in countries that have ratified them. The legal framework should protect those rights.

The employer should not be informed by the occupational health professional of the diagnosis or medical condition of an employee or even details of the disability, except a conclusion regarding fitness for duty (expressed as "fit," "unfit," or "fit with accommodation/modification") and the accommodations or modifications required in the event of a disability. There should be mechanisms for appeal of fitness-for-duty decisions on new hires or return to work. (This is not the norm in many countries.)

There are a few, rare, special cases in which the occupational health professional may need to act in the interest of society above the interest of the individual worker or employer. Occupational health professionals must respect trade secrets but recognize a higher duty to health protection in those rare instances when a secret needs to be disclosed (for example, to save someone's life or to make a diagnosis in a serious illness). The occupational health professional must report serious risks to management or to a competent governmental authority, notwithstanding the personal risk. On the other hand, the risk must be truly "serious," and such action has to be appropriate to the circumstances.

Where employees may be a threat to themselves or to others in the workplace, they should be informed of the risk and given an opportunity to change jobs or ask for reassignment. ("Safety-sensitive" workers, such as truck drivers, airplane pilots, and police are held to a higher standard of fitness and reliability, for the protection of others.) Sometimes, the occupational health professional must violate confidentiality and notify management or the appropriate government authority if the worker does not choose a course of action that protects others. Again, the threshold for notifying management and government regulatory agencies is quite high: the situation must exceed the usual degree of risk in any workplace, which implies risk of serious injury or death. Legal advice should always be sought in such situations, of course.

Prepared by Tee L. Guidotti

Safety and Health Standards

The ILO Conventions and Recommendations on occupational safety and health define the rights of the workers and allocate duties and responsibilities to the competent (government) authority, the employers, and the workers in the field of occupational health and safety. They serve as targets for achievement for the national authorities that put their policies and approaches into action.

ILO occupational safety and health standards exert considerable influence on the laws and regulations of countries because of their status being grounded in international law. The texts of laws in many countries have been modeled on the relevant provisions of ILO instruments. Drafts of new legislation or amendments are often prepared with ILO standards in mind in order to ensure compliance with ratified Conventions or to permit the ratification of other Conventions. Trade unions use ILO standards to support their arguments in collective bargaining and in promoting legislation. National governments frequently consult the ILO about the compatibility of proposed texts with international labor standards.

Occupational safety and health standards from the ILO fall broadly into four categories:

- policy guidance
- worker protection, by risk
- worker protection, by industry sector
- special measures

The first category provides the policy guidance by the ILO on occupational health and safety. It is essentially contained in three international Conventions and their accompanying Recommendations. The ILO Occupational Safety and Health Convention, 1981 (No. 155) and Recommendation 1981 (No. 164) provide for the adoption of a national occupational health and safety policy and prescribe the progressive application of comprehensive preventive actions and measures at the national and enterprise levels to ensure worker protection and to improve the work environment. They establish the responsibility of employers for making work and equipment safe as well as establishing the duties and rights of workers. In 2002, the ILO adopted a new Protocol to the C. 155 Convention and Recommendation No. 194 updating the list of occupational diseases. The Protocol requests ratifying Member States to establish and review requirements and procedures for the recording and notification of occupational accidents and diseases, dangerous occurrences, and commuting accidents. The Protocol also requests Member States to publish annual statistics following classification guidelines that are compatible with the latest international schemes of the ILO or other relevant international organizations. The Recommendation No. 194 requests Member States to establish a national list of occupational diseases for the purpose of prevention, recording, notification, and compensation.

The ILO Occupational Health Services Convention, 1985 (No. 161) and the Recommendation 1985 (No. 171) provide for the establishment of occupational health services that comprise preventive functions, are responsible for advising employers and workers on maintaining safe and healthy work environments, and adapting work to the capabilities of workers. Occupational health services also contribute to the implementation of national occupational health policies and perform their functions at the enterprise level. The emphasis of these international instruments is on roles, best use of resources, and cooperation between all those concerned with workers' health.

Recently, the ILO has adopted the Promotional Framework for Occupational Safety and Health Convention, 2006 (No. 187) providing for a comprehensive promotional framework for occupational safety and health (OSH). The Convention calls for the promotion of national preventive safety and health culture and periodic review of the measures for implementation and ratification of ILO Conventions in the field of occupational safety and health (OSH). The systematic improvement of national OSH practice should be achieved through the formulation of national OSH policy, a national OSH system, and establishment of national OSH programs. These programs are strategic time-bound programs that focus on specific national priorities for OSH, are based on analyses of the situations in the countries concerned, and should be preferably summarized as national OSH profiles. Programs should be developed and implemented following tripartite consultations between government, employers, and workers and endorsed by the highest government authorities. Programs need clear objectives, targets, and indicators and should aim at strengthening the national OSH systems to ensure sustainability of improvements and the development of a preventive safety culture.

The second category provides for the protection of workers against specific risks, including chemical hazards, ionizing radiation, benzene, asbestos, occupational cancer, air pollution, noise and vibration, and other hazards arising out of the use of machinery.

The third category provides protection in certain sectors of economic activity, such as construction, mining, commerce and clerical work, dock work, prevention of major industrial accidents, safety and health in agriculture, and others.

The fourth category encompasses special measures, such as medical examinations of young workers, maximum load weights to be transported by a single worker, accident prevention on board ships, and others.

The ILO Conventions and Recommendations dealing with occupational health and safety matters have the status of standards, which once adopted on the national level are mandatory in the country. Further guidance on how to improve occupational health and prevent occupational injuries and diseases is provided in the ILO Codes of Practice, which are used for formulating detailed national regulations in this field. The Codes of Practice suggest practical solutions for the application of the ILO international standards.

ILO Codes of Practice are prepared in the form of detailed technical specifications that are intended to assist governments and employers' and workers' organizations in drawing up national regulations and guidelines, work regulations, and collective agreements. The Codes of Practice cover different sectors of activity (e.g., mining, agriculture, forestry, construction, iron and steel production, shipbuilding, dock work) or particular risks (e.g., industrial accidents, ionizing radiation, chemical substances, asbestos, noise and vibration, ambient factors, exposure to airborne substances) as well as transfer of technology and recording and notification of occupational accidents and diseases. Codes of Practice indicate "what should be done." They are prepared during ILO tripartite technical meetings of experts, and the ILO Governing Body approves their publication.

The overall objective of the use of international standards in the field of occupational health and safety is to:

- reduce the number of occupational accidents and diseases, which represent a serious burden for national economies
- adapt the work environment, equipment, and work practices to the physical and mental capacity of the worker
- enhance the physical, mental, and social well-being of workers in all occupations, including the informal sector and agriculture
- encourage the establishment of national policies and prevention programs on occupational health that contribute to the achievement of sustainable development

The challenge today is to find practical solutions and robust approaches to achieve expanded worker protection in rapidly changing national situations due to globalization of the world economy. The ILO international instruments on occupational health and safety constitute viable standards that are instrumental in shaping national laws and regulations. They promote the principles of "decent work" and guarantee fundamental rights, including the right to a safe and healthy work environment.

27

OCCUPATIONAL HEALTH SERVICES

Tee L. Guidotti

Occupational health practice requires an organizational structure, basic equipment, procedures, and facilities for providing care as well as trained people to provide the care. An organization that provides treatment, monitoring, and prevention for individual workers and for the workforce in general is called an *occupational health service*. *Providers* is a general term for professionals who deliver care of various types, including physicians, nurses, hygienists, and many other types of occupational health professionals and technicians.

In English, the word *service* (as in occupational health service) means a department or organization that "serves" workers and employers by providing such care. The same word, *service*, can also mean the individual task or care that is provided, such as a medical evaluation, setting a broken bone, sewing up a laceration, putting on an educational program, conducting a laboratory test, or counseling a worker with a mental health problem. In context, it is usually clear what is meant, but the reader should be aware that the word *service* can mean either the specific type of care that is provided or the organization that provides it.

Occupational health services can be provided through the primary health-care system or in specialized facilities and organizations.

OCCUPATIONAL HEALTH INTEGRATED WITH PRIMARY HEALTH CARE

Much of the delivery of occupational health services takes place within the system of primary health care where suitably trained generalist health-care providers may be the first professionals to identify a workplace problem. The early detection of workplace hazards or clusters of workplace disease or injury is both an ethical obligation for health professionals as well as one of the most useful methods available for identifying interventions to prevent further morbidity and mortality. Medical surveillance and biological monitoring of exposed workers can be integrated readily into district-based primary health-care services. The World Health

Organization model for Basic Occupational Health Services assumes that primary health-care services provide a comprehensive approach to disease prevention and treatment and that they will be able to address the role of workplace hazards together with environmental hazards, such as lack of sanitation, clean water, and disease control.

For many years, the World Health Organization has had a policy of emphasizing *primary care*. Occupational health may be provided as an essential part of the primary care system. To understand how this works, and the challenges of doing so, requires an understanding of primary care itself.

Primary care is the provision of basic services of diagnosis and medical treatment, basic levels of sanitation, and essential medical services for prevention, such as immunization. Primary care is usually provided by physicians and nurses and, for sanitation, public health workers who live in the community they serve. Sometimes this care is provided by health workers who are trained as technicians or health-care assistants. These primary care providers are usually not trained to provide specialized services or advanced levels of care, although they may have training in greater depth in problems common in their communities, such as malaria. They are, however, trained to recognize more serious or complicated problems that require referral to hospitals or to specialized practitioners.

Primary care providers deal with common injuries and illnesses and childbirth where this is not assisted by midwives. They provide immunizations, contraception, health education, basic medicines, and mental health care. They may conduct inspections and advise on public health measures, such as clean water and sanitation for the community, as well.

Primary care providers may have their own clinics and offices or, in rural areas, they may move from one community to another. The services they provide generally match the health-care needs of the community but do not include highly advanced care or require expensive or special equipment.

Primary care practitioners are needed in all communities. In developed countries, such as the United Kingdom, primary care practitioners serve as the *gatekeepers*, which means that they evaluate the needs of the patient and decide whether the patient needs advanced levels of care. If an advanced level of care is required, they make the necessary referrals to specialists or arrange for transfer to hospitals. In developing countries and in rural, disadvantaged, or remote areas of developed countries, primary care practitioners may be the only health workers available.

The World Health Organization views primary care providers as the backbone of the health-care system in all countries. They provide the essential first level of care. For most people, this level of care is sufficient. For those who need more, the primary care provider is the first contact and can guide the patient to the right health care and services that are required. Funding for health at the national level has the best results when invested in primary care because it brings needed health care to the most people and provides prevention, which reduces illness and reduces the need for more advanced care.

However, bringing primary care to all people presents big challenges. One major challenge is geographical distribution. Most physicians and nurses usually prefer to live in larger communities and to have access to more technically sophisticated equipment and laboratories. Life is much better when a health professional can take time off and can trade working hours with other health professionals. Working in isolated or rural communities can be very demanding, and there may be little or no opportunity to take time off. For these reasons, health-care workers often do not locate where they are needed most. This leaves large areas with few practitioners to serve them. There is almost always a severe shortage of health-care providers in rural areas in every country.

Another challenge is professional satisfaction. Health workers who are ambitious usually want more advanced training to refine their professional skills. They may prefer to specialize in order to become very good at what they do. It is difficult to keep the best health-care workers satisfied when they are obliged to stay in one place and can perform only routine services or see common problems.

Another challenge is economic. Primary care providers usually do not earn as much money as specialists. In countries where patients must pay for their care, the health-care provider may not be paid by patients who are poor and sick. Where health care is paid for by the government, the primary care provider usually does not earn as much as the specialist. There may be little governmental or private money to pay for medicines, vaccines, and medical equipment. Sometimes preventive care, such as immunizations, is paid poorly or not paid at all.

Primary care is also demanding. The primary care provider usually must deal with a wide variety of problems, has little time to spend on any one patient, works long hours, and is often very stressed. Demands on the practitioner can be overwhelming, because he or she must constantly make difficult decisions about whether to give priority to one patient over another or to spend time on one problem or another. Taking care of families and neighbors can be very rewarding, but if something goes wrong it is difficult to escape bad feelings, especially in a small community.

On the other hand, primary care has many rewards. The community is usually grateful. The practitioner has the opportunity to get to know families. There is satisfaction in meeting the needs of the community and knowing that one's work has made a difference in the lives of people one knows personally.

Integrating occupational health with primary care is a major goal but is difficult in practice. Primary care providers often lack the training to provide occupational health services and have little time to learn. Occupational health services of a preventive nature may seem to be a low priority compared to providing urgently needed care. If occupational health services are well paid, there may be resentment if the practitioner spends time on those issues instead of taking care of community residents.

On the other hand, providing occupational health services can be a source of needed income to primary care practitioners. This form of practice is often easier to manage than a busy clinic and may be a welcome relief in the day. It is interesting and diverse and builds relationships with local employers and workers. It provides opportunities for prevention and improving the health of workers, who with their families may also be served by the practitioner in their primary care practice.

To help solve these problems and to promote the integration of occupational health and primary care, WHO has developed training programs and manuals to help primary care providers learn about and provide occupational health services at the community level. For example, the Eastern Mediterranean Regional office of WHO has produced a manual for primary care providers that can be used in training or as a guide to providing occupational health services to workers at local employment sites.

Specialized Occupational Health Services

Larger and more complex organizations require specialized occupational health services to meet their needs. These may include:

- large employers with many employees in different jobs posing a variety of hazards
- corporations with many locations or locations in many countries, which have a need to coordinate their services
- enterprises, public or private, that are engaged in unusually hazardous activities, such as blasting, or that handle hazards requiring special expertise, such as radioactive sources
- enterprises in which the health of workers is a particularly sensitive issue, such as airlines, which must be concerned with the wellness of their pilots and their fitness to fly
- collections of enterprises, sharing specialized resources in order to get maximum benefit

Specialized Occupational Health Professions

The various occupational health professions developed from different historical traditions, perform different duties, and offer different essential skills and knowledge, or *core competencies*. Even so, occupational health professions all have certain core competencies in common and a common ethical framework (see Box 26.1). In general, these competencies are reflected in the content of this book. It is therefore reasonable to expect that occupational physicians, occupational nurses, occupational hygienists, most safety officers, and many other technical occupational health personnel will have a working knowledge of most of the concepts and facts mentioned in this book. Thus, one way to evaluate an occupational health professional before hiring is to use this book to frame questions to determine their understanding of common problems.

Another important characteristic of all occupational health professionals, regardless of their specific profession, is that they are able to think of both individual cases and populations. In general, physicians, nurses, and technicians are trained to deal with specific cases and the investigation of particular problems. However, occupational physicians, occupational nurses, and occupational hygienists are also trained to look at the big picture, to see patterns in the workplace. This may mean understanding workers both as individuals and as a population (mainly through the application of epidemiology) or understanding the pattern of hazards

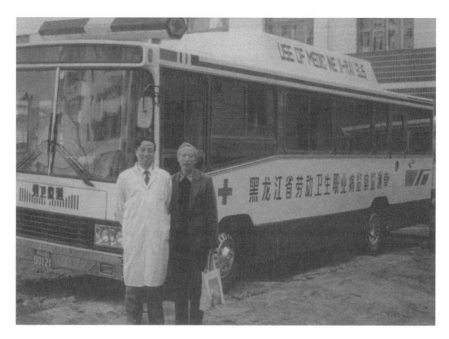

Figure 27.1 Mobile X-ray unit of the Heilongjiang Provincial Occupational Health Institute, Harbin (China), in 1987, with the director at that time, Dr. Feng Keyu, and Liu Shuchun, professor of toxicology at the institute. (Photograph by Tee L. Guidotti, University of Alberta.)

in a workplace (where they are most likely to occur, where they are likely to be most severe). This versatility becomes particularly important when the time comes to conduct detailed investigations or to put protective measures into place.

A third common characteristic of specialized occupational health professionals is that they are trained to manage programs for the delivery of services. Monitoring the health of workers, evaluating hazards, and tracking the resolution of problems requires good management skills, the ability to supervise people, and accurate record-keeping skills. A good occupational health professional will be able to formulate a budget, evaluate equipment acquisitions, put together at least a simple organizational framework for an office or administrative department, and set up a filing system that will keep track of individual workers and important problems.

An important concern of occupational health professionals is the necessity of keeping up with new developments in both their health profession and in the industry in which they are working. One way of doing this is to participate in *continuing education* programs when they are available. Another is to belong to organizations that inform their members of new developments and provide opportunities for networking and learning. The international organization of occupational health professionals is the International Commission on Occupational Health (ICOH), which has scientific committees on almost all aspects of occupational health. Membership in ICOH or in large national organizations indicates that the occupational health professional is at least connected to others in the profession and is exposed to new developments in his or her field.

However, occupational health professionals also have skills and resources that reflect their special training. Physicians and nurses, in particular, are often active in their professional societies in the local community and often work in local hospitals, which gives them the opportunity to establish professional relationships, to learn which community practitioners are best for a particular medical need or referral, to make sure that local hospitals and practitioners are equipped to meet the needs of the workers under their care, to make fast arrangements for transfer to hospitals when necessary, and to understand the needs of workers in the context of the community in which they live.

This section describes occupational health professions using Canada as an example of how each is organized in one exemplary country.

Occupational Physicians Occupational physicians are medical doctors who have received special training or who have benefited from specialized experience in *occupational medicine*. This special training usually follows graduation from medical school and is often undertaken in formal programs similar to other medical specialties. However, many occupational physicians enter the practice of occupational medicine after they have been in medical practice for some time. They may even specialize in another area of medicine first and become occupational physicians later in their careers. In such cases, they usually obtain their training informally through continuing education courses and through on-the-job experience.

In most countries, occupational physicians have their own training programs, organizations, and specialty certification or recognition systems. Canada is a good example and has a particularly well-developed and straightforward system. In Canada, there are formal training programs, accredited by the Royal College of Physicians and Surgeons of Canada (RCPSC), for physicians who enter the specialty. After this training, which may take as long as five years (less if they have already completed some relevant training in another specialty), these physicians take an examination and, if they pass, are awarded a particular specialty credential, Fellow of the Royal College of Physicians of Canada (FRCPC). However, many physicians cannot take time out of their careers to do this if they make the decision to go into occupational medicine later. For them, there is another certifying body, the Canadian Board of Occupational Medicine (CBOM). These physicians have the opportunity to request an evaluation of their experience, after which they are supervised in practice for a period of time and then take a series of examinations and demonstrations of competence, which leads to a different credential, the Certificate of the CBOM (CCBOM). (There is also a higher level—a "Fellow.") The existence of these two pathways allows occupational physicians in Canada to specialize later in their careers, gives them a way to show their specialized expertise, and provides an easy way for employers to tell the difference. Both groups usually belong to the national organization, the Occupational and Environmental Medical Association of Canada (OEMAC). Becoming a member of OEMAC provides these physicians with a convenient way of learning about new developments, keeping in touch with their colleagues, and presenting their opinions to

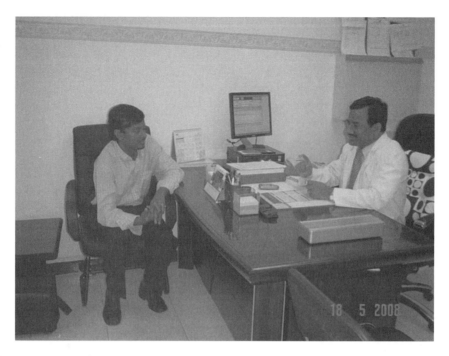

Figure 27.2 A worker in Kuwait being interviewed by Dr. Madhava Rao, medical director of the Shuaiba Occupational Medical Centre, a government-operated occupational health facility that serves workers in an area west of Kuwait City. Employers in this area are involved in oilfield services, construction, manufacturing, and municipal government. (Photograph courtesy of the Shuaiba Occupational Medical Centre, Ministry of Health, Kuwait.)

government and employer groups. Continuing education in the specialty is provided by OEMAC, the RCPSC, by local medical schools, and sometimes by other specialty organizations, such as the Canadian Thoracic Society.

Occupational physicians may work in individual plants as *plant physicians* providing medical care for an employer's individual facilities, as *medical directors* supervising health-related affairs for large organizations, as *contract physicians* providing services for many employers in a given area, or as *consultants* called in to address specific problems or issues. Most occupational physicians are able to provide diagnosis and treatment for individual cases, yet also manage programs for the entire workforce.

In the United States, there is also a health profession called *physician's assistants*. These are health workers who are specially trained in providing specific types of medical treatment and performing various duties in occupational medicine under the supervision of a physician. Many of them work in occupational medicine.

Occupational Health Nurses *Occupational health nurses* (OHNs) often have a system similar to that of occupational physicians, but these systems tend to vary more by country. Many countries have formal programs for certifying OHNs as specialists in occupational health nursing; others consider occupational health nursing to be a field within community health nursing.

Programs for training OHNs can be formal programs in which the nurse takes classes and are supervised for a period but are more often based on alternative models of training. For example, many OHNs in Canada study for their certification by long-distance education. On completion of the training program, they are eligible to take an examination that, if they pass, certifies them as a Certified Occupational Health Nurse (COHN). This certification examination is administered by the Canadian Nurses Association. Many nurses in Canada practice occupational health nursing without certification, but the system sets a high standard of practice expected for everyone, not only COHNs. Their national organization is the Canadian Occupational Health Nurses Association. There are also associations in the various provinces, such as the Ontario Occupational Health Nurses Association. Becoming a member of these associations provides OHNs with a convenient way of learning about new developments, hearing about job opportunities, keeping in touch with their colleagues in the local area and nationally, and presenting their opinions and concerns to government and employer groups.

There are many more nurses in occupational health than there are physicians. Nurses are commonly hired by individual facilities and have responsibility for conducting routine periodic health surveillance, providing basic treatment to injured workers at the site, providing care for workers who have personal health problems that would otherwise require them to leave their workplace to get care, and managing programs required to show compliance with regulations. Although nurses are required to have a physician authorize their work, there are many procedures and treatment plans that the nurse can perform when the physician is not present once *standing orders* have been issued. Thus, OHNs have an unusual degree of professional freedom within the nursing profession.

In some countries, particularly the United States, *nurse practitioners* are nurses trained to a high level who can take on many of the tasks of a physician without supervision.

Occupational Hygienists *Occupational hygienists* are specialized technical professionals who study workplace hazards. A trained occupational hygienist is able to identify a probable hazard, measure the level of exposure of workers to the hazard, evaluate the magnitude of the health risk, and design a means of controlling the hazard or protecting the worker. The occupational hygienist, therefore, is the primary professional who performs the duties outlined in Chapter 4 of this book.

Hygienists vary in their training and preparation more than occupational physicians or nurses. Some hygienists are engineers or chemists. Others are trained in special graduate programs, usually after they receive university degrees, and may receive a master's degree, licentiate, or engineering degree or its equivalent on completion. They may then take an examination for a certification in the field. In Canada, to continue this example, this is the Canadian Registration Board for Occupational Hygiene, and the official designation is the Registered Occupational Hygienist (ROH). However, occupational hygiene is not yet as well-standardized worldwide as occupational medicine or occupational health nursing. Some countries still do not recognize occupational hygiene as a specialty. Others recognize the official designations of the American Industrial Hygiene Association (Certified Occupational Hygienist or COH) or the multilevel system of the British Occupational Hygiene Society (Fellow, Member, or Licentiate) or their own national systems (e.g., Japan). There are many occupational hygiene associations in various countries as well as the International Occupational Hygiene Association. In addition, hygienists often represent their interests through other organizations and sections of organizations devoted to engineering or occupational health.

Hygienists are often employed by large corporations and become very skilled in dealing with problems characteristic of a particular industry. Often, they are employed as consultants. Because much of occupational hygiene involves collecting samples and placing monitors for evaluating hazards, many organizations hire *occupational hygiene technicians*, who do this work under the supervision of hygienists.

Safety Professionals Safety professionals are a more diverse group and have many of the same skills as occupational hygienists. In general, they emphasize physical hazards, such as those outlined in Chapter 6, but also have a working knowledge of toxic hazards.

Safety professionals are often trained informally through short courses or continuing education, but in recent years there has been a trend toward making their preparation more formal. Some university programs exist, and where they do they are often connected to schools of engineering. Certification programs for safety professionals tend to vary more than other occupational health professions. In Canada, there is a Canadian Registration Board of Occupational Safety Professions, which functions as a sister organization to the hygienists' board described above. The world standard, however, is the National Examination Board for Occupational Safety and Health (NEBOSH) in the UK, which accredits formal safety training programs.

Some safety technicians are given responsibility in their organizations without special training and are expected to learn on the job. This is not the best way, but it is very common. Membership in the Canadian Society of Safety Engineers provides professional support.

Ergonomists *Ergonomists* are specialists in how work is performed, the physical and psychological characteristics of the workplace, and how well they match or do not match the capacity of the worker. Ergonomists work mostly as consultants in evaluating problems in the workplace or in designing machines, work stations, or tools that are efficient, easy to use, unlikely to cause injury, easy to understand and monitor, and free of unnecessary stresses that may cause musculoskeletal disorders. The field of ergonomics is described in the section on chemical hazards in Chapter 2 and in Chapter 7. Ergonomists vary widely in their preparation, from highly trained engineers to technicians who have taken short courses. Some countries have certification systems for ergonomists, such as the Canadian College for the Certification of Professional Ergonomists.

Other Occupational Health Professionals Other professional fields are also specialized for work in occupational health. These professions usually do not have formal certification or registration programs. They are not present in every country, but they are widely recognized around the world.

Occupational psychologists specialize in mental health issues in the workplace, including depression (a leading cause of absence from work), poor relations with coworkers, stress, and substance abuse. They are experts in many of the fields discussed in Chapters 11 and 18. Many occupational psychologists specialize in administering and interpreting tests of mental capacity and brain function, as described in Chapter 11.

Employee assistance professionals are experts in substance abuse (drugs and alcohol), behavioral addictions (often including gambling and credit card debt), and managing workers who have personal problems. Employee assistance programs are described in Chapter 11.

Epidemiologists are scientists who study patterns of disease, health-related behavior, and determinants of injury and disease in populations. Occupational epidemiologists specialize in the type of epidemiology described in Chapter 3, which is focused primarily on finding the causes of occupational injury and disease. Their training usually requires several years and begins after university.

Toxicologists are scientists who study the effects of chemicals on the body. Their field is described in Chapters 2 and 9. Their training also requires several years and begins after university.

Health physicists are radiation health specialists. They are trained to measure exposure to radiation and in ways to prevent exposure in the workplace. Their field is described in the section on radiation in Chapter 8.

Hearing conservationists or hearing protection technicians (the name varies) are trained to measure exposure to noise, conduct screening tests for hearing loss, and manage noise control and hearing protection programs, as described in Chapter 8. This usually requires a short course. *Audiologists*, on the other hand, are health practitioners who possess advanced degrees. They specialize in more advanced testing for the diagnosis of hearing loss, fitting hearing aids, and protecting workers from noise exposure. *Acoustical engineers* specialize in how sound waves are generated, absorbed, and reflected and in measures to reduce noise exposure.

Injured workers may require the assistance of specialists in various rehabilitation fields in order to regain the strength, coordination, skills, and abilities they had before the injury. *Rehabilitation therapists* are professionals in restoring the ability to function after an injury. They may use exercises, electrical stimulation of nerves across the skin, deep heating, or other measures to do this. They also teach injured workers how to protect themselves from a second injury. *Occupational therapists* are specialized professionals who train injured people or help them relearn how to perform various tasks that are useful in daily life or on the job after an injury or illness has impaired their ability. (Despite the name, which refers to the mode of therapy rather than its application to work-related injuries, occupational therapists may treat any person who needs their help, not only injured workers.)

Vocational counselors are specialists in evaluating the skills that workers may have and in determining what they can do. These professionals are sometimes called in to help injured workers decide what to do next if they cannot return to their usual job. The vocational counselor will determine what is possible, what additional training they may require, and whether there is a job market for their skills.

There are many other professions that have some connection with occupational health, although they may not consider themselves to be occupational health professionals. In certain countries, such as Sweden and Finland, there is a very rich tradition in many professions of specializing in occupational health. In others, particularly in developing countries, the health-care system may not recognize a professional specialization in occupational health, or it may be difficult to earn a living from occupational health care alone.

THE EMPLOYEE HEALTH SERVICE:

Occupational Health Services at the Local Level

Occupational health services are provided at the local level through plant- or facility-based employee health services or by local practitioners in their own offices and clinics. In this and the following section, the word *service* also means the department or organization that provides care, in addition to the type of care that is being provided.

Occupational health services at the local level can be organized in many ways. What form is best in a particular situation depends on many factors:

- If the plant or facility is large and employs many workers, and especially if it is remote from other sources of health care, it is most efficient to have a small clinic, often called an infirmary, on site and staffed with a physician, at least one nurse, and technicians as required.
- If the plant or facility has special hazards, such as radiation, it may be necessary to have full- or part-time professionals who are specialized in that hazard as part of the staff.
- If the plant or facility is small or medium-sized, it may not require this level of staffing and may require only a single nurse.
- If the plant or facility is located in a large community where health care is nearby and readily available, it is often preferable for the employer to enter into contracts with local practitioners to provide the care and to limit the services at the plant itself to a nurse who can supervise care for injured workers who need more than first aid.
- If a community has many employers, none of which are very big, a single or a few occupational health practitioners usually have contracts with many employers and either see injured workers at their own office or spend some time every week or month at each location.
- If a community is small and has one big employer, that employer often hires a physician and nurse and makes arrangements with the community and, often, other employers in the area to provide help when the community needs it.

These arrangements are called *mutual assistance agreements*. For example, some big companies allow their ambulances to transport community residents when they are not in use at the plant.

- When one big employer frequently contracts with other employers to provide services at their site, the larger employer often provides occupational health services for contractors' employees. Sometimes, the larger employer also provides training for the workers and writes requirements for safe work practices into the contracts.
- In areas where health services are poor or difficult to access and workers live with their families, large employers often have complete health-care organizations, including hospitals. These serve the employees and their families. Frequently, these systems later form the basis for community health care as towns and communities grow up around the plant. Sometimes they are absorbed into social insurance systems, especially if the employer is the government or a public agency.

A large, well-designed employee health service typically employs a physician and as many nurses as are required to serve the needs of the workforce. The physician is usually, but not always, the manager of the employee health service as well as the chief provider of medical care. Usually, the center of the employee health service is a clinic, but it is sometimes an office where the nurse or physician can evaluate the injured worker to determine what care is needed and where to send him or her. The clinic or infirmary is best located where workers can walk in and can get care easily. Those workers who are not seriously injured may be able to return to work right away. Workers who come to the employee health center for routine periodic health surveillance or training will also be able to return to work quickly, reducing lost time.

Usually, such clinics have a small waiting area, treatment rooms where physicians and nurses can see the worker in privacy, and a small area with a few beds where injured workers can rest after treatment or wait for an ambulance to take them to a hospital. Medications are kept in locked cabinets, both to prevent theft and to ensure that drugs are not abused. There is usually an office and a conference room for training and where cases are discussed and reviewed. Records are kept at the clinic in an area or room that can be locked for security when the clinic is closed.

Employee assistance programs, on the other hand, are usually better placed away from the workplace or out of sight in the back of the regular health service, in locations where workers can seek help without seeing other workers. This protects confidentiality and makes them more likely to seek the help they need. (See the section on employee assistance programs in Chapter 11.)

The smooth operation of an employee health service requires constant attention. Waiting should be kept to a minimum, and the level of treatment that is provided should be limited. For example, if the injuries that a worker has experienced cannot be treated quickly or are too extensive for adequate treatment at the clinic, the physician or nurse should concentrate on evaluating the situation quickly, determining what care will be required, and arranging for the worker to be taken by car or ambulance to a nearby hospital as quickly as possible, accompanied by copies of records to help the treating physicians to know what to do. The process of quickly determining what level of care is required is called *triage*.

Most employee health services also provide medical care on a limited basis for minor illnesses or workers who have chronic diseases. For example, a worker with high blood pressure may have his or her blood pressure checked periodically by the employee health service. A worker with diabetes may have his or her blood sugar checked. Sometimes the employee health service will monitor whether a worker is taking medications that have been prescribed. A worker who has allergies or a common illness may get single treatments or basic care. The objective of providing this type of care for problems that are not related to the job is to ensure that the worker gets the care required without having to take time away from the job. However, few employee health services provide extensive medical care. They do not replace or substitute for the worker's own physician, unless they are part of a larger health service for employees and their families as described above.

In addition to treating injured workers, employee health services typically provide periodic health surveillance, worker education and training, and fitness-to-work evaluations to determine when an employee is ready to return to work. They are usually involved in formulating emergency plans for their facilities. Employee health services have to maintain extensive and accurate records and must keep these records confidential.

Employee health services usually have their own budgets and are managed locally but report to the senior management of the enterprise.

The Corporate Health Service: Occupational Health Services at the Enterprise Level

Many large employers, public and private, have occupational health departments. These are often called medical departments. They have responsibility for coordinating occupational health services throughout the organization, ensuring the quality and uniformity of care in the plants and facilities operated by the employer, advising on health-related affairs that affect the employer, and monitoring the health of workers throughout the organization. They often manage special problems through a staff of specialized professionals or hire consultants when there is a need. Corporate health services often have a close relationship with the human resources departments of their employers and advise on hiring standards, health insurance, and policies on when workers may return to work or when they are considered disabled. They manage programs to reduce injuries or occupational diseases, training programs, and programs for health promotion. They usually manage preparations for business-related travel and handle health problems among executives in the enterprise. They are expected to be well informed about health issues and to know about epidemics or health problems in parts of the world where the enterprise operates. They are responsible for ensuring that the employer complies with health-related laws and regulations and occupational health standards in each country.

Corporate health services are located at the headquarters of the employer and report to the senior managers, usually the chief executive officer (the president) or a vice president. They are usually led by a medical director, who is always a physician, or a senior manager, who may be a health professional or a senior executive with health experience. When they are operated by a senior manager, there is almost always a part-time physician available on contract to advise on medical matters. The staff usually travels a great deal, dealing with problems at every plant and facility that the enterprise operates.

Different enterprises organize their corporate health departments in different ways. In most, physicians and nurses are in one department, which may include occupational hygienists. Safety professionals may work in this department but usually are housed in a separate department or are posted to individual plants. Many employers have one department to cover occupational health, occupational safety, environmental issues, and product-related safety issues.

Corporate occupational health departments have budgets and their own policies that govern confidentiality, record keeping, procedures for investigating serious incidents or disease outbreaks wherever they occur, and communications with government representatives, media, and local health professionals. They supervise contracting with local health professionals and set standards for training and health care.

28

DELIVERING HEALTH CARE

Tee L. Guidotti

Occupational health services in industry provide health care and prevention services in order to maintain the health of all employees, not just those who were at one time injured or exposed to a hazard while on the job. The term *occupational health service* is used in two senses. When singular, the term usually refers to a facility or a department or other administrative unit charged with responsibility for occupational health as well as safety. This use of the term is analogous to a *service* in a hospital. When plural or when specified as one of several opportunities, the term usually means an activity, program, or function, in the sense of a service to be provided. Occupational health services in this sense may also be divided into two categories, ameliorative and preventive. Ameliorative services are intended to cure or limit disease or to manage existing problems. (Amelioration means to improve the situation; it is used here instead of "curative" because diseases and serious injuries often cannot be completely cured.) Preventive services seek to avoid exposure to hazards, detect disorders at an early and potentially curable stage, and limit disability. Both types are provided in industry, but the emphasis is usually on prevention. Employers are increasingly outsourcing curative-oriented treatment or rehabilitation to off-site health-care providers.

Occupational health services in industry can be divided into *in-plant* and *off-site* facilities and services. A plant physician or occupational health nurse oversees in-plant services. On the corporate level, a corporate medical director may oversee the in-plant services or coordinate and supervise the delivery of care by off-site contract physicians, or a combination of both.

Although clinical aspects of occupational health care are similar to a general medical practice, preventive services, administration, and communications are more obviously part of the day-to-day practice in occupational medicine. A real opportunity exists to prevent injury and disease and to promote good health through preventive action. The physician, nurse, or other healthcare provider never acts alone in an occupationally related case. Each action is reviewed and discussed behind the scenes and often generates multiple decisions and communications in the form of telephone authorizations, claims, chart reviews, and requests for clarification. Thus, an essential aspect of occupational health care is communication. Maintaining confidentiality requires great care and attention because some parties to the case are entitled to full information and others may not be. (See Box 26.1.)

CORPORATE OCCUPATIONAL HEALTH SERVICES

Occupational health services do not exist as an end in themselves but as a means to an end. They are created to prevent an unnecessary interference with the primary mission of the organization, whether that mission is to create wealth, provide a needed service, or protect the interests of a community of people. Organizations as disparate as small businesses, corporations, government agencies, and the military have similar needs for effective occupational health services. Occupational health care is a process, not an outcome, and the success and quality of a service providing such care is measured by the absence of problems rather than by a specific end point. It therefore follows that a commitment to sound occupational health practices must be ongoing and not limited to a specific problem-solving exercise, such as narrowly focusing on a particular hazard, employee assistance program, drug testing, or health promotion. The decision makers within an organization must accept this fundamental principle before a commitment to provide occupational health services begins to make sense and the value of such services becomes apparent.

A successful occupational health service is appropriate to the needs of the organization it serves, efficiently managed, ethical, and respectful in treatment of the worker. The offerings of the health services marketplace are limitless but may be inflexible and ill-suited to a particular workplace or workforce. A successful service is rarely found "off the shelf." Obtaining the right system to meet the needs of the employer requires careful analysis and good planning. The variety of "packaged" occupational health programs for sale in the marketplace does not obviate the need for planning and evaluation because many of these package deals may be of little or no value to the employer and may not provide a service of acceptable quality for the worker. They may be poorly conceived, badly implemented, inflexible, or unsuitable to the employer's particular situation. Lacking a plan and carefully considered expectations, an employer can easily fall into the trap of paying for a system or program that fails to meet the real need.

Providing occupational health services to a corporate employer requires an understanding of how such organizations work. All large organizations have a common basic structure. The line of authority extends from the top leader to the employee at the lowest level. All management decisions and orders relating to the goods or services that are the business of the organization are conveyed along this line. The staff line, perpendicular to the line of authority, supports it by providing necessary services such as financial, legal, human resources, and occupational health and safety. Thus, occupational health and safety supervision is intrinsically a staff rather than a line management function, but its practice during production must necessarily be on the line of *responsibility* if safe work practices are to be followed consistently. The occupational health safety staff cannot be in all places at all times and cannot know the workplace as well as the workers who are regularly assigned there. If staff, in an advisory capacity, bears the primary corporate responsibility for occupational safety and health, the line managers may not be as responsive or interested. Individual managers and supervisors must be individually responsible for the safety performance or injury experience in their areas and should be individually evaluated for performance just as they are on productivity.

Large employers, by definition, have more than 1,000 employees and usually need a full-time, in-house corporate medical department. Sometimes this corporate service acts primarily to coordinate a network of individual healthcare providers at scattered workplaces, either plant physicians or community physicians receiving employees at their own facilities. The department should have a close working relationship with the safety and occupational hygiene functions.

In a company this size, the occupational health service will often be part of the human resources department, although this is not ideal. A direct reporting relationship at the highest possible level is much better. Employees often mistrust health services that are too closely tied to personnel departments, fearing that confidential information may be shared. A soundly run occupational health service can reduce absence due to incapacity, but involving it in personnel issues such as absence monitoring and disciplinary action destroys the delicate balance. Under these circumstances, the occupational health service becomes an extension of the personnel manager. When workers view the occupational health service as the means by which management reviews their attendance and singles them out for discipline, cooperation and goodwill promptly evaporate and are seldom, if ever, regained. The physician in such a position becomes labeled as just another management functionary, and medical judgments from the occupational health service are viewed as untrustworthy and prejudicial to the worker. Having taken the occupational health service this far down the road, insensitive managers may press even further for the physician to become a "team player" siding with management inappropriately or request violations of confidentiality.

Safety and hygiene staff usually report to an operating manager, who often has other responsibilities for risk and loss control. Once a company has grown to approximately 3,000 employees, a single administrative grouping of health, safety, and hygiene should usually be formed under a senior manager, preferably the medical director, if the medical director has management skills for the responsibility. (A common arrangement is for companies to have a manager for "HSE" – health, safety, and environment – which these days often includes monitoring compliance with environmental regulations and achieving sustainability.)

All organizations benefit from an explicit occupational health and safety policy to specify their responsibilities to their employees and their employees' responsibility for safe work practices. A model occupational and environmental health policy, one that could apply to any company large enough to have a corporate medical department, will confirm the company's commitment to protect the health and safety of its employees and to persons living or working near company operations and assign responsibility for the actions and decisions required to maintain this commitment.

Each employer has its own pattern of labor/management relationships, unionized or not. Sometimes there is a mixture of both, as when a union represents some workers, but others in another division or job are not organized. The responsibility for protecting worker health rests squarely with management, as an ethical imperative. (See Box 26.1.) In the non-unionized setting, management must fulfill this obligation with no less diligence than when it has a union looking over its shoulder. Effective policies and procedures to protect employee well-being should be in place regardless. These should be based on the moral commitment that protecting employee well-being is a fundamental principle of doing business.

COMMUNITY-BASED SERVICES

Increasingly in developed countries, occupational health services are being delivered in the community by physicians, small medical groups, and clinics that serve several employers and that are available for individual workers who seek care. The business model varies greatly around the world. In Kuwait, for example, the Shuaiba Occupational Medical Centre is a full-service occupational health center providing medical services, laboratory, occupational hygiene, and consultation in one location supported by the Ministry of Health. In the United States and Canada, many occupational health services are private clinics and provide only limited service, such as medical care without occupational hygiene. In France, many occupational health services provide mandatory surveillance and screening but do not provide medical treatment.

Hospitals and large clinics often sponsor occupational health services. They may be part of government-supported occupational health care in some areas, such as Québec, or private, as is common in the United States.

Most occupational health care is probably still provided through the general medical care system, such as medical offices and hospital emergency departments. It is common for primary care physicians to treat occupational injuries without involving occupational physicians or nurses, and in many countries these specialized health professionals are simply not available in the community. The World Health Organization and the International Labour Organization encourage the provision of occupational health care through the primary care health system in developing countries and have defined a set of "Basic Occupational Health Services" that represents essential services for workers and employers in all countries.

OCCUPATIONAL HEALTH PROFESSIONALS

An *occupational physician* is a medical doctor practicing occupational medicine predominantly or exclusively. *Occupational medicine specialists* are trained in the specialty and may or may not hold the usual certification for specialists that is customary in the country where they live and practice. Most physicians entering the field do so in mid-career rather than at the beginning of their career. Some physicians are *corporate medical directors* and have responsibilities for health issues

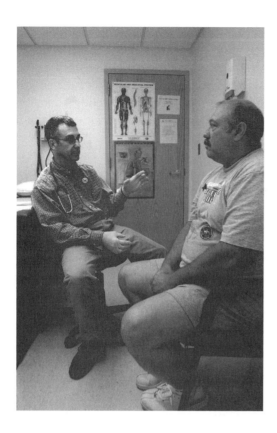

Figure 28.1 An occupational physician with a community-based practice discusses a health issue with a worker in a clinic in West Virginia (USA). (Photograph by © Earl Dotter, all rights reserved.)

in their companies. Others are *plant physicians* who take care of workers in one facility or complex. Many are in practice in the community. Some work for government or in medical training centers.

An *occupational health nurse* is a nurse specializing in occupational health services. The occupational health nurse usually works in an in-plant setting. There are national certification systems in many countries, emphasizing skills in health education, occupational health and disease recognition, rehabilitation, and administration. The specialty is highly attractive within the nursing profession for its relative autonomy and level of responsibility.

An *occupational hygienist* is a technical expert, often an engineer, specializing in the recognition, evaluation, and control of occupational health hazards. Training in occupational hygiene includes extensive study in ventilation, analytical chemistry, mathematics, and toxicology. The profession is in high demand in industry as consultants. In the United States they are called industrial hygienists.

A *safety engineer* is a professional with training in the recognition and control of safety hazards. Safety education is usually not at the graduate level; many safety professionals have obtained their training in short-term, intensive institutes or seminars.

An *audiologist* is engaged in the evaluation of hearing disorders and performs audiometric evaluations on workers exposed to noise.

Other occupational health professionals include toxicologists, epidemiologists, acoustical engineers, ergonomists, analytical laboratory technicians, health physicists (radiation hazard control experts), and many others. These occupational health professionals often work as consultants to many industries on a project-by-project or an as-needed basis.

STAFFING

Some large companies have staffing formulae for assigning personnel to their occupational health service, and staffing formulae are written into law or regulation in some countries. For industries without particular physical or chemical hazards, there are rough guidelines that may be followed. A safety officer is generally sufficient for a site with less than 200 employees; an occupational health nurse is usually placed on site for more than 300 employees and for every additional 750 employees; an occupational hygienist becomes justified as a permanent position at approximately 500 employees; and a plant physician on at least a part-time basis becomes cost-effective at approximately 1,000 employees and on a full-time basis for more than 2,000. These guidelines have little empirical basis other than general acceptance in industry but have remained relatively unchanged for many years. Companies with unusual workplace hazards or risk, or in locations far from medical care, may need to modify these general guidelines.

FACILITIES AND EQUIPMENT

The siting and design of the clinical facility itself should be undertaken with care and preferably designed after close examination of a successful model. The floor plan should allow good traffic flow for both emergency and routine cases. It is impossible to describe a design that meets the needs of all organizations, however. Advice from consultants in both architecture and occupational health and visits to other facilities are always good ideas before committing to construction and equipment purchase.

Medications to be stocked are the minimum needed for the symptomatic relief of common occupational disorders or personal illnesses affecting employees on the job. Because of the liability, security, and logistical problems associated with handling narcotics and other restricted medication, these should be avoided unless the worksite is remote from accessible health care and the risk of injury is high.

Although occupational physicians cannot substitute for family physicians in providing comprehensive care, it is not unreasonable to be able to treat common complaints in order to prevent unnecessary time off work. It is usually not cost-effective for occupational health clinics to maintain clinical laboratory apparatus beyond a bench centrifuge, microscope, and simple office testing supplies unless the clinic is located in a remote area and must function as a self-contained infirmary. When the volume of tests is relatively low, the overhead cost to provide a complete testing capacity on site can be quite high, the cost of quality assurance may become disproportionate to the expense of operations, and such capacity is often unnecessary. It is usually not cost-effective to acquire X-ray equipment unless the industry is one at high risk for serious injuries and the site is a large one. Maintaining quality assurance for laboratory and radiological services can be a serious problem when the volume of cases is low, and costs can be driven up by unwarranted utilization in an effort to justify use of the equipment. Usually, a local clinic or hospital can provide such services as needed at a much lower total cost, even if fees are high for individual tests, and provides some guarantee of quality assurance and without an incentive to over-order tests. An occupational health service should be able to provide a realistic cost/benefit analysis for the organization of which it is a part or which uses it for health-care services.

RECORD KEEPING

An occupational health service must maintain at least two types of records, personal health records and exposure records. Medical records contain confidential information and should never be accessible to unauthorized personnel, including management. Exposure records are the results of environmental monitoring or group data on personal exposure; they are not necessarily confidential unless they identify individuals. These records:

• document significant exposures sustained by the worker
• match the worker's health and fitness to job placement requirements
• document the worker's health on entry for fitness-to-work determinations
• summarize the results of periodic health surveillance
• comply with regulatory requirements

Some countries, such as the United States, require that medical records and exposure records be kept for *all* workers, even those exposed to little or no toxic substances in the usual work environment, for long periods of time (30 years in the U.S.). Workers have access to their own exposure and medical records, with copies to be provided free of charge. Both records are normally the property of the employer or whoever caused the record to be created in the first place. However, workers must consent to the release of any information that could identify them as individuals, even to their own union. Anonymous data (with all identifiers deleted) and group exposure data may be shared, but not personal medical records, which cannot be individually reviewed by any party other than the worker or an authorized health professional. Management representatives are not entitled to view the record, even if identifiers are removed. Only the worker can authorize release of health information from the medical record and sharing of the information with other parties. An exception to this general rule is when records are subpoenaed for litigation or become part of a disputed workers' compensation claim or are requested under the legal authority of a regulatory agency. These legal requirements vary from country to country, and local regulations should be reviewed and followed closely.

Certain exemptions to the record access regulation have been made. Medical research is usually permitted, but individual identification of workers is not allowed without explicit permission. Employee assistance records are considered separate from the medical record if they are maintained in a different file; they should always remain confidential unless there is a legally enforceable order or command to produce them. Also, employees who leave the employer after less than one year of employment without a claim for compensation may be given their medical record to take with them, and then copies do not have to be retained and stored by the employer.

Employers are responsible for ensuring that the procedures are followed and for requiring health-care providers outside their organization to follow these same regulations. In the present climate of increasing litigation, it is wise to be prudent and to obtain indisputable authorization for all transfers of confidential information.

CLINICAL MANAGEMENT

Acute care refers to the provision of care for both occupational disorders and non-occupational disorders occurring in the workplace. Acute care of the injured worker is the most basic form of occupational medical care and usually involves the treatment of injuries.

In occupational medicine, the diagnosis is often the beginning rather than the end of the evaluative process. This is particularly true for occupational illnesses due to workplace exposures and for repetitive motion injuries. The related but distinct questions of the responsible exposure, the work-relatedness of the condition, and the expected degree of disability are sometimes more important than a precise diagnosis, because the answers to such questions determine eligibility for compensation, prognosis for rehabilitation, fitness for future work, and prevention actions to be taken for the protection of other workers.

Workers' compensation is a compulsory, no-fault form of insurance for workers injured in the course of employment. In a workers' compensation system, workers surrender their right to take legal action against their employer for negligent acts, but they are compensated for injuries or illness sustained at work regardless of fault. Employers pay the insurance and compensation costs on a pooled basis, with premiums calculated on the industry experience and past claims against the employer.

In many jurisdictions, the employer is also required by law to report any work-related injury that results in a worker or workers losing time from the job (one to three days) and all fatalities. For example, the U.S. Occupational Safety and Health Administration (OSHA) has uniform requirements for all employers to report injuries and to keep first aid logs, called "OSHA 300 Logs." These are sometimes misleading because employers often misclassify injuries or bring injured workers back to work on paper in order to make their performance look better. Physicians are also required to report occupational injuries and illnesses.

Prompt and effective treatment of the injured worker can save that individual from unnecessary permanent disability. An early return to work, when medically indicated, can also assist in rehabilitation. However, acute care in an occupational health-care setting is more than a simple service function as it might be in a hospital emergency room. Opportunities exist within a well-organized occupational health-care system to use the lessons learned from each injury, either singly or as aggregate statistical data, to prevent future injuries. The ultimate goal of an occupational health intervention, obviously, is to control the hazard that led to the problem in the first place.

Conventional medical practice emphasizes the identification, evaluation, and treatment of a disorder. Correcting the underlying problem causing the disorder is of equal importance in situations where a hazard persists and may affect others. In occupational medicine, the physician must often be concerned that seeing a worker with an occupational disorder means that a health hazard continues to exist. However, in most cases of cancer or other chronic diseases with long latency periods, the exposure that caused the illness is often long gone. Without special training or expertise in occupational health, the physician is not technically qualified to recommend or advise on specific corrective measures and therefore should concentrate on clearly stating the problems. However, the physician can serve as a valuable member of a team that includes industrial hygienists and engineers devoted to problem solving.

In such cases, consultants are brought in under contract. The medical director may provide a valuable service monitoring the activities of consultants and ensuring that they stay on track.

EVALUATION OF PROGRAMS AND PROJECTS

There is a growing movement in industry to have occupational health services externally reviewed and formally accredited. *Accreditation* means approval and certification as adequate by an outside organization after review of facilities, policies, and procedures.

Effective evaluation depends on good record keeping and the cooperation of all concerned. The following are some practical measures that facilitate effective evaluation.

- The need for a given program should be clearly documented before a program is begun. Baseline data is essential, as is the selection of the appropriate measurements to be employed.
- The record-keeping system should be systematic and easy to use. All pertinent data should be recorded in an easily retrievable format, whenever possible on computer or at least in a standardized form, and kept in a central location. The amount of data collected that does not directly relate to the program should be kept to a minimum to facilitate handling.
- Someone other than the project staff should formulate the criteria to be used for evaluation well before the evaluation is conducted.
- Subjective response in matters such as user satisfaction should be considered very carefully. Often expressions of dissatisfaction or lack of understanding signal grave problems that lie below the surface and are not being expressed clearly or because of some other concern.

Evaluation allows the physician or nurse-manager to pinpoint problems and to act to correct them. It allows the service to adapt by adding equipment, staff, or space or by cutting back in some areas for more efficient operation. It permits the physician and occupational health nurse to plan for continuing education of the staff based on the needs of the practice or weaknesses in their own preparation. It helps reduce liability by highlighting problem areas that require better control, safer procedures, referral, or further training on the part of the provider.

Occupational health care serves the interests of both the worker and the employer, but only if a high quality of service is provided to both. Monitoring the quality of care and periodically evaluating the effectiveness of the service helps to ensure this.

29

ECONOMIC BURDEN

Liang Youxin

In spite of substantial advances in occupational health and safety, working conditions for the majority of people do not meet the minimum standards and guidelines set by the International Labour Organization (ILO) and the World Health Organization (WHO) for occupational safety, health, and social protection. Only 5% to 10% of workers in developing countries and 20% to 50% of workers in industrialized countries (with a few exceptions) are estimated to have access to adequate occupational health services. Even in advanced economies (for example, in the United States), 40% of a workforce of approximately 130 million people do not have such access, and a large proportion of work sites do not regularly inspect for occupational health and safety problems.

According to ILO and WHO, poor occupational safety and health lead worldwide to 250 million accidents, 335,000 fatalities, and 60 to 150 million occupational diseases, which together result in 1.2 million work-related deaths a year. Adverse and substandard conditions of work constitute an enormous and unnecessary health loss, great suffering, and economic loss amounting to 4% to 5% of GDP of countries.

In 1992, in the countries of the European Union, the direct cost paid out in compensation for work-related diseases and injuries reached €27, 000 million. (WHO 1999) In 1994, the overall cost of all work accidents and work-related ill health to the British economy was estimated between £6,000 and £12,000 million. According to the U.S. National Institute of Occupational Safety and Health (NIOSH 2000), each day an average of 9,000 American workers sustain disabling injuries on the job, 17 workers die from an injury sustained at work, and 137 workers die from work-related diseases. The economic burden of this continuing toll is high. Data from one NIOSH-funded study revealed a loss of US$171 billion annually in direct and indirect costs of occupational injuries and illnesses ($145 billion for injuries and $26 billion for diseases). These costs compare to $33 billion for AIDS, $67.3 billion for Alzheimer's disease, $164.3 billion for circulatory diseases, and $170.7 billion for cancer.

The health status of the workforce in every country has an immediate and direct impact on national and world economies. Total economic losses due to occupational illness and injuries are enormous, although today's picture is almost certainly underestimated. WHO estimates that in Latin America, for example, only between 1% and 4% of all occupational diseases are reported; in other words, the great majority are not reported at all. Even in industrialized countries, reporting systems are sometimes fragmented (Lehtinen 2000). As a result, the burden of disease due to occupational exposures is normally underestimated. Nevertheless, such losses are a serious burden on economic development, which should be a matter of special concern. Thus, apart from health considerations, the improvement of working conditions is a sound economic investment.

WORKER PRODUCTIVITY

Health at work has an influence on economic factors at all levels of economy, both direct and indirect. For example, work-related ill health results in lost productive time, financial compensation, and medical care costs, whereas healthy workers contribute to better productivity and quality. However, the implications for the stakeholders (workers, employers, policy makers, governments, and collective resources) are not fully understood.

The costs attributed to employee health problems are usually measured in terms of direct health-care costs, such as medical care, insurance, disability compensation, and pension claims. As important but seldom measured is the decrease in productivity for much larger group of employees whose health problems have not necessarily led to absenteeism and the decrease in productivity for the disabled group before and after sick leave. For example, an employee suffering from low back pain may be limited in the weight he or she can lift or in the postures that he or she can be expected to maintain. An employee with carpal tunnel syndrome may be limited in the amount of keyboard work that can be performed. To better estimate the role of health risk factors and diseases on economic losses, Burton and colleagues (1999) recommended using the following three measurements as an indicator of indirect health costs; the time lost to employee absenteeism, the time lost to disability, and the actual decrease in the productivity of employees while they are on the job. These measurements can be combined to produce a Worker Productivity Index (WPI) (Burton et al. 1999).

The Worker Productivity Index

The WPI is composed of two major measures of lost productivity—time away from the job due to illness and time lost due to a failure to maintain the productivity standard (Burton et al. 1999). The measure of time lost away from work included the time lost because of scattered illnesses and short-term disability absences. This is generally called *absenteeism*, although some authors prefer the term *absence*. The second measure was an estimate of the time lost because of lowered productivity while the employee was on the job—a measure of so-called *presenteeism*.

The absenteeism component was compiled as the ratio of total illness hours plus total short-term disability (STD) hours to the number of weeks employed during the study period (A):

- Lost hours per week due to absenteeism (A) = Total illness hours + total STD hours/weeks employed
- Lost hours per week due to failure to meet productivity standard (B) = [100% − (overall score [if < 0.5])/(0.5)] × Average weekly staffing hours
- Total lost hours per week (C) = Lost hours per week due to absenteeism + Lost hours per week due to failure to meet productivity standard

The presenteeism ratio again made use of the overall productivity standard. If the employee's overall score was greater than or equal to 0.5, he or she was rated as meeting the standard (as above) and considered to have lost 0 hours per week. Scores of less than 0.5 were evaluated as a proportion of 0.5 and subtracted from 100%. For example, an overall score of 0.4 produced a ratio of 20% (1 − [0.4/0.5] × 100% = 20%). This percentage was then multiplied by the employee's average weekly staffing time as an estimate of the hours per week that the employee was not attaining the productivity standard (B). The total amount of time lost in an average week was determined by adding the absenteeism and the presenteeism ratios (C). The WPI serves as an indicator of the total amount of time per full-time workweek (40 hours) that an employee is effectively productive. To compute the WPI, the total lost hours per week were divided by the scheduled hours worked and subtracted from 100%. For example, a full-time employee who averaged 8 lost hours per week would be given a WPI of 80% (100% − [8/40, %] = 80%).

Health Risks and The Compliance Rate of Productivity Standard The WPIs of 564 telephone customer service agents were correlated with the employees' number and types of health risks, measured by a health risk appraisal (HRA) questionnaire. Health risks that were significantly related to a failure to attain the productivity standard included general distress ($p \leq 0.01$), diabetes ($p \leq 0.05$), and BMI (body mass index) ($p \leq 0.05$). As the overall number of health risks increased, the likelihood of meeting the productivity standard decreased, although this did not reach statistical significance (Table 29.1).

Health Risks and Work Time Lost The results also show the relationship between health risks and the amount and type of work time lost. Those employees who identified themselves as diabetic showed significantly more hours lost to illness absence ($p \leq 0.05$), to STD absence ($p \leq 0.001$), and to failure to meet the productivity standard ($p \leq 0.01$). Those with high general distress scores showed significantly more illness hours ($p \leq 0.05$) and lost hours due to failure to meet the productivity standard ($p \leq 0.05$). Employees with at-risk BMI scores also showed significantly more illness hours ($p \leq 0.05$) and lost hours due to failure to meet the productivity standard ($p \leq 0.05$). Again, the health risk status, such as the type and number of health risks, is closely associated with the work time lost. In particular, workers with two health risks showed significantly more illness hours

TABLE 29.1

RELATIONSHIP BETWEEN HEALTH RISKS AND PRODUCTIVITY STANDARD

Risk parameter	Total # employees		Met productivity standard		Did not meet productivity standard		P valueb
	n	%	n	%	n	%	
Total with HRA	564	100	386	68.40	178	31.60	
Selected health risks							
Lifestyle							
Current smokers	108	19.1	77	19.9	31	17.4	0.477
Physical activities (<1/week)	104	18.4	75	19.4	29	16.3	0.372
Seatbelt usage(<90%)	104	18.4	79	20.5	25	14.0	0.068
Encountered violent event	22	3.9	14	3.6	8	4.5	0.631
Perception							
Distress	179	31.7	109	28.2	70	39.3	0.009**
Biological risks							
Diabetes	15	2.7	6	1.6	9	5.1	0.016*
High blood pressure	48	8.5	32	8.3	16	9.0	0.782
Cholesterol	26	4.6	16	4.1	10	5.6	0.438
BMI at risk§	168	29.8	104	26.9	64	36.0	0.03*
Number of risks							
Low (0 to 1 risk)	340	60.3	241	62.4	99	55.6	
Medium (2 risks)	137	24.3	91	23.6	46	25.8	0.339
High (3+ risks)	87	15.4	54	14.0	33	18.5	0.113

§BMI: Body mass index; * $p < 0.05$, **$P < 0.01$

(p ≤ 0.05 and p ≤ 0.01, respectively), and those with three or more health risks showed significantly more time lost due to STD absence (p ≤ 0.05). The WPI ratings reinforce the valid use of the productivity variable in reflecting the profound effects associated with various health-risk categories (see Table 29.2).

Lost Productivity and Disease States The WPI ratings for the disease states are noteworthy for their generally low levels, compared with the WPI ratings for the health risks. It is logical to assume that the presence of a manifested disease state should produce greater productivity loss than the presence of health risk. Those with digestive disorders and mental health STD episodes showed the lowest WPI ratings (62% and 67%, respectively). With regard to the total lost time, employees with STD episodes from digestive disorders and mental disorders showed the greatest overall loss of productivity. Employees with digestive disorders showed significantly greater time lost due to a failure to attain the productivity standard (Table 29.3).

TABLE 29.2

WORKER PRODUCTIVITY INDEX (WPI) FOR HEALTH RISK (HOURS/WEEK)

Risk parameter	Total time lost (mean)	WPI (%)
Total with HRA	4.431	89
Selected health risks		
Lifestyle		
Current smokers	4.147	90
Physical activities (< 1/week)	3.238	92
Seatbelt usage (< 90%)	3.443	91
Encountered violent event	5.772	86
Perception		
Distress	5.396	87
Biological risks		
Diabetes	11.364	72
High blood pressure	5.068	87
Cholesterol	6.128	85
BMI at risk	5.790	86
Number of risks		
0 to 1 risk factor	4.059	90
2 risk factors	4.635	88
3+ risk factors	5.565	86

TABLE 29.3

WORKER PRODUCTIVITY INDEX FOR SELECTED DISEASE STATES (HOURS/WEEK)

STD disease state	Total time lost (mean)	WPI (%)
Mental Health	13.189	67
Respiratory	9.246	77
Injury	8.433	79
Digestive	15.964	60
Musculoskeletal	8.242	79
Cancer	6.582	84
Other	7.488	81

The Rationale of the Study

In overall health risk status, as the number of health risks increased for an employee, the overall productivity decreased. In particular, workers with two health risks and those with three or more health risks showed significantly more illness hours, and those with three or more health risks showed significantly more time lost due to STD absence. The WPI ratings for the various health-risk categories reinforce the profound effect of diabetes on worker productivity. These employees had the lowest WPI rating (72%) (Table 29.2).

This study has demonstrated not only that health risks and diseases are associated with decreased productivity, but also that different disease states affect the WPI in different patterns. Data of this sort are essential in designing corporate responses to health management costs. Wellness programs need to be targeted toward health risks that are specific to a given workforce and must be evaluated in light of the specific cost pattern the risks produce. This sort of study also points to the primary role that occupational health intervention and consultation can play in increasing the productivity of a workforce.

BOX 29.1

Economic Burden of Silicosis: A Case Study in China

China is the world's most populous country, at approximately 1.3 billion people. The working population exposed to silica-containing dusts may be as large as 12 million. Silicosis has long been the most serious and prevalent occupational lung disease in this country, consisting of 72.5% of the total reported 10,228 cases of occupational diseases in 1997. These represent 7,418 new cases of pneumoconiosis (72.5%), 598 cases of acute poisoning (12.8%), 1,313 cases of chronic poisoning (12.8%), and 899 others (8.8%). According to the statistics, the cumulative number of pneumoconiosis cases recorded in China between 1949 and 1996 reached 524,759. The majority of the pneumoconiosis occurred in mining industries, particularly coal mining, resulting in anthracosilicosis, which accounted for about 40% of the disease incidence. Of those affected, 134,674 (25.7%) had died, and 390,089 (74.3%) were alive [as of 1996]. Moreover, a nationwide survey conducted in 1986 found that an even greater number—around 600,000 workers—exposed to dust were classified with suspected cases of silicosis. (Liang 1998, Zhou 1997)

Silicosis is known as a progressive and irreversible fibrogenic lung disease that results in not only human suffering but also crushing socioeconomic burdens. The examples provided below illustrate the economic liability of silicosis in terms of medical costs, production loss, and pension/compensation for premature retirement and death and show the benefit from investment in preventive measures.

Data from the selected examples were collected from the official report, Nationwide Epidemiological Survey on Pneumoconiosis and Silicosis, published by the Chinese Ministry of Health (1986) and from articles published in Chinese medical periodicals from the mid-1980s. The national data, obtained from dozens of factories and mining facilities, were calculated to estimate the economic loss associated with silicosis in terms of direct and indirect costs. The data that appeared in the journals provided a more complete picture and facilitated a rough estimation of economic burden from disease and the expected benefit from the investment for dust control and silicosis prevention in machinery manufacturing in Shanghai.

Estimates based on the National Survey provide strong evidence to show that silicosis is one of the costliest occupational diseases. The national survey from dozens of enterprises (1986 and 1996) revealed that the average economic losses, in terms of direct and indirect costs, were 2,869 and 12,896 yuan/person/year, respectively (Table 29.4).

It was estimated that there were 310,000 cases of silicosis in China in 1986. Based on the above estimates, the total yearly economic losses would have reached 5 billion yuan RMB after 1986. However, it should be noted that according to the market value replacement, the value of 1 yuan RMB in the late 1990s was valued at about one-fifth of that in the mid-1980s. Therefore, the annual economic losses associated with silicosis will increase from 5 billion to 25 billion RMB. This stunning figure represents 0.4% of China's total national product (around 6,000 billion yuan RMB or US$750 billion in 1999).

TABLE 29.4

ESTIMATED ECONOMIC LOSSES OF SILICOSIS FROM DIRECT AND INDIRECT COSTS (YUAN/PERSON) IN 1986

Data Source	Direct Costs	Indirect Costs	Funeral Expenses
20 plants, Shanghai	2,623	30,732	1,627
10 provinces or cities, other parts of China	3,030	8,925	5,133
13 coal mines, other parts of China	2,620	6,892	5,195
4 nonferrous metal mines, other parts of China	3,202	5,035	—
Average	2,869	12,896	3,985

BOX 29.2

A Study in Shanghai

In 1992, an important study was conducted among 2,164 foundry workers who had been exposed to dust for over one year in a machinery factory in Shanghai. The number of existing cases of silicosis in the factory between 1988 and 1992 were 80 to 84, for a prevalence rate of about 3789/100,000, which is very high. To maintain that high a prevalence implies a very high incidence rate of new cases, to make up for patients that die or are forced to leave the workplace every year.

Direct economic losses resulted from medical costs, work leave losses, and the management expenses for existing patients during the period between 1988 and 1992. The average direct economic losses for existing patients of pneumoconiosis between 1988 and 1992 were estimated at 3,736 yuan/person/year (Table 29.5).

In addition, the fatalities of pneumoconiosis during that period were another source of direct economic losses, which included death compensation and funeral expenses. It was estimated that the average cost per death was 3,285 yuan RMB (Table 29.6).

TABLE 29.5

DIRECT ECONOMIC LOSSES OF EXISTING PATIENTS DURING 1988–1992

Year	# of Cases	Medical Costs (in 10,000 yuan)	Work Leave Losses (in 10,000 yuan)	Management Expenses (in 10,000 yuan)	Subtotal (in 10,000 yuan)	Yuan Person/Year
1988	80	7.84	5.44	0.77	14.06	1,756
1989	83	15.43	6.52	0.93	22.88	2,757
1990	82	21.22	6.72	1.12	29.06	3,544
1991	85	30.73	7.80	1.33	39.86	4,689
1992	84	37.56	9.19	2.06	48.81	5,811
Total	414	112.78	35.67	6.21	154.66	3,736

TABLE 29.6

DIRECT COSTS OF FATALITIES FROM PNEUMOCONIOSIS (YUAN) (1988–1992)

Year	# of Deaths	Death Compensation	Difference of Funeral Expenses*	Total	Yuan/ Death
1988	0	0	0	0	0
1989	1	1,812	97	1,909	1,909
1990	4	8,717	2,491	11,208	2,808
1991	6	15,460	5,153	20,613	3,436
1992	1	8,971	1,715	5,686	5,686
Total	12	29,960	9,456	39,416	3,285

* Note: According to a governmental regulation, funeral expenses for a fatal case of silicosis would include an extra subsidy of one month's regular salary.

The indirect economic losses included the production and profits/tax losses due to work leave. According to the registry, approximately 50% of the workers suffering from pneumoconiosis in the factory had to quit their work, which caused a tremendous decrease of production and profits/tax for the industry (Table 29.7). Moreover, the remaining 50% of the workers with early or middle stage took approximately 105 absentee days yearly, which resulted in one third of the production and profits/tax losses.

The results indicated that the indirect economic losses resulting from a reduction of productivity, industry profit, and state tax of a patient with advanced disease would have reached up to 19,800 + 4,609 = 24,499 yuan RMB/person/year. For patients at early or middle disease stages who were still employed, the indirect losses would be roughly one-third (i.e., 8,166 yuan/person). Therefore, on average, the indirect economic losses resulting from a worker suffering from silicosis will be (24,499 + 8,166 yuan/person)/2 = 16,288 yuan/person/year.

TABLE 29.7

INDIRECT ECONOMIC LOSSES DUE TO WORK LEAVE ASSOCIATED WITH
PNEUMOCONIOSIS (1988–1892)

Year	# Leaving Work	Production Loss (in 10,000 yuan)		Profits/Tax Losses (in 10,000 yuan)	
		Total	Per person	Total	Per person
1988	38	62.91	1.66	20.12	5,295
1989	37	68.50	1.85	18.88	5,103
1990	35	68.61	1.96	16.86	6,003
1991	34	71.44	2.10	16.74	4,897
1992	25	63.24	2.53	5.42	2,168
Total	169	334.70	1.98	77.90	4,609

The yearly total economic losses from silicosis will be the sum of direct costs and indirect costs resulting from the existing cases of silicosis in addition to the death compensation and funeral expenses for patients who died in the fiscal year.

The total yearly economic losses associated with silicosis will be the number of existing cases in the year × (direct + indirect costs) + number of deaths in the year × (death compensation + funeral expenses).

According to the statistics, there were 390,089 silicosis patients who survived. The annual death rate from silicosis was about 1.2%, implying that yearly deaths from silicosis may total 5,000. Therefore, based on the Shanghai survey, the total annual economic losses to China as a result of silicosis reached 7.83 billion yuan (US$978 million) during 1988 to 1992. This figure accounted for 0.4% of the total national production in 1992 (2,022.3 billion yuan in 1992), as calculated from the following equation:

390,089 × (3,736 yuan + 16,288 yuan) + 5,000 × 3,285 yuan = 7.83 billion yuan/year.

Benefits of Prevention

So what benefits might be expected from a strategy of prevention? The working conditions in the foundry workshops of machinery factories were quite poor in the 1960s, with an average air concentration of silica-containing dust of 130.1 mg/m^3, 65 times more than the maximum allowable concentration (MAC)—2 mg/m^3—adopted in China. After dust control measures were taken, the dust concentration at workplaces dropped from 130.1 mg/m^3 in 1963 to 3.9 mg/m^3 in 1992. Therefore, 2,164 foundry workers would have been exposed to much higher dust levels, resulting in 664 expected cases of silicosis if the control measures had not been implemented in 1963. In fact, the total number of observed cases of silicosis was only 108, implying that 556 workers had avoided contracting the disease due to the reduction of dust exposure (Table 29.8).

TABLE 29.8

THE DIFFERENCE BETWEEN EXPECTED AND OBSERVED CASES OF SILICOSIS IN
MACHINERY MANUFACTURING IN SHANGHAI (1988–1992)

Dust Exposure (mg/year)	# Workers	Adjusted Cumulative Prevalence (%)	# Expected Cases	# Observed Cases	Difference Expected/ Observed Cases
0	28	0.83	0	4	−4
200	138	1.59	2	15	−13
400	73	2.89	2	18	−26
600	157	4.94	8	17	−9
800	60	8.05	5	16	−11
1,000	108	12.45	13	7	6
1,200	92	18.28	17	9	8
1,400	172	25.58	44	6	38
1,600	113	34.17	39	3	36
≥ 1,800	1,223	43.67	534	3	531
Total	2,164		664	108	556

Thus, the economic benefit from the reduction in silicosis cases can be calculated as follows:

- Benefit from avoiding direct loss (medical costs only): $556 \times 3,736$ yuan = 2.08 million.
- Cumulative savings after dust control were calculated to be 8,896 yuan/person/year.
- Benefits from avoiding indirect loss (profits/tax): 8,896 yuan/person/year $\times$ 16,288 = 145 million.
- Total benefits from the intervention: 2.08 million + 145 million = 147 million yuan.

Costs of the Preventive Measures Taken

The cumulative costs invested in prevention were 10,187 million yuan during the period between 1963 and 1992. The investment in preventive measures was positive as seen from the cost-benefit analysis (Table 29.9). The ratio of benefit to the cost reached up to 145 million yuan/10.19 million = 14.2 Y.

Conclusions

The preliminary conclusions drawn from both the nationwide and Shanghai surveys have been similar. It is remarkable that the estimated economic losses to China associated with silicosis alone accounted for 0.4% to 0.5% of the GNP. Therefore, this anthropogenic disease has brought not only human suffering but

TABLE 29.9

CUMULATIVE COSTS INVESTED IN DUST CONTROL (IN 10,000 YUAN) (1963–1992)

Year	Dust Control Facilities	Electricity Consumed	Maintenance	Management	Subtotal
1963	8.16	16.63	0.21	2.52	27.52
1966	26.70	49.64	0.64	4.39	81.37
1971	31.09	41.07	0.40	7.72	80.28
1976	30.17	24.41	4.13	10.26	68.97
1981	76.41	93.95	28.80	22.37	221.53
1986	168.50	153.38	34.88	5.99	362.75
1991–92	64.29	53.51	7.75	50.75	176.30
Total	405.32	432.59	76.81	104.00	1,018.72

also significant socioeconomic burdens to the society. Neither the health consequences nor the economic burden is affordable. In the absence of effective curative treatment for silicosis, the only reasonable protection of workers' health is to control dust exposure levels for workers in dust-generating workplaces. As shown by the Shanghai data, although the investments for preventive measures are costly, the benefits generated can be expected to dramatically exceed the costs. This work on cost-benefit and cost-effectiveness analysis of occupational health services strongly supports the case for promoting silicosis prevention.

It is worthwhile to demonstrate the relationship between health and productivity/efficiency and the economic impact of occupational health and safety on the nation's development. Unfortunately, for the majority of the relevant stakeholders, occupational health and safety have been seen only as a financial burden for industry and for the nation. But the recent economic appraisals show a totally different scenario. Occupational health and safety activities have been found to be profitable, and the cost-benefit ratios in some countries have been high. It is important to publish such results in order to increase the awareness of both political and economic decision makers of the benefits of occupational health and safety. Organizing occupational health services for each worker in the world according to Western European standards would cost about US$120 billion, i.e., approximately 0.4% of the total GDP of the world, while the economic losses from occupational accidents and disease are estimated to comprise 4% of the GNP.

The economics of occupational safety and health can demonstrate interesting incentives to business. It has become clear that both industrial and national (or regional) economies can benefit from better occupational safety and health (both in reducing costs and improving productivity and innovation). Much must be done to solidify the evidence and to develop methods that will help decision makers.

30

EMERGING ISSUES
IN THE NEW ECONOMY

Jorma Rantanen

Occupational health occupies a unique economic role. It encompasses all of the following somewhat contradictory statements simultaneously:

- an investment that pays off in increased productivity and health for the whole society
- a cost that employers seek to minimize because it does not directly increase production or profits in the short term
- a protection for the employer against catastrophic loss and the cost of serious injury and loss of business reputation
- an ethical imperative that is an accepted part of business for modern societies
- a legal and regulatory responsibility of employers toward their workers that comes at a time when most employers would prefer to avoid government regulation
- a means of improving the level of health of the population in general through education, health promotion, and control of hazards
- a cost that some employers feel will make them unsuccessful when they try to sell their products in competition with other enterprises that do not spend as much for occupational health
- a public responsibility that is carried out largely by private employers
- a specialized area of health care where experts are in short supply
- the means of preventing a major burden of disability, incapacity, and health-care costs in every country
- a short-term cost to employers when employers in many countries are shielded from the economic burden of the failure of occupational health due to insurance and health-care financing (or lack of same)
- a means of controlling unnecessary risks at a time when some promote risk taking as a good thing that advances society and an individual's own interests

Because of these contradictions, support for effective occupational health varies widely from country to country, depending on attitudes and political and economic trends. Nevertheless, the positive case for effective occupational health is really very simple:

- A safe working environment is a recognized human right that all people would want for themselves and their families.
- Protecting the health of workers and their families is a sound investment in public health.
- Preventing disability due to occupational disorders removes a major cause of suffering, economic insecurity, and lost economic productivity.
- Society becomes more productive and equitable when unnecessary risks are controlled. All occupational disorders can be prevented.
- Occupational health services are a shared responsibility of the public and private sectors and require government supervision.
- Occupational health services are best viewed as an investment in the foundations of society, not as a benefit to workers or a luxury.

Changing trends in the economy have a great influence on occupational health services. This chapter will review some of these recent trends and the effects they have had.

GLOBALIZATION

Working life has changed rapidly since the 1980s ended the era of a stable economy dominated by the manufacturing industry. A new step in the progress of globalization was taken with the closure of the General Agreement on Tariffs and Trade (GATT) Uruguay Round in 1994. Its successor, the World Trade Organization (WTO), was given a special mission to promote free trade and simultaneously generate agreements and rules for global economic operations. Globalization was also promoted by the worldwide introduction of new information and communication technologies that have radically changed the time and space dimensions of global economies, including work life.

The impact of globalization is universal; the process of globalization affects every workplace in the world either positively or negatively. Numerous positive effects (e.g., growth of world trade, new employment opportunities, closer international collaboration, vulnerability to a global recession) are already visible, but a number of adverse consequences have also occurred (e.g., high unemployment, growing economic gaps between and within countries, and overwhelming domination of economic values over social values). There is a common view among globalization scholars that the world, on average, has become wealthier, and some developing countries have been positively impacted, but the gaps between the richest and the poorest have widened. New global governance is needed to make the world of work more human-oriented, to balance the development, and to share the benefits of globalization more equally as proposed by the United Nations' former Secretary-General, Mr. Kofi Annan (1998).

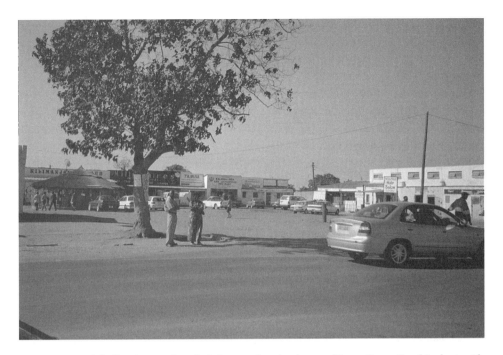

Figure 30.1 Globalization and trade bring modernization and benefits to Zambia, but with them come costs and social change.(Photograph by Tee L. Guidotti, George Washington University.)

CHANGES IN ENTERPRISE STRUCTURES

Two opposing trends in how businesses are organized have taken place at the same time:

- consolidation—as companies in the private sector grow to greater size
- fragmentation—as operating units become less cohesive

Consolidation is the result of a management philosophy that holds that companies need to expand in order to achieve efficiencies of scale, to operate globally, and to compete against multinational giants. Mergers of multinational companies, and large corporations within countries that want to become multinational, are accomplished to reach the size needed for global-scale operations. Such large global companies often introduce corporate-wide policies and standards for all operation sites, including occupational health and safety. Such policies have a positive impact on working conditions in many industrialized and developing countries. Unfortunately, there are also negative examples in which occupational health and safety standards have been compromised in order to achieve greater competitiveness.

Fragmentation has been occurring at the same time because of a management philosophy that encourages decision making at the lowest practical level in the organization in order to be able to adapt quickly to changing circumstances and to hold managers accountable for very specific, well-defined operations. This trend has included management innovations called *decentralization, delayering,* and *outsourcing.*

In decentralization, companies are fragmented into smaller units, managers of each make the important decisions rather than a central office, and each unit is held accountable for its own performance. For example, an enterprise with operations in different countries would give more authority to the manager in each country to make key decisions, such as borrowing loan money, purchasing supplies, and pricing the product, instead of dictating these decisions from headquarters.

In delayering, enterprises remove layers of management so that there are fewer positions in management or managers supervising the person actually doing the work. This management philosophy works both as a means of obtaining the greatest efficiency and to ensure that managers are in close touch with real problems being faced in operating the organization. Unfortunately, delayering has largely removed the upper-level supervisors and managers in benefits and human resources who were most familiar with occupational health services and the value they add to the company.

In outsourcing, any activity that is not directly relevant to the core business is contracted out to be done by another company or vendor. For example, a company that formerly ran its own food services for employees and shipped its own products directly to consumers may now contract with a food services company to run the cafeteria and a fulfillment company to ship out product orders. This frees the company to concentrate on developing and making the product, to do what it presumably does best. Most major companies in developed countries have outsourced their occupational health services to external service units. Outsourcing, particularly, has had major consequences for occupational health and safety. In addition to outsourcing health services, large enterprises have given business to, created or stimulated the creation of many smaller contracting enterprises to service the needs of the larger entity. This has given rise to a paradox: proliferation of small enterprises at the national level during an era of consolidation among large companies at the global level.

It is more difficult to provide occupational health services in this changing environment. As contacts between vendors and contractors and their customer or contracting companies get looser, discontinuities in quality and goals may occur (Rantanen et al. 1994). It is sometimes more difficult for external services to have the same impact on work hazards and the work environment as in-company services. Companies providing these outsourced services, which are themselves small enterprises usually serving several employers, may be at risk of becoming less specialized than workplace-oriented services, which weakens prevention activities (Rantanen 1999). Warnings about hazards must be communicated from the outside providers to the managers of companies, which is generally achieved by provision of a written summary called a *safety data sheet* (SDS; *material safety data sheet*, MSDS, in the US and Canada) but the occupational health providers are not often involved in correcting the problem. It is easy in such situations for problems to be overlooked or ignored.

The trend toward fragmentation is likely to continue. Presently, over 90% of all business enterprises in the world are small, but these small enterprises employ the vast majority of employees (over 85% of European Union workers are employed or self-employed in small facilities). (See Chapter 22.)

EMPLOYMENT AND OCCUPATIONS

While globalization has increased economic activities and employment in some areas, it has also cut off employment and eliminated jobs in many countries, local communities, and economic sectors. Dozens of occupations have become obsolete and have disappeared, and fewer new occupations have been created. The world has a total of 800 million unemployed or underemployed people, and many sectors continue to lose jobs. The types of employment have also changed through the growing prevalence of short-term and fixed-term work contracts and the increasing number of self-employed and precarious workers. For occupational health services, this sets up discontinuities in the client-service provider relationship. Serving higher numbers of smaller, scattered workplaces or solitary workers results in lower efficiency as higher costs and more time and effort are needed to improve working environments and conditions. Again, this trend tends to focus occupational health activities toward the individual worker, as if it were a medical problem, instead of the overall work environment and working conditions, as problem of prevention and public health.

In view of such structural changes, a search for new service provision models is under way in many countries, including such innovations as delegating the provision of occupational health services to primary health-care units (e.g., Italy and Finland), connecting smaller enterprises that need services to larger networks (the Netherlands), and generating new forms of services for groups of enterprises that operate on a not-for-profit basis. In some countries, a new trend is the organization of countrywide private companies providing occupational health services, especially those which serve a special branch of the economy or all types of enterprises (Hämäläinen et al. 2001).

The workers who are protected by occupational health services are also changing. In industrial societies, the vast majority of employees held blue-collar manufacturing or tradesmen jobs or worked in primary production (mining, forestry, agriculture, fishery, etc.) or did manual labor. In post-industrial societies, the mechanization and automation of production has reduced the numbers of such workers in many industries by 70% to 90%, and the remaining workers often operate complex machines rather than perform heavy physical work. This is a huge change; in Finland, for example, the blue-collar/white-collar ratio in the workforce was 7:3 in the 1970s; today it is 3:7.

Changes in occupational organizations impact occupational health concerns and activities. Although the traditional musculo-manual hazards cannot be forgotten, the new challenges of expert-type work, the psychological issues of work, and the new work organizations now must be considered as part of the mainstream of occupational health. Global economic change is having a strong impact on the demands and the skills required in occupational health.

DEMOGRAPHIC CHANGES

Many demographic changes in the workforce are taking place in the global economy:

- rapid aging of the workforce, particularly in developed countries, but also in many developing countries
- growing numbers of female workers in work life
- the challenge of providing equal opportunities for handicapped and migrant workers
- the gradual elimination of child labor
- multi-ethnic work communities reflecting immigration patterns and the internationalization of work
- challenges of maintaining equity, providing support for vulnerable groups, and preventing discrimination

Occupational health experts should take an active role in supporting and facilitating these special groups to get them well integrated into work life by promoting their employability, ensuring the availability of occupational health services for all, and promoting the modification of work and work environments as necessary. Specific good-practice guidelines are needed for occupational health services to meet these new challenges.

TIME MANAGEMENT

The first working time limit regulations were enacted over 100 years ago to adjust working hours to reasonable amounts, first from a norm of 12 to 16 hours/day, to 10 hours/day, and later, in the early decades of the 20th century, to 8 hours/day. The number of holidays has also increased in many countries. The total number of annual working hours has consequently been reduced by 50% over this 100-year period. There is a wide variation in the length of average working time in different countries; in the United States and Japan, working times are about 10% to 20% longer than in the European countries.

High demands on the worker for productivity in the new economy increase exposure to stress. Industrial activities have become adjusted to a 24-hour, 7-day work schedule. This makes time management more and more difficult for a growing number of workers as it has had an impact on the working hours throughout the world. For example, in Finland, one-third of the workforce works over 45 hours a week (the upper 8% works 60–85 hours a week); another third works about the normal 40 ± 5 hours a week; and one-third are working less than 30 hours a week (many of whom are the so-called "underemployed", who would prefer to work a full day).

In addition to the growing variation in the length of the workday (or workweek), the increased prevalence of unconventional work hours, evening work, weekend work, and two-shift work now affects about one-third of the workforce. In countries where low-paid jobs are common, a substantial proportion of the workforce must hold two jobs to sustain their families.

Unconventional work hours (night shifts and two-shift work) have been associated with elevated accident risk, increased risk of cardiovascular disorders, stress, and psychophysiological exhaustion (chronic overwork). Sleep debt is surprisingly common (12% of workers in Finland suffer, on the average, from a constant 2-hour sleep deficiency), which has an impact on accident risk and human errors. Occupational health experts should work toward the minimization of unconventional work hours and emphasize the importance of human psychophysiological diurnal rhythms in following the health and safety of workers in relation to work schedules.

THE STRESS EPIDEMIC

Increasing global competition, growing productivity demands, and continuous work changes, together with job insecurity, are associated with increased stress in the work life. Up to 30% to 50% of workers in different countries and different economic sectors report high time pressure and tight deadlines, preventing them from doing their job as well as they would like and causing psychological stress. Psychological stress is particularly likely if high demands on workers are associated with little opportunity to self-regulate the work itself. Stress, if continuous, has been found to be detrimental to physical health (cardiovascular disorders), mental health (psychological burnout), safety (accident risks), and musculoskeletal disorders (particularly hand-arm and shoulder-neck syndrome). Stress also causes substantial economic losses due to absenteeism, work disability, and a lower level of quality products and services.

Stress prevention should include not only actions directed to the individual worker, but measures directed at the work organization, moderation of the total workload, competence building, and collaboration within the workplace. Support from foremen and a supervisor is of crucial importance in stress management programs.

MOBILITY OF WORKERS

International Mobility

Today, workers travel around the world far more than in the past, and that mobility is likely to continue to grow in globalizing economies for the following reasons.

First, big multinational companies often provide job opportunities for their employees abroad. Such workers are offered occupational health and safety services, which usually follow a high corporate standard. The ILO has provided an international guideline for good practices for multinational companies, and the Organisation for Economic Co-operation and Development (OECD) has provided general principles for the operation of multinationals.

Second, other workers migrate or travel to obtain employment or better living standards (employment and economic migration). Although some of these workers are professionals and are well compensated, others are poor or struggling and require jobs for economic security and to send money home to their families. The ILO estimates the number of migrant workers in the world to be approximately 100 million. Some research shows that the unprivileged and underserved position of migrant workers includes a higher risk of occupational accidents and a lower use of occupational health services and health services in general than domestic workers. The conflict between the role of the female worker in modern work life and the traditional role of woman in the original culture causes problems. Special occupational health measures are needed to meet the health needs of migrant workers.

A third group of workers migrate because of political or environmental pressures in their home areas or war or civil conflict. These include migrants officially designated as refugees and others who are simply fleeing a difficult situation. Sometimes, these migrant workers must live in refugee camps. They are usually not welcomed into local society and may find it difficult to adjust. These migrants often find it difficult to find and keep jobs, may be paid very little, and have lost the status and security they once had in their home communities.

Local Mobility

Getting around in rural areas is often slow and uncertain. Getting around in cities is usually easier, but as cities grow in population and complexity, basic transportation tends to slow and become more congested.

Growing urbanization is one of the most consistent trends worldwide. Commuting between home and the workplace requires more and more time, particularly in big urban centers in newly industrialized and developing countries. If public transport is not efficient, commuting traffic presents a substantial risk to safety and health. In some countries, the risk of fatal and severe accidents is higher from commuting traffic than in the workplace, and in rapidly urbanizing developing countries, public transportation is usually inadequate, heavily loaded, and risky. In many countries, the time needed for commuting may be two hours in one direction, making the total length of the workday 12 hours. Improving commuting traffic safety is an important target for the overall safety of working people, particularly in newly industrialized and developing countries. Improving public transportation, appropriate city planning, and industrial siting policies are important measures to reduce commuting time and thereby moderate the length of the workday.

SOLUTIONS: CORPORATE SOCIAL RESPONSIBILITY AND PUBLIC SECTOR RESPONSIBILITY

Corporate social responsibility is a popular phrase, particularly in view of sustainable environmental development and responsibility toward the community. Good care, safety, health, and well-being of the company's own workers are, however, the priority issues in view of a company's social responsibility, sustainability, and credibility. Part of social responsibility is organizing competent, high-quality occupational health and safety services for the company's personnel. If appropriately trained, such occupational health representatives can play a key role in environmental health services as well and thus contribute to a company's responsibility to its community.

Role of the Public Sector

Due to the globalization of economic activities, the public sector is challenged by demands of higher economic efficiency, better client service, higher-quality products, and flexibility despite smaller budgets than ever before. Together with a constricting public budget, global competition rules have a strong privatizing effect on public services, including health services. Governments want to encourage turning public enterprises into private enterprises when they can, and private enterprises would rather use private suppliers, vendors, and contractors than relying on public services.

Occupational health services are usually funded by employers. Even when public services are available, big and medium-sized companies usually prefer to use private service providers. This new trend increases the commercialization of occupational health services and stimulates the formation of new enterprises to meet the demand, as discussed above regarding outsourcing. Commercialization weakens the utilization of total comprehensive services and favors individually priced services, which targets individual workers. It is much easier to see the benefit and to budget for treating work-related injuries and managing individual health problems than it is to anticipate occupational health problems and to take action to prevent them. It is particularly difficult to practice prevention when the occupational health service is external to the enterprise, as in outsourced services. Thus, commercialization tends to work against the objective of a comprehensive occupational health program that strives for a balanced approach to workers, the work environment and work community, and work organizations.

It is certain that many workers will never be provided with adequate private occupational health services if left solely to market mechanisms. The weakened role of the public sector is certain to result in fewer programs for underserved groups, small-scale enterprises, the self-employed, such as agricultural and informal sector workers, and workers in sparsely populated areas because commercial services are not sustainable—their costs cannot be recovered and no profit is possible. Therefore, the public sector has a permanent role and a continuing responsibility for provision of services to underserved groups, even in a market-oriented, globalized economy.

Action by Occupational Health

In most countries of the world, the trends discussed above are already well advanced. Occupational health has many challenges ahead; some of the issues raised in this chapter include:

- to provide services for everyone, in an economic system that differentiates among workers by employer, sector, and operating unit
- to find ways to provide services for mobile workers

- to provide services for workers in fragmented workplaces, small and medium-sized enterprises, the self-employed, and workers in the informal sector and other underserved groups
- to expand the content of services to cover psychological and psychosocial aspects of work, which have become of increasing importance
- to develop the connection between occupational health and work ability in order to achieve better employability

A summary of the challenges and actions of occupational health in the changing work life is presented in Table 30.1.

Occupational health services should be a basic right of working citizens, as recognized by international organizations and the constitutions of most democratic states.

TABLE 30.1

EMERGING ISSUES IN THE NEW ECONOMY

Emerging Trend	Work Life Challenge/Health Impact	Occupational Health Actions Needed
Globalization as a whole	Growing competition More mobility Higher job demands Growing flexibility	Adjustment of work life and job demands to human work ability Introducing human and social dimensions as equal principles with economic dimension Supporting international organizations in humanization of work life
Introduction of new technologies	Computerization of work Need to reorganize the work New competence and skill demands New ergonomic problems Repetitive strain injury from VDTs Telework	Guidelines for organization and ergonomics of VDT work to optimize the visual, cognitive, and manual interfaces Training workers in the use of communication technology Good-practice guidelines for telework
Merging and fragmentation of enterprises and work organizations	Business re-engineering Mergers Fusions Downsizing Outsourcing Replacements Unemployment Uncertainty Lowered job security	Support to personnel administration and workers to prepare for organizational changes Mental health and social support for laid-off workers Preparation in activities for job-seeking and employability Introducing health aspects into re-engineering programs Consulting for crisis management
New modes of employment and occupations	Short-term and fixed-term employment with high turnover, no continuity, and no job security Self-employment, small and medium-sized enterprises, informal employment Disappearing old occupations leading to unemployment, emergence of new occupations with new job demands	Development of services for scattered and discontinuous workplaces Strengthening workers' self-management of occupational health and safety issues Initiating intensive retraining programs Introduction of job-securing skills Initiating special programs and actions for employability

(Continued)

TABLE 30.1 (Contd.)

Emerging Trend	Work Life Challenge/Health Impact	Occupational Health Actions Needed
Demographic changes	Aging of the workforce	Identification of health and social needs of different groups and individuals
	Higher participation of female workers	Adjustment of work to the needs and capacities of specific groups and individuals
	Growing numbers of migrant and mobile workers	Ensuring good health care responding to individual needs
	Handicapped and young workers	Supporting and promoting health and work ability
	New ethnic pluralism	Good-practice guidelines
Time management	Unconventional working hours	Instruction of superiors and management on better planning and organization of work
	24/7 economies	Better dimensioning of the workforce in relation to needs
	Unreasonable working hours and working weeks	Guidance regarding physiological time rhythms
	Time pressures	Moderation of working hours
	Sleep debt or sleep disturbances	Guidance in time management
	Additional safety and health risks	
	Problems with family life	
	Double burden of female workers	
Psychological stress	New epidemic: occupational stress due to inadequate time budgeting and management	Identification of sources of stress and overload
	Physical and mental health impact	Advice on good organization of work
	Productivity loss	Ensuring the competence and skills of workers
	Poor work climate	Moderation of workload
	Poor quality of products and services	Stress management programs
	Burnout	Interventions and support in treating burnout cases
	Sickness absence (absenteeism)	

Commuting	Growing need for commuting in large urban areas	Development of city and industrial planning
	Density of commuting traffic with traffic jams and high accident risks	Development of public transportation
	Increasing time needed for commuting with extra burden on workers	Promotion of walking and biking to work, safe traffic routes
	Increasing air pollution with adverse health and environment impacts	Satellite offices
		Telework
		Flextime
Corporate and public sector responsibility	Constriction of tax revenues and public services	Corporate social responsibility
	Privatization and outsourcing of public services	Developing basic regulations on public services and occupational health services in particular
	Overwork and demotivation of public-sector workers	Provision of model contents for outsourced service producers
		Good-practice guidelines and standards
		New organizational models for occupational health services and primary health care

31

THE FUTURE

Jorma Rantanen

The early pioneers of public health and occupational health believed that once effective preventive actions had been implemented and problems were corrected, the occupational health professions would disappear. History has proven that assumption incorrect. New problems are created constantly, old problems reappear in new industries and operations, and the economy is always changing, bringing new challenges to the workplace. The need for occupational health will exist as long as human work is done. In the changing world of work, the field of occupational health and the expertise of occupational health experts must continuously develop to meet new challenges and opportunities in modern work life.

Since the beginning of the 1990s, the world's economies have moved faster than ever in innovation, trade, and change. They have integrated into a global economic system, which has become more dynamic than ever before. The globalization process affects the lives of people in every corner of the world, especially in the work environment, resulting in both positive and adverse effects. Changes in employment and working conditions are now driven by the changes in global economies. These changes have had a huge impact on the practice of occupational health and safety. The process of globalization will continue and even accelerate in the next few decades and will lead to a new world economic and social order. This chapter attempts to present a vision from today's perspective of what to expect for the next 10 to 15 years of occupational life, although these are, of course, only predictions.

FUTURE CHANGES IN THE WORLD OF WORK

The most important new trends in the world of work that will have an impact on working conditions will probably be the following:

- Globalization of economies, which is occurring through the liberalization of world trade, deregulation, and free movement of capital, goods, and services across national borders.

- New technologies, new information and communication technologies, automation, nanotechnologies, mobile communications, intelligent living and working environments, biotechnologies and bioinformatics, space technologies, and new energy options affecting work life.
- New occupational exposures and hazards as hundreds of new substances are introduced into the workplace every year to join the 50,000 to 100,000 chemicals now in use as the world's consumption of chemicals per capita grows steadily.
- Big changes in economies, enterprises, communities, and regions, including growing urbanization and megacities, new macro-, meso-, and microstructures in communities, including changes in structure, business operations, and the invention of new types of enterprises.
- Big demographic changes in the workforce include aging workers, increased participation of female workers, growing mobility of workers, demands for higher levels of skill and competence, longer life expectancy, better health for most (but pockets of ill health, e.g., individuals living with HIV/AIDS and other emerging diseases), and unanticipated changes in social habits and working cultures.
- New patterns of employment, which will include more short-term contracts, fixed-time contracts, temporary and agency workers, part-time jobs, persistent and high rates of unemployment, and growing numbers of self-employed and informal sector workers.
- High rates of worker turnover, so that workers will come to expect numerous changes of occupations and jobs throughout a working career.
- New types of work organization, including an increasing use of flexible production programs, teamwork, telework, self-steered jobs, mobile workers equipped with mobile technologies, and working from home.
- Jobs based on strength alone, the so-called musculo-manual and physical jobs, will become fewer and fewer. Although the proportion of manual workers will decline, they are not likely to disappear. There is work that cannot be mechanized and where human labor is needed (e.g., elder care).
- The proportion of mentally demanding, specialized expert occupations will increase and may outstrip the supply of trained workers required.
- The proportion of service occupations at all levels of skill will increase.
- Middle-paying jobs may become scarce while both high-paying and low-paying jobs become more common; this appears to be happening in many post-industrial economies.
- Unconventional working hours will become increasingly common. The old pattern of seven- or eight-hour workdays or shifts will become less common. New work schedules will have increased variability: some may be very short (e.g., bus drivers often work two half-shifts during hours of peak traffic) and others very long (some employers, particularly in remote locations, allow their workers to work 12 hours or more for several days and then give them days or weeks off). Shift work and weekend work in workplaces that stay open for business around the clock will become even more common in the global "24/7" economy.

- Workers will live much longer and will need to continue to earn an income, resulting in postponed retirement.

While traditional occupational health and safety regulation is still needed, new areas of regulation and worker protection—such as equity, workers' participation, prevention of violence and harassment, protection of work ability, training, and education—are being introduced and will be fundamental to workers' rights in the future. New social security schemes recognize workers' improved overall health and higher life expectancy.

The impact of these changes in work will inevitably be felt in the worker's personal life. There is growing concern about the relationship between work and family life and the impact of occupational factors on individual private lives and lifestyles.

CHANGE IN THE WORKPLACE

Change in the practice of occupational health is inevitable because there have been and will continue to be massive changes where occupational health services are provided—in the workplace, in large enterprises, in public-sector organizations, in small enterprises, among the self-employed, on farms, and in the homes of home industry workers. New types of work organizations, including teleworking from home and centralized call centers, will make the workplace an idea more than an actual location. The interdependence, management, and structures of all these work sites are more dynamic than ever. Some of these changes can be predicted, but others will surprise occupational health professionals.

The trends described in Chapter 30 will follow their natural progressions and may transform into novel ways of doing business. In the contemporary globalized economic system, about 50,000 multinational corporations determine the major international trends in big enterprises. Policies of fragmenting local workplaces into smaller and smaller units and outsourcing numerous formerly in-house activities, such as accounting, maintenance, and company services such as cleaning, will continue and may even accelerate. Today, in many organizations and perhaps most companies in North America, occupational health services are generally outsourced—companies buy the services as they feel they need them, without retaining health professionals on their permanent staff. The outside services that result have looser links to the company or workplace than the in-house occupational health activities they replace. The staff of these services cannot know the workplace as well and have less opportunity to influence the general policy and strategy of the enterprise.

Outsourcing has stimulated the growth of contract services. Individuals and groups of occupational health professionals, usually at a senior level, have always worked as consultants and under contract to enterprises to do certain jobs. Now, even routine services are provided under contract, so occupational health professionals often have many clients but can give only a small amount of time and attention to each. Enterprises like this arrangement because they do not have to pay the salary and benefits for a full-time worker, and they can discharge the contract worker easily whenever the job is finished or if they do not like the result.

This market for occupational health services leaves much undone. Microenterprises, small and medium-sized enterprises, the self-employed, home workers, agricultural workers, and informal sector workers cannot afford to purchase occupational health services. To protect the health of workers in these sectors, occupational health services need to be offered free of charge or at very low cost as a part of the community's general public health services. As the fragmentation process increases the number and proportion of small workplaces, as described in Chapter 30, the rapid changes of work life will increase the need for occupational health services. However, this increased need will not necessarily, and does not now, create a market for occupational health services. Despite real needs, if health and safety issues are not recognized and considered important, no funds will be allocated to provide the services.

Access is also a growing problem, although it has always been difficult to provide for the needs of remote, agricultural, or small enterprises. The workplaces of the self-employed and teleworkers will become especially difficult to reach. Given their size, tendency to have a high turnover of workers, and economic uncertainty, employees of small enterprises may face interruptions in occupational health service and may not have their problems solved or their working conditions properly evaluated. An employer may decide not to pay for justified periodic health evaluations because of occupational exposures that occurred earlier in another workplace owned by a different employer. New innovative strategies need to be developed for providing these workers with adequate occupational health services.

A key characteristic in the global economy is flexibility. Flexibility is required to satisfy market needs and to survive in more competitive environments. This requirement will only increase. Human labor is the most flexible production factor, even in modern work life. Table 31.1 lists a number of ways in which flexibility in human work input is increased. Many of these organizational and technical solutions will become standard features in the future globalized economy.

Due to increased competition and relentless pressure to reduce costs and to do more with less, employers are driven to increase productivity, i.e., how much an individual worker can produce. Productivity gains observed in industrialized countries during the past decade have been the result of the escalation of the number of work-hours per worker rather than the use of other productivity factors (e.g., increasing and better technology or work efficiencies). In the future, increasing productivity gains are likely to come from increased flexibility in the use of workers. Human flexibility, in particular, refers to the availability of workers to work when and where they are needed. The availability of workers depends on several factors:

- regulations
- employment contracts, unions, and labor agreements
- educational level, skill, and competence
- cultural attitudes and practices

TABLE 31.1

TYPES OF FLEXIBILITY IN MODERN WORK LIFE

Human Work Input

- Working hours and shifts
- Flexibility through adapting to work intensity
- Flexibility through competence and skills development
- Flexible salary systems
- Modes of employment, full time, part time
- Flexibility through mobility
- Flexible employment contracts and agency work

Organizational and Technical

- Work organization
- Flexible managerial systems
- Flexible technology
- Flexible manufacturing systems (FMS)
- Fast production systems
- Network organizations
- Subcontracting

- family obligations
- entitlement to leave time, holidays, and time off
- workforce organization
- location and distance between the jobs and the worker
- health and safety measures to protect the worker
- work capacity and the burden of disability and illness

Availability is heavily affected by the work schedule regulations and agreements, gender, the age structure of the workforce, the accumulation of seniority on the job (*seniority* is a priority for job assignments or job security that derives from the length of time an employee has been with the employer), sickness absence, and pension policies.

Availability also means that workers have the capacity to do the job. The higher the education and skill required in the job, the more critical will be ensuring the availability of production workers. Poor work ability, substandard working conditions, badly organized work, poor social climate, low work motivation, and exposures to occupational hazards (e.g., accidents and diseases) increase sickness absence (absenteeism) and work disability and reduce the capacity and hence the availability of workers.

Obviously, enhancing worker availability can go only so far. The worker has a personal life, lives in a community, has a family, and has other commitments in society. His or her life does not belong to the employer. The tendency to require longer hours, harder work, and working "as needed" will reach a limit, but the relentless pressure will continue. Modern work life already shows signs of reaching human physiological limits in terms of working hours and work intensity that can be sustained over a long time. Taken to extremes, these trends may turn out to be counterproductive and detrimental to health and safety in the long term. Occupational health and safety personnel need to understand these trends and the limits of working life in order to advise employers on moderation and physiologically sound work arrangements, including working hours.

Although the impact of globalization is not completely positive for occupational health, it is not completely negative either. Globalization does provide considerable promise for the future. Occupational health is included in the list of global common goods to be promoted through effective global governance exercised by the United Nations and its specialist organizations, the WHO and the ILO. As multinational enterprises establish production facilities with uniform practices, standards for worker protection are spreading around the world. Economic development is generating the investment base and increasing wages and health-care costs so that enterprises and governments have more financial incentives to protect the health of workers. Technology is leading to safer ways of doing more dangerous work. As globalization puts pressure on managers to emphasize cutting costs and push for greater production, it also provides the opportunity for greater worker protection and health promotion.

FUTURE CHALLENGES TO OCCUPATIONAL HEALTH

The developments described above present numerous challenges to occupational health professionals. They must be addressed by focused research and by innovation in practice. Here are some ideas of what should be done (Takala 2002a; WHO 1995).

New structures for providing services need to be developed, and the infrastructure at the national level needs to be rationalized in every country. First, the two billion-plus working people who currently do not have access to occupational health services need to be provided with such an opportunity. Promotion of occupational health among big and medium-sized companies is needed in all countries. Scattered agricultural workers, self-employed workers, microenterprises, and small enterprises need to be covered by some sort of public occupational health services system. Effective strategies for the follow-up of health and safety of mobile, short-, and fixed-term workers need to be developed. The health and capacity of the unemployed needs to be considered and obstacles to employability removed. To reach these objectives, stronger actions are needed at international, national, and local levels.

Occupational Health Practice

The need for occupational health services in their present form has not disappeared in the world, but how it is practiced has changed. The so-called traditional health and safety hazards such as toxic chemicals, hazardous physical and biological factors, and the problems of heavy and ergonomically incorrect work can be met with existing occupational health and safety strategies, such as risk identification and assessment, hazardous exposure prevention and control, and consequence management, directed to both working people and the work environment. The subject matter of this book will always be needed, whether it is perceived as being of great or little value.

However, the future will demand that occupational health professionals confront new problems and adapt to the new realities. New health and safety problems related to new technologies, new work organizations, or new work practices will require different approaches. Ideally, occupational health professionals will be involved in the design, development, and decision making regarding change of work conditions and will be in a position to introduce health and safety criteria to create healthy workplaces within every new plant or workplace. This will require new skills in collaboration, diplomacy, communication, business management, and problem solving on the part of occupational health practitioners.

Moreover, the social aspects of the workplace cannot be ignored. To ensure the smooth operation of the enterprise, teamwork, new management methods, and new job demands for innovations and continuous learning at work, the occupational health professional must be perceived as someone who can solve problems. Employer-employee relationships and dialogue, managerial and working cultures, and psychological and social quality of work need to be developed to a new, higher level. Obviously, occupational health professionals do not (usually) run the enterprise and do not control the relationship between employers and workers and their representatives, but they can help facilitate communication and can act as honest advisors. Occupational health personnel can provide expert advice and assist in the development of the psychosocial quality of the workplace. Again, the skill and competence needed in this area should include aspects of psychology in the training curricula of occupational health personnel. Often, a multidisciplinary occupational health and safety team is needed to implement such new strategies.

Occupational health professionals cannot cover the wide range of issues now emerging in occupational health without help from colleagues in other disciplines. A multidisciplinary and multiprofessional approach might include specialists in toxicology, occupational hygiene, safety, psychology, ergonomics, medicine, and other fields in addition to occupational health generalists. Although it makes sense to address problems this way, the team approach is not easy to organize. It requires that these specialists be available in the first place, that they understand the problem, that they understand each other, and that somebody pay for the work to be done. In various countries, multidisciplinary problem-solving teams have been organized through universities, state organizations, workers' compensation or other insurance systems, or by private foundations. However, there are limits to what can be done. Even the largest enterprises rarely hire large multidisciplinary teams (numbering 5 or more experts), even for their biggest industrial problems, and when they do they do not support the team for longer than is necessary to address the immediate problem. The only practical means of building a team and keeping it together to address problems has been public sponsorship, through government-supported occupational health service provision units (as in the Netherlands) or regional institutes of occupational health (as in Finland).

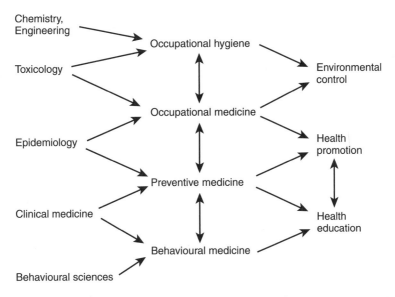

Figure 31.1 Relationships among the disciplines that make up occupational health.

Research

Research in occupational health will be as important as it has ever been. Many new technologies, working methods, and work organizations are introduced in the workplace without prior testing. Sometimes these innovations work well and sometimes not so well, and they may cause new occupational health problems. It is important to develop rapid methods for risk assessment and risk prediction to ensure that workers are protected and that the enterprise meets its objectives. Research has to cover many more complex problems than before, including multiple exposures, disorders that result from causal factors, and workers who change jobs frequently during their working lives. A wide range of outcomes, such as psychological overload, needs to be included in research efforts. In short, occupational health, and occupational health research, is growing more complex.

The role of research, which has always been central to occupational health, is growing even greater in importance. In addition to continued research on specific risk factors, hazards, mechanisms, and outcomes, more insightful studies are needed on issues of organization and occupational health services, such as:

- the best structures, functions, and models for occupational health service provision
- the quality of work environment, health, and work ability of workers
- the economic impact of occupational health services
- international occupational health, including the challenges faced by developing societies
- models for predicting the effects of new developments in workplace organization

Challenges to occupational health are challenges for active professionals in occupational health to adapt and to innovate.

Occupational health services will have to follow a multidisciplinary approach in the future, as occupational health problems will have a much wider scope than in the past. For example, occupational medicine will need support and closer collaboration with other key professions in occupational health such as nursing, occupational hygiene, ergonomics, safety, and psychology. At the same time, a high level of specific competence will be expected of every occupational health personnel.

Continuous change calls for continuous professional development. The professions active in occupational health need to update their knowledge and skills to keep pace with rapid changes in work life. The reorganization and reshaping of training curricula is inevitable, and complementary training needs to be strengthened.

As globalization changes the key features of work life in a more universal direction, occupational health experts must take a more comprehensive approach in order to predict future changes and challenges and to be able to operate in expanded international environments. Occupational health professionals from around the world need to be able to work together, learn from each other, and understand that the practice of occupational health does not stop at the borders of any country or any economic sector.

Occupational health is an information-rich activity. Occupational health professionals can make effective use of information and communication technologies. Facility in information and communication technology will be a key to success in occupational health practice, as these modern technologies provide new opportunities for providing services more efficiently, more accurately, and more quickly. Modern information technology, such as relational databases, allow data to be correlated and turned into a more complete picture; this information, over time, leads to new knowledge and insights into the workplace, patterns of health, and tools to anticipate and prevent problems in new situations. Inter-institutional networks can be easily generated, if the motivation is there, among key partners, such as enterprises sharing information with their vendors or sub-contractors, rapid reporting to government agencies for surveillance, or real-time studies conducted by research institutions.

Ethics is a crucial issue for occupational health, as it is for business and for all society. Strengthening ethical conduct in the rapidly changing world of work is an important challenge to all occupational health professionals. Numerous pressures from modern work life threaten the professional ethics of occupational health experts. In addition to traditional (Hippocratean) professional ethics, ethical principles in the globalization of work life must be considered. Determining and safeguarding ethical principles and professional independence are key issues in ensuring the sustainable future and credibility and trust for occupational health professions. The Code of Ethics of the International Commission on Occupational Health (1992) provides authoritative guidance for the occupational health professions. (See Box 29.1.)

SUMMARY

A majority of the world's workers still live and work in conditions that do not meet the minimum health and safety standards defined by the International Labour Organization (ILO). Occupational health, as a field, has established and effective ways of solving these problems. Despite this, basic protection still has not been extended to most of the world's workforce.

Even in countries where traditional occupational health hazards and their consequences—occupational accidents and diseases—have been effectively controlled, new problems and challenges will emerge due to the process of globalization itself, the introduction of new technologies, new work organizations, and new work practices. Although many problems will be effectively eliminated or controlled, new problems for health and safety will arise. This can be seen in the global stress epidemic, problems with working hours and ergonomics, and hazards related to new technologies and new substances.

The future requires a more comprehensive and multidisciplinary approach to occupational health. Such an approach would obviously include prevention, control, and curative treatment but also health promotion and economic development. Occupational health professionals will be challenged to maintain and expand their competence and skills, to adopt a multidisciplinary work culture, and to safeguard ethical principles and professional independence.

REFERENCES AND
RECOMMENDED READING

This is a textbook and not a reference work or a monograph. References are cited selectively in the text where the author considered it essential, for example, to document a study or number.

Those readers who wish to read more on a particular topic are directed to these reference sources as their first resort for a general briefing:

- *The ILO Encyclopaedia of Occupational Health*. Geneva, International Labour Organization. Use current edition (at the time of writing, 4/ed, 1998; a fifth edition is in progress).
- Websites of the World Health Organization, International Labour Organization, the International Commission on Occupational Health, and the major occupational health and safety regulatory agencies and research agencies. Information available over the internet from authoritative bodies such as these is much more up to date than a print publication can manage.
- International Commission on Occupational Health. ICOH Code of Ethics for Occupational Health Professionals. Rome. [www.icohweb.org.] Essential reading for all occupational health professionals.
- Profiles of individual hazards, which are available from the following sources:
  - International Programme on Chemical Safety (WHO) [http://www.who.int/ipcs/publications/en/]
  - Agency for Toxic Substances and Disease Registry (USA) [http://www.atsdr.cdc.gov/toxpro2.html]
  - Many national occupational health and safety agencies, such as the UK Health and Safety Executive and the National Institute of Occupational Safety and Health (part of the U.S. Centers for Disease Control and Prevention).
  - Commercial publications. There are many good guides to health and safety of specific hazardous substances.
  - Occupational exposure standards, which are of two types:
    - Mandated, from regulatory agencies, such as the European Agency for Safety and Health, Occupational Safety and Health Administration (USA), Health and Safety Executive (UK), Deutsche Forschungsgemeinschaft (Germany), and others.
    - Recommended or advisory, such as the American Conference of Governmental Industrial Hygienists (U.S.-based but international),

National Institute of Occupational Safety and Health (U.S.), British Standards Institute, International Organization for Standards, and others, among them professional associations, standards-setting bodies, and research agencies.

The reader who wishes to explore various topics is advised to search the current academic literature systematically rather than relying on text references and to explore the topic on the Internet, as authoritative Web sites are more likely to be up to date than any print text can be. For the most part, this book addresses itself to general principles, not material that quickly goes out of date.

Beyond this general guidance, there are far too many books and articles in the field of occupational health than can be cited here. All of the contributors to this book have published important contributions of their own, but it would be unfair to favor the works of authors who have contributed to this book over other equally fine contributors who did not have this opportunity.

Some authors of chapters in this book provided reference lists that they would like to share with readers. The first drafts of some of the chapters in this book were produced around 2001, and the references reflect this. The chapters have been updated several times and edited since then, but the reference lists were not and are now out of date as a guide to the current literature. Some of the references remain useful, however, as a record of sources that informed the thinking that the authors brought to their work and of valuable material that might otherwise be lost or overlooked.

The following recommended readings were selected from the original reference lists provided by these authors, with the addition of a few works that authors brought to our attention later. They should not be considered a complete bibliography or a systematically compiled list of readings. Many of these references document case studies outlined in the boxes. Others are of historical or professional interest because of their influence on the field.

The list is consolidated, rather than provided by chapter, to avoid duplication. Items that were clearly out of date but of no historical interest have been omitted. Works cited by more than one author are given only once, and when works of several authors were cited from one monograph, only the major work has been listed. The sources given in this list are all in English, only because this book is written in English and so it is obviously the common language of all readers. There are, of course, many more reference sources in other languages.

SUGGESTED READINGS BY TOPIC

Some of these references are mentioned in the text or boxes. They are not necessarily current but all have in one way or another informed the work and the authors would like to bring them to the readers' attention.

Future of Occupational Health (General)

Alli, B. O. 2001. *Fundamental principles of occupational health and safety*. Geneva: International Labour Office.

Annan, K. A. 1998. Occupational health and safety—A high priority on the global, international and national agenda. Editorial. Työterveiset, *Newsletter of the Finnish Institute of Occupational Health* 1:3.

Cassou, B., F. Derriennic, Y. Iwatsubo, and M. Amphoux. 1992. Physical disability after retirement and occupational risk factors during working life: A cross sectional epidemiological study in the Paris area. *J Epidemiol Comm Health* 46:506–511.

Chia, S. E. 1989. A study of the usage of respirators among granite quarry workers in Singapore. *Singapore Medical Journal* 30:269–272.

Ferrie, J. E., M. G. Marmot, J. Griffiths, and E. Ziglio, eds. *Labour market changes and job insecurity: A challenge for social welfare and health promotion.* WHO Regional Publications, European Series, No. 81. Copenhagen: World Health Organization, Regional Office for Europe, 11–30.

Freeman, C., and L. Soete. 1994. Work for all or mass unemployment. *Computerised technical change into the 21st Century.* London: Pinter Publishers.

Hämäläinen, R-M, K. Husman, K. Räsänen, P. Westerholm, and J. Rantanen. 2001. Survey of the quality and effectiveness of occupational health services in the European Union and Norway and Switzerland. In *People and Work, Research Reports* 45. Eds. Suvi Lehtinen, Kimmo Räsänen, Kaj Husman, Jorma Rantanen. Helsinki: Finnish Institute of Occupational Health.

Health and Safety Commission. 2000. *Occupational Health Advisory Committee report and recommendations on improving access to occupational health support.* London: Health and Safety Commission.

ILO. 1999. *Decent work.* Report of the Director-General. International Labour Conference, 87th Session 1999. Geneva: International Labour Office.

Kaul, I., I. Grunberg, and MA Stern, eds. 1999. *Global public goods.* UNDP (United Nations Development Programme). Oxford University Press.

Last, J. M., ed. 2007. *A dictionary of public health.* Oxford: Oxford University Press. (This title is expected to be revised periodically in the future: use most current edition.)

Leavell, H. R., and E. G. Clark. 1965. *Preventive medicine for the doctor in his community,* 3rd ed. New York: McGraw-Hill.

Lee, H. S., W. H. Phoon, S. Y. T. Wang, and K. P. Tan. 1996. Occupational respiratory diseases in Singapore. *Singapore Medical Journal* 37:160–164.

Lehtinen, S. 2000. ICOH 2000 in Singapore and the millennium message. *Asian-Pacific Newsletter on Occupational Health and Safety* 7(3):66–68.

Leigh, J. P., and J. F. Fries. 1992. Disability in occupations in a national sample. *Am J Public Health* 82:1517–1524.

Leow, S. B. 1973. *Investigation into the dust emission from granite quarries in Singapore and Pulau Ubin.* Singapore Institute of Standards and Industrial Research.

Letourneux, V. 1997. *Precarious employment and working conditions in the European Union.* Dublin: European Foundation for the Improvement of Living and Working Conditions.

Lo, F-C, Y-M Yeung, eds. 1998. *Globalization and the world of large cities.* Tokyo-New York-Paris: United Nations University Press.

National Institute for Occupational Safety and Health. 2000. *National Occupational Research Agenda: 21 priorities for the 21st century.* Washington, D.C.: NIOSH, Centers for Disease Control and Prevention.

Rantanen, J., ed. 1990. *Occupational health services: An overview.* Copenhagen: World Health Organization, European Region.

Rantanen, J. 1999. Impact of globalization on occupational health. *Eur J Oncol* 4(2):111–9.

Rifkin, J. 1996. *Technology, jobs and your future: The end of work. The decline of the global labor force and the dawn of the post-market era.* New York: G.P. Putnam's Sons.

Sauter, S., and L. Rosenstock. 1998. Consequences of new patterns of work organisation. In *The Changing World of Work,* 60–2. Conference Proceedings, Bilbao 19–21 October 1998.

Suzuki,Y. 1998. Inaugural address: Global ageing and the World Health Organization. In *Ageing and health. A global challenge for the 21st century*, 13–8. Proceedings of a WHO symposium, Kobe, 10–13 November 1998. World Health Organization, Belgium 1999.

Takala, J. 2002a. Introductory report: Decent work—safe work. Paper presented at the 16th World Congress on Safety and Health, Vienna, May 27.

Takala, T., and P. Pallab. 2002b. Individual, collective, and social responsibility of the firm. *Business Ethics* 9(12):109 –118.

Theorell, T., ed. 1997. Future worklife—special issue, in honor of Lennart Levi. *Scand J Work Environ Health* 23 (suppl. 4).

WHO. 1995. *Global strategy on occupational health for all.* Geneva: World Health Organization.

Agriculture

Antle, J. M., and S. M. Capalbo. 1994. Pesticides, productivity, and farmer health—Implications for regulatory policy and agricultural research. *Am J Agr Econ* 76:598–602.

Choudhry, A. W. 1989. Occupational health in agriculture. *East African Newsletter on Occupational Health and Safety* 3:16–19.

Forastieri, V. 2001. Challenges in providing occupational safety and health services to workers in agriculture. *Afr Newslett on Occup Health and Safety* 11:33–8.

Kishi, M. 1999. Indonesian farmers' perceptions of pesticides and resultant health problems from exposure. *Epidemiology* 10: 3540.

Myers, M. L. 1998. Health problems and disease patterns in agriculture. In *ILO encyclopaedia of occupational health and safety.* 4th ed. Ed. J. M. Stellman, 64.60–64.65. Geneva: International Labour Office.

Pratt, D., and J. May. 1994. Agricultural occupational medicine. In *Occupational medicine.* 3rd ed. Eds. C. Zenz, O. B. Dickerson, and E. P. Horvath Jr. St. Louis: Mosby-Year Book Inc.

Schilling, R., and N. Andersson. 1986. Occupational epidemiology in developing countries. *J Occup Health Safety—Aust NZ* 2:468–478.

Sekimpi, D. 1992. Occupational health services for agricultural workers. In *Occupational health in developing countries.* Ed. J. Jeyaratnam, 31–61. Oxford: Oxford University Press.

Sekimpi, D. K. 1993. Changes in the social culture of work in Africa: Implications for Occupational Health and Safety. *African Newsletter on Occupational Health and Safety* 3:66–68.

Biological Hazards

Wright, W. E. 2009. *Couturier's Occupational and Environmental Infectious Diseases.* 2nd ed. Beverly Farms, Massachusetts (USA): OEM Press.

Common Chemicals

Agency for Toxic Substances and Disease Registry. *Toxicological Profiles.* www.atsdr.cdc.gov

Bowler, R. M., and J. E. Cone. 1999. *Occupational Medicine Secrets.* Philadelphia: Hanley & Belfus.

Harbison, R. D. 1998. *Hamilton & Hardy's Industrial Toxicology.* 5th ed. St. Louis: Mosby.

Hathaway, G. J., N. H. Proctor, and J. P. Hughes. 1996. *Proctor & Hughes' chemical hazards of the workplace.* 4th ed. New York: Van Nostrand Reinhold.

Patnaik, P. 1999. *A comprehensive guide to the hazardous properties of chemical substances.* 2nd ed. New York: Wiley.

Toxicology

Aldridge, W. N., ed. 1996. *Mechanisms and Concepts in Toxicology.* London: Taylor & Francis Ltd.

Borm, P. J. A, and P.T. Henderson. 1996. Occupational toxicology. In *Toxicology. Principles and Applications.* Eds. R. J. M. Niesink, J. de Vries, J. Hollinger, and M. A. Hollinger. Boca Raton, FL: CRC Press, Inc.

Klaassen, C. D., ed. 2009. *Casarett & Doull's toxicology: The basic science of poisons,* 7th ed. New York: McGraw-Hill Company. (Updated periodically: use current edition.)

Deichmann, W. B., D. Henschler, B. Holmstedt, and G. Keil. 1986. What is there that is not poison? A study of the third defense by Paracelsus. *Arch Toxicol* 58:207–213.

Doll, R., T. Peto, K. Wheatley, R. Gray, and I. Sutherland. 1994. Mortality in relation to smoking: 40 years' observations on male British doctors. *Brit Med J* 309:901–911.

Feron, V. J., R. B. Beems, P. G. J. Reuzel, and A. Zwart. 1996a. Respiratory toxicology; pathophysiology, toxicological pathology and mechanisms of toxicity. In *Toxicology. Principles and Applications.* eds R. J. M. Niesink, J. de Vries, J. Hollinger, and M. A. Hollinger. Boca Raton, FL: CRC Press, Inc.

Feron, V. J., R. B. Beems, P. G. J. Reuzel, and A. Zwart. 1996b. Inhalatory exposure and methodological aspects. In *Toxicology. Principles and Applications.* Eds. R. J. M. Niesink, J. de Vries, J. Hollinger, and M. A. Hollinger. Boca Raton, FL: CRC Press, Inc.

Hard, G. C. 1998. Recent developments in the investigation of thyroid regulation and thyroid carcinogenesis. *Environ Health Perspect* 106(8):427–436.

Hill, R. N., T. M. Crisp, P. M. Hurley, S. L. Rosenthal, and D. V. Singh. 1998. Risk assessment of thyroid follicular cell tumors. *Environ Health Perspect* 106(8):447–457.

Hurley, P. M., R. N. Hill, and R. J. Whiting. 1998. Mode of carcinogenic action of pesticides inducing thyroid follicular cell tumors in rodents. *Environ Health Perspect* 106(8):437–445.

International Agency for Research on Cancer. IARC monographs on the evaluation of carcinogenic risks to humans. Lyon, France: International Agency for Research on Cancer. Current edition, check Web site for list of monographs available.

Kane, A. B., P. Boffetta, R. Saracci, and J. D. Wilbourn, eds. 1996. *Mechanisms of fibre carcinogenesis.* IARC Scientific Publications No. 140, Lyon, France: International Agency for Research on Cancer.

Klaassen, C. D., ed. 1996. *Casarett & Doull's toxicology: The basic science of poisons.* New York: McGraw-Hill Company.

Pelin, K., A. Hirvonen, M. Taavitsainen, and K. Linnainmaa. 1995a. Cytogenetic response to asbestos fibers in cultured human primary mesothelial cells from 10 different donors. *Mutat Res* 334:225–233.

Pelin, K., P. Kivipensas, and K. Linnainmaa. 1995b. Effects of asbestos and man-made vitreous fibers on cell division in cultured human mesothelial cells in comparison to rodent cells. *Environ Mol Mutag* 25:118–125.

Purchase, I. F. H. 1994. Current knowledge of mechanisms of carcinogenicity: Genotoxins versus non-genotoxins. *Human Exp Tox* 13:17–28.

Savolainen, K., and J. Kangas. 1995. Strategies for biological monitoring of workers exposed to pesticides. In *Bioindicators of Environmental Health. Ecovision World Monograph Series.* Eds. M. Munawar, O. Hänninen, S. Roy, N. Munawar, L. Kärenlampi, and D. Brown. Amsterdam: SPB Academic Publishing.

Schaper, M. 1993. Development of a database for sensory irritants and its use in establishing occupational exposure limits. *Am Ind Hyg Assoc J* 54:488–544.

van Delft, J. H. M, R. A. Baan, and L. Roza. 1998. Biological effect markers for exposure to carcinogenic compound and their relevance for risk assessment. *Crit Rev Toxicol* 28(5):477–510.

Whorton, M. D., R. M. Krauss, and T. H. Milby. 1977. Infertility in male pesticide workers. *Lancet* 2:1259–261.

Brisman, S. J., and Järvholm, B. G. 1995. Occurrence of self-reported asthma among Swedish bakers. *Scand J Work Environ Health* 21:487–493.

Checkoway, H. A, N. E. Pearce, and D. J. Crawford-Brown. 1989. *Research methods in occupational epidemiology*. New York: Oxford University Press.

Friedenreich, C. M. 1993. Methods for pooled analyses of epidemiological studies. *Epidemiology* 4:295–302.

Heederik, D., and M. Attfield. 2000. Characterisation of dust exposure for the study of chronic occupational lung disease: A comparison of different exposure assessment strategies. *Am J Epidemiol* 151:982–90.

Hernberg, S. 1981. "Negative" results in cohort studies—How to recognise fallacies. *Scand J Work Environ Health* 7 (suppl. 4):121–6.

Hernberg, S. 1992. *Introduction to occupational epidemiology*. Chelsea (MI): Lewis Publishers, Inc.

Hill, A. B. 1965. The environment and disease: Association or causation. *Proc Roy Soc Med* 58:295–300.

Karjalainen, A., L. Aalto, R. Jolanki, H. Keskinen, I. Mäkinen, and A. Savela. 2001. *Occupational Diseases in Finland in 1999*. Helsinki: Finnish Institute of Occupational Health.

Karjalainen, A., K. Kurppa, R. Martikainen, Klaukka, and J. Karjalainen. 2001. Work is related to a substantial portion of adult-onset asthma incidence in the Finnish population. *Am J Respir Crit Care Med* 164:565–8.

Kennedy, S. M., N. Le Moual, D. Choudat, and F. Kauffmann. 2000. Development of an asthma specific job exposure matrix and its application in the epidemiological study of genetics and environment in asthma (EGEA). *Occup Environ Med* 57:635–641.

Kivimäki, M., M. Elovainio, and J. Vahtera. 2000. Workplace bullying and sickness absence in hospital staff. *Occup Environ Med* 57:656–660.

Knutsson, A., J. Hallquist, C. Reuterwall, T. Theorell, and T . Åkerstedt. 1999. Shiftwork and myocardial infarction: A case control study. *Occup Environ Med* 56:46–50.

Koskinen, K., J.-P. Rinne, A. Zitting, A. Tossavainen, J. Kivekäs, K. Reijula, P. Roto, and M. S. Huuskonen. 1996. Screening for asbestos-induced diseases in Finland. *American Journal of Industrial Medicine* 30(3):241–251.

Kromhout, H., D. Heederik, L. M. Dalderup, and D. Kromhout. 1992. Performance of two general job-exposure matrices in a study of lung cancer morbidity in the Zutphen cohort. *Am J Epidemiol* 136:698–711.

Porta, M., ed. 2008. *A dictionary of epidemiology*, 5th edition. Oxford: Oxford University Press. (Revised periodically: use most current edition.)

Pearce, N., and J. Crane. 1996. Epidemiological methods. In *Occupational and Environmental Respiratory Disease*. Eds. P. Harper, M. B. Schenker, and J. R. Balmes. St. Louis (Missouri): Mosby.

Pekkanen, J., and N. Pearce. 1999. Defining asthma in epidemiological studies. *Eur Respir J* 14:951–957.

Petitti, D. B. 1994. Meta-analysis, decision analysis and cost-effectiveness analysis. In *Methods for Quantitative Synthesis in Medicine*. New York, Oxford: Oxford University Press.

Pukkala, E. 1995. *Cancer risk by social class and occupation: A survey of 109,000 cancer cases among finns of working age*. Basel: Karger.

Strauss, R. E, W. S. Richardson, P. Glasziou, and R. B. Haynes. 2005. *Evidence-based medicine*. Edinburgh: Churchill Livingstone.

Son, P. H., L. V. Trung, T. N. Lan, M. Keifer, and S. Barnhart. 2000. Use of geographical information system to identify silica risks and plan prevention strategies. 26th International Congress on Occupational Health. August 27–September 1, 2000, Singapore.

Torén, K., J. Brisman, and B. Järvholm. 1993. Asthma and asthma-like symptoms in adults assessed by questionnaires. *Chest* 104:600–608.

Uitti, J., Nordman, L. Halmepuro, and J. Savolainen. 1997. Respiratory symptoms, pulmonary function and allergy to fur animals among fur farmers and fur garment workers. *Scand J Work Environ Health* 23:428–34.

Ursin, G., M. P. Longnecker, R. W. Haile, and S. Greenland. 1995. A meta-analysis of body mass index and risk of premenopausal breast cancer. *Epidemiology* 6:137–41.

Venables, K. M. 1994. Epidemiology. In *Occupational Lung Disorders*. 3rd ed. Ed. W.R. Parkes Oxford: Butterworth-Heinemann.

Venables, K. M. 1989. Survey design. In *Occupational Health Practice*. Ed. H. A. Waldron. Kent (England): Butterworths.

Weed, D. L. 1997. Methodologic guidelines for review papers. *J Natl Cancer Inst* 89:6–7.

Wulff, H. R., and P.C. Gotzsche. 2000. *Rational diagnosis and treatment: Evidence-based clinical decision-making*. 3rd ed. Bodmin (Cornwall): MPG Books Ltd.

Zitting, A., A. Karjalainen, O. Impivaara, A. Tossavainen, T. Kuusela, J. Mäki, and M.S. Huuskonen. 1995. Radiographic small lung opacities and pleural abnormalities as a consequence of asbestos exposure in an adult population. *Scand J Work Environ Health* 21:470–7.

Ergonomics

Bjorkstein, M. G., B. Almby, and E. S. Jansson. 1994. Hand and shoulder ailments among laboratory technicians using modern plunger-operated pipettes. *Applied Ergonomics* 25:88–94.

Caple, D. 2000. Ergonomic tools to objectively assess workplace risks. In *Moving in on occupational injury*. Ed. D. Worth. Oxford: Butterworth.

Drills, R. J. 1963. Folk norms and biomechanics. *Human Factors* 5:427–41.

Hendrick, H. W. 1999. Ergonomics: An international perspective. In *The occupational ergonomics handbook*. Eds. W. Karwowski and W. Marras. New York: CRC Press LLC.

Hopsu, L., V. Louhevaara, O. Korhonen, and M. Miettinen. 1994. *Ergonomic and developmental intervention in cleaning work*. Proceedings of the 12th Triennial Congress of the International Ergonomics Association, Vol. 6: General Issues, Toronto, Canada.

IEA Triennial Report 1997–2000. 2000. Santa Monica: International Ergonomics Association Press.

Ilmarinen, J., and V. Louhevaara, eds. 1999. FinnAge—Respect for the ageing: Action programme to promote health, work ability and well-being of ageing workers, 1990–1996. *People and Work, Research Reports 26*. Helsinki: Finnish Institute of Occupational Health.

Jastrzebowski, W. 1857. An outline of ergonomics or science of work based upon the truths drawn from the science of nature 1857. In *An outline of ergonomics or the science of work*. Ed. D. Koradecka. 2000. Warsaw: Central Institute of Labour Protection.

Kirvesoja, H. 2001. Experimental ergonomic evaluation with user trials: EEE product development procedures. *Acta Universitatis Ouluensis, C Technica* 157, Oulu, Finland.

Kontogiannis, T., and D. Embrey. 1997. A user-centered design approach for introducing computer-based process information systems. *Applied Ergonomics* 28:109–19.

Lintula, M., and N. Nevala. 2006 Ergonomics and the usability of mechanical single-channel liquid dosage pipettes. *Int J Ind Ergon* 36:257–263.

Louhevaara, V. 1999. Participatory ergonomics as a measure for maintaining work ability. In FinnAge—Respect for the ageing: Action programme to promote health, work ability and well-being of ageing workers, 1990–1996. Eds. J. Ilmarinen and V. Louhevaara. *People and Work, Research Reports 26*. Helsinki: Finnish Institute of Occupational Health.

Louhevaara, V., M. Miettinen, P. Mäkinen, E. Viikari-Juntura, E-P Takala, E. Kuosma, E. Toppila, and P. von Nandelstadh. 1996. Ergonomic intervention for reducing postural load of aging vehicle inspectors. Proceedings of the XIth Annual International Occupational Ergonomics and Safety Congress, Zurich, Switzerland.

Lu, M-L, T. James, B. Lowe, M. Barrero, and Y-K A. Kong. 2008. An investigation of hand forces and postures for using selected mechanical pipettes. *Int J Ind Ergon* 38:18–29.

Marmaras, N., G. Poulakakis, and V. Papakostopoulos. 1999. Technical note: Ergonomic design in ancient Greece. *Applied Ergonomics* 30:361–8.

Nevala-Puranen, N., and M. Lintula. 2001. Ergonomics and usability of Finnpipettes. In *Promotion of Health through Ergonomic Working and Living Conditions. Outcomes and methods of research and practice. Publications 7.* Proceedings of NES 2001. University of Tampere, School of Public Health, Tampere, Finland.

Oborne, D., R. Branton, F. Leal, P. Shipley, and T. Stewart, eds. 1993. *Person-centered ergonomics. A Brantonial view of human factors.* London: Taylor & Francis.

Pheasant, S. T. 1996. *Bodyspace: Anthromometry, ergonomics and the design of work.* 2nd ed. London: Taylor & Francis.

Pohjonen, T. 2001. *Perceived work ability and physical capacity of home care workers. Effects of physical exercise and ergonomic intervention on factors related to work ability.* PhD Diss., Kuopio University Publications D. Medical Sciences 260. Kuopio, Finland.

Pohjonen, T., A. Punakallio, O. Korhonen, and V. Louhevaara. 1998. Participatory ergonomics for reducing load and strain in the home care work. *Int J Ind Ergon* 21:345–52.

SFS-EN ISO 9241-11. Ergonomic requirements for office work with visual display terminals (VDTs). Part 11: Guidance on usability.

Wichansky, A. M. 2000. Usability testing in 2000 and beyond. *Ergonomics* 43:998–1006.

Vilkki, M., C-H Nygård, V. Louhevaara, and M. Mattila. 1999. Reducing the physical work load of ageing operators in the production of welding wire (Fundia). In FinnAge—Respect for the ageing: Action programme to promote health, work ability and well-being of ageing workers, 1990–1996. Eds. J. Ilmarinen and V. Louhevaara. *People and Work, Research Reports 26.* Helsinki: Finnish Institute of Occupational Health.

Wilson, J. R. 1995. A framework and context for ergonomics methodology. In *Evaluation of human work. A practical ergonomics methodology.* Eds. J. R. Wilson and N. Corlett. London: Taylor & Francis.

Wilson, J. R. 1998. Task analysis and work design. In *Work organization and ergonomics.* Eds. Di Matino and N. Corlett. Geneva: International Labour Office.

Wood, D. D., R. O. Andres, and N. E. Laurie. 1997. Micropipettes: An ergonomic product evaluation. In *Advances in Occupational Ergonomics and Safety II.* Eds. B. Das and W. Karwowski. IOS Press and Ohmsha.

Health Promotion, Prevention, and Wellness

Dias, E., and R. Mendes. 2002. *Contribuição à Ampliação e Operacionalização dos Conceitos de Promoção da Saúde no Trabalho e de Locais de Trabalho Saudável.* Belo Horizonte. Working document prepared for the Pan American Health Organization.

Downie, R. S., C. Tannahill, and A. Tannahill. 1996. *Health promotion: Models and values.* 2nd ed. Oxford:Oxford University Press..

Fielding, J. E. 1998. Worksite health promotion. In *Encyclopaedia of occupational health and safety.* 4th ed., Volume I. Ed. J. M. Stellman, 15.8–15.12. Geneva: International Labour Office.

Guidotti, T. L., L. Ford, and M. Wheeler. 2000. The Fort McMurray Demonstration Project in Social Marketing: Theory, design and evaluation. *American Journal of Preventive Medicine* 18(2):163–169.

National Quality Institute and Health Canada. 2000. *Canadian healthy workplace criteria.* Ottawa: National Quality Institute.

Pan American Health Organization. 1996. *Health promotion: An anthology.* Scientific Publication No. 557. Washington, DC: PAHO/WHO.

Schilling, R. S. F. 1984. More effective prevention in occupational health practice? *J Soc Occup Med* 34:71–79.

Scutchfield, F. D., and C. W. Keck. 1997. *Principles of public health practice*. Albany: ITP.

Warshaw, L. J., and J. Messite. 1998. Health protection and promotion in the workplace: An overview. *ILO encyclopaedia of occupational health and safety*. 4th ed. Ed. J. M. Stellman. Geneva: International Labour Office.

Woolf, S. H., S. Jonas, and R. S. Lawrence. 1996. *Health promotion and disease prevention in clinical practice*. Baltimore: Williams & Wilkins.

World Health Organization. 1984. *Health promotion: A discussion document on the concepts and principles*. Copenhagen: WHO Regional Office for Europe.

World Health Organization. 1988. *Health promotion for working populations: Report of a WHO expert committee on health promotion in the work setting*. Technical Report Series No. 765. Geneva: WHO.

World Health Organization. (1997) *WHO's Global Healthy Work Approach*. Geneva: WHO.28 p.

Industries, Occupations, and Hazard Control

Ng, T. P., W. H. Phoon, H. S. Lee, and K. T. Tan. 1992. An epidemiological survey of respiratory morbidity among granite quarry workers in Singapore: Radiological abnormalities. *Annals Academy of Medicine Singapore* 21:305–311.

Tan, K. T. 1979. A review of dust control in granite quarries. *Singapore Community Health Bulletin* 20:34–349.

Zober, A., M. Nasterlack, and D. Pallapies. 1998. In *Exposure-based hazards: Chemical international occupational and environmental medicine*. Eds. J. A. Herzstein, W. B. Bunn III, L. E. Fleming, J. M. Harrington, J. Jeyaratnam, and I. R. Gardner, 483–492. St. Louis: Mosby.

Musculoskeletal Disorders

Armstrong, T. J., P. Buckle, L. J. Fine et al. 1993 A conceptual model for work-related neck and upper-limb musculoskeletal disorders. *Scand J Work Environ Health* 19:73–84.

Bergenudd, H., and B. Nilsson. 1988. Back pain in middle age; occupational workload and psychologic factors: An epidemiologic survey. *Spine* 13:58–60.

Bergenudd, H., and B. Nilsson. 1994. The prevalence of locomotor complaints in middle age and their relationship to health and socioeconomic factors. *Clin Orthop* 308:264–70.

Bongers, P. M., de C. R. Winter, M. A. Kompier et al. 1993. Psychosocial factors at work and musculoskeletal disease. *Scand J Work Environ Health* 19:297–312.

Malmivaara, A., U. Häkkinen, T. Aro, M. L. Heinrichs, L. Koskenniemi, E. Kuosma, S. Lappi, R. Paloheimo, C. Servo, V. Vaaranen, et al. 1995. The treatment of acute low back pain—Bed rest, exercises, or ordinary activity? *New England Journal of Medicine* 332(6):351–5.

Nachemson, A., E. Egon Jonsson, eds. 2000. *Neck and back pain: The scientific evidence of causes, diagnosis, and treatment*. Philadelphia: Lippincott Williams & Wilkins.

Westgaard, R. H., and J. Winkel. 1997. Ergonomic intervention research for improved musculoskeletal health: A critical review. *Int J Ind Ergon* 20:463–500.

Occupational Health Nursing

Oakley, K. 2008. *Occupational health nursing*. Wiley.

Occupational Medicine and Related Topics

Aw, T-C, K. Gardiner, J. M. Harrington. 2007. *Pocket consultant: Occupational health*. Oxford: Blackwell.

Guidotti, T. L. 2010. *The Praeger handbook of occupational and environmental medicine*. Santa Barbara, California (USA): Praeger/ABC CLIO.

Koh, D., C. L. Seng, and J. Jeyaratnam. 2001. *Textbook of Occupational Medicine Practice*. 2nd ed. Singapore: World Scientific.

Levy, B. S., D. L. Wegman, S. L. Baron, and R. K. Sokas. 2005. *Occupational and environmental health*. 5th ed. New York: Oxford University Press.

Rogers, R., and T. L. Guidotti. 1995. Indoor air quality and building-associated outbreaks. In *Environmental Lung Disease*. Eds. E. Cordasco, S. Demeter, and C. Zenz, 179–207. New York: Van Nostrand Reinhold.

Rüdiger, H. W. 1999. Biomonitoring. Chapter 42. In *Occupational Medicine Toxicology*. Eds. H. Marquardt, S. G. Schäfer, R. D. McClellan, and F. Welsch, 1027–1040. Academic Press.

Small Enterprises

Bohle, P., and M. Quinlan. 2000. *Managing occupational health and safety*. 2nd ed. Melbourne: MacMillan Publishers Australia.

Herford, M. E. 1950. An experimental group service for small plants. *American Journal of Public Health* 40:1529–1533.

Howell, J., J. Spickett, and K. Hudson. 1998. The management of hazardous substances in small business in Western Australia. *The Journal of Occupational Health and Safety* 14:457–463.

Rantanen, J., S. Lehtinen, and M. Mikheev, eds. 1994. Health protection and health promotion in small-scale enterprises. Proceedings of the Joint WHO/ILO Task Group 1–3, November 1993. Helsinki: World Health Organization, Finnish Institute of Occupational Health.

Stress

Bosma, H., R. Peter, J. Siegrist, and M. Marmot. 1998. Two alternative job stress models and the risk of coronary heart disease. *Am J Pub Health* 88(1):68–74.

Caplan, R. D., S. Cobb, J. R. P. French, R. V. Harrison, and S. R. Pinneau. 1975. *Job demands and worker health: Main effects and occupational differences*. HEW publications No. (NIOSH) 75-160, NIOSH, Cincinnati.

Cohen, S., D. A. J. Tyrrel, and A. P. Smith. 1991. Psychological stress and susceptibility to the common cold. *N Eng J Med* 325(9):606–612.

Elden, M. 1986. Socio-technical systems ideas as public policy in Norway: Empowering participation through worker-managed change. *J Appl Behav Science* 22(3):239–55.

Elovainio, M., M. Kivimäki, and K. Helkama. 2001. Organizational justice evaluations, job control, and occupational strain. *Journal of Applied Psychology* 86:418–424.

European Agency for Safety and Health at Work. 2002. *How to tackle psychosocial issues and reduce work-related stress*. Bilbao: European Communities.

European Commission. 2000. *Guidance on work-related stress—Spice of life or kiss of death?* Luxembourg: Office for Official Publications of the European Communities.

European Foundation for the Improvement of Living and Working Conditions. 1994. *Stress at work: Causes, effects and prevention (Guide for small and medium size enterprises)*. Luxembourg: Office for Official Publications of the European Communities.

Hendrix, W. H., B. A. Spencer, and G. S. Gibson. 1994. Organizational and extraorganizational factors affecting stress, employee well-being, and absenteeism for males and females. *J Business Psychol* 9(2):103–28.

Hoshuyama T., S. Saeki, K. Takahashi, and T. Okubo. 1993. A matched case-control study of sudden unexpected death among Japanese workers. *Journal of Epidemiol* 3:29–34.

Hurrell, J. J. Jr, and M. A. McLaney. 1988. Exposure to job stress—A new psychometric instrument. *Scand J Work Environ Health* 14 Suppl 1:27–8.

Hurrell, J. J. Jr, and L. R. Murphy. 1996. Occupational stress intervention. *Am J Ind Med* 29(4):338–41.

Hurrell, J. J. Jr, D. L. Nelson, and B. L. Simmons. 1998. Measuring job stressors and strains: Where we have been, where we are, and where we need to go. *J Occup Health Psychol* 3(4):368–89.

Israel, B. A., J. S. House, S. J. Schurman, C. A. Heaney, and R. P. Mero. 1989. The relation of personal resources, participation, influence, interpersonal relationships and coping strategies to occupational stress, job strains and health: A multivariate analysis. *Work and Stress* 3(2):163–94.

Israel, B. A, et al. 1996. Occupational stress, safety, and health: Conceptual framework and principles for effective prevention interventions. *Journal of Occupational Health Psychology* 1(3):261–86.

Jemmott, J. B, and S. E. Locke. 1984. Psychosocial factors, immunologic mediation and human susceptibility to infectious diseases: How much do we know? *Psychological Bulletin* 95(1):78–108.

Johnson, J. V, and G. Johansson, eds. 1991. *The psychosocial work environment: Work organization, democratization and death*. Amityville, New York: Baywood Publishing Company.

Johnson, J. V, W. Stewart, et al. 1996. Long-term psychosocial work environment and cardiovascular mortality among Swedish men. *American Journal of Public Health* 86(3):324–31.

Johnson, J. V., and E. M. Hall. 1988. Job strain, work place social support, and cardiovascular disease: A cross-sectional study of a random sample of the Swedish working population. *Am J Public Health* 78(10):1336–42.

Jones, F., and J. Bright. 2001. *Stress: Myth, theory and research*. London: Prentice Hall.

Kaplan, M., and T. Rankin. 1993. *Quantitative measures from organizations undergoing major change in the way work is performed: A survey of 18 Canadian workplaces*. Toronto, Ontario: Government of Ontario.

Karasek, R. A. 1979. Job demands, job decision latitude, and mental strain: Implications for job redesign. *Administrative Science Quarterly* 24:285–307.

Karasek, R., D. Baker, F. Marxer, A. Ahlbom, and T. Thorell. 1981. Job decision latitude, job demands and cardiovascular disease: A prospective study of Swedish men. *American Journal of Public Health* 71(7):694–705.

Karasek, R., and T. Thorell. 1990. *Healthy work: Stress, productivity, and the reconstruction of working life*. New York: Basic Books.

Karasek, R. A. 1979. Job demands, job decision latitude, and mental strain: Implications for job redesign. *Adm Sci Q* 24:285–307.

Karasek, R., D. Baker, F. Marxer, A. Ahlbom, and T. Theorell. 1981. Job decision latitude, job demands, and cardiovascular disease: A prospective study of Swedish men. *Am J Public Health* 71(7):694–705.

Karasek, R., C. Brisson, N. Kawakami, I. Houtman, P. Bongers, and B. Amick. 1998. The Job Content Questionnaire (JCQ): An instrument for internationally comparative assessments of psychosocial job characteristics. *J Occup Health Psychol* 3(4):322–55.

Karasek, R., and T. Theorell. 1990. *Healthy work*. New York: Basic Books, Inc.

Kiecolt-Glaser, J. K, and R. Glaser. 1995. Psychoneuroimmunology and health consequences: Data and shared mechanisms. *Psychosomatic Medicine* 57:269–74.

Kivimäki, M., M. Elovainio, and J. Vahtera. 2000. Workplace bullying and sickness absence in hospital staff. *Occup Environ Med* 57:656–660.

Kohn, M. L, and C. Schooler. 1978. The reciprocal effects of substantive complexity of work and intellectual flexibility: A longitudinal assessment. *American Journal of Sociology* 84:24–52.

Levi, L., S. L. Sauter, and T. Shimomitsu. 1999. Work-related stress—It's time to act. *J Occup Health Psychol* 4(4):394–6.

Lindström, K., T. Leino, J. Seitsamo, and I. Torstila. 1997. A longitudinal study of work characteristics and health complaints among insurance employees in VDT work. *International Journal of Human-Computer Interaction* 4:343–368.

Schaufeli, W., and D. Enzmann. 1998. *The burnout companion to study and practice: A critical analysis.* London: Taylor & Francis.

Matthews, K. A., et al. 1987. Stressful work conditions and diastolic blood pressure among blue collar factory workers. *American Journal of Epidemiology* 126(2):280–291.

Melamed, S., et al. 1989. Ergonomic stress levels, personal characteristics, accident occurrence and sickness absence among factory workers. *Ergonomics* 32(9):1101–10.

Muntaner, C., and P. J. O'Campo. 1993. A critical appraisal of the demand/control model of the psychosocial work environment: Epistemological, social, behavioral and class considerations. *Social Science and Medicine* 36(11): 1509–17.

Murphy, L. R. 1996. Stress management in work settings: A critical review of the health effects. *Am J Health Promot* 11(2):112–35.

National Institute for Occupational Safety and Health. 1999. *Stress... at work.* DHHS (NIOSH) Publication No.99-101, NIOSH, Cincinnati.

Peter, R., and J. Siegrist. 2000. Psychosocial work environment and the risk of coronary heart disease. *Int Arch Occup Environ Health* 73 Suppl:S41–5.

Quick, J. C., L. R. Murphy, and J. J. Hurrell Jr, eds. 1992. *Stress and well-being at work: Assessments and interventions for occupational mental health.* Washington, DC: American Psychological Association.

Quick, J. C., J. D. Quick, D. L. Nelson, and J. J. Hurrell Jr., eds. 1997. *Preventive stress management in organizations.* Washington, DC: American Psychological Association.

Sauter, S. L., S. Y. Lim, and L. R. Murphy. 1996. Organizational health: A new paradigm for occupational stress research at NIOSH. *Sangyo Seishin Hoken* (Occupational Mental Health) 4(4):248–254.

Schnall, P. L., P. A. Landsbergis, and D. Baker. 1994. Job strain and cardiovascular disease. *Annu Rev Public Health* 15:381–411.

Selye, H. 1976. *The stress of life.* New York: McGraw-Hill.

Shannon, H. S, et al. 1996. Workplace organizational correlates of lost-time accident rates in manufacturing. *American Journal of Industrial Medicine* 29:258.

Shehadeh, V., and M. Shain. 1990. *Influences on Wellness in the Workplace: Technical Report.* Ottawa: Health and Welfare Canada.

Siegrist, J. 1996. Adverse health effects of high-effort/low-reward conditions. *J Occup Health Psychol.* 1(1):27–41.

Siegrist, J., and R. Peter. 2000. The effort-reward imbalance model. *Occup Med* 15(1):83–87.

Sokegima, S., and S. Kagamimori. 1998. Working hours as a risk factor for acute myocardial infarction in Japan: Case-control study. *British Medical Journal* 317:775.

Steptoe, A., O. Evans, and G. Fieldman. 1997. Perceptions of control over work: Psychophysiological responses to self-paced and externally-paced tasks in an adult population sample. *International Journal of Psychophysiology* 25(3):211–20.

Theorell, T., A. Tsutsumi, J. Hallquist et al. 1997. Decision latitude, job strain and myocardial infarction: A study of working men in Stockholm. *American Journal of Public Health,* 88(3):382–8.

Theorell, T., and R.A. Karasek. 1996. Current issues relating to psychosocial job strain and cardiovascular disease research. *J Occup Health Psychol* 1(1):9–26.

Uehata, T. 1991. Long working hours and occupational stress-related cardiovascular attacks among middle-aged workers in Japan. *Journal of Human Ergology* 20:147–153.

Videman, T., H. Rauhala, S. Asp, K. Lindström, G. Cedercreutz, M. Kämppi, S. Tola, and J. D. G. Troup. 1989. Patient-handling skill, back injuries, and back pain. An intervention study in nursing. *Spine* 14:148–156.

Warr, P. B. 1990. Decision latitude, job demands, and employee well-being. *Work and Stress*, 4(4):285–94.

Westgaard, R.H., and J. Winkel. 1997. Ergonomic intervention research for improved musculoskeletal health: A critical review. *International Journal of Industrial Ergonomics* 20: 463–500.

Williams, S., and C. L. Cooper. 1998. Measuring occupational stress: Development of the pressure management indicator. *J Occup Health Psychol* 3(4):306–21.

Burden of Disease

Burton, W. N., D. J. Conti, C.-Y. Chen, A. B. Schultz, and D. W. Edington. 1999. The role of health risk factors and disease on worker productivity. *J Occup Environ Med* 41(10):863–877.

Liang, Y. X., H. Fu, and X. Q. Gu. 1998. Provision of occupational health services in China. *Asian-Pacific Newsletter on Occupational Health and Safety* 5(2):34–39.

WHO. 1999. Proceedings of the Fourth Network Meeting of the WHO Collaborating Centers in Occupational Health, June 7–9 1999, Espoo, Finland. In *Protection of the human environment, occupational and environmental health series*, 26–28. Geneva: World Health Organization.

Zhou, C. Q., Y. Gao, Q. Y. Ma. 1997. Pneumoconiosis in China. *Asian-Pacific Newsletter on Occupational Health and Safety* 4(2):44–49.

INDEX

Dichlorodiphenyltricholoroethane
(DDT), 186
DIH. *See* Department of Industrial Health
(DIH)
Dimethylbenzene. *See* Xylene
Direct-reading noise meter, 77
Disability, 273, 337
calculation, 275
functional capacity, 274
in insurance sense, 274–75
prevention of, 273–74
types, 275
Disaster management, 108
Disease prevention, 344
employers' responsibilities, 349
opportunities for, 348
primary, 345
secondary, 345
strategies, 345
tertiary, 345–46
Diseases, 259
determinants of, 43
general, 301
multicausal, 38
work-related, 44
Dislocations, 267
Disorders, 259, 265
cardiovascular, 327
immune, 196
liver, 327
male fertility, 325
neurological, 182, 316–17
Distributive justice, 6
Diurnal cycle, 207
Dose meters, 77
Dose-response effect, 24
Drainage water, 464
Droplet nuclei, 228
Drugs, 359
Dynamic populations, 47, 48
Dysautonomias, 316

E
3E's formulation, 110
EAP. *See* Employee assistance program
(EAP)
Earmuffs, 235
Earplugs, 235
Economic development

in China, 490
cycle, 490
disease economic burden, 490–91
disruptions, 487–88
effects on population health, 500
export-driven development, 489
health care cost, 491
human rights, 493
illness implications, 502, 503
market-driven development, 489
mercantilism, 489
mixed economies, 489
model of, 492
occupational health in, 486–87
population and resource issues, 493–94
process elements, 492–93
public health issues, 501
self-sufficiency, 489
socialism, 489
strategies for, 488–89
transitions, 488–89
urbanization, 494–96
worker protection and, 488
Economy
emerging issues, 557–59
global, 563
Eczema, 302
Efferent fibers, 294, 316
Effort-reward model, 201
EHF. *See* Extremely high frequencies
(EHF)
Electrical safety, 108
electricians, 463–64
electricity generation, 376–77
Electromagnetic
radiation, 142
spectrum, 146, 147
Electromagnetic fields (EMF), 145–46
Electromyography (EMG), 137, 317
Electronic noise suppression devices, 235
Electronics, 366
chemical hazards, 368–69
microelectronic components, 367
microelectronic industry, 367
physical hazards, 368
and semiconductor manufacturing, 367
Electroplating, 378
Emergency medical service (EMS),
467, 472

Emergency medical technician
(EMT), 472
Emerging infections, 191, 402
avian influenza, 403
pandemic influenza, 403
severe acute respiratory syndrome,
402–3
EMF. *See* Electromagnetic fields (EMF)
EMG. *See* Electromyography (EMG)
Employee assistance professionals, 521
Employee assistance program (EAP), 213
Employee health service, 522
assistance programs, 523
clinic, 523
health services, 522
health surveillance, 524
medical care, 524
operation, 523–24
physician, 523
Employee health service. *See* Occupational
health services
Employment, 551
Empowerment, 349
EMS. *See* Emergency medical service
(EMS)
EMT. *See* Emergency medical technician
(EMT)
Endocrine
disorders, 328
mimics, 325
Endogenous dermatitis, 302. *See also*
Dermatitis
Endotoxins, 425
Energy, 369
biomass fuels, 377
coal, 370–72
cogeneration, 370
electricity generation, 376–77
natural gas, 373–74
nuclear, 375
oil sands, 374–75
oil shale, 374
petroleum, 372–73
sources, 370
technologies, 369
thermal power, 376
Engineering controls, 218, 220. *See also*
Administrative controls
housekeeping and hygiene, 221

preventive maintenance, 220
safe work practices, 220–21
Enterprise structure, 549
consolidation, 549
fragmentation, 549–50
management innovations, 550
Environmental
degradation, 498–99
hazards, 513
protection, 365–66
Epicondylitis, 282
Epidemiologists, 521
Equity, 6
Ergonomics, 131, 132
applied, 133–34
core knowledge, 133
goals, 131, 134, 139
macro-level, 135
modern, 132
participatory, 138–39, 140–41
principles, 133
as science, 132
solving workplace problems, 134
and usability, 139, 141
Ergonomists, 135, 520
background requirement, 135, 136
competency, 136, 138
in research laboratory, 136–37
Ethidium bromide, 358, 359
Ethylene dichloride, 387
Ethylene oxide (EtO), 403
EtO. *See* Ethylene oxide (EtO)
Excretion, 21, 23–24
Executive physical evaluation, 353
Export-driven development, 489
Exposed subjects, 52
Exposure assessment, 64–65, 72, 73
analysis, 75, 78, 79
building-associated illness, 79–82
control standards, 364–65
German MAK-values, 364
planning, 75
possibilities for, 73
problems in, 82, 88
records, 532
standardizing risk classification, 87–88
Exposure-response effect. *See* Dose-
response effect
Extremely high frequencies (EHF), 149

Health-related outcomes, 499
Hearing conservationists, 521
Hearing protection technicians. *See*
    Hearing conservationists
Heat
  exhaustion, 156
  fatigue, 156
  stress, 155–57
  stroke, 156
  syncope, 156
Heating, ventilation, and air conditioning
    workers (HVAC workers), 466
Heavy
  equipment operators, 463
  metals, 327
Helmets, 235
Hepatitis B, 401. *See also* HIV/AIDS
Hepatitis B virus (HBV), 194
Hepatitis C, 401
Hepatitis C virus (HCV), 194–95
Hepatotoxicity, 327
Herbicides, 187–88
  paraquat, 187
  triazines, 187
Herd immunity, 402
Hertz (Hz), 315
Hexachlorocyclohexanes (HCH), 186
HF. *See* Hydrofluoric acid (HF)
High altitude sickness, 155
Historical cohort study, 52
HIV. *See* Human immunodeficiency
    virus (HIV)
HIV/AIDS, 401, 402
Honeymoon effect, 211
Hospitals
  anesthetic gases, 405
  antineoplastic agents, 404–5
  chemical hazards, 403, 404
  exposures, 397, 408
  hazard zones, 397
  health services, 410, 411
  infectious threats, 402
  latex allergy, 405
  laundry and contamination, 398
  methicillin-resistant Staphylococcus
    aureus, 402
  occupational injury, 409
  pathogens, 399
  prevention, 408
  stress, 410

  violence, 409–10
HRA. *See* Health risk appraisal (HRA)
HSE. *See* Health, safety, and environment
    (HSE)
Human flexibility, 563
Human immunodeficiency virus
    (HIV), 195
Human rights, 493
  child labor, 497
  employment opportunities, 498
  relationships, 496
  women in societies, 497
  work environment, 504
HVAC workers. *See* Heating, ventilation,
    and air conditioning workers (HVAC
    workers)
Hydrazine, 358
Hydroelectric energy, 370
Hydrofluoric acid (HF), 356, 358, 369
Hydrogen cyanide, 172–73
  health effects, 172–73
  uses and sources, 173
  Hydrogen sulfide, 172, 427
  health effects, 172
  uses and sources, 172
Hypernephroma, 389
Hypersensitivity, 28
  pneumonitis, 197, 308–9, 425, 426
Hz. *See* Hertz (Hz)

I

IARC. *See* International Agency for
    Research on Cancer (IARC)
ICOH. *See* International Commission on
    Occupational Health (ICOH)
IEA. *See* International Ergonomics
    Association (IEA)
Illumination, 148
ILO. *See* International Labour
    Organization (ILO)
Immune reactions
  allergic responses, 28
  immune responses, 27–28
Immunization, 194, 197, 403
Impairment, 274, 337
  partial, 274
  permanent, 273
  temporary, 272–73
  total, 274
Implantable lenses, 502

Impulse
  meters, 151
  noise, 315
Incidence density ratio. *See* Rate ratio
Incident, 108
Industrial hygiene. *See* Occupational
    hygiene
Industry
  biomedical research, 356–57
  biotechnology, 358–59
  chemical, 359
  electronics, 366
  energy technologies, 369–77
  environmental protection, 365
  metal fabrication, 377–80
  mining, 380
  occupational hazards, 355
  paper and pulp, 383–86
  pharmaceuticals, 359
  plastics, 386–87
  revolution, 487
  rubber, 386–88
  smelting, 382
  steel, 388–89
  transportation, 389–92
  wood products, 392
Inferential statistics, 42. *See also*
    Descriptive statistics
Inflammation, 25
Influenza, pandemic, 403
Informal
  sector, 440–43, 456–57
  work, 446, 448
Infrared radiation, 148
Injury, 259
  crush, 268, 269
  minor, 126
  needlestick, 401
  prevention, 111, 122–23, 126
  pyramid, 111–12
  risk situations of, 123
  serious, 126
  soft-tissue, 267, 269
Insulation workers, 466
International Agency for Research on
    Cancer (IARC), 165–66, 174, 206, 319
International Commission on
    Occupational Health (ICOH), 17,
    506, 516
  code of ethics, 506–7

duties and obligations, 507–9
International Ergonomics Association
    (IEA), 18, 132
International Labour Organization (ILO),
    4, 10, 17, 95, 159, 340, 419, 504
  codes of practice, 511
  conventions, 505
  functions, 505
  mandate, 505
  measures, 510
  objectives, 7
  policy guidance, 509–10
  safety and health, 509, 536
  tripartite structure, 505
  worker protection, 510
International Occupational Hygiene
    Association (IOHA), 18
International Program on Chemical Safety
    (IPCS), 175
Interstitium, 305
Investment, 489
IOHA. *See* International Occupational
    Hygiene Association (IOHA)
Ionizing radiation, 142. *See also*
    Non-ionizing radiation
  exposure to, 144
  instruments, 144
  measurements, 144
  sources, 143
  types, 142
IPCS. *See* International Program on
    Chemical Safety (IPCS)
Ironworkers, 464
Irritants, 303
Irritation, 25

J
JEM. *See* Job exposure matrix (JEM)
Job, 446
  casual, 491
  demand-control model, 475
  description, 335
  injured workers return, 338
  seniority, 564
Job burnout, 210, 475
  deskilling, 211
  frustration effect, 210–11
  honeymoon effect, 211
  interventions, 476
  personality characteristics, 212

Maximum workplace concentration
(MAK), 361
MCPA. *See* 5-chloro-
2-methylphenoxyacetic acid (MCPA)
Medical
certification, 252
departments, 524
directors, 518
Melanoma, 304
Meltdown, 375
Mercantilism, 489
Mercurial erethism, 183–84
Mercury, 183–84
health effects, 183–84
uses and sources, 183
Mesothelioma, 312–13
Meta-analysis, 59, 70
Metabolism, 21, 23
Metal fabrication, 377
assembly work, 378
electroplating, 378
hazards, 377
machining, 377
manufacturing, 377, 379
occupational dermatitis, 377
pickling, 378
shipbuilding, 378
stamping, 379
Methicillin-resistant Staphylococcus
aureus (MRSA), 402
Methylcyclopentadienyl manganese
tricarbonyl (MMT), 182
Micro business. *See* Small business
Microbial allergies, 196
agents, 189
asthma, 196, 197
extrinsic allergic alveolitis, 197
Microwave, 149
radiation, 408
transmissions, 149
Mineral dusts. *See* Fibrogenic dusts
Mining, 380
coal, 381
explosives, 381
hazards, 381
radon daughters, 382
roof falls, 381–82
tunneling and shoring, 381
underground, 381

Mixed economies, 489
Mixed-connective tissue disease, 387
MMT. *See* Methylcyclopentadienyl
manganese tricarbonyl (MMT)
Mobilization, 23
Molecular epidemiology, 38. *See also*
Occupational epidemiology
Monitoring, 245
environmental, 95
ethics and social issues, 104, 106
guidelines for, 105
workers, 94
Monomers, 360–61, 387
Mortality, 52, 53
Motor neuropathies, 317
MRI. *See* Magnetic resonance imaging
(MRI)
MRSA. *See* Methicillin-resistant
Staphylococcus aureus (MRSA)
MSDS. *See* Material safety data sheet
(MSDS)
Multifactoral diseases. *See* Diseases,
multicausal
Multiple trauma, 269
Muscle relaxant, 288
Musculoskeletal disorders, 265, 277.
See also Occupational health
case study, 295–96
characteristics, 297
diagnosis, 281
evaluation, 279
muscle tension and spasm, 281
nerve damage, 283
patterns, 281
physical findings, 280
prevalence, 277, 278
prevention, 298–99
prognosis, 290–92
risk factors, 278
repetitive strain injury, 283–84
social influences, 297
syndromes, 284–88
tendonitis, 282
tenosynovitis, 282
treatments, 288–89
types, 278, 279
vascular compromise, 283
worker's setbacks, 289, 290

Occupational lung disease (*cont'd*)
obstructive disease, 305
occupational asthma, 306
pneumoconiosis, 309
radon daughters, 382
restrictive disease, 305
steel, 389
toxic inhalation, 308
types, 305–6
wood, 395–96
Occupational medicine, 356
role, 29
specialists, 529
Occupational safety and health (OSH),
510
Occupational Safety and Health
Administration (OSHA), 439, 533
Occupational skin diseases, 301
categories, 302
treatment, 304
Odds ratio (OR), 57
Odors, 91
ODTS. *See* Organic dust toxic syndrome
(ODTS)
OECD. *See* Organization for Economic
Cooperation and Development
(OECD)
OEL. *See* Occupational exposure level
(OEL)
OEMAC. *See* Occupational and
Environmental Medical Association of
Canada (OEMAC)
Office workers, 466
OHN. *See* Occupational health nurse
(OHN)
On-condition maintenance, 220
OP insecticides. *See* Organophosphorus
insecticides (OP insecticides)
Opacity, 310
Open-pit mines, 380
OR. *See* Odds ratio (OR)
Organic dust toxic syndrome (ODTS), 425
Organic solvents, 327
Organization for Economic Cooperation
and Development (OECD), 30,
370, 553
Organized labor, 445
Organochlorine compounds, 185–86
Organophosphate pesticides, 426

Organophosphorus insecticides (OP
insecticides), 186
OSH. *See* Occupational safety and
health (OSH)
OSHA. *See* Occupational Safety and Health
Administration (OSHA)
Osteoarthritis, 287–88
Ottawa Charter, 348
Outreach program, 448
assimilation degree, 449
community identification, 449
educational level, 450
family ties, 450
health trends, 451
immigration status, 449
language and literacy, 449
legal status, 450
living standard, 450
religion, 450
social class, 450
social organization, 449
social status, 449–50
urbanization, 449
Outsourcing, 550, 562
Overhaul, 468
Overuse syndrome. *See* Repetitive
strain injury (RSI)

P
Pain, 269, 280, 292
afferent and efferent fibers, 294
analgesics for, 288
in musculoskeletal disorders, 292–93
neuropeptide uses, 294–95
nociceptive, 293
nociceptor use, 293–94
research, 293
treatment, 292
types, 293
Paper and pulp, 383
algal control, 386
chemical exposures, 385
Kraft, 384
lignin, 383
occupational disorder, 385–86
papermaking, 385
pulp-making processes, 384
sulfite, 384
thermomechanical process, 384–85